Pathology of Occupational Lung Disease

❖ **Second Edition**

Pathology of Occupational Lung Disease

❖ **Second Edition**

Andrew Churg, MD
Professor of Pathology
The University of British Columbia
Pathologist
Vancouver Hospital
Vancouver, British Columbia

Francis H. Y. Green, MD
Professor of Pathology
The University of Calgary
Calgary, Alberta

Williams & Wilkins
A WAVERLY COMPANY

BALTIMORE • PHILADELPHIA • LONDON • PARIS • BANGKOK
BUENOS AIRES • HONG KONG • MUNICH • SYDNEY • TOKYO • WROCLAW

Editor: Charles W. Mitchell
Managing Editor: Grace Miller
Marketing Manager: Peter Darcy
Production Coordinator: Raymond E. Reter
Project Editor: Ulita Lushnycky
Text and Cover Designer: Graphic World, Inc., St. Louis, Missouri
Illustration Planner: Lorraine Wrzosek
Typesetter: Maryland Composition Co., Inc., Glen Burnie, Maryland
Printer & Binder: R.R. Donnelley & Sons Co., Crawfordsville, Indiana
Digitized Illustrations: Maryland Composition Co., Inc., Glen Burnie, Maryland

351 West Camden Street
Baltimore, Maryland 21201-2436 USA

Rose Tree Corporate Center
1400 North Providence Road
Building II, Suite 5025
Media, Pennsylvania 19063-2043 USA

Accurate indications, adverse reactions, and dosage schedules for drugs are provided in this book, but it is possible that they may change. The reader is urged to review the package information data of the manufacturers of the medications mentioned.

Printed in the United States of America

First Edition, 1988, by IGAKU-SHOIN Medical Publishers, Inc.

Library of Congress Cataloging-in-Publication Data

Pathology of occupational lung disease / [edited by] Andrew Churg.
Francis H.Y. Green. — 2nd ed.
p. cm.
Includes bibliographical references and index.
ISBN 0-683-30386-4
1. Lungs—Diseases. 2. Occupational diseases. 3. Lungs—Dust diseases. I. Churg, Andrew. II. Green, Francis H. Y.
[DNLM: 1. Lung Diseases—pathology. 2. Occupational Diseases—chemically induced. WF 600 P297 1998]
RC756.P37 1998
616.2′4—dc21
DNLM/DLC
for Library of Congress 97-33344
CIP

To purchase additional copies of this book, call our customer service department at **(800) 638-0672** or fax orders to **(800) 447-8438.** For other book services, including chapter reprints and large quantity sales, ask for the Special Sales department.

Canadian customers should call **(800) 665-1148,** or fax **(800) 665-0103.** For all other calls originating outside of the United States, please call **(410) 528-4223** or fax us at **(410) 528-8550.**

Visit Williams & Wilkins on the Internet: **http://www.wwilkins.com** or contact our customer service department at **custserv@wwilkins.com**. Williams & Wilkins customer service representatives are available from 8:30 am to 6:00 pm, EST, Monday through Friday, for telephone access.

97 98 99 00 01
1 2 3 4 5 6 7 8 9 10

To the late *Charles B. Carrington*,
teacher and friend.

❖

Preface to the Second Edition

In this second edition of *Pathology of Occupational Lung Disease* we have attempted both to separate areas that we believe need more emphasis and to incorporate advances and controversies in thinking that have developed in the 10 years since the first edition.

A separate chapter on clinical features of occupational lung diseases, written by an experienced clinician, has been included. We have also separated and expanded the chapter on pathologic reaction patterns in an attempt to provide a visual impression of the various morphologic patterns of occupational lung disease and their differential diagnosis. Advances in molecular biologic analysis are beginning to shed light on the pathogenesis of mineral dust-induced disease, particularly silicosis and the asbestos-related diseases, and we have provided more detailed information on these processes.

The chapter on extrinsic allergic alveolitis and occupational asthma has been completely redone, in part to reflect the continuing increase in asthma as a major cause of morbidity and mortality in both occupational and nonoccupational settings. Occupational asthma is believed to be today's most commonly compensated occupational lung disease, and the chapter on Legal Considerations for the Pathologist contains a section on occupational asthma.

There remain no end of controversies, and some have become sharper, if anything, in the past 10 years; many have been considered in more detail in this edition. One such controversy is whether exposure to dust causes nonasthmatic chronic airflow obstruction. New information on the structural abnormalities that appear to be associated with dust-induced airflow obstruction and on their functional correlates has been incorporated into the chapters on coal, silica, and metals.

There has also been a slow but steady increase in the number of substances classified as occupational pulmonary carcinogens, and more space has been devoted to this topic. Many of these classifications are quite controversial; the recent decision by the International Agency for Research on Cancer to classify silica as a carcinogen is a good example. The issue of occupational asbestos exposure and its relation to carcinoma is still divided between those who believe that carcinoma in this setting is related to the presence of asbestosis and those who believe it is not. The diagnosis of mesothelioma, while still a problem in some instances, is becoming somewhat easier as more cases accumulate and more specific immunohistochemical testing becomes available; on the other hand, separation of benign and malignant mesothelial reactions continues to be extremely difficult in some instances. Information on the risks of relatively low level exposure to asbestos, risks that have caused some countries to ban the use of asbestos while others still permit its use, has been updated. The chapter on the effects of man-made mineral fibers has been extensively revised.

Last, we have consciously maintained an emphasis on pathologic reaction patterns and differential diagnosis while providing enough background to allow the pathologist to understand the clinical and epidemiologic settings of the various entities we discuss.

We wish to thank Marnie Cudmore for help in preparation of the manuscript.

Andrew Churg
Francis H. Y. Green

Preface to the First Edition

This book arises from our experience as pathologists involved with occupational lung disease. Although there are excellent books that describe the clinical and radiographic features of occupational lung disease, no equivalent pathologic reference exists. Instead, the pathologic literature is widely scattered, and, particularly for uncommon conditions, pathologic descriptions are often poorly defined, obscure, confusing, outdated, and not infrequently contradictory. An additional motivation for the preparation of this volume was the current and apparently increasing legal involvement of the pathologist in many areas of occupational medicine, an involvement that sometimes forces him or her to extremes of diagnostic subtlety (and occasionally imagination!) not needed in other areas of pathology.

We emphasize the pathologic features of occupational lung disease. We assume that the reader already has a working knowledge of pulmonary pathology, and we do not attempt to define such basic terms as *interstitial fibrosis, honeycombing,* and *emphysema.* Our emphasis is on the diagnostic-pathologic features of occupational lung disease at the gross and microscopic levels and on adjunctive methods needed for the pathologist to arrive at a diagnosis. We point out areas of controversy or uncertainty to make the reader aware of their existence.

The less detailed information on mineralogy, occupations at risk, and clinical, radiographic, and functional changes is intended to provide enough background for the nonexpert pathologist to put his or her observations into clinical and occupational context, but this de-emphasis is not meant to belittle the importance of such data. As we note in Chapter 1, clinical information is crucial when rendering a diagnosis.

Because of our emphasis, we have ignored or given only minimal space to several areas. Occupation-associated infections have not been covered at all, since most such infections generally have no features specific to the occupational setting. The same reasoning applies to our brief treatment of occupational lung cancers, which, as a rule, have no features that allow the investigator to determine an occupational etiology on the basis of pathologic observations. The extremely important problem of occupational asthma, which probably accounts for more lung disease in the occupational setting than that produced by all types of mineral dusts, is only briefly considered since such cases are never biopsied, and the associated pathologic reactions, if any, are virtually unknown.

We have included a certain amount of information on "environmental" lung disease for several areas in which the reactions seen after environmental exposure are similar to those seen in the occupational setting; namely, certain aspects of asbestos disease, extrinsic allergic alveolitis, and effects of intravenous drug injection. There are obviously many other "environmental" agents that range from cigarette smoke to air pollution to radiation and they are of importance in pulmonary disease, but they are mentioned only in so far as they confound or modify the pathologic features of occupational lung diseases.

We are especially grateful to the numerous pathologists who have contributed case material used in this book, to the National Institute for Occupational Safety and Health (NIOSH) for providing access to study material, to M. Schultz for help in preparing the manuscript, and to L. DePaoli and M. Skromeda for photographic assistance.

Andrew Churg
Francis H. Y. Green

Contributors

Raymond Bégin, MD, FCCP

Professor of Medicine, Pulmonary Service, CUSE Fleurimont, Sherbrooke, Quèbec, Canada

Andrew Churg, MD, PhD, FRCPC

Professor of Pathology, The University of British Columbia, Pathologist, Vancouver Hospital, Vancouver, British Columbia, Canada

Thomas V. Colby, MD

Consultant in Surgical Pathology, Mayo Clinic, Scottsdale, Arizona, Professor of Pathology, Mayo Medical School, Rochester, Minnesota

Allen R. Gibbs, DD, MD, ChB

Consultant Pathologist, Department of Histopathology, Llandough Hospital, Penarth, Wales, United Kingdom

Francis H. Y. Green, MD

Professor of Pathology, The University of Calgary, Calgary, Alberta, Canada

Stephen I. Richman, BS, JD

Richman and Smith, Washington, Pennsylvania

Carl J. Smith, Jr., BA, JD

Richman and Smith, Washington, Pennsylvania

Val Vallyathan, PhD

Team Leader, National Institute for Occupational Safety and Health, Professor of Pathology, West Virginia University, Morgantown, West Virginia

J. C. Wagner, MD, FRCPATH

Retired MRC Pneumoconiosis Unit, Llandough Hospital, Penarth, Wales, United Kingdom

J. L. Wright

Professor of Pathology, University of British Columbia, Vancouver, British Columbia, Canada

Contents

Color Plates

Plate 1

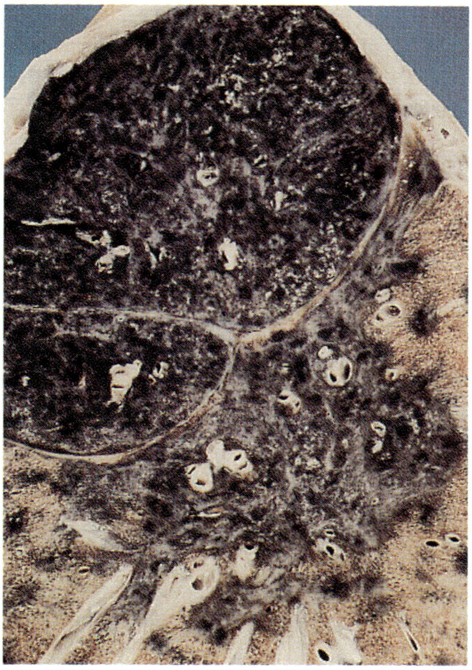

Plate 1. Progressive Massive Fibrosis (PMF). The upper lobe is completely replaced by coal dust and fibrous tissue. The lesions were bilateral. Cor pulmonale was noted at autopsy. The miner was 54-years-old at death and had worked for 16 years in underground coal mines as a roof bolter.

Plate 2 (Parts A-L)

Plate 2. (**A–C**) Various forms of asbestos body seen in Millipore filter preparations. Note the clear straight central cores (best seen in A) and the branched forms. (Originals, ×160).

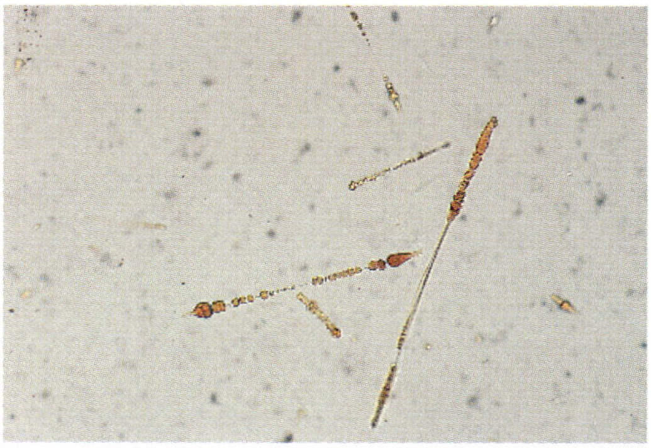

A

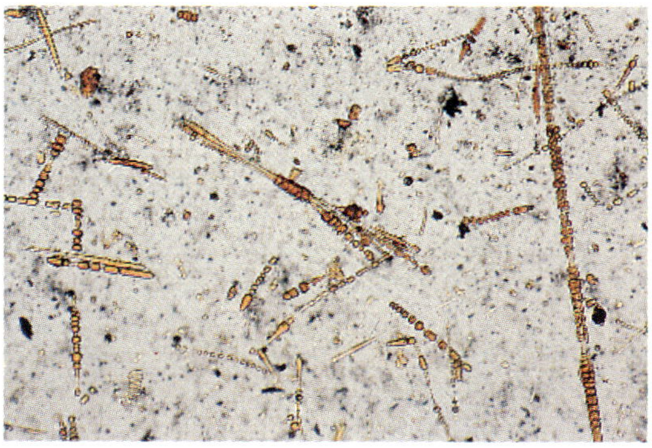

B

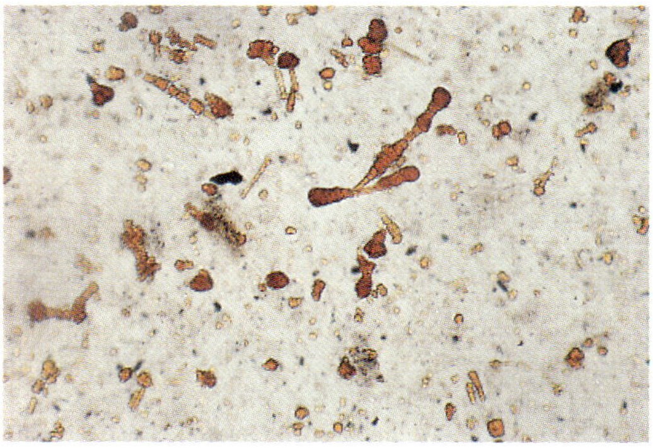

C

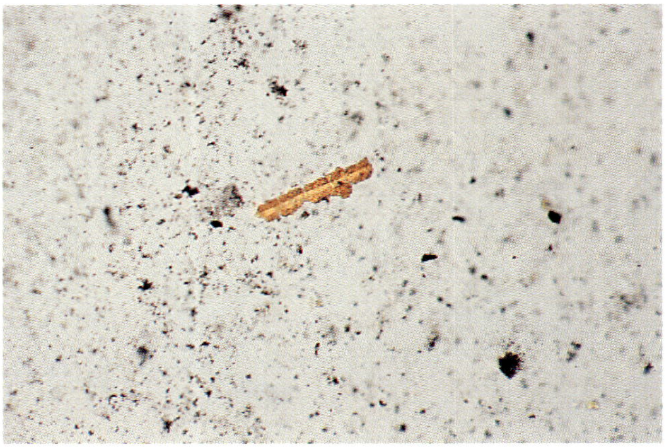
D

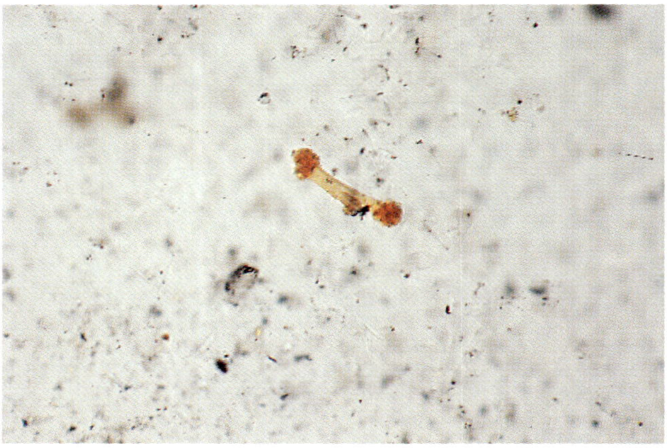
E

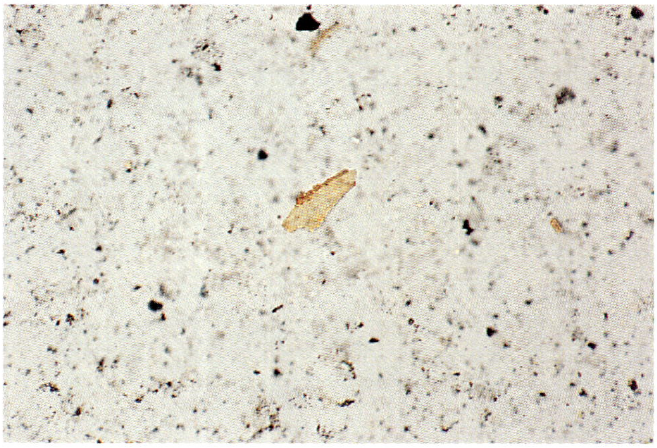
F

Plate 2. ***Continued***
(**D–F**) Various forms of sheet silicate body seen in Millipore filter preparations. Parts D and E show forms that have broad fibrous cores that could be confused with asbestos bodies; however, the cores are distinctly yellow (whereas asbestos cores are clear) and much wider than asbestos cores. Part F shows a plate-like form. These bodies are usually formed on talc or mica. (Originals, ×160).

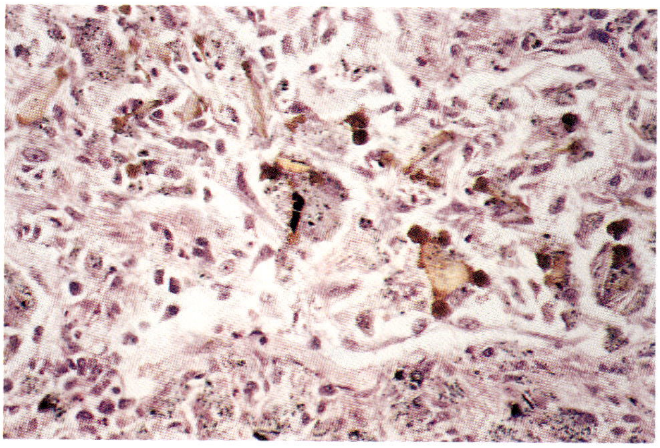

G

Plate 2. ***Continued***
(**G**) Sheet silicate (talc and mica) bodies in tissue section. A black-cored body, probably formed on carbon, is also present. From the lung of a roofing materials maker. (Original, ×160).

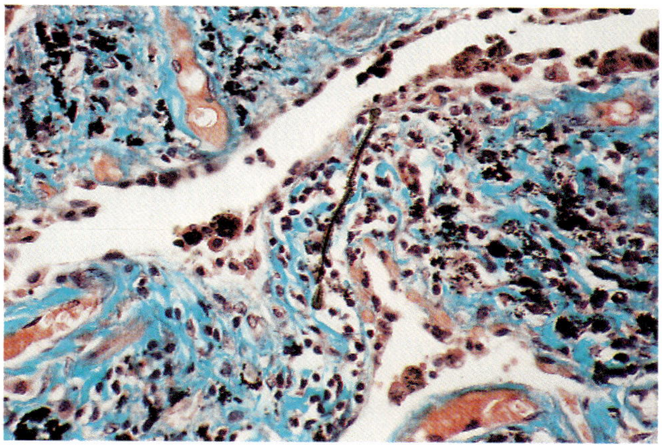

H

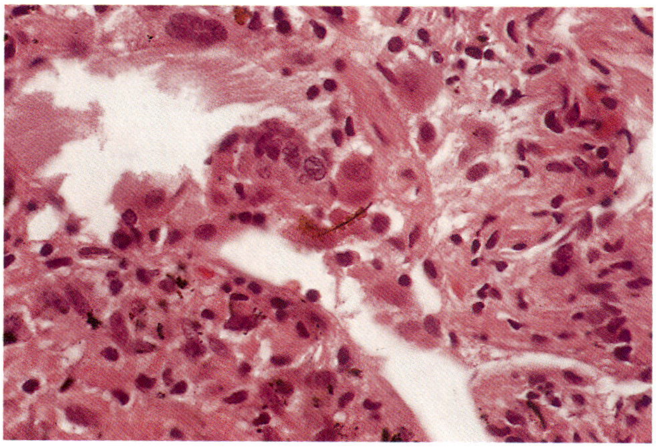

I

Plate 2. ***Continued***
(**H** and **I**) Bodies with black fibrous cores. Part H shows a body with a core of rutile from a hard rock miner (rutile contaminates quartz). Part I shows a body with an iron core from a worker in an iron-processing operation (courtesy Dr. R. Dodson). (Originals, ×160).

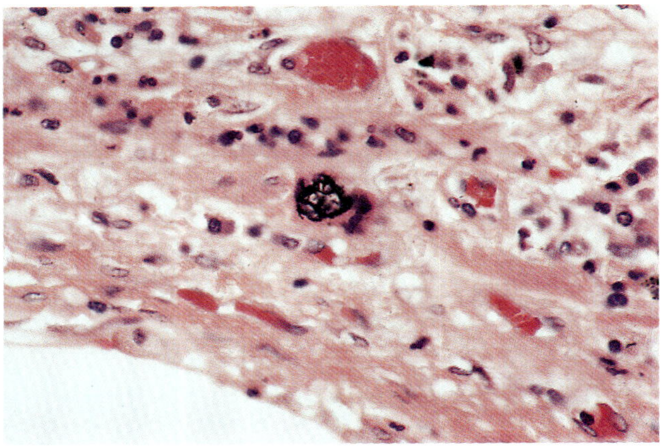

J

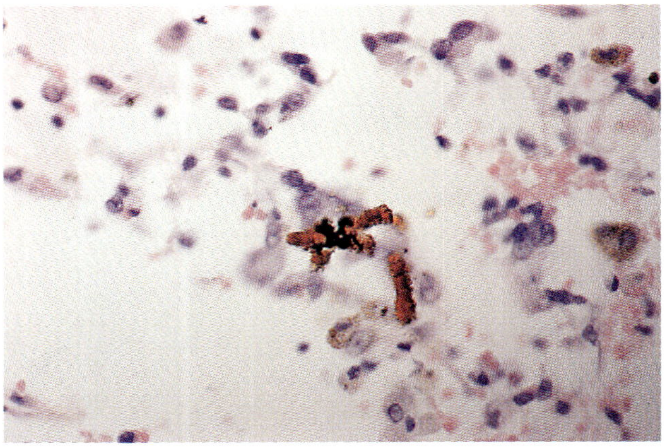

K

Plate 2. *Continued*
(**J** and **K**) Forms of coal fly ash seen in tissue section. Part J shows a partially dissolved fly ash sphere in a macrophage. Part K shows a more disintegrated sphere with a ferruginous coat. (Originals, ×160).

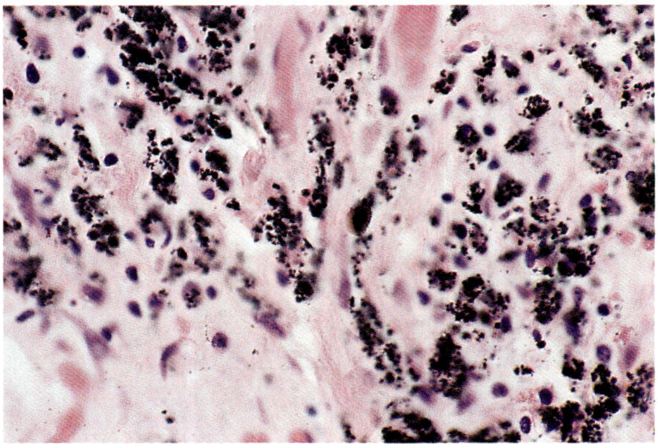

L

Plate 2. *Continued*
(**L**) Round ferruginous bodies, probably formed on iron. From the lung of an arc-welder. (Original, ×160).

CHAPTER 1

Clinical Evaluation of the Patient with Occupational Lung Disease

❖ Raymond Bégin

GENERAL CONSIDERATIONS

This chapter considers clinical data for diagnosis, assessment of impairment and disability, and compensation of occupational lung diseases. It emphasizes the history of occupational and environmental exposure, physical examination, use of lung function testing in the documentation of a work-related disease and impairment evaluation, and the contribution of the chest radiograph to the overall assessment of occupational lung diseases. Clinical interventions by physicians with workers at risk or with pneumoconiosis are also briefly discussed.

OCCUPATIONAL HISTORY

The detailed, complete, and chronologic history of the person's occupation and an understanding of the job tasks and exposures are invaluable in the establishment of a diagnosis of occupational lung disease. At times exposures to asbestos, silica, and other minerals are readily known and acknowledged by the patient, but in many cases the substances at work that could contribute to disease are largely unknown or relate to exposure that is forgotten unless specifically questioned. In that regard the review of material safety data sheets (MSDS) of all products used in the workplace, past and present when possible, should permit identification of substances possibly associated with lung diseases. A communication with the industrial hygienist or safety officer in the plant may clarify workers' exposures. Hazards in the workplace can be verified in reference sources such as National Institute of Occupational Safety and Health Publication 77–181 (1), ILO Encyclopedia of Occupational Health and Safety (2), and recent textbooks on occupational asthma (3).

Hazards of exposure to hobby or other nonoccupational activities should be sought carefully, as they may clarify the cause of an allergic alveolitis, extrinsic asthma, or mineral dust disease.

The smoking history from adolescence to the time of consultation should be obtained, as it may be a cofactor in diseases such as occupational chronic obstructive pulmonary disease (COPD), byssinosis, and lung cancer.

SYMPTOM HISTORY

The symptom history plays an important role in establishing the diagnosis and in evaluating impairment and disability. The relation of symptoms and their severity to the workplace should be assessed at initial evaluation. The circumstances of onset of the respiratory symptoms should be clearly described. The course, evolution, and aggravating factors should be known. The patient's knowledge of any allergies and their relation to agents in the workplace should be sought. Dust control and other protective methods used in the workplace, treatments used to relieve symptoms, and the effectiveness of these treatments should be sought. The development of similar symptoms in coworkers should be questioned at the initial interview.

Dyspnea is a common complaint in many occupational lung diseases. Dyspnea should be characterized and the British Medical Research Council questionnaire (Table 1.1) used to grade its severity (4). Other respiratory symptoms, in particular cough, chest pain, and exercise intolerance, should be identified.

The medical, surgical, and accident history, smoking status and history, family history, medications used, and allergies also provide additional clues to differentiate an occupational from a nonoccupational lung disease.

Medical records of all previous hospitalizations or emergency room visits and workplace infirmary visits should be reviewed, particularly for cases of suspected occupational airway disease in association with accidental exposures.

PHYSICAL EXAMINATION

Physical examination is important both for diagnosis and for assessing the severity of conditions such as emphysema and fibrosis. Evidence of dyspnea, cough, and wheezing, common findings in many types of occupational lung disease, should be sought. Adventitious lung sounds should be noted; fine rales at the bases suggest an interstitial fibrotic or inflammatory process. Clubbing may also be observed with advanced fibrosis, for example in asbestosis, but neither rales nor clubbing is pathognomonic of an occupational lung disease. The evolution of the characteristics of the rales in asbestosis and other fibrotic diseases can indicate progression or stability of the process. Signs of right heart failure can be found late in the disease in the patient who has developed cor pulmonale sec-

TABLE 1.1
Classification of Dyspnea on Exertion

QUESTIONNAIRE MODIFIED FROM THE BRITISH MEDICAL RESEARCH COUNCIL (4)	
QUESTIONS	**GRADE OF DYSPNEA IF ANSWER IS YES[a]**
A. Are you troubled by shortness of breath when hurrying on level ground or walking up a slight hill?	Grade 2
B. Do you get short of breath walking with other people of your own age on level ground?	Grade 3
C. Do you have to stop for breath when walking at your own pace on level ground?	Grade 4
D. Do you get breathless on dressing or on washing?	Grade 5

[a] If the patient complaints of shortness of breath on exertion but answers no to question A, dyspnea Grade 1 should be recorded.

ondary to complicated pneumoconiosis due to coal, silica, or silicates and in diffuse fibrotic diseases such as asbestosis.

Physical examination may reveal systemic disorders that may be related to occupation (for example, scleroderma in workers with silica exposure) as well as diseases that are not related to occupation. Physical examination is also important in the assessment of disability in the worker with occupational lung disease (see next section).

SPECIFIC INVESTIGATIONS

Skin Prick Tests and Specific Immunoglobulins

These tests are clinical adjuncts that help in the recognition of exposure and reactivity to a suspected workplace agent. Skin reactivity and serologic tests for specific immunoglobulins to high-molecular-weight agents can be used to establish sensitization to an agent but not necessarily the presence of a disease. For example, the specific immunoglobulins to *Mycopolyspora faeni* are often high in farmers without allergic alveolitis. However, the association of a positive test with clinical features of allergic alveolitis strongly suggests the disease. A detailed review of these tests is provided in a recent guideline proceeding (5) and further comments in a consensus statement of the American College of Chest Physicians (6).

Chest Radiography

Radiologic examinations are particularly useful in establishing the diagnosis, documenting extent, and monitoring progression of anatomic lesions in pneumoconioses and in differentiating them from cancers, old scars, and other lesions. They have limited value in the evaluation of functional impairment. The International Classification of Chest Radiographs provided by the International Labor Organisation (ILO 1980 classification) (7) is largely used for interpretation of the radiograph. It provides a glossary of descriptive terms and a set of 22 standard radiographs illustrating pleuropulmonary changes that can be found in the pneumoconioses. The system is purely descriptive and makes no pathologic correlation. It reduces variability between trained readers and facilitates comparison over time, particularly when prior films are not available. In addition, the scoring of the disease on the ILO classification provides a useful clinical indicator of disease severity on radiologic grounds that is useful in attributing the cause of death, particularly in the absence of an autopsy.

The chest radiographs should be standard high-kilovoltage posteroanterior (PA) and lateral views taken at maximal inspiration, as detailed in the recommendations of the ILO (7). The readings of chest radiographs are done on the PA views. The technical quality should be good and the radiographs taken under conditions for optimal visualization of the lung parenchyma.

Technical quality is graded on a four-point scale: 1, good; 2, acceptable, with no technical defect likely to impair classification; 3, poor, with some technical defect, still acceptable for purpose of classification; 4, unreadable.

Parenchymal Abnormalities. The opacities are recorded for shape and size. The shapes are either rounded or irregular. In each case three sizes are differentiated: The letters p, q, and r are for rounded opacities, where p is the diameter of individual opacities up to about 1.5 mm; q is the diameter exceeding 1.5 and up to 3 mm; r is the diameter exceeding 3 mm and up to 10 mm. The letters s, t, and u are for irregular opacities with a similar size scale.

The profusion (number) of opacities is scored according to the ILO grading system and the viewer's assessment of the concentration of opacities compared with the standard radiographs. This classification recognizes the existence of a continuum of change from no opacity to the most advanced category. The scores can be converted to a linear scale of 0 to 10 (12 grades) as follows: ILO grade 0/- (clearly normal) and 0/0 (normal after a good look) equals 0 on the linear scale; ILO grade 0/1 equals 1; 1/0 equals 2; 1/1 equals 3; 1/2 equals 4; 2/1 equals 5; 2/2 equals 6; 2/3 equals 7; 3/2 equals 8; 3/3 equals 9; 3/4 equals 10. The profusion of opacities is scored so as to weigh the usual six areas of the lung—upper, middle, and lower left and right lung fields—seen on the chest radiograph, with emphasis on the abnormalities detected, as recommended by the ILO report (7).

In the ILO classification, to group patients with similar diseases, four categories are defined on the basis of the same profusion scores:

0, profusion scores 0/-, 0/0, 0/1
1, profusion scores 1/0, 1/1, 1/2
2, profusion scores 2/1, 2/2, 2/3
3, profusion scores 3/2, 3/3 and 3/4

Grouping of opacities or confluence is classified as coalescence (ax) when the confluence is less than 10 mm in diameter and as large opacities (complicated pneumoconiosis, progressive massive fibrosis) when larger than 10 mm in diameter. Category A represents an opacity having a greatest diameter exceeding 10 mm up to and including 50 mm or several opacities, each exceeding 10 mm, the sum of whose greatest diameter does not exceed 50 mm. Category B represents one or more opacities larger than those in category A, whose combined area does not exceed the equivalent of the right upper lung field (one-third of lung height). Category C represents one or more opacities whose combined area exceeds the equivalent of the right upper lung field. Chest radiographs with accompanying ILO grades are shown in Figures 7.1, 7.2, and 9.13*A*.

Pleural Abnormalities. Pleural changes are classified by width and extent according to the ILO system. For chest walls, the width categories are ***a***, ***b***, and ***c*** and the extent scores, ***1***, ***2***, and ***3***. Diaphragmatic and costophrenic angle lesions are classified as present or absent. Pleural calcification is also noted (7).

A simple total score of pleural changes has been developed (8, 9) to scale the asbestos pleural abnormalities as follows: each diaphragm and each costophrenic angle change is scored as 1 (maximum of 4); pleural plaques en face are scored as 1; the circumscribed pleural plaques classified as ***a1***, ***a2***, ***b1*** are scored as 1; the ***a3***, ***b2***, ***c1***, as 2; and the ***c2*** and ***c3*** as 3 for each side of the thorax. The pleural changes classified as diffuse are scored at twice the score of circumscribed pleural changes for the same type of ILO classification as given earlier (e.g., a diffuse pleural change of ***b2*** ILO classification would be scored as 4 when diffuse). With this scale scores of pleural disease vary between 0 and 16.

Other Abnormalities. Finally, symbols are used to note changes suggesting abnormalities that may or may not have occupational origin.

ax, coalescence of small pneumoconiotic opacities
bu, bulla

ca, cancer of lung or pleura
cn, calcification of small pneumoconiotic opacities
co, abnormality of cardiac size or shape
cp, cor pulmonale
cv, cavity
di, marked distortion of the intrathoracic organs
ef, effusion
em, definite emphysema
es, eggshell calcification of the hilar or mediastinal lymph nodes
fr, fractured rib(s)
hi, enlargement of hilar or mediastinal lymph nodes
ho, honeycomb lung
id, ill-defined diaphragm
ih, ill-defined heart outline
kl, septal (Kerley) lines
od, other significant abnormality
pi, pleural thickening in the interlobar fissure of mediastinum
px, pneumothorax
rp, rheumatoid pneumoconiosis
tb, tuberculosis

Reporting sheets have been developed by ILO, NIOSH, and the Ontario Workers' Compensation Board. Their use facilitates the classification of chest radiographs according to the ILO scheme (7). Table 1.2 presents a summary of ILO classification for pleuropulmonary readings.

Chest Tomodensitometry

In recent years chest tomodensitometry (computed tomography, or CT), of the thorax has become an additional tool for diagnosis and assessment of the severity of lesions. Technical advances have allowed improvement of imaging, with thick and thin slices, high resolution, and appropriate windows as noted in the more recent publications (8–14). Several studies have demonstrated that CT scan is more sensitive than standard chest radiograph for evaluation of pneumoconioses and asbestos-related pleural diseases (6–12). CT can be used in the initial diagnosis and also in early detection of conglomeration in silicosis. Unfortunately, there is still no widely accepted standard of readings of CT images at this time, but the same principles as the ILO 1980 system for radiograph classification can be applied to reading CT images (8, 14).

A brief description of the usual radiologic changes seen in the pneumoconioses is presented in Table 1.3. There is more descriptive and illustrative information in clinical textbooks on the pneumoconioses (15, 16).

Pulmonary Function Tests

Spirometry. The measurement of forced expiratory volumes and related indices of airflow rates, including forced vital capacity (FVC), forced expiratory volume in 1 second (FEV_1), and the ratio of FEV_1 to FVC gives the minimum information needed to assess functional respiratory deficit. On the forced expiratory flow curve one can usually determine that the limitation is restrictive or obstructive. Restrictive deficits should be confirmed by full lung volume measurements. The apparatus and procedure for measurement of forced expiratory

TABLE 1.2
ILO Classification of Chest Radiographs

A. SMALL OPACITIES			
PROFUSION	**CATEGORY**	**MINOR CATEGORIES**	
	0 (normal)	0/−, 0/0, 0/1	
	1 (mild)	1/0, 1/1, 1/2	
	2 (moderate)	2/1, 2/2, 2/3	
	3 (severe)	3/2, 3/3, 3/+	
TYPE OR SHAPE	**SIZE**	**ROUNDED**	**IRREGULAR**
	<1.5 mm	p	s
	1.5–3 mm	q	t
	3–10 mm	r	u

B. LARGE OPACITIES		
	CATEGORY	**SIZE**
	A	10–50 mm
	B	>A, <right upper lobe
	C	>right upper lobe

C. PLEURAL ABNORMALITIES

Pleural thickening — type: circumscribed or diffuse
Diaphragmatic plaque and Costophrenic angle — present or absent, right and/or left side
Chest wall circumscribed thickening (plaques) or diffuse thickening or en face thickening (extent only) right and/or left side

	WIDTH	**EXTENT**
	a ≤ 5 mm	1 ≤¼ of chest wall
	b = 5–10 mm	2 >¼ and <½ of chest wall
	c = 10 mm	3 >½ of chest wall

Pleural calcification
Chest wall, diaphragm, and other sites (mediastinum or pericardium) right and/or left side

	EXTENT	**SIZE**
	1	≤20 mm
	2	20–100 mm
	3	>100 mm

Film quality and symbols are also recorded.

volumes should be in accordance with the American Thoracic Society recommendations (17).

Parameters of early disease of the small airways, such as the maximum mid-expiratory flow rate (MMEF) and expiratory flow rates at fixed levels of the FVC_{25-75}, are not routinely used in assessment of functional deficit (18). Although more sensitive, these parameters have large variability and poor repro-

TABLE 1.3
Usual Radiologic Changes in the Pneumoconioses

DISEASE/AGENT	RADIOLOGIC CHANGES
Asbestosis	Irregular opacities at bases Interlobular bands of fibrosis (crow's paw) Lung masses (tumors) Transient pleural effusion Pleural plaques, calcified or not, limited or diffuse Rounded atelectasis Pleural fibrosis Irregular pleural thickening (mesothelioma)
Coal workers' pneumoconiosis	Rounded opacities at apices Confluence of opacities; large opacities in advanced disease
Silicosis	Alveolar filling; ground glass in acute silicoproteinosis Rounded opacities in most cases Hilar node enlargement ± eggshell calcifications Confluence of opacities; large opacities in advanced disease
Silicatosis	Rounded and/or irregular opacities in mid-lower fields Confluence of opacities; large opacities in advanced disease
Rheumatoid pneumoconiosis	Rapidly enlarging opacities ± cavitation in any field Mild or absent simple pneumoconiosis
High-density "inert" dust (iron, tin, barium, antimony, zirconium, chromium, silver)	Dense rounded opacities in most cases, some irregularities
Low-density "inert" dust (limestone, cement, marble, gypsum, silicon carbide)	Soft rounded opacities in most cases; some irregularities Dense round opacities suggest silica exposure Pleural plaques in silicon carbide workers
Berylliosis	Alveolar filling; ground glass in acute phase Irregular nodules; honeycombing later
Allergic alveolitis (hypersensitivity pneumonitis)	Alveolar filling; ground glass in acute phase Irregular nodules; honeycombing later
Asthma, bronchitis, byssinosis	Usually no change
Fumes	Alveolar filling; ground glass in acute phase Bronchiolitis obliterans; opacities ± irregularities

ducibility. Their ability to predict obstructive airway disease has never been documented. Finally, the demonstrated correlations between reduction of FEV_1 and dyspnea have not been found for the small airway disease parameters.

The interpretation of the forced expiratory volumes and related indices of airflow rates must take into account the shape or form of the flow–volume curve. In addition one should be careful in the interpretation of a slightly reduced ratio of FEV_1 to FVC when the FEV_1 is normal and/or the FVC is above predicted values. The use of appropriate reference values is important. At present the CECA reference values (19) appear adequate for most patients with European ancestry. Corrections should be applied (0.85 or 0.9 times the usual prediction), when dealing with subjects of Asian, Afro-American, and some other ancestries (18, 20).

Lung Volumes. The measurement of FEV and related indices of airflow rates do not fully characterize functional impairment. Lung volumes are also important.

Total lung capacity (TLC), functional residual capacity (FRC), slow vital capacity (SVC or VC), and residual volume (RV) are the commonly used measurements. They are necessary to confirm a restrictive syndrome, characterized by reduction in TLC. Lung volumes are also useful to assess the volume of air trapping in obstructive diseases. An increase in FRC can contribute to dyspnea as well as a reduction in FEV_1. Total body plethysmography is preferred to the helium dilution method for these measurements, as the latter can seriously underestimate the lung volume in obstructive lung diseases (21).

Carbon Monoxide Diffusing Capacity. Carbon monoxide diffusing capacity (DL_{co}) assesses gas transfer between lungs and the bloodstream. The single-breath method should be used (22). The DL_{co} can be severely reduced in emphysema, interstitial lung fibrosis, and pulmonary hypertension. After correction for alveolar volume it is often normal in asthma, chronic bronchitis, and chest wall restriction.

A major limitation of most of these lung function tests is that they are done at rest, while the major complaint of an active worker is usually during activity. The resting DL_{co} is the exception, as it can predict exercise desaturation with modest accuracy.

Exercise Testing. The standard exercise test is the most appropriate way of directly and accurately evaluating the performance of the respiratory and cardiovascular systems during exercise. It is used to assess the nature of the functional limitation and to provide a rational basis to determine the capacity of a person to accomplish a level of exertion required for various jobs (23, 24). The recommended protocol uses a progressive workload as the standard (25, 26). Measured parameters are workload in watts per minute, minute ventilation, respiratory frequency, tidal volume, electrocardiogram, cardiac frequency, oxygen consumption, carbon dioxide production, and respiratory exchange ratio (carbon dioxide elimination divided by oxygen consumption).

If one suspects exercise carbon dioxide retention or desaturation, the exercise protocol should include gas exchange and arterial blood gas measurements at rest and exercise. The results of exercise tests can be checked against reference tables that allow conversion of workloads to equivalent energy output units: kilocalories per hour, watts, kilograms per meter, or oxygen consumption in liters per minute (24–27). In the interpretation of exercise tests only the limitations associated with respiratory dysfunction should be used for rating respiratory disability. Generally the level of exercise sustainable over the long term at work is always below 50% of the maximal intensity achieved in the JONES stage 1 test (26).

Arterial Blood Gases. The analysis of blood gases can be used to measure the partial arterial pressure of oxygen and carbon dioxide ($Pao2$, $Paco2$), the level of hemoglobin, the percentage of oxyhemoglobin saturation ($Sao2$), the arterial content of oxygen and carbon dioxide, and the different parameters of acid–base balance. The measurements can be made both at rest and on exercise. Along with measurements of expired gases, an analysis of blood gases allows the measurement of the alveoloarterial oxygen gradient ($A - aO_2$) and physiologic dead space (Vd/Vt). Certain abnormalities may become evident only on exercise.

Can noninvasive techniques such as oxymetry and transcutaneous carbon dioxide pressure (PCO_2) replace the measurements of blood gases? For values over 90% the accuracy of oxygen saturation measurement is reliable to within 1 to 2%. Because of the shape of the oxyhemoglobin dissociation curve, oxymetry is less sensitive to variations of PO_2 and may hide important falls during exercise. Steady-state measurements of transcutaneous PCO_2 are reliable, but their response time is too slow to make them useful on exercise. The measurement of arterial blood gases remains the best method when available, particularly for the evaluation of impairment and disability.

SPECIAL TESTS FOR BRONCHIAL ASTHMA

Asthma has intermittent and paroxysmal characteristics that call for particular evaluations. Asthma symptoms are related to bronchial obstruction and to bronchial hyperresponsiveness. Allergy to various common antigens affects more than 50% of patients with adult asthma. The results of allergy skin tests to specific agents in the workplace are important to the diagnosis. Apart from the usual pulmonary function tests, evaluation of asthma necessitates specialized tests recommended in recent reviews (3, 5, 6).

Nonspecific Bronchial Provocation Tests. The purpose of nonspecific bronchial provocation tests is to measure the degree of bronchial responsiveness to nonspecific stimuli. The tests use histamine or methacholine to induce bronchoconstriction according to the Cockcroft's protocol (28). Nonspecific irritants, such as dusts, fumes, and gases (e.g., sulfur dioxide (SO_2), nitrogen dioxide), and important changes in the physical characteristics of the surrounding air (cold, heat, humidity, dryness) can bother asthmatics who have significant nonspecific bronchial hyperresponsiveness.

Specific Bronchial Provocation Tests. Occupational asthma is the result of sensitization to a specific substance in the workplace that is generally characteristic of that type of work. Specific bronchial provocation tests are helpful to establish the diagnosis of occupational asthma (29, 30). As much as possible the test laboratory should simulate the usual working conditions. The subject is exposed first to a placebo and afterward to the suspected sensitizing agent or agents. Forced expiratory curves are monitored for 8 hours following exposure. Recommended procedures have been published (31, 32).

Work Site Investigation. It is not always possible to reproduce in the laboratory the usual working conditions. In this situation changes in nonspecific bronchial hyperreactivity and the monitoring of expiratory flow curves in the work site are alternative methods. This is traditional in cotton textile mills and is preferred in industries in which specific sensitizing agents are multiple, difficult to reproduce in the laboratory, or unknown.

IMPAIRMENT AND DISABILITY EVALUATION

General Considerations. Several rating schemes have been proposed to assess impairment and disability resulting from occupational respiratory diseases (33–38), but much variation persists between the different systems (see Chapter 13 for a discussion of medicolegal issues related to impairment and disability).

Pulmonary function testing measures the degree of lung dysfunction induced by a disease. Functional impairment brings about symptoms, mainly dyspnea, that can interfere with activities and thus cause some degree of disability to the individual. However, in addition to dyspnea, cough, and chest pain, symptoms related to hypoxia or hypercapnia may contribute to a patient's disability and should be taken into account. Pulmonary function tests at rest are poor predictors of the working capacity, which is better assessed by exercise testing.

Anatomic lesions, independent of respiratory impairment, can affect the worker. Radiographic abnormalities in silicosis can prevent access to the workplace. This factor should also be considered in the assessment of disability.

Bronchial asthma is a condition that is intermittent and partially reversible. Specific findings are required to make the diagnosis and assess the impairment related to occupational asthma (37). Frequency and severity of exacerbations, intolerance to specific substances at work, and the aggravating role of nonspecific bronchial hyrresponsiveness must be taken into consideration.

Described next is a rating scheme developed for the Workmen's Compensation Board (WCB) of Québec (38). It integrates numerous variables used in the assessment of disability for all occupational respiratory disorders. This scheme has the advantage of being usable for all occupational lung diseases, and the deficit is proportional to severity of impairment. Alternative schemes can be consulted (33–37).

Definitions. A few fundamental notions must be clearly defined when dealing with workers' compensation. They include diagnosis, impairment, disability, and imputability.

Diagnosis. The diagnosis of a suspected occupational respiratory disease should be documented as much as possible. The contributions of pathologists and mineralogists are of the utmost importance for mineral dust diseases, when lung tissues samples are available. Any disease and its functional consequences should be evaluated. As part of the medical evaluation of a worker, symptoms must be considered in relation to both the diagnosis and the associated functional consequences. It is the latter that may lead to disability. The functional consequences are often the same for different diseases. One must further distinguish two concepts: respiratory functional impairment and disability (33, 34).

Respiratory Impairment. Respiratory impairment results from loss of respiratory function, which influences the capacity of a person to execute tasks of daily living. Respiratory impairment is evaluated by lung function and exercise tests in comparison with predicted values for subjects of same age, height, and sex. Most guidelines classify the degree of abnormality of functional parameters by progressive severity (33–35). The functional respiratory impairment is a global assessment of lung dysfunction, expressed usually as a percent. Exercise tests establish a link between performed oxygen consumption and energy expenditure needed for various activities of daily living or work (39–42).

Disability. Disability is the inability to perform remunerative work because of a disease and/or loss of integrity. The respiratory impairment plays an essential but not exclusive role in disability. Assessment should include variables such as exercise limitation, nature of work, prognosis of disease, and in some cases cultural and social conditions such as alternative work, worker training, schooling, and education. In practical terms disability, either temporary or permanent, can be divided into two categories: (*a*) *total disability*, or the inability to perform any remunerative work and (*b*) *partial or specific disability*, or the inability to do a specific job.

Imputability. The causal attribution of asbestosis or mesothelioma to asbestos exposure is obvious in many cases. At times more than one factor contributes to symptoms or impairment of lung function. Occupational and personal factors may contribute to diseases with multifactorial causes such as COPD, asthma, and bronchogenic cancer. Then a global judgment without consideration for the respective contributions of occupational and personal factors can cause two types of errors: (*a*) *undercompensation* and absence of recognition of an occupational disease if personal factors are considered dominant or (*b*) *overcompensation* if one attributes the disease only to occupational factors and ignores personal factors such as smoking history and atopy, which can also contribute to the genesis of COPD, lung cancer, and asthma. The fair solution is to evaluate reasonably all contributing factors and apportion their role or roles accordingly.

Compensation is usually considered when a causal association is proved beyond reasonable doubt for groups of workers exposed to an offending agent in the workplace. The concept of probability of causation (PC), or attributable risk percentage, usually applies when it is more than 50%, meaning the worker's risk is more than twice that of the general population; in this situation workers should be eligible for compensation. PC is determined as the risk of disease in exposed persons (Re) and unexposed (Ru), both otherwise having same risk factors as cases (Re′). Then, Pc equals Re minus Ru divided by Re′, the excess risk divided by the total risk in exposed persons. Dividing top and bottom of the equation by Ru′ permits expression of relative risk of exposed versus unexposed, or RR equals Re divided by Ru (43, 44).

Although compensation decisions are the domain of public administration, physicians are often requested to provide input. Expert opinions should be based on adequate medical, epidemiologic, and scientific information on the matter. In spite of the difficult nature of the task, one can objectively proceed to apportion responsibilities and establish the percentage of deficit attributable to the occupational component of the disease whenever possible.

Questions to Be Addressed. The procedure for evaluating respiratory impairment and disability should address the following questions:

1. What is the diagnosis?
2. Is disease causally related to work?
3. What is the resulting degree of functional impairment?
4. Is the disease and/or functional impairment a cause of inability to perform the specific job?
5. To what extent does the disease limit ability to do other work?
6. Are aggravating factors or other conditions interfering with working capacity?

General Evaluation Procedures

The medical evaluation is based on several elements, some obligatory, some optional: medical and work history, physical examination, chest radiography, pulmonary function tests, exercise tests, and in the case of asthma, nonspecific and specific airway reactivity tests.

Diagnosis and Minimal Deficit. Significant functional abnormalities do not always exist at the time of diagnosis of occupational respiratory disease, but an irreversible, potentially progressive illness is itself a prejudice. Opacities on the chest radiograph of a patient with silicosis or the occupational sensitization to a substance may reduce the possibility of finding a job or buying life insurance. To compensate for these disadvantages, it is reasonable to allow a minimal impairment, such as 5%, at the time the diagnosis is established.

Global Anatomic and Physiologic Impairment. The global impairment is obtained by adding the minimal impairment related to disease recognition to the percentage of functional impairment as evaluated in Table 1.4 and the appropriate aggravating factors of Tables 1.5 and 1.6 up to a maximum cumulative sum of 100%.

Functional Assessment. Selection of the tests is a matter of medical judgment. Investigation includes all tests needed for establishment of the impairment

TABLE 1.4
Classification of Impairment of Respiratory System

CLASS	I	II	III	IV	V
FVC or SVC (% prediction)	>80	70–80	60–69	50–59	<50
FEV_1 (% prediction)	>80	70–80	55–69	40–54	<40
FEV_1/FVC (% prediction)	>90	80–90	70–79	54–69	<55
TLC (% prediction)					
(in restriction)	>85	75–85	65–74	60–64	<60
	or	or	or	or	or
(in obstruction)	<115	115–125	126–135	136–140	>140
DLco (% prediction)	>75	60–75	50–69	40–49	<40
VO_2MAX (male, 70 kg)					
(mL/min)	≥2000	2000	1500	1000	500
(mL/min/kg)	≥30	25–30	15–24	10–14	<10
Respiratory	None	Slight	Moderate	Severe	Very severe
Impairment	0%	5–20%	25–55%	60–100%	100%

Respiratory impairment should be rated according to parameters most pertinent to the person's condition (e.g., parameters for asbestosis are not same as for emphysema). For asthma, values of FEV_1 should be acquired after use of a bronchodilator. FVC, forced vital capacity; SVC, slow vital capacity; FEV_1, forced expiratory volume in 1 second; FEV_1/FVC, ratio; TLC, total lung capacity; DLco, diffusion capacity for carbon monoxide; VO_{2MAX} maximal intake of oxygen, a measure of fitness.

Bégin R, Desmeules M, Gauthier JJ, Ostiguy G. Évaluation de l'invalidité respiratoire: barème proposé à la Commission de la Santé et de la Sécurité au Travail du Québec, Comité spécial des présidents. Québec Workers' Compensation Board, October 1994; with permission.

Adapted from Bégin R, Desmeules M, Gauthier JJ, Ostiguy G. Évaluation de l'invalidité respiratoire: barème proposé à la Commission de la Santé et de la Sécurité au Travail du Québec, Comité spécial des présidents. Québec Workers' Compensation Board, October 1994.

TABLE 1.5
Aggravating Factors

A. ANATOMICAL

ABNORMALITY/SURGERY	DEFICIT ADDED
Thoracopulmonary anatomic abnormality	
slight	5%
moderate	10
severe	15
Thoracotomy or thoracoscopy	5
Lobectomy	5
Bilobectomy	10
Pneumonectomy	20

B. HYPOXEMIA

CLASS	Pao_2 (mm Hg)	GRADIENT (A − ao_2)	SaO_2 (%)	DEFICIT ADDED
Normal	>85	≤119	>94	0%
Slight	70–84	20–34	93–94	0
Moderate	60–69	35–44	90–92	5
Severe	<60	≥45	<90	10

C. HYPERCAPNIA

CLASS	$Paco_2$ (mm Hg)	DEFICIT ADDED
Normal	≤46	0%
Slight	47–50	5
Moderate	51–60	10
Severe	>60	15

The aggravating factors listed above are used to further adjust the total deficit of a person initially evaluated with Table 1.3

Bégin R, Desmeules M, Gauthier JJ, Ostiguy G. Évaluation de l'invalidité respiratoire: barème proposé à la Commission de la Santé et de la Sécurité au Travail du Québec, Comité spécial des présidents. Québec Workers' Compensation Board, October 1994; with permission.

Adapted from Bégin R, Desmeules M. Gauthier JJ, Ostiguy G. Évaluation de l'invalidité respiratoire: barème proposé à la Commission de la Santé et de la Sécurité au Travail du Québec, Comité spécial des présidents. Québec Workers' Compensation Board, October 1994.

classes presented in Table 1.4. The tests also provide information on functional deficit, residual function, and exercise tolerance of the person evaluated. This provides a sound basis for the description of the type of work adapted to the claimant's condition if a change of job is required.

Aggravating Factors. Respiratory function testing per Table 1.5 does not always completely delineate the anatomic damage resulting from respiratory disorders. The conglomerates of silicosis or sequelae of a chest trauma or surgical lung resection affect disability, which may not be readily assessed by lung function tests. Similarly, hypoxemia and hypercapnia are indicators of disease severity that must be considered beyond the functional assessment of Table l.4. Table

TABLE 1.6
Aggravating Factors in Asthma

A. BRONCHIAL INSTABILITY

CLASS	REVERSIBILITY (% INCREASE IN FEV_1)	HYPERREACTIVITY (PC_{20} IN MG/ML)	DEFICIT ADDED
Normal	<10	>8	0%
Slight	10–19	1–8	0
Moderate	20–29	0.125–1	5
Severe	≥30	<0.125	10

B. CLINICAL SEVERITY

CLASS	CLINICAL SEVERITY	DEFICIT ADDED
Normal	Asymptomatic most of time Intermittent Bd once in a while over 1 yr Normal PEF	0%
Slight	Intermittent symptoms, <2/week Nocturnal symptoms <2/month Bd prn, <2/week, low-dose inhaled steroids PEF > 80% predicted, variability 20–30%	5
Moderate	Exacerbations >2/week Nocturnal symptoms >2/month Bd daily; high-dose inhaled steroids daily PEF 60–80% predicted; variability 20–30%	10
Severe	Frequent day or night exacerbations Persistent symptoms limiting activities History of hospitalization for asthma or status asthmaticus Long-acting Bd needed for night coverage Bd daily; high-dose inhaled steroids daily Frequent use of systemic steroids PEF <60% predicted; variability >30%	15

Reversibility = percent increase in FEV_1 = improvement of FEV_1 after inhalation of 2 puffs of a β2 bronchodilator microaerosol administered through an aerochamber (Bd). PC20, provocative concentration of methacholine that induces a 20% fall of FEV_1. Slight bronchial instability is not considered an aggravating factor here, as it is already included in the baseline deficit of occupational asthma. Clinical severity is a scale derived from the International Consensus Report on Diagnosis and Treatment of Asthma (45). PEF, peak expiratory flow, to be used when available. For inhaled steroids, low dose ≤1000 μg beclomethasone or 800 μg Budesonide, considered the minimal daily dose required to stabilize asthma.

Bégin R, Desmeules M, Gauthier JJ, Ostiguy G. Évaluation de l'invalidité respiratoire: barème proposé à la Commission de la Santé et de la Sécurité au Travail du Québec, Comité spécial des présidents. Québec Workers' Compensation Board, October 1994; with permission.

Adapted from Bégin R, Desmeules M. Gauthier JJ, Ostiguy G. Évaluation de l'invalidité respiratoire: barème proposé à la Commission de la Santé et de la Sécurité au Travail du Québec, Comité spécial des présidents. Québec Workers' Compensation Board, October 1994.

1.5 provides a grid that can be used to consider these aggravating factors. Similarly, in asthma, bronchial instability and clinical severity are not appropriately evaluated by the functional assessment of Table 1.4. Table 1.6 provides a grid that can be used to consider these aggravating factors in asthma.

TABLE 1.7
Classification of Workers' Functional Limitations

CLASS OF WORK	VO_{2MAX} (ML/MIN/KG)	REQUIRED ENERGY (VO_2 IN ML/MIN)	EXAMPLES OF JOBS
I Heavy	>30	($VO_2 \geq 2000$) Lift a 100-lb load or carry a 50-lb load	Heavy manual labor Miners, lumberjacks, farmers, building foundry workers, dockers, masons, bricklayers, pipefitters
II Moderate	25–30	($VO_2 = 2000$) Lift a 50-lb load or carry a 20-lb load	Moderate manual labor Post office workers, factory workers, household maintenance, nursing, auto body workers
III Light	15–25	($VO_2 = 1500$) Lift or carry frequently a maximum 10-lb load	Light manual labor Active professional work, sales business, hairdressers, hotel workers, restaurant employees
IV Sedentary	10–15	($VO_2 = 1000$) No physical effort usually required; carry occasionally a 10-lb load	Sedentary labor Receptionists, janitors, secretaries, administrators, professionals
V None	<10	($VO_2 \leq 500$) Totally disabled for any job	No labor

VO_2, oxygen consumption or uptake in milliliters per minute.

Evaluation of Occupational Asthma. The definition of occupational asthma differs among authors and countries(3). One sound definition proposed by the Canadian Thoracic Society (29) described occupational asthma thus: "Variable airways obstruction along with bronchial hyperreactivity caused by sensitisation to a specific substance present in the workplace."

The nonspecific airway responsiveness of an asthmatic varies with respiratory infections, seasonal allergies, drugs, working environment, and so on. Assessment of the respiratory impairment of an asthmatic should be done under optimal conditions, that is, stable clinical condition with optimal medication and without infection. Several months may be needed for the bronchial reactivity of an occupational asthmatic to stabilize after the removal of the responsible substance. Thus disability evaluation should be carried out some 2 years after last exposure to the offending agent.

Functional Assessment. The clinical severity of the illness takes into account the frequency, intensity, and duration of symptoms; the daily variations of expiratory flows; daily regular medication; and adjustments of therapy as required by exacerbations. It avoids the tedious scoring system proposed in the American Thoracic Society guidelines (34).

Reversibility of Airway Obstruction. In asthmatics, airway obstruction being variable, postbronchodilator values should be used to grade the impairment in Table 1.4 because the use of medications is taken into account in considering the aggravating factors of Table 1.6.

Nonspecific Hyperreactivity. Airway hyperreactivity is found in most asthmatics. According to its severity, it may contribute to symptoms, limit exercise tolerance of the person to the working environment, and thus contribute to respiratory disability. This bronchial hyperreactivity is subject to considerable overlap between asthmatic and nonasthmatic subjects. Reference values that give more weight to specificity than sensitivity are used for airway hyperreactivity in the deficit assessment of Table 1.6.

Clinical Severity of the Illness. In most guides to evaluation of respiratory disability it is recommended to take into account the clinical severity of the illness (34, 37, 45). This approach has recently been validated (46). The scale presented in Table 1.6 is derived from the International Consensus on Asthma (47). In this table reference to drugs and their dosages is applied only if they are required for optimal treatment. Appropriate corrections for undertreatment or overtreatment should apply. Table 1.5 can be consulted when chronic hypoxemia and/or hypercapnia are aggravating factors.

Evaluation of Chronic Obstructive Pulmonary Disease. Evaluation of COPD can be established readily via Table 1.4. However, as the cause of these diseases is multifactorial, it is often difficult to identify the causative factors. Establishing the role played by occupational exposure may be problematic. Clinical features of both COPD and asthma can be present in reactive airway dysfunction syndrome (RADS). If airway obstruction is clinically variable or highly responsive to bronchodilators, Table 1.6 can be used.

Evaluation of Cancer of the Lung and Pleura. Respiratory function disorders resulting from cancers of the lung and pleura should be assessed through the recommended general procedure. These diseases are frequently associated with numerous symptoms and serious degradation of the patient's general condition. Moreover, the situation often deteriorates rapidly, and the bad prognosis of the disease should also be taken into consideration. The following procedures are recommended:

1. For resectable cancers and those in which a curative resection has been done, the use of the general assessment to establish the degree of respiratory impairment is recommended. Severity of clinical features should be used as a modulator in ascribing disability.
2. For unresectable cancers treated with radiation therapy or chemotherapy, one should presume that the respiratory impairment is very severe, corresponding to class V on Table 1.4. These patients should be considered totally disabled, as they generally have severe symptoms and poor prognosis. Side effects associated with treatment add to their predicament.

Evaluation of Tuberculosis, Fungal Infections, and Other Occupational Respiratory Infections. Most respiratory infections can be separated into two phases: an early active phase with or without treatment and a late stable phase with or without sequelae.

Active Phase. In the active phase the clinical features of the disease change rapidly, and it is not appropriate to assess respiratory functional impairment. Temporary total disability may be justified as long as treatment is administered or the condition is not stabilized.

Phase of Sequelae. Identifying the end of the active phase and determining whether the condition is stable are a matter of judgment by the physician. In practical terms stabilization of the condition usually corresponds to the end of active treatment. The general diagnostic procedures should be used to assess respiratory impairment and the resulting disability.

Evaluation of Functional Limitation and Ability to Work. Once respiratory impairment and disability have been fixed, the degree of functional limitation is established precisely to define the remaining ability to work. Data gathered from exercise testing are particularly helpful to this end. Table 1.7 provides a list of jobs derived from the classification of professions (39–42, 48). It is based on required energy output estimated from oxygen consumption at exercise. Examples of trades classified in five categories are presented.

WORKPLACE HYGIENE AND PREVENTION

In all workplaces that harbor the risk of occupational lung diseases, recognition of the use of substances potentially injurious to one's health is the cornerstone of application of appropriate industrial hygiene programs, with the support of legislative measures that establish the permissive exposure level (PEL) for most substances of concern in the workplace. These PELs are promulgated and enforced by the Occupational Safety and Health Administration under the Department of Labor in the United States and by the WCB in Canada. The PELs are available through the Registry of Toxic Effects of Chemical Substances and available on CD-ROM computer format (49).

Prevention is based on effective engineering controls that may include reduction or substitution of hazardous substances in the workplace, adequate exhaust ventilation systems, and regular revision of hazardous processes and practices. Also the development, implementation, and periodic revision of safe standard operating procedures (safe work practice programs) are effective preventive measures. The use of respirators should be encouraged during hazardous practices (unavoidable situations that expose workers to levels above PEL). Practical information on hazardous substances in the workplace should be made available to the workers. PEL should also be observed for sensitizing substances, but the level of exposure that induces asthma in sensitized persons is often well below PEL.

For accidental exposures emergency procedures should be developed and frequently practiced to prevent and mitigate the effects of industrial accidents, which still remain an important cause of occupational lung diseases.

SURVEILLANCE

Medical surveillance programs are legislated for most workplaces with a midsize to large workforce and hazardous substances in the workplace. Medical practice consists essentially of pre-employment evaluation of health, periodic evaluation of health and work practice, and when appropriate, temporary retirement from work and referral to specialists for full evaluation of workers. Pre-employment evaluation may include physical examination, chest radiograph, spirometry, and when appropriate, bronchial reactivity testing. Periodic re-examinations are often regulated for most traditional pneumoconioses and require examinations similar to those for pre-employment. In the case of cotton workers, spirometry before and after the work shift is required. Similar approaches, with addition of immunologic monitoring in some, are recommended for occupational asthma (6).

TREATMENT AND PATIENT MANAGEMENT

Medical treatment to improve work exposure tolerance is not generally recommended. The approach of choice is complete removal from exposure to the offending substance in the workplace, which is possible for some workers but not all. In the traditional pneumoconioses, for workers with minimal disease resulting from past high exposures, workplace exposure to hazardous substances below the PEL (usually less than one-third PEL) may be considered on an individual basis and subject to close follow-up. For workers with more than minimal disease, complete removal from exposure remains mandatory.

Many patients with occupational lung disease need medical help for maximal functional status; for advice on reasonable workplace accommodation, exercise training, nutrition, and sexuality; for smoking cessation programs, and for medical treatments of persistent symptoms. The usual medical practice to provide curative, supportive, preventive, and rehabilitative therapies applies equally to persons with occupational lung disease as to the general population, given the particular considerations specific for each occupational lung disease. Further details on these matters are more completely developed in clinical textbooks of occupational lung disease (2, 3, 15, 16).

REFERENCES

1. Key MM, Butler AF, Ligo RN, et al. Occupational diseases: a guide to their recognition. US DHEW (NIOSH) Publication No. 77–181, 1977.
2. L. Parmeggiani, ed. Encyclopedia of Occupational Health and Safety. 3rd ed. Geneva, Switzerland: International Labor Organisation. ILO Publication 92–2-103289–2, 1983.
3. Bernstein IL, Chan-Yeung M, Malo JL, Bernstein DI. Asthma in the workplace. New York: Marcel Dekker, 1993.
4. Medical Research Council (1960, UK). Short questionnaire on respiratory symptoms. In: Lloyd Davies TA, ed. Respiratory disease in foundrymen: report of a survey. London: Department of Employment, 1971.
5. Bernstein IL, ed. Proceedings of the Taskforce on Guidelines for Standardizing Old and New Technologies Used for the Diagnosis and Treatment of Allergic Diseases. J Allergy Clin Immunol 1988;82:488–99.
6. Chan-Yeung M, ed. Assessment of asthma in the workplace. ACCP Consensus Statement. Chest 1995;108:1084–1117.
7. International Labor Organization. Guidelines for the Use of ILO International Classification of Radiographs of Pneumoconioses. Occupational Safety and Health Series, No. 22, ILO, Genève, 1980.
8. Bégin R, Ostiguy G, Fillion R, et al. Computed tomography in the early detection of asbestosis. Br J Ind Med 1993;50:689–698.
9. Ostiguy G, Vaillancourt C, Bégin R. Respiratory health of workers exposed to metal

dusts and foundry fumes in a copper refinery. Occup Environ Med 1995;52: 204–210.
10. Bégin R, Boctor M, Bergeron D, et al. Radiographic assessment of pleuropulmonary disease in asbestos workers: P-A, 4-view films and computed tomography of the thorax. Br J Ind Med 1984;41:373–383.
11. Bégin R, Bergeron D, Samson L, et al. CT assessment of silicosis in exposed workers. Am J Roentgenol 1987;148:509–514.
12. Staples CA, Gamsu G, Ray CS, Webb WR. High-resolution computed tomography and lung function in asbestos exposed workers with normal radiographs. Am Rev Respir Dis 1989;139:1502–1508.
13. Rémy-Jardin M, Degreef JM, Buscard R, et al. Coal-workers' pneumoconiosis: CT assessment in exposed workers and correlations with radiographic findings. Radiology 1990;177:363–371.
14. Bégin R, Ostiguy G, Filion R, Colman N. Computed tomography scan in the early detection of silicosis. Am Rev Respir Dis 1991;144:697–705.
15. Parkes WR, ed. Occupational lung disorders. 3rd ed. Oxford, UK: Butterworth-Heinermann, 1994.
16. Harber P, Schenker MB, Balmes JR, eds. Occupational and environmental respiratory disease. St Louis: Mosby, 1996.
17. Morris AH, Kanner RE, Crapo RO, Gardner RM. Clinical pulmonary function testing. 2nd ed. Intermountain Thoracic Society, 1984.
18. American Thoracic Society. Lung function testing: selection of reference values and interpretative strategies. Am Rev Respir Dis 1991;144:1202–1218.
19. European Community for Coal and Steel. Ph H Quanjer, ed. Standardized lung function testing: report of working party: standardization of lung function tests. Bull Eur Physiopathol Respir 1983;19(Suppl 5):1–95.
20. Clausen JL. Prediction of normal values. In: Clausen JL, ed. Pulmonary function testing guidelines and controversies. New York: Academic Press, 1982:51–61.
21. Dubois AB, Bothelo SY, Bedell GN, et al. A rapid plethysmographic method for measuring thoracic gas volume. J Clin Invest 1956;35:322–326.
22. Cotes JE, Chinn DJ, Quanjer PHH, et al. Standardization of the measurement of transfer factor (diffusing capacity). Report of Working Party. Standardization of lung function tests, 1993 update. Eur Respir J 1993;6(Suppl 16):41–53.
23. Oren A, Sue DY, Hansen JE, et al. The role of exercise testing in impairment evaluation. Am Rev Respir Dis 1987;135:230–235.
24. Cotes JE. Rating respiratory disability: a report on behalf of a working group of the European Society for Clinical Respiratory Physiology. Eur Respir J 1990;3: 1074–1077.
25. Jones NL, Campbell EJM. Clinical exercise testing. 3rd ed. Philadelphia: WB Saunders, 1987.
26. Jones NL, Makrides L, Hitchcock C, et al. Normal standards for an incremental progressive cycle ergometer test. Am Rev Respir Dis 1985;131:700–708.
27. Åstrand PO, Rodahl K. Textbook of work physiology. New York: McGraw-Hill, 1970.
28. Cockcroft DW, Killian DN, Mellon JA, Hargrave FE. Bronchial reactivity to inhaled histamine: a method and clinical survey. Clin Allergy 1977;7:235–243.
29. Malo JL. L'asthme professionnel: rapport du comité de la société de thoracologie du Canada. Le Clinicien 1988;Mars 57–84.
30. Pepys J, Hutchcroft BJ. Bronchial provocation tests in the aetiologic diagnosis and analysis of asthma. Am Rev Respir Dis 111:829–859, 1975.
31. Sterk PJ, Fabbri LM, Quenjer PH, et al. Airway responsiveness: standardized challenge testing with pharmacological, physical and sensitizing stimuli in adults. Eur Respir J 1993;6 (Suppl 16):53–83.
32. Cartier P, Bernstein IL, Sherwood Burge P, et al. Guidelines for bronchoprovocation in the investigation of occupational asthma: report of the subcommittee on bronchial provocation for occupational asthma. J Allergy Clin Immunol 1989;84:823–29.

33. Doege TC, Houston TP, eds. Guides to the evaluation of permanent impairment. 3rd ed. American Medical Association, 1993.
34. Renzetti AD, Bleecker ER, Epler G, et al. Evaluation of impairment/disability secondary to respiratory disorders. Am Rev Respir Dis 1986;133:1205–1209.
35. Gaensler EA, Wright GW. Evaluation of respiratory impairment. Arch Environ Health 1966;12:146–189.
36. Ostiguy G, ed. Summary of task force report on occupational respiratory disease (pneumoconiosis). Can Med Assoc J 1979;121:414–421.
37. American Thoracic Society. Guidelines for the evaluation of impairment/disability in patients with asthma. Am Rev Respir Dis 1993;147:1056–61.
38. Bégin R, Desmeules M, Gauthier JJ, Ostiguy G. Évaluation de l'invalidité respiratoire: barème proposé à la Commission de la Santé et de la Sécurité au Travail du Québec, Comité spécial des présidents. Québec Workers' Compensation Board, October 1994.
39. Gordon EE. Energy costs of activities in health and disease. Arch Intern Med 1958; 101:702–13.
40. Tennessee Heart Association. Physicians handbook for evaluation of cardiovascular and physical fitness, 1972.
41. Canadian Medical Association. Proceedings of the international symposium on physical activity and cardiovascular health. In: Can Med Assoc Journal 1967;96: 695–915.
42. Morehouse LE, Miller AT. Physiology of exercise. St Louis: Mosby, 1971.
43. Bond V. The cancer risk attributable to radiation exposure: some practical problems. Health Physics 1981;40:108–11.
44. Rothman KJ. Modern epidemiology. Boston: Little, Brown, 1986.
45. Disability evaluation under social security. Washington: Department of Health and Human Services, SSA Publication 05–10089, 1986.
46. Blanc PD, Jones M, Besson MS, et al. Work disability among adults with asthma. Chest 1993;104:1371–1377.
47. International consensus on diagnosis and treatment of asthma. Bethesda, MD: National Institutes of Health NHLB Institute, Publication 92–3091, 1992.
48. Canadian Classification of Professions. Government of Canada publication 1971. (This document is largely derived from references 40 and 41.)
49. Canadian Centre for Occupational Health and Safety. CCINFO disk. Series C2 (RTECS) [CD-ROM]. MS-DOS version. Ontario, Canada.

CHAPTER 2

Pathologic Features of Occupational Lung Disease

❖ Francis H. Y. Green
❖ Andrew Churg

GENERAL CONSIDERATIONS

This chapter provides an approach for the pathologic examination of suspected cases of occupational lung disease and illustrates the basic patterns of nonneoplastic pathologic changes in the lung. The conditions discussed in this book are for the most part produced by inhalation of dust particles. Although detailed knowledge of the factors that govern the deposition and clearance of such particles and of the interaction of particles with cells and tissues is not essential to diagnosis, some familiarity with these topics can be useful in understanding the mechanisms whereby particles produce disease (1–5). The pathogenesis of the occupational lung diseases covered in this book is discussed in the chapters that follow. Techniques for the identification of inhaled materials and their quantification are described in Chapter 3.

An important point in assessing any kind of lung disease is that interpretation of pulmonary pathology, more than many other fields of pathology, requires some familiarity with clinical lung disease, pulmonary function, and radiographic appearances (see Chapter 1). Attempts to render a diagnosis of occupational lung disease in a pathologic vacuum, when all one has is a piece of tissue and no clinical information, are guaranteed to result in serious errors. Thus the tables of various pathologic reactions listed in this chapter are intended only as guidelines; the pathologist must obtain appropriate clinical and historical information before making a final diagnosis.

Many workers are likely to be exposed to any given agent, but *the fact of exposure is not synonymous with disease*. Most agents cause clinically apparent disease in only a relatively small proportion of those exposed (6). The relation between exposure and a suspected occupational lung disease is complex and depends on such factors as cumulative exposure (dose), clearance and dissolution, latency, individual susceptibility, interactions with host factors (e.g., smoking) and biologic plausibility. All of these factors should be considered before rendering an opinion on specific causation.

Making a diagnosis and establishing exposure are separate processes. Furthermore, some pathologic observations have no or little clinical importance but nonetheless have broader implications. An example is the presence of pleural plaques. These lesions produce no functional abnormalities, nor are they premalignant. They are, however, important markers of exposure to asbestos (see Chapter 9).

The presence of more than one disease process in a given patient is not unusual. The best example is lung cancer. Most patients show evidence of other smoking-related lung diseases (chronic bronchitis, small airway disease, emphysema) and a small minority also have asbestosis. To assess for other diseases it is necessary to take representative samples of lung well away from the tumor.

Although population studies reveal a moderate or good correlation between pathology and the physiologic and radiographic findings (see Chapter 6), in a given individual this relationship may be less than perfect. As a general rule pathology is more sensitive than routine pulmonary function or standard chest radiographs in its ability to detect disease. Thus mild forms of disease that are apparent to the pathologist may not be associated with functional or radiologic abnormalities. This is true particularly for diseases that have a distinct anatomic correlation, for example dust macules associated with extensive deposition of dusts such as the radiodense metals iron, tin, and barium, which produce a markedly abnormal chest radiograph with few or no clinical or functional changes. It is less likely to be true for diseases that primarily involve pathophysiologic mechanisms, for example occupational asthma, industrial (chronic) bronchitis, and pulmonary hypertension. In these cases it is possible to have severe impairment with relatively few anatomic findings.

Advances in technology, for example computed tomography (7, 8), functional tests for small airway disease (9), and morphometry (10) are improving our understanding of the relationship between pathologic and radiographic or functional changes, but these comments about the role of pathology still apply.

Finally, it is important to distinguish impairment, which is what the physician measures, from disability, which in its simplest and most practical term is a measure of lost wages. A physician may be able to function quite adequately with a mild degree of asbestosis; a heavy laborer may not. Determination of disability is essentially a legal and administrative rather than medical judgment (See Chapters 1 and 14).

THE IMPORTANCE OF THE OCCUPATIONAL AND ENVIRONMENTAL HISTORY

The occupational history is in many respects the cheapest, quickest, and most reliable indicator of the agent or agents, hence the disease or diseases to which the patient may be subject: "A good exposure history, carefully taken, remains the most powerful of the chest physician's tools" (11). The usefulness of such histories depends, of course, on the patient's or the physician's knowledge of specific exposures in specific occupations. Four important limitations of occupational history must be stressed:

1. *The patient may be unaware of the exposure.* This can come about either because he or she does not know in detail the nature of the materials used or because the constituents of the processes or products are industrial secrets. Asbestos and agents causing occupational asthma are the worst problems in this regard. It has been estimated that in the past at least 3000

products contained asbestos (12). Similarly, a wide variety of agents may produce occupational asthma (see Chapter 12), and more are reported all the time. When a suspected agent is found in lung tissue, it may be helpful to obtain materials from the workplace to be sure that these match the materials in the lung. However, failure to obtain a match does not always indicate a lack of workplace exposure, since most of the diseases in question have long latencies (20 to 30 years), and industrial processes and agents may change. Sometimes considerable detective work is necessary to turn up a historical sample relevant to the case or even to find out what is in current workplace materials.

2. *The history may not be sufficiently thorough.* Histories found in routine medical charts are particular offenders, the most common occupation being "retired." Because of the long latency for many pneumoconioses, elicitation of a current job may not be adequate; discovery of remote exposures in occupations completely unrelated to the patient's present employment can be critical to the diagnosis. Asbestos is the most obvious culprit in this regard: some individuals now presenting with mesotheliomas were exposed during shipyard employment in World War II and since that time have had completely different jobs that did not entail asbestos exposure. One solution to this problem is to take sequential occupational histories starting with first employment and continuing to the present (see Chapter 1). Another source of problems in this area is bystander exposure; i.e., an employee worked next to someone using a particular substance but did not use it himself.
3. *Exposure to more than one agent may have occurred.* For example, substantial amounts of crystalline silica commonly accompany ores and minerals, so that persons with ore-handling occupations are at risk for silicosis. Another example is talc, which may contain not only silica but asbestos; at least in the past the product sold as talc was sometimes more asbestos than talc (see Chapter 8). Thus some disease in talc workers may be a manifestation of exposure to asbestos rather than talc.
4. *Exposures to hazardous agents occur outside the workplace.* It is often useful to solicit information on hazardous hobbies and do-it-yourself interests, including home renovation, and the nature of the spouse's job. Exposure of family members to toxic materials brought home on work clothes is a well-recognized hazard (13). Occasionally disease is found in persons living around a factory or dump.

The Natural History of Occupational Lung Disease

In general the risk of developing an occupational lung disease is directly related to the target-specific dose (amount of the toxin that interacts with a cell or organ system) and cumulative exposure (average exposure times the years exposed). With the exception of acute lung injuries resulting from exposure to toxic gases and fumes (see Chapter 4) and some forms of occupational asthma (see Chapter 12), almost all occupational lung diseases have latency periods ranging from several months to many decades. The concept of latency is important for diagnosis, as it is rare to develop a chronic pneumoconiosis or occupational lung cancer within 15 years of first exposure, and some diseases, for example mesothelioma, often have latencies exceeding 40 years (see Chapter 10). Latency is influenced by exposure; in general, the greater the cumulative expo-

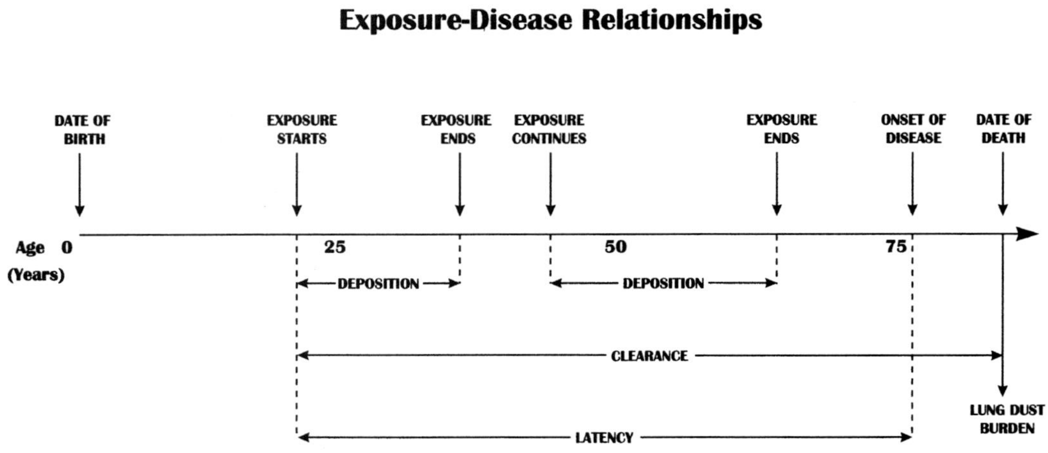

FIGURE 2.1
Temporal relationships between exposure and disease onset for a hypothetical case of an occupational lung disease, assuming that exposure was intermittent. Lifetime cumulative exposure, a common index of exposure in epidemiologic studies, is calculated from the exposure concentration (for example, milligrams per cubic meter) for the number of years exposed. The lung dust burden, a common index of dose in pathologic studies, equals the total amount of dust deposited in the lung minus the dust that has been cleared.

sure, the shorter the latency. The best example of this is silicosis, which manifests three distinct forms according to cumulative exposure and intensity of exposure. Acute silicosis develops within months of intense exposure to crystalline silica and shows a pathologic picture of alveolar lipoproteinosis. Moderate exposures result in a granulomatous and interstitial pneumonitis (subacute silicosis), and chronic lower-level exposures lead to the formation of classic nodular silicosis (see Chapter 7).

The timing of the exposure may also be important. Relatively brief and relatively low-level exposure to asbestos in younger individuals does not result in asbestosis but may put the individual at risk for mesothelioma many decades later (see Chapter 10). Finally, the residence time must be considered. In the previous example residence time is important because of the durability and long retention of amphibole asbestos fibers in the lung. Residence time is also important in the natural history of progressive massive fibrosis (PMF) and in the continuing increased rate of decline of forced expiratory volume in 1 second (FEV_1) in retired coal miners (see Chapter 6). The relationships among age, exposure history, latency, and progression of disease are shown in Figure 2.1.

PATHOLOGIC EXAMINATION

Legal Requirements for Notification

In many countries, including the United Kingdom, Australia, South Africa, and parts of the United States and Canada, the law requires that occupational lung diseases be reported to the coroner, medical examiner, or local health authority, and pathologic examination of such cases may be performed in a central laboratory. In the United States there is also a voluntary national autopsy program for coal miners. The pathologist should be aware of any such local requirements.

Choice of Specimen Type

Except in the patient with carcinoma, transbronchial biopsies have limited value to the pathologist when dealing with suspected occupational lung disease. Transbronchial biopsies are limited in two ways:

1. The small size and randomness of the sample tends to miss specific small lesions, and even if such lesions are found, it is often unclear from a transbronchial biopsy whether the finding accounts for the problem that brought the patient to medical attention. For example, one would not normally think of performing a transbronchial biopsy on a hard-rock miner with a fine nodular pattern on the chest radiograph (presumed silicosis) without clinical or radiographic reason to believe that an additional process such as tuberculosis or carcinoma was present.
2. Transbronchial biopsy is totally inadequate when dealing with diseases that have a component of interstitial fibrosis and inflammation and that are identified in large part by their characteristic low-power microscopic pattern. The evaluation of interstitial fibrosis and inflammation in transbronchial biopsies is difficult at best because the parenchyma is collapsed. Wall et al. (14) have shown that the use of a transbronchial biopsy to determine the presence or absence of nonoccupational chronic interstitial pneumonias such as usual interstitial pneumonia (UIP) is inaccurate. Exactly the same conclusions apply to occupational diseases such as asbestosis and talcosis, which are morphologically similar forms of chronic interstitial lung diseases.

The usefulness of pleural needle biopsies is also limited. Such biopsies can produce high yields in cases of tuberculosis and malignancy (15), but it is usually difficult to be certain of the diagnosis of mesothelioma on a pleural needle biopsy; larger pieces of tissue from pleuroscopy or thoracotomy are preferred.

Open lung biopsy or larger specimens obtained from resections or autopsies remains the gold standard for most types of parenchymal lung disease. However, even open biopsy has its limitations. The presence, type, and severity of emphysema are best judged in a whole lobe or lung. Because many forms of interstitial fibrosis are more severe in the periphery of the lung, open biopsy can overestimate the degree of disease that is actually present. *It is extremely important, therefore, to correlate the presumptive pathologic diagnosis, particularly in regard to severity, with the clinical findings*. For example, if severe fibrosis and honeycombing are found in an open biopsy but the patient has no functional or radiographic evidence of diffuse disease, it is virtually certain that the patient does not have diffuse interstitial fibrosis; most likely the biopsy sample comes from a local scar.

Specimen Handling

In general, open and thoracoscopic biopsies, lobes, and lungs can be handled much as for nonoccupational lung disease. Formalin is probably the best fixative; it does not add heavy metals to the specimen and does not interfere with analytic procedures. It is critical that all specimens be fixed by inflation; interpretation of any kind of lung biopsy or lobe is made vastly more difficult if the specimen is collapsed (16). Open biopsies can be inflated by inserting a needle into the parenchyma and gently infusing formalin with a syringe (17); after brief fixation the biopsy is blocked to give the largest possible pieces. When it is necessary to perform a frozen section on an open or thoracoscopic biopsy, inflation of the specimen with diluted frozen-section mounting medium before freezing produces sections that are much easier to read. If an analytic procedure of some kind may be needed, it is preferable to retain material in formalin rather than embedding it.

Inflation of lobes or lungs is conveniently carried out by placing a formalin tank on a shelf and running a hose from tank to bronchus. The inflation time and pressure are not critical; many laboratories use a pressure of approximately 25 cm of water. After fixation the specimens should be sliced in a midsagittal plane. *Gross photography of medicolegal specimens is highly recommended.*

Gross Examination

A large amount of information can be gleaned from gross examination (Table 2.1), even examination of open lung biopsies. Macules (nonfibrotic collections of mineral dust deposited around small airways) and nodules (fibrotic lesions with rounded or stellate borders in the lung parenchyma or perivascular or subpleural connective tissues) are usually easily seen, although nodules sometimes blend into the parenchyma and are better appreciated by palpation. The color of nodules or macules is often helpful in identifying the dust (Table 2.1), but black macules are found in many lungs as a result of breathing polluted urban air and/or cigarette smoke. The nodular or macular lesions of silicosis, silicatosis, and coal workers' pneumoconiosis are more prominent in the upper zones. Progressive massive fibrosis or complicated pneumonoconiosis, defined as nodular fibrotic lesions larger than 1 cm in diameter, also tends to be upper or mid zonal and is usually bilateral.

Emphysema caused by cigarette smoke, mineral dust, or both is seen in persons with occupational dust exposures, and the nature, extent, and severity of emphysema are best judged on gross examination rather than on microscopic slides.

Interstitial fibrosis tends to be obvious on cut sections of open biopsies or resection specimens if they have been inflated. Again, gross examination provides a much better idea of the extent of fibrosis than does the microscopic section. Evaluation of the distribution of lesions in lobes or lungs also yields valuable information. Most types of mineral dust–induced diffuse interstitial fibrosis or honeycombing (e.g., asbestosis, talcosis) are more severe in the lower zones. Honeycombing in upper zones may be caused by chronic berylliosis or aluminum-induced fibrosis, although nonoccupational causes such as sarcoidosis, eosinophilic granuloma, and tuberculosis are considerably more common. Extrinsic allergic alveolitis may produce either upper or lower zonal disease. Hard metal disease tends to be mid to lower zonal.

Mesotheliomas of the pleura or peritoneum surround viscera, and this again is a useful finding. But mesotheliomas may spread into the lung parenchyma, and carcinomas can also spread along the pleura, so the diagnosis must be determined by microscopic examination.

Definitions of Lesions and Their Microscopic Features

The combination of gross and histologic examination is the basic routine tool for classifying occupational lung diseases; general microscopic features are listed in Table 2.2. Definitions and representative illustrations of the more common le-

TABLE 2.1
Gross Evaluation of the Pathology Specimen

GROSS OBSERVATION	AGENT AND DISEASE
Consolidation in pattern of adult respiratory distress syndrome	Many agents, including fumes, gases, and smoke
Emphysema	Cigarette smoke Simple coal worker's pneumoconiosis Silica and some metal oxide exposures
Macules	
Black	Coal, carbon, graphite, cigarette smoke
Red to brown	Iron
Gray	Aluminum, some silicates
White	Titanium dioxide
Brown	Some silicates
Nodular fibrosis	Coal worker's pneumoconiosis Silicosis Mixed-dust fibrosis Silicate pneumoconioses
Diffuse interstitial fibrosis (lower zone predominant)	Asbestosis Talcosis and diffuse fibrosis produced by other sheet silicates (e.g., mica) Hard-metal disease (sometimes mid-zonal) Some cases of extrinsic allergic alveolitis
Diffuse interstitial fibrosis (upper zone predominant)	Some cases of aluminum-induced fibrosis Some cases of extrinsic allergic alveolitis Chronic berylliosis Silica
Mass lesions in lung	Carcinomas Massive fibrosis (complicated pneumoconiosis)
Discrete pleural nodules	Silica
Diffuse visceral pleural fibrosis	Asbestos Talc, possibly as a result of asbestos contamination Kaolin and other silicates
Parietal pleural plaques	Asbestos Talc, probably as a result of asbestos contamination Refractory ceramic fibers

sions are given later in the chapter. Greater detail can be found in the specific chapters that follow.

Dust resides in the lungs of all individuals, particularly cigarette smokers and those living in polluted environments. This dust is typically found around small airways and blood vessels and in the subpleural and interlobular connective tissues. In those with occupational dust exposure, fairly large numbers of particles may be seen in these locations. These findings must not be overinterpreted: the diagnosis of pneumoconiosis requires the identification of specific lesions. If dust is present, color and birefringence are also useful albeit limited methods of identification (Table 2.2; see Chapter 3).

TABLE 2.2
Microscopic Evaluation of the Pathology Specimen

MICROSCOPIC PATTERN	AGENT AND DISEASE
Dust accumulation in pleura, interlobular septa, and around small vessels, airways	All dusts
Diffuse alveolar damage	Many fumes, gases, and smoke
Airway epithelial necrosis	Many fumes, gases, and smoke
Bronchiolitis obliterans	Many fumes, gases, and smoke
Small airway disease	Many dusts (asbestos, silicates) Cigarette smoke
Dust macules	Many "inert" metals such as iron, tin Silicate minerals such as talc, mica Coal dust Other mineral dusts on occasion
Nodular fibrosis	Silica, silicate, and mixed-dust fibrosis
Progressive massive fibrosis	Silica, coal, silicates, and Caplan's lesions
Granulomas	
Sarcoid type	Berylliosis
Hypersensitivity type	Extrinsic allergic alveolitis
Foreign body type	Sheet silicates
Fibrotic nodules in hilar or intrapulmonary lymph nodes	Silica, coal (*not* a pneumoconiosis)
Diffuse interstitial fibrosis, inflammation	Asbestosis (asbestos bodies required) Talcosis from other sheet silicates, e.g., mica Hard-metal disease Aluminum-induced fibrosis Extrinsic allergic alveolitis Berylliosis Silica Coal Local scarring of no diagnostic significance around mass lesions such as carcinomas
Emphysema	Cigarette smoke Simple coal worker's pneumoconiosis Silica and some metal oxide exposures

Diffuse Alveolar Damage. For all practical purposes diffuse alveolar damage from occupational causes is identical to that from nonoccupational causes. It shows hyaline membranes in alveolar ducts in the early stages and intra-alveolar and intra–small airway granulation tissue in later stages. An interstitial inflammatory infiltrate and interstitial edema are usually present; see Chapter 4).

Small Airway Disease. There are three major forms of small airway disease: bronchiolitis obliterans, bronchiolitis associated with cigarette smoking, and mineral dust–associated small airway disease.

Bronchiolitis obliterans is a clinicopathologic syndrome involving progressive small airway injury with a variable onset from acute to chronic and in the severe case, marked airflow obstruction. In symptomatic cases the chest radiograph may be normal but more usually shows bilateral hyperinflation with subtle (bibasilar) micronodular infiltrates. Physical examination reveals dry crackles over the lower lobes, particularly on inspiration, and a midexpiratory squeak. Pulmonary function tests in the early stages show obstructive changes and a mottled distribution of defects on the ventilation–perfusion scan. Two morphologic patterns are seen (18). Morphology characterized by granulation tissue plugs (proliferative bronchiolitis) in small airways is closely akin to bronchiolitis obliterans organizing pneumonia (BOOP) and generally resolves without sequelae; it typically is not associated with obstructive changes. The form characterized by circumferential collagenous scarring with narrowing or obliteration of the airway lumen (constrictive bronchiolitis) tends to lead to irreversible airflow obstruction. Bronchiolitis obliterans has a variety of causes; in the field of occupational lung disease both proliferative and constrictive bronchiolitis may be seen after exposure to oxidant and irritant gases such as nitrogen oxides, ammonia, and chlorine) (see Chapter 4). Proliferative bronchiolitis may be seen as part of extrinsic allergic alveolitis (see Chapter 12).

Bronchiolitis associated with cigarette smoking and respiratory bronchiolitis with interstitial lung disease (RB-ILD) are covered here because they should be distinguished from mineral dust–associated airway disease, discussed later in the chapter. Cigarette smoke–induced bronchiolitis (commonly called small airway disease) is associated with chronic airflow obstruction when the process is severe. The membranous bronchioles and to a much lesser extent the more distal respiratory bronchioles show a variable combination of airway wall fibrosis and distortion with a chronic inflammatory infiltrate and often mucus metaplasia of the epithelium. Often pigmented macrophages (smoker's macrophages) are found in the lumens of respiratory bronchioles and alveolar ducts. These airway lesions are extremely common in cigarette smokers (Figs. 2.2 and 2.3).

An uncommon variant is RB-ILD in which changes in the small airways are associated with interstitial fibrosis. In RB-ILD the clinical features are cough, dyspnea, and rales. The chest radiograph may be normal, but bronchial wall thickening, prominence of the perivascular interstitium, small regular and irregular opacities, and small peripheral ring shadows have been described (19). Pulmonary function tests reveal a mixed obstructive and restrictive pattern, often with an increased residual volume (RV). Gas diffusion (DLco) may be normal or mildly reduced. Histopathologic changes are characteristic: chronic inflammation of the terminal bronchioles, respiratory bronchioles, and alveolar ducts is associated with mild fibrosis of their walls and adjacent alveoli (9, 20). There is also variable smooth muscle hyperplasia and accumulation of tan macrophages (smoker's macrophages) in the respiratory bronchioles and adjacent air spaces.

Mineral dust–associated small airway disease is also a distinct pathologic entity (21) caused by exposure to both fibrous (21) and nonfibrous mineral particles (22). It is characterized by deposition of mineral dust in the walls of small airways and alveolar ducts, with some accentuation at airway bifurcations (Fig. 2.3). In most instances mineral dust particles can be observed on light microscopy or polarization microscopy. Although cigarette smoke and mineral dust affect the same anatomic location, they can be distinguished on qualitative and quantitative criteria. A study by Wright (23)shows that mineral dusts produce small airway fibrosis above and beyond that caused by cigarette smoke.

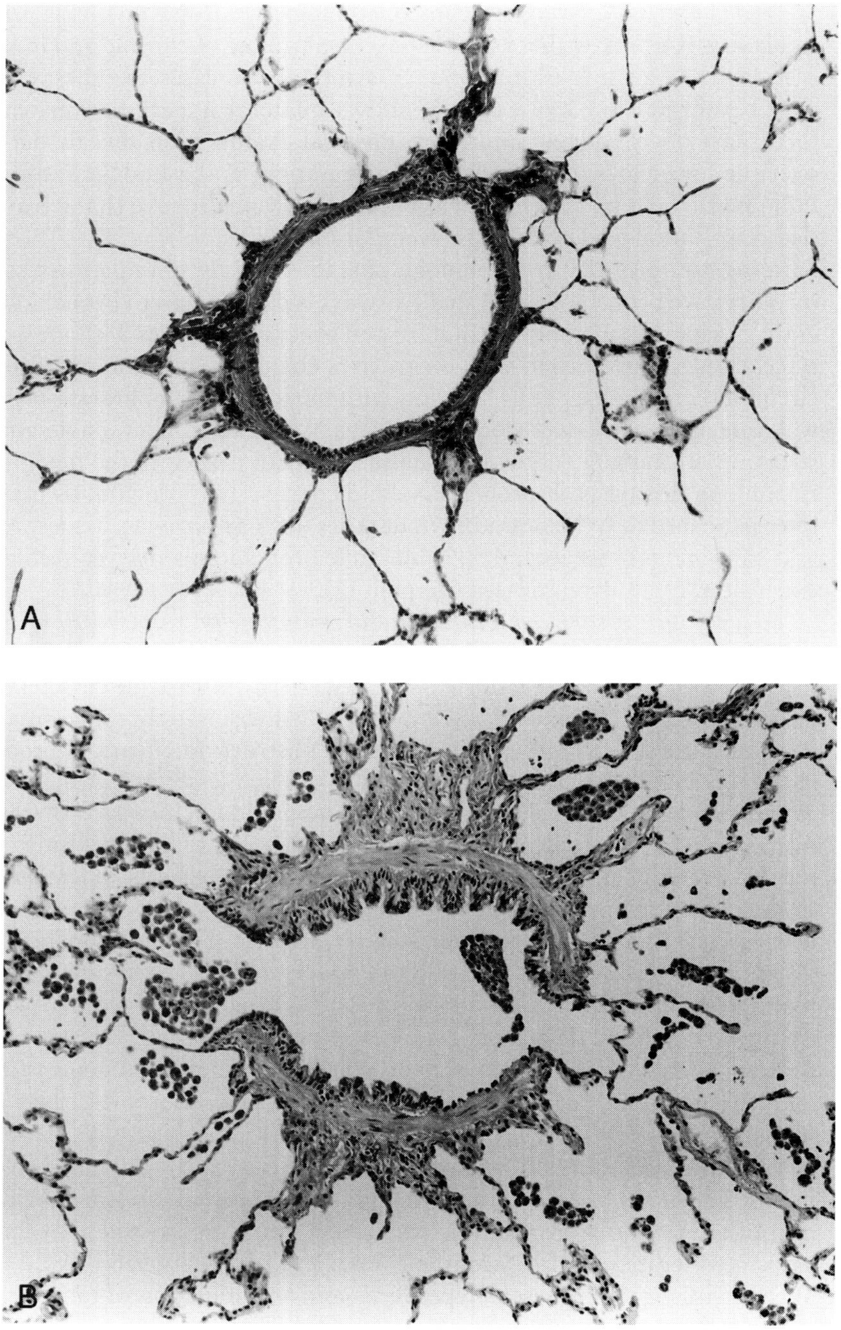

FIGURE 2.2

A. Normal membranous bronchiole. The small airway shown has a thin spiral wall of smooth muscle and is lined by cuboidal ciliated epithelial cells. A small amount of black pigment is seen in the adventitia. **B.** Membranous bronchiolitis associated with cigarette smoking. The section shows a terminal bronchiole at the respiratory bronchiolar junction from a young male cigarette smoker. There is smooth muscle hyperplasia, adventitial fibrosis, inflammation, and hyperplasia of the bronchiolar epithelium. Clusters of tan macrophages (smokers' macrophages) are seen in the adjacent alveoli.

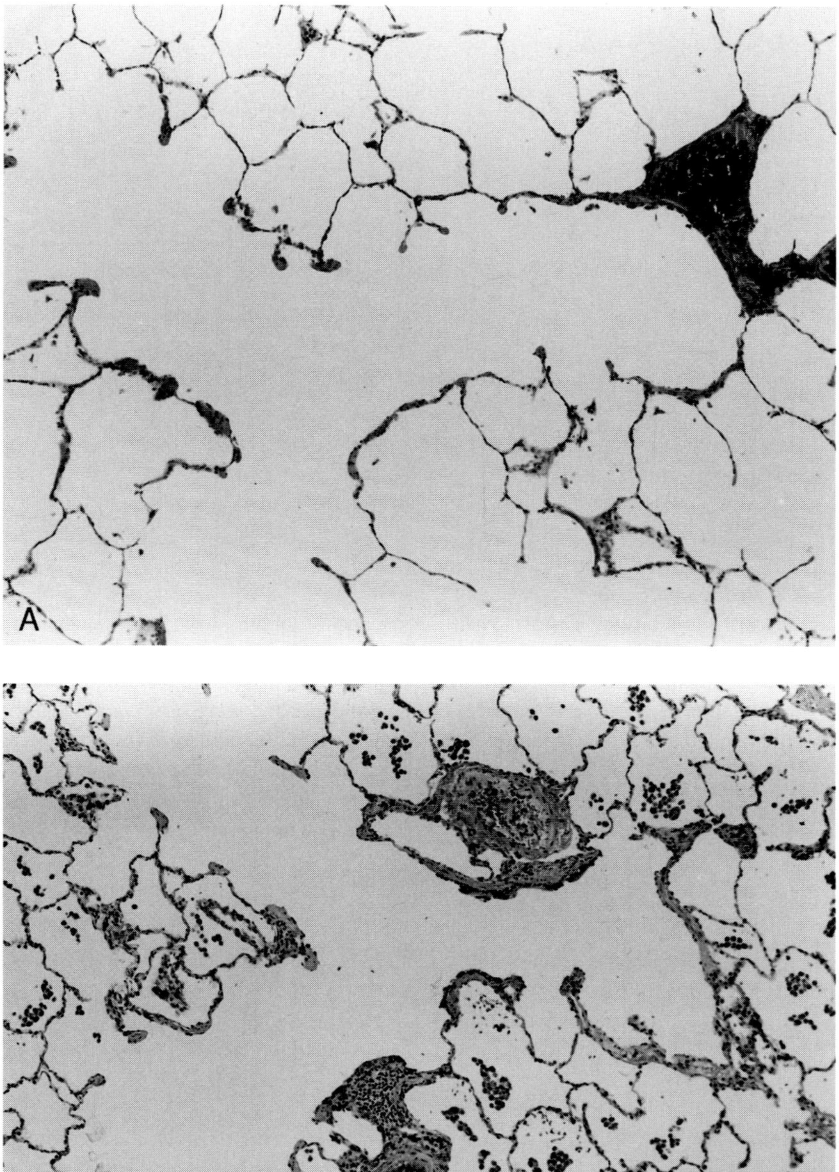

FIGURE 2.3

A. Normal respiratory bronchiole. Microscopic section of lung from young nonsmoking man showing the first two divisions of respiratory bronchioles and adjacent alveoli. The walls of the respiratory bronchioles are alveolated. The areas of thickening of the walls of the respiratory bronchioles are due to the normal focal distribution of smooth muscle and elastic fibers. **B.** Mild respiratory bronchiolitis associated with cigarette smoking. Microscopic sections of lung from a young male cigarette smoker. The walls of the respiratory bronchiole are slightly thickened by an increase in collagen and smooth muscle. There is a mild chronic inflammatory cell infiltrate of the respiratory bronchiole's wall, and the lining epithelium is hyperplastic. Black pigment is seen around the small blood vessels. Clusters of tan macrophages (smokers' macrophages) are seen in the adjacent alveoli.

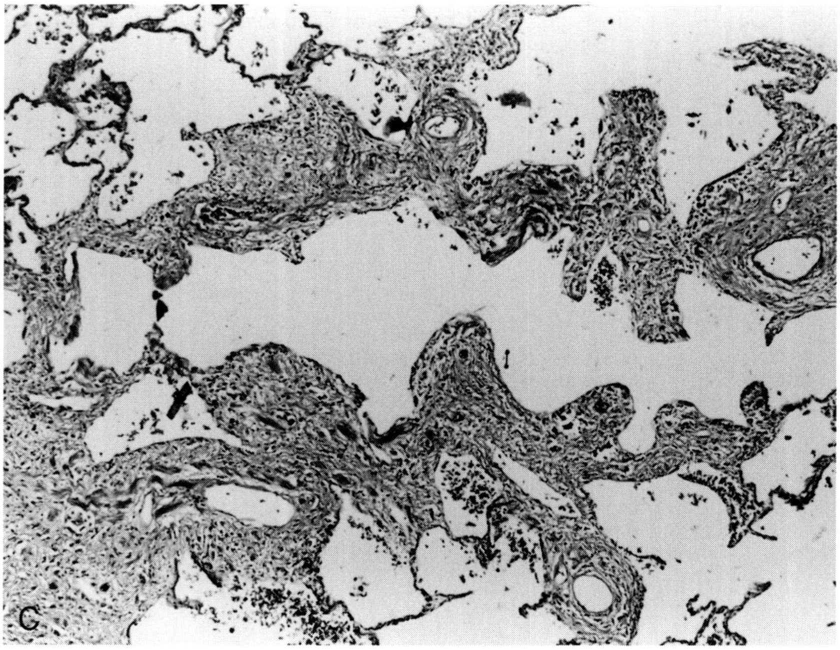

FIGURE 2.3 ***(continued)***

C. Mineral dust small airway disease. Microscopic section of lung from male miner exposed to both silica (quartz) dust and asbestos. The wall of the respiratory bronchiole is distorted, narrowed, and greatly thickened by fibrosis. Black pigment and macrophages are not prominent in this lesion. Asbestos bodies and particles of silica and silicates were observed in the fibrotic wall by light and polarizing microscopy, respectively. (Case C is courtesy of Dr. Dominic Spagnolio, Department of Pathology, Queen Elizabeth II Hospital, Perth, Western Ontario.)

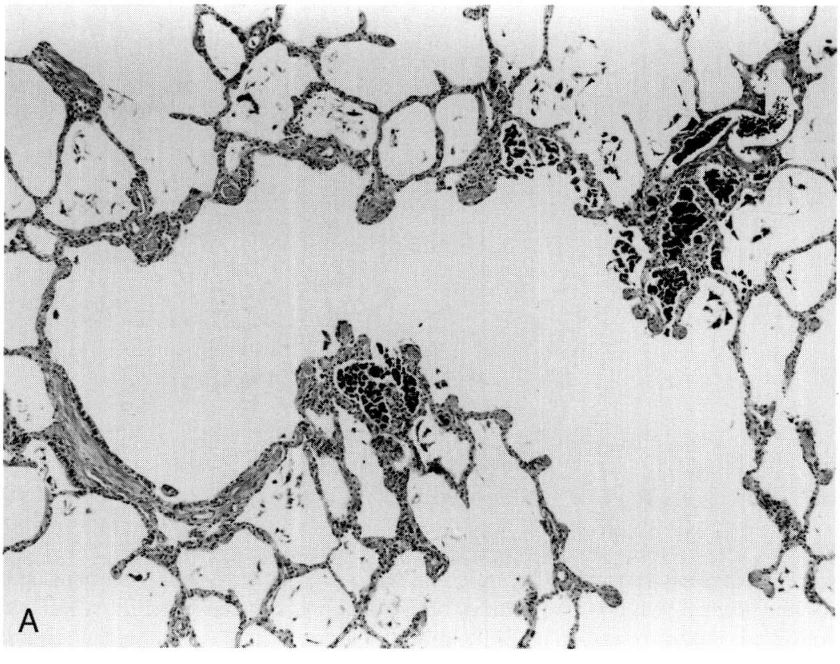

FIGURE 2.4

A. Evolution of the dust macule. Section of respiratory bronchiole from a young coal miner actively employed at the time of death. Clusters of black macrophages are seen in alveoli adjacent to the respiratory bronchiole. At this stage the dust has not been incorporated into the wall of the respiratory bronchiole.

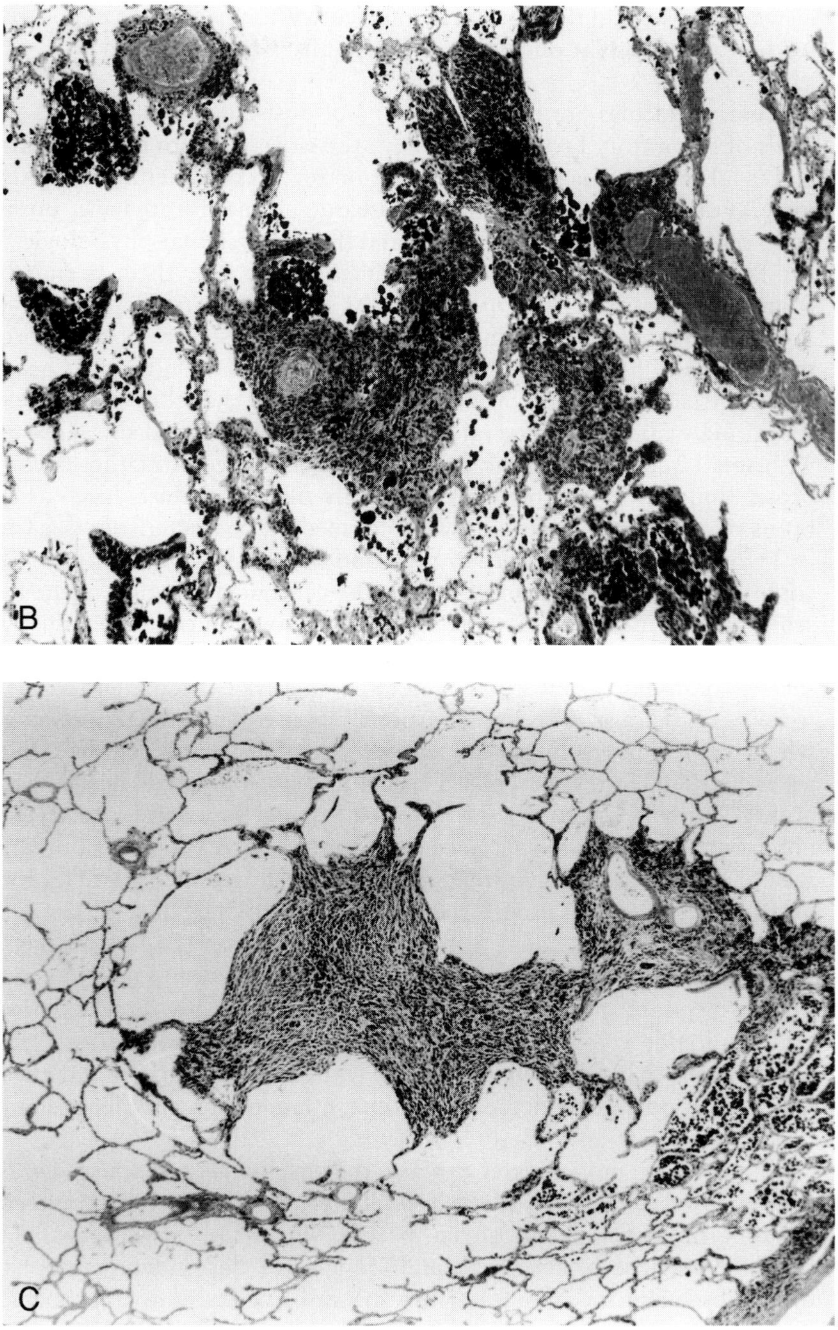

FIGURE 2.4 *(continued)*

B. Section of lung from a 31-year-old coal miner killed in an underground explosion. Black pigment is seen in macrophages within alveoli and within the walls of the respiratory bronchioles. Focal emphysema is not present. **C.** Section of lung from older active coal miner showing classic appearances of the coal dust macule with associated focal emphysema.

Furthermore, cigarette smoke rarely produces marked abnormalities of the respiratory bronchioles, the characteristic lesion of mineral dust–associated small airway disease, and the fibrosis associated with mineral dust exposure may extend into the alveolar ducts (Fig. 2.3) (see also Chapters 5 and 9).

Macules. Macules are focal collections of dust-laden macrophages within the walls of respiratory bronchioles. They are associated with mild reticulin fibrosis and focal emphysema (24). This definition reveals considerable overlap between mineral dust–induced small airway disease and the dust macule. Both are centered on the respiratory bronchiole, and they have similar physiologic correlates (9). Perhaps the most meaningful distinction is to view them as ends of a spectrum of changes. The term *macule* is best applied to large deposits of weakly fibrogenic dusts (e.g., coal and carbon) in the walls of respiratory bronchioles with mild and predominantly reticulin fibrosis and a tendency to be associated with centriacinar dilation or focal emphysema. At the other end of the spectrum the strongly fibrogenic mineral dusts, such as asbestos and silica, are associated with small quantities of visible dust, a predominance of mature collagenous fibrosis, and airway narrowing. Moderately fibrogenic dusts, such as the nonfibrous silicates, produce lesions with intermediate characteristics (see Chapter 8).

Two major theories, *sequestration* and *overload*, have been proposed to account for the accumulation of dust in the centriacinar region of the lungs. The sequestration model predicts that a constant fraction of inhaled dust will enter the interstitium of the lung and be retained for a long period. In this model the severity of disease is linearly related to cumulative exposure and to the inherent toxicity of the dust. This model probably best explains small airway disease in which a constant fraction of mineral dust particles that reach the small airways are sequestered into their walls. This model may apply to all dusts inhaled at relatively low concentrations. The overload model was developed to explain the nonlinearity of alveolar clearance in relation to increasing dust burden. Experimental studies have shown that the clearance of retained particles by alveolar macrophages becomes progressively impaired until lung dust burden increases at a rate approximately equal to the rate of deposition (25, 26). It has been observed in a number of animal species (rats, hamsters, and mice) exposed to insoluble respirable particulates, including carbon (27, 28), diesel exhaust (29), titanium dioxide (27, 28), and mineral dusts (30). This model better explains the observations that relatively inert dusts (e.g., coal and carbon black) can stimulate a disproportionate degree of chronic inflammation and fibrosis at high dust burdens (31–33).

The overload model better explains the development of severe disease in persons exposed to relatively inert dusts. It also provides a better model for understanding the development of the macule, which can be viewed as developing from the collapse of alveoli around sequestered dust-laden macrophages with their subsequent incorporation into the walls of respiratory bronchioles (Fig. 2.4). These two primary models for dust accumulation in the interstitium of the lung are shown in Fig. 2.5.

Regardless of the mechanism for the sequestration of dust within the interstitium, dust accumulation provides the stimulus for the initiation of inflammatory and fibrogenic processes. Dust-activated macrophages release reactive oxygen species (34), platelet-activating factor (PAF) (35), transforming growth factor-β, platelet-derived growth factor (PDGF), type I insulinlike growth factor (IGF-1) (36), tumor necrosis factor (TNF) (37), arachidonic acid, and its metabolites

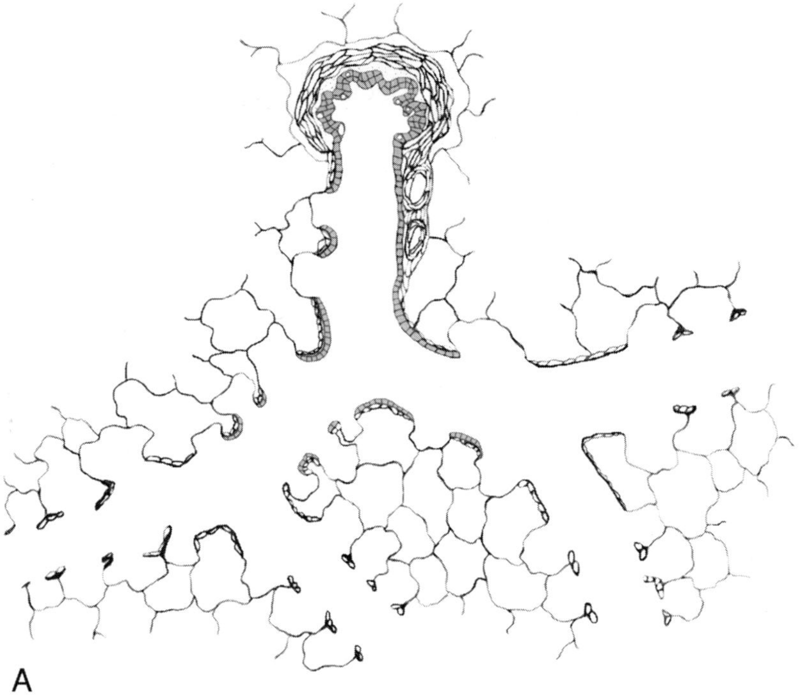

A

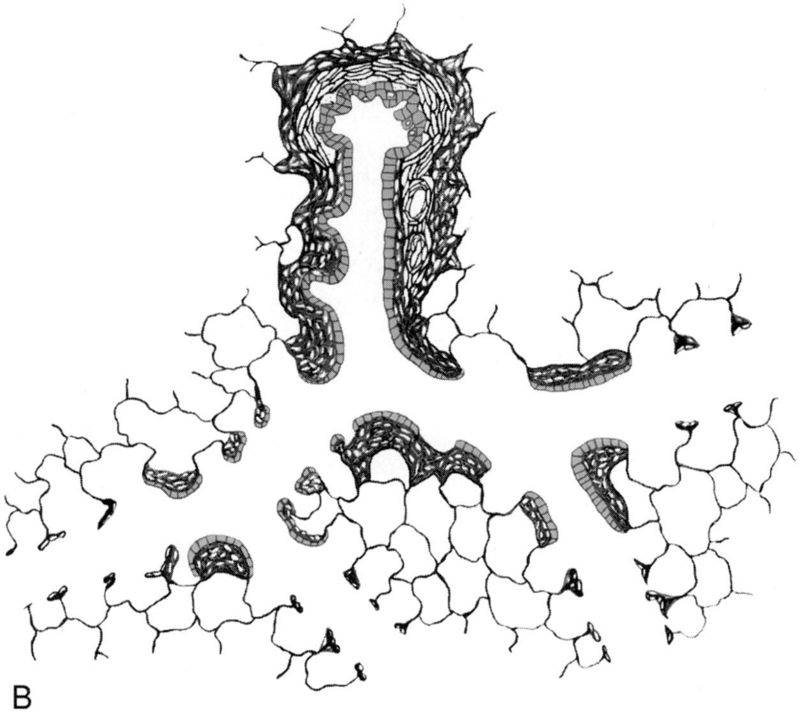

B

FIGURE 2.5

A. Normal terminal bronchiole with three generations of respiratory bronchioles. The walls of the respiratory bronchioles become progressively more alveolated from the first- to third-order bronchiole. There is also a progressive diminution in the amount of smooth muscle in the walls. The nonalveolated surface of the respiratory bronchioles is lined with ciliated cuboidal epithelium proximally and flattened alveolar epithelium distally. **B.** Mineral dust small airway disease. The walls of both the terminal bronchiole and proximal respiratory bronchioles are thick-

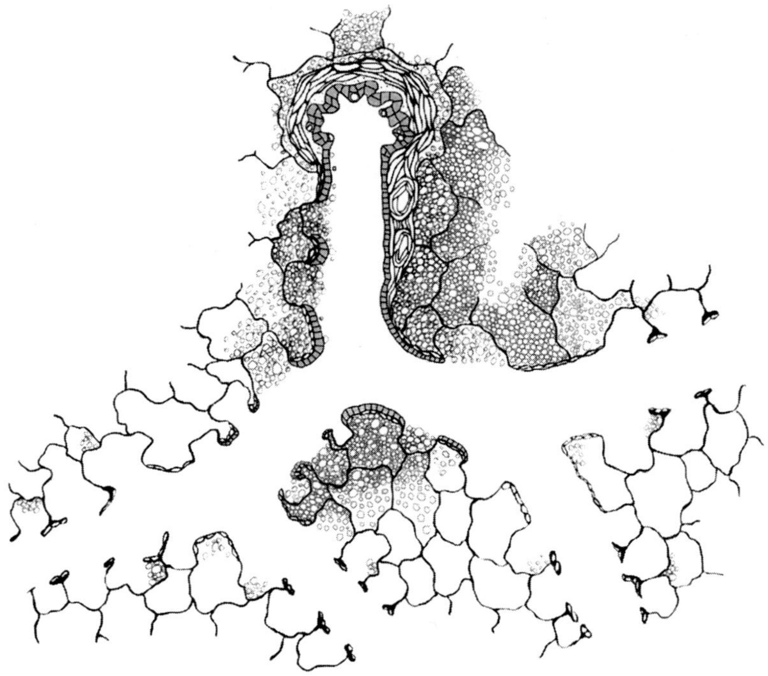

C

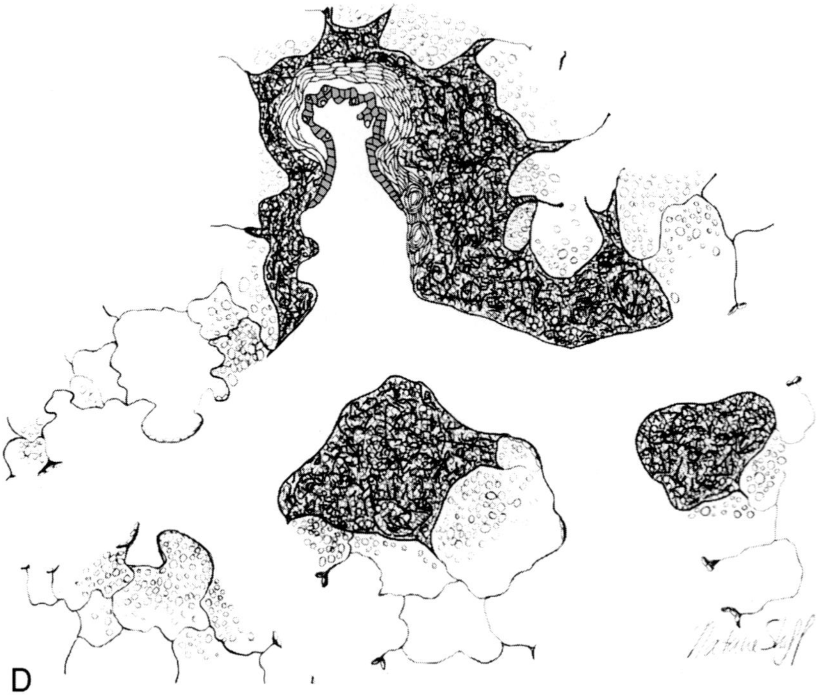

D

FIGURE 2.5 ***(continued)***
ened by a combination of increased connective tissue and smooth muscle. The bronchiolar epithelium is hyperplastic and extends deeper into the acinus. The lumen of the respiratory bronchiole narrows slightly and eventually becomes distorted (not shown). The fibrosis is marked at the bifurcations of the airways, the sites of maximum impaction of inhaled particles. This lesion is thought to evolve primarily through the incorporation of fibrogenic dusts into the walls of the respiratory bronchioles with an associated inflammatory and fibrogenic response. **C.** The dust overload in a person heavily exposed to a relatively nonfibrogenic dust, for example

(38). All of these factors have been shown to influence fibrogenesis either directly or indirectly (39, 40).

The type of dust and its surface characteristics influence the cellular response. Freshly fractured particles of silica or coal are more cytotoxic than aged particles of the same composition and size because of the formation of free radicals at the fractured surface (41). Occlusion or coating of the surface of a particle can also reduce its toxicity (42–45).

Emphysema. Emphysema is defined in anatomic terms as a permanent enlargement of the airspaces distal to the terminal bronchiole associated with destruction of the airspace walls (46). The types of emphysema include centriacinar, focal, panacinar, paraseptal, scar or irregular, senile, and bullous. However, centriacinar and panacinar are by far the most common types and are the two most commonly associated with cigarette smoking and mineral dust exposure. When associated with macules, the emphysema is termed focal but is for all practical purposes identical to ordinary centriacinar emphysema (Fig. 2.4). Emphysema is best appreciated on gross examination; good examples of the different types of emphysema can be found in Chapter 6.

Nodules. Nodules are characteristic of the response to silica (quartz) (see Chapter 7), silicate minerals (see Chapter 8) and to mixtures of dust containing free silica and other less fibrogenic dusts (mixed-dust pneumoconiosis) (see Chapters 6, 7, and 8). Nodules vary in size from a few millimeters to 1 cm across, are rounded and firm to palpation, and like macules, have a predilection for the upper lung zones. They may be found throughout the interstitium, including the subpleural area and adjacent to bronchovascular structures. Emphysema of the irregular or scar type is often seen at the periphery of the nodule. Microscopically nodules have three basic patterns, silicotic, mixed dust, and giant cell granulomatous.

Silicotic Nodule. The silicotic nodule is a generally sharply circumscribed nodular lesion with a whorled collagenous center and variable amounts of dust, usually around the nodule periphery (Fig. 2.6*A*; see Chapter 7).

Mixed-Dust Nodule. The mixed-dust nodule is a stellate (medusa head) lesion, often with less collagen than a typical silicotic nodule; the collagen is arranged in interlacing bundles or randomly rather than in a concentric pattern. Most examples contain large amounts of dust (Figs. 2.6, *B* and *C*; see Chapters 6 and 8).

FIGURE 2.5 ***(continued)***
coal or carbon black. Dusty macrophages accumulate in the alveoli adjacent to the respiratory bronchioles. This drawing shows a person currently exposed to high concentrations of dust for a relatively short period. The macrophages are sequestered in the alveoli because of overloading of the clearance mechanism. **D.** The situation associated with long-term dust overload. The lesion illustrates a macule in which dusty macrophages with mild fibrosis are incorporated into the walls of the respiratory bronchioles and are seen as a mantle around the terminal bronchiole. One mechanism whereby these lesions may form is collapse of the alveoli containing sequestered macrophages. As the macule forms, the alveolar walls break down, probably because of release of proteolytic enzymes by activated macrophages, and the respiratory bronchioles dilate as a result (focal emphysema). Comparison of Figures 2.5*B* and 2.5*D* indicates that the overload-associated macule and the mineral dust–induced small airways associated with fibrogenic dusts eventually have a very similar anatomic distribution. (Drawings by Natalie Shiff.)

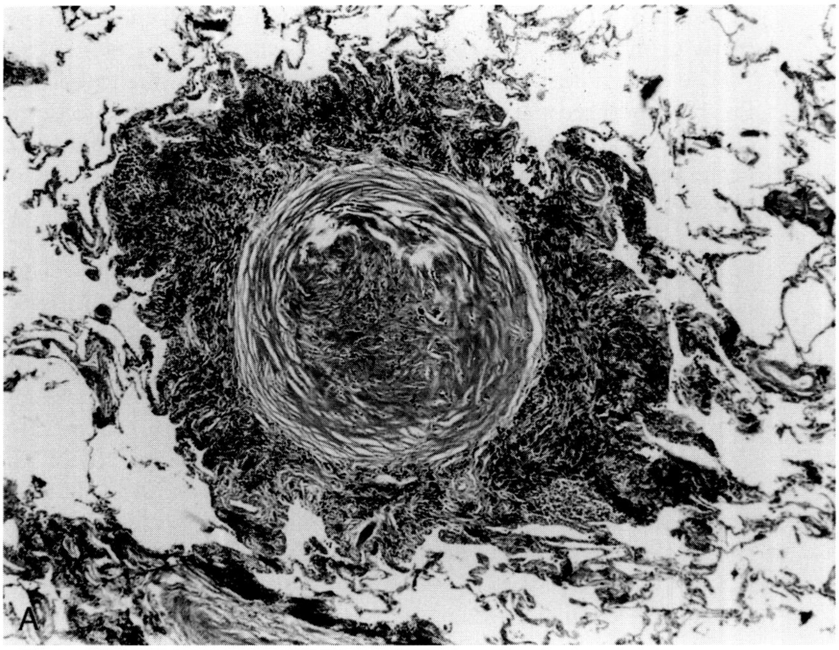

FIGURE 2.6
A. Silicotic nodule in a coal miner. The nodule shows a whorled collagenous center with a mantle of black pigmented macrophages. Polarizing microscopy revealed numerous weakly birefringent particles in the center of the lesion (consistent with quartz) and large numbers of brightly birefringent needle-shaped particles at the periphery (consistent with silicate minerals). **B.** Mixed-dust nodule. This lesion shows less distinct whorling of the collagen fibers. Much of the collagen is arranged in interlacing bundles, and the periphery of the lesion has a stellate outline. **C.** Mixed-dust nodule. This lesion shows much less fibrosis and more dust than seen in **A** and **B.** (The central pale area is a blood vessel.) The fibrosis consists of randomly arranged fibers of collagen and reticulin interspersed with dust particles. There is marked emphysema adjacent to the nodule.

Giant-Cell Granulomatous Nodule. More cellular and the least fibrotic of the three types, giant-cell granulomatous nodules are composed of histiocytic cells and giant cells with large quantities of intracellular birefringent dust particles. They are commonly seen in association with exposures to talc and other sheet silicates (see Chapter 8 and Fig. 13.2).

Diffuse Interstitial Fibrosis. Diffuse fibrotic interstitial lung disease is characterized by a proliferation of mesenchymal cells within the interstitium and the progressive deposition of connective tissue elements. Inflammation and edema are variable in severity and extent and may be transient. Initially the fibrosis, which includes collagens, elastic fibers, and smooth muscle cells, extends in linear fashion within the alveolar walls (Fig. 2.7). In later stages the lung architecture is remodeled, with formation of thick-walled cystic spaces, so-called honeycomb lung (Fig. 2.8). It is seen in association with exposures to asbestos, silica, silicates, coal, and some metals.

When dust exposure is present, specific indicators such as numerous birefringent crystals (for example in talcosis) or ferruginous bodies (asbestos bodies in asbestosis) are required for the specific diagnosis. In hard metal disease diffuse

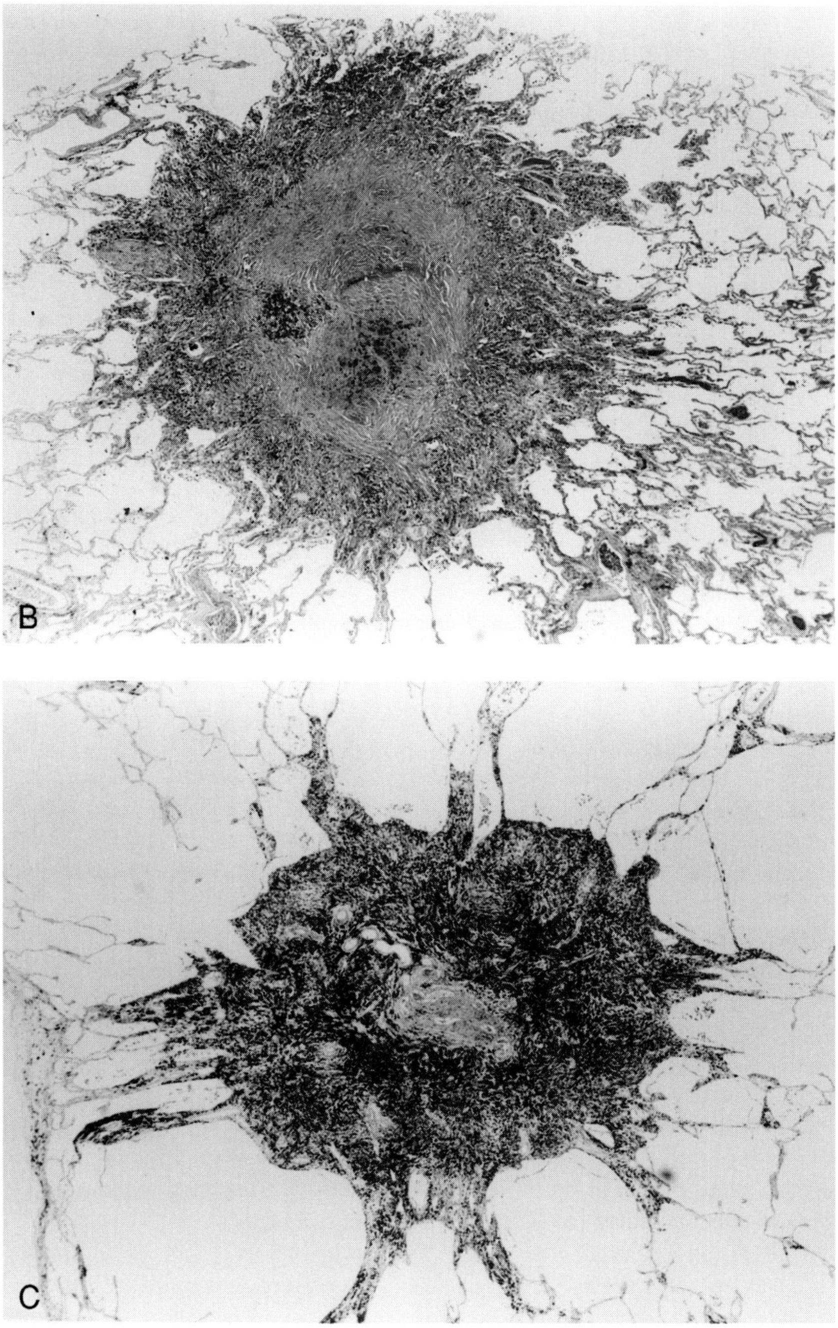

FIGURE 2.6 *(continued)*

fibrosis is accompanied by numerous alveolar giant cells and macrophages (see Chapter 5 for illustrations).

Progressive Massive Fibrosis. Progressive massive fibrosis (PMF), also called complicated pneumoconiosis, usually occurs against a background of simple pneumoconiosis (macules and nodules). PMF is associated with disability and

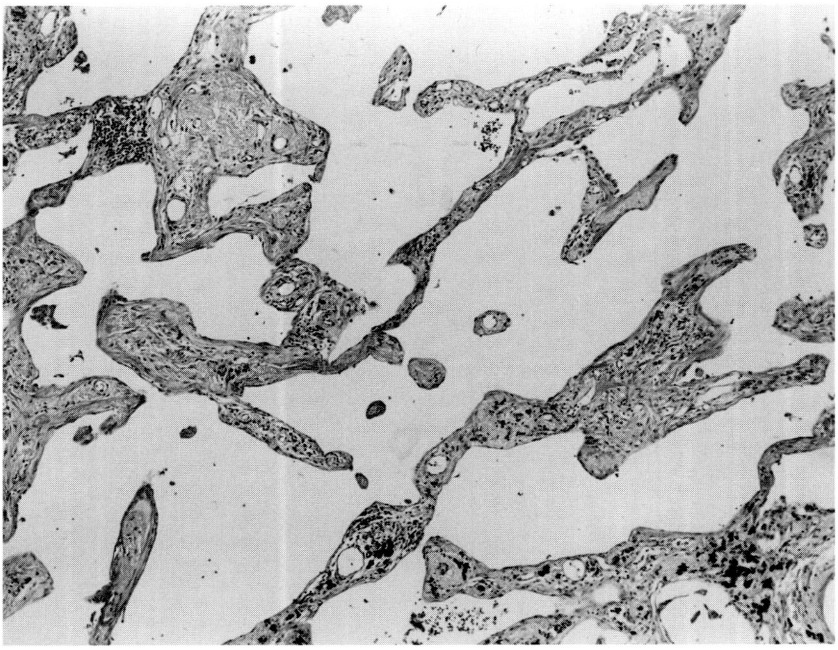

FIGURE 2.7
Diffuse interstitial fibrosis. Section of lung showing diffuse thickening of the alveolar interstitium by collagen fibers. There is a variable amount of chronic inflammation and visible pigment.

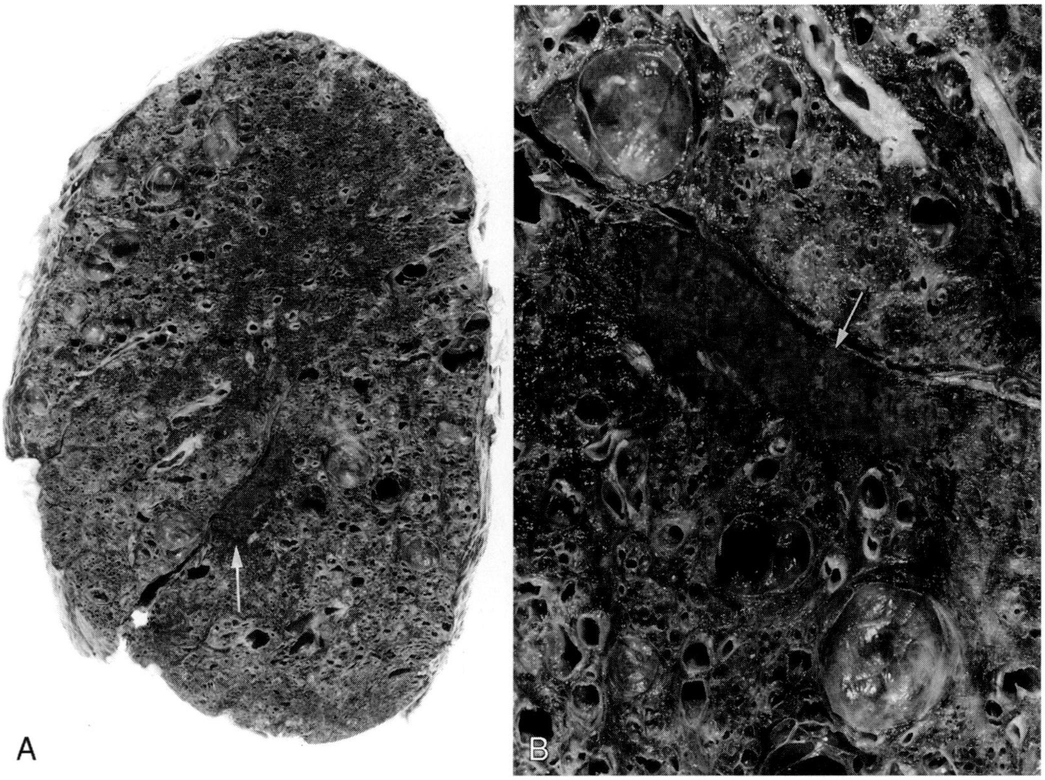

FIGURE 2.8
A. Interstitial fibrosis with honeycombing and PMF. Whole lung section from miner exposed to silicates and silica (quartz). The lung shows advanced interstitial fibrosis with honeycombing, nodules, and early PMF (*arrow*). The honeycomb fibrosis is most severe at the periphery of the lung. **B.** Close-up of the PMF lesion (*arrow*) adjacent to the interlobar fissure. The PMF lesion shows pale silicotic nodules. Details of the honeycomb cysts are also apparent.

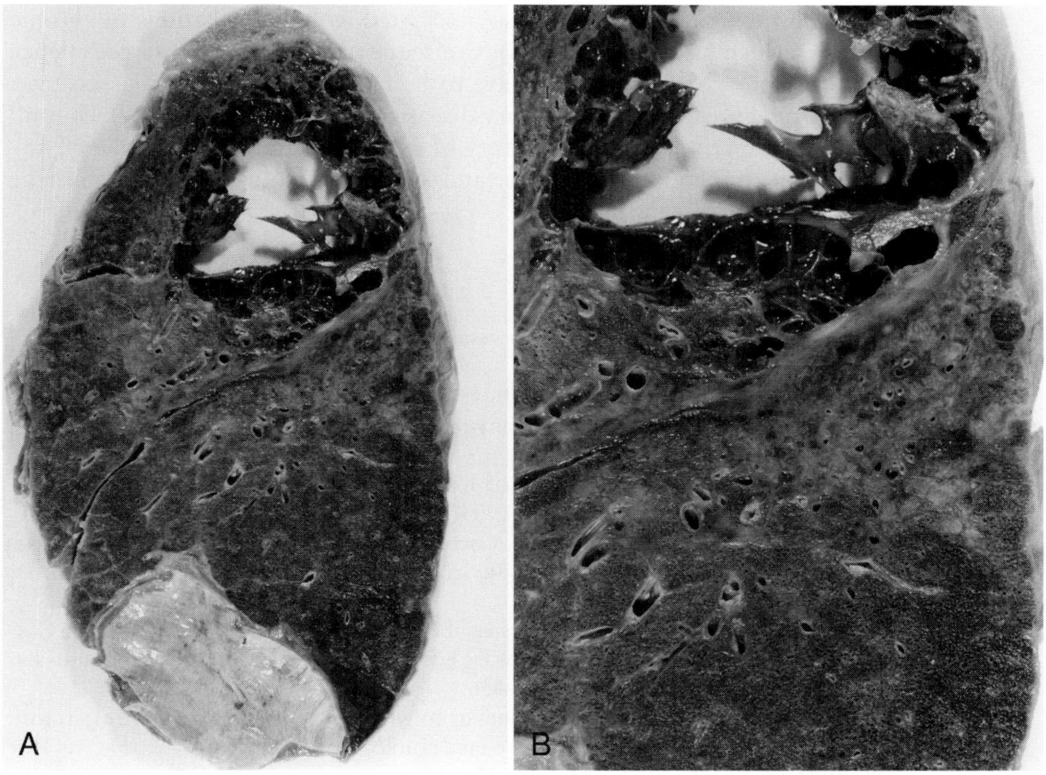

FIGURE 2.9
A. Cavitary PMF lesion replacing most of the upper lobe in a worker exposed to silica. **B.** Close-up of the lung shown in **A.** Note the individual silicotic nodules in the superior segment of the lower lobe; these are becoming confluent to form the PMF lesion.

premature death and tends to progress in the absence of further exposure. The lesions, defined on the basis of a size greater than 1 cm, are most common in the upper and posterior portions of the lung and are usually bilateral. They have been described in association with exposure to silica, nonfibrous silicates, coal mine dust, and carbon black. On cut surface the lesions are usually pigmented and firm to rubbery in consistency, and they may contain cavities filled with pigmented fluid (Figs. 2.8, 2.9, and Fig. 8.5). Superimposed infection with tuberculosis or atypical mycobacteria may occur but is less common today.

CONFOUNDERS: EFFECTS OF CIGARETTE SMOKE, AIR POLLUTANTS, AND COEXISTING DISEASE

With a few exceptions most of the patterns just described and illustrated are not specific to patients with occupational lung disease. Cigarette smoke, for example, is the major cause of both emphysema and small airway disease, and the distribution of smoke-related pigment is similar to that seen in the dust macule. Similarly, diffuse alveolar damage, bronchiolitis obliterans, and diffuse interstitial fibrosis have many causes that are not related to occupation. Even old healed infectious granulomas and nonspecific scars from old pneumonia may resemble the nodular lesions of pneumoconiosis.

Air pollutants, such as ozone, oxides of nitrogen (NOx), sulfur dioxide

(SO_{20}), and fine particulates, are also associated with exacerbations of chronic lung disease such as asthma (47, 48). Consequently, air quality and prevalence of disease in the community may have to be taken into account in assessing a case of chronic obstructive pulmonary disease or occupational asthma. Thus all available information, including history of exposure, latency requirements, any accepted epidemiologic associations, and specific pathologic features must be used to arrive at a diagnosis.

REFERENCES

1. Mossman BT, Sesko AM. In vitro assays to predict the pathogenicity of mineral fibers. Toxicology 1990;60:53–61.
2. Brain JD, Godleski J, Kreyling W. In vivo evaluation of chemical biopersistence of nonfibrous inorganic particles. Environ Health Perspect 1994;102(Suppl 5): 119–125.
3. Churg A, Wright JL. Persistence of natural mineral fibers in human lungs: an overview. Environ Health Perspect 1994;102(Suppl 5):229–233.
4. Oberdorster G, Ferin J, Lehnert BE. Correlation between particle size, in vivo particle persistence and lung injury. Environ Health Perspect 1994;102(Suppl 5): 173–179.
5. Kane AB. Questions and controversies about the pathogenesis of silicosis. In: Castranova V, Vallyathan V, Wallace WE , eds. Silica and silica-induced lung diseases. Boca Raton: CRC Press, 1996:121–136.
6. American Thoracic Society. Guidelines as to what constitutes an adverse respiratory health effect, with special reference to epidemiologic studies of air pollution. Am Rev Respir Dis 1985;131:666–668.
7. Gevenois PA, Pichot E, Dargent F, et al. Low grade coal worker's pneumoconiosis: comparison of CT and chest radiography. Acta Radiol 1994;35:351–356.
8. Remy-Jardin M, Degreef JM, Beuscart R, et al. Coal worker's pneumoconiosis: CT assessment in exposed workers and correlation with radiographic findings. Radiology 1990;177:363–371.
9. Wright JL, Cagle P, Churg A, et al. Diseases of the small airways. Am Rev Respir Dis 1992;146:240–262.
10. Bolender RP, Hyde DM, Dehoff RT. Lung morphometry: a new generation of tools and experiments for organ, tissue, cell and molecular biology. Am J Physiol 1993; 265(Lung Cell Mol Physiol 9):L521–L548.
11. Becklake M. Asbestos-related diseases of the lung and pleura. Am Rev Respir Dis 1982;127:187–194.
12. Hendry NW. The geology, occurrences, and major uses of asbestos. Ann N Y Acad Sci 1965;135:12–22.
13. Report to Congress on Workers' Home Contamination Study Conducted under the Workers' Family Protection Act (29 U.S.C 671a). Cincinnati, OH: National Institute for Occupational Safety and Health, 1997.
14. Wall CP, Gaensler EA, Carrington CB, Hayes JA. Comparison of transbronchial and open biopsies in chronic infiltrative lung diseases. Am Rev Respir Dis 1981;123: 280–285.
15. Von Hoff DD, LiVolsi V. Diagnostic reliability of needle biopsy of the pleura. A review of 272 biopsies. Am J Clin Pathol 1975;64:200–205.
16. Thurlbeck WM. Examination of the lung: autopsy. In: Thurlbeck WM, Churg AM , eds. Pathology of the lung. 2nd ed. New York: Thieme, 1995:129–136.
17. Churg A. An inflation procedure for open lung biopsies. Am J Surg Pathol 1983;7: 69–72.
18. Colby TV, Carrington CB. Interstitial lung disease. In: Thurlbeck WM, Churg AM, eds. Pathology of the lung. 2nd ed. New York: Thieme, 1995:589–737.
19. Holt RM, Schmidt RA, Godwin JD, Raghu G. High resolution CT in respiratory

bronchiolitis-associated interstitial lung disease. J Computer Assisted Tomogr 1993; 17:46–50.
20. Adesina AM, Vallyathan V, McQuillen EN, et al. Bronchiolar inflammation and fibrosis associated with smoking. Am Rev Respir Dis 1991;143:144–149.
21. Wright JL, Churg A. Morphology of small-airway lesions in patients with asbestos exposure. Hum Pathol 1984;15:68–74.
22. Churg A, Wright JL. Small airway lesions in persons exposed to nonasbestos mineral dust. Hum Pathol 1983;14:688–693.
23. Wright JL. Small airway disease: its role in chronic airflow obstruction. Semin Respir Med 1992;13:72–84.
24. Kleinerman J, Green FHY, Harley R, et al. Pathology standards for coal workers' pneumoconiosis: report of the Pneumoconiosis Committee of the College of American Pathologists to the National Institute for Occupational Safety and Health. Arch Pathol Lab Med 1979;103:375–431.
25. Morrow PE. Dust overloading of the lungs: update and appraisal. Toxicol Appl Pharmacol 1992;113:1–12.
26. Mauderly JL, Cheng YS, Snipes MB. Particle overload in toxicological studies: friend or foe? J Aerosol Med 1990;3(Suppl 1):169–188.
27. Muhle H, Bellmann B, Greutzenberg O, et al. Dust overloading of lungs after exposure of rats to particles of low solubility: comparative studies. J Aerosol Sci 1990;21: 374–377.
28. Muhle H, Greutzenberg O, Bellmann B, et al. Dust overloading of lungs: investigation of various materials, species differences and irreversibility of effects. J Aerosol Med 1990;3(Suppl 1):S111–S128.
29. Wolff RK, Henderson RF, Snipes MB, et al. Alterations in particle accumulation and clearance in lungs of rats chronically exposed to diesel exhaust. Fundam Appl Toxicol 1987;9:154–166.
30. Vincent JH, Johnston AM, Jones AD, et al. Kinetics of deposition and clearance of inhaled mineral dusts during chronic exposure. Br J Ind Med 1985;42:707–715.
31. Morrow PE. Possible mechanisms to explain dust overloading of the lungs. Fundam Appl Toxicol 1988;10:369–384.
32. Muhle H, Bellmann B, Creutzenberg O, et al. Pulmonary response to toner upon chronic inhalation exposure in rats. Fundam Appl Toxicol 1991;17:280–299.
33. Driscoll KE, Maurer JK, Crosby LL. Overload of lung clearance is associated with activation of alveolar macrophage tumor necrosis factor and fibronectin release. J Aerosol Med 1900b;3(Suppl 1):S83–S91.
34. Wallaert B, Lassalle P, Fortin F, et al. Superoxide anion generation by alveolar inflammatory cells in simple pneumoconiosis and in progressive massive fibrosis of nonsmoking coal workers. Am Rev Respir Dis 1990;141:129–133.
35. Kang JH, Van Dyke K, Pailes WH, Castranova V. Potential role of platelet-activating factor in development of occupational lung disease: action as an activator or potentiator of pulmonary phagocytes. In: Frantz RL, Ramani RV, eds. Proceedings of the Third Symposium on Respirable Dust in the Mineral Industries. Littleton, CO: Society for Mining, Metallurgy and Exploration, 1991:183–190.
36. Vanhee D, Gosset P, Wallaert B, et al. Mechanisms of fibrosis in coal workers' pneumoconiosis: increased production of platelet-derived growth factor, insulin-like growth factor type 1, and transforming growth factor β and relationship to disease severity. Am J Respir Crit Care Med 1994;150:1049–1055.
37. Driscoll KE, Maurer JK, Crosby LL. Overload of lung clearance is associated with activation of alveolar macrophage tumour necrosis factor and fibronectin release. J Aerosol Med 1990;3(Suppl):S83–S91.
38. Demers LM, Kuhn DC. Influence of mineral dusts on metabolism of arachidonic acid by alveolar macrophages. Environ Health Perspect 1994;102(Suppl 10):97–100.
39. Lapp NL, Castranova V. How silicosis and coal workers' pneumoconiosis develop: a cellular assessment. Occup Med: State Art Rev 1993;8:35–56.
40. Borm PJA, Schins R, Janssen YMW, Lenaerts L. Molecular basis for differences in

susceptibility to coal workers' pneumoconiosis. Toxicol Lett 1992;64/65:767–772.
41. Vallyathan V, Shi X. The role of oxygen free radicals in occupational and environmental lung diseases. Environ Health Perspect 1997;105(Suppl 1):165–177.
42. Kriegseis W, Scharmann A. Specific harmfulness of respirable dusts from West German coal mines: 5. Influence of mineral surface properties. Ann Occup Hyg 1982;26: 511–525.
43. LeBouffant L, Addison J, Bolton RE, et al. Compared in vitro and in vivo toxicity of coalmine dusts: relationship with mineralogical composition. Ann Occup Hyg 1988; 32(Suppl 1):611–620.
44. Wallace WE, Vallyathan V, Keane MJ, et al. Suppression of inhaled particle cytotoxicity by pulmonary surfactant and retoxification by phospholipase. Ann Occup Hyg 1988;32(Suppl 1):291–298.
45. Cilento EV, Georgellis GB. The effects of dipalmitoyl lecithin coated fresh quartz on superoxide release from alveolar macrophages in vitro. In: Frantz RL, Ramani RV , eds. Proceedings of the Third Symposium on Respirable Dusts in the Mineral Industry. Littleton, CO: Society of Mining Engineering, 1991:313–315.
46. Fletcher CM, Pride NB. Definitions of emphysema, chronic bronchitis, asthma and airflow obstruction: 25 years on from the Ciba symposium. Thorax 1984;39: 81–85.
47. Health effects of outdoor air pollution. Committee of the Environmental and Occupational Health Assembly, American Thoracic Society. Am J Respir Crit Care Med 1996;153:3–50.
48. Health effects of outdoor air pollution: 2. Committee of the Environmental and Occupational Health Assembly, American Thoracic Society. Am J Respir Crit Care Med 1996;153:477–498.

CHAPTER 3

Analytic Methods for Identifying and Quantifying Mineral Particles in Lung Tissue

❖ Andrew Churg
❖ Francis H. Y. Green

INTRODUCTION

Analysis of lung tissue to demonstrate the presence or amount of an element or mineral may have diagnostic, research, and/or medicolegal value. In general such techniques are time-consuming and expensive and are mostly used as research procedures. *Beyond simple light microscopic observation and polarization, as a rule analytic techniques are not required in the diagnosis of most cases of occupational lung disease*, and in the diagnostic setting they should only be employed to answer specific questions.

APPLICATIONS OF MINERALOGIC ANALYSIS OF LUNG TISSUE

Confirmation or exclusion of a putative diagnosis by demonstration of the presence and amount of a specific element or mineral in lung is the most frequent application of mineralogic analysis. As a general rule quantitative or semiquantitative methods are required because everyone has some mineral dust in the lungs (1–6) (see "Lung Mineral Dust in the General Population," later in the chapter). The mere qualitative demonstration that a given element or mineral is present usually has no value unless it is rarely or never found except in occupationally exposed individuals; an example of the latter is tungsten, which as a practical proposition is seen only in the lungs of those exposed to hard metal (Chapter 5).

However, quantitative analysis of beryllium content is required to confirm the diagnosis of berylliosis in a patient whose biopsy shows sarcoidlike granulomas (see Chapter 5). Also, to confirm the asbestos causation of a mesothelioma, one must digest the lung tissue and determine the concentration of extracted asbestos bodies or fibers (see Chapter 9). Expected background levels are necessary for both of these analyses (6). For asbestos the issue is even more complex, because different asbestos-induced diseases are associated with different fiber burdens (see Chapter 9); for example, an amphibole fiber burden some five times maximum background is satisfactory to implicate asbestos as the cause of a mesothelioma but not as a cause of diffuse interstitial fibrosis of unknown cause, since development of asbestosis (asbestos-induced diffuse interstitial fibrosis) necessitates extremely high fiber burdens.

Most important, the demonstration of any amount of an element or mineral in the lung is confirmation of exposure, not disease; determining whether the element or mineral is responsible for a disease process depends on appropriate clinical and pathologic findings.

The second application is *as a guide to the diagnosis of an unknown process.* Identification of an unknown particulate seen in histologic sections or extracted from lung can sometimes be useful when the diagnosis is uncertain. For example, Goldbach et al. (7) identified talc crystals in a biopsy of a mass lesion and on this basis retrospectively obtained a history of talc inhalation, eventually establishing the diagnosis of talc pneumoconiosis. Similarly, the finding of asbestos bodies in histologic sections in a case of diffuse interstitial fibrosis should suggest asbestosis (see Chapter 9). But this approach is fraught with danger, since many particles have no diagnostic significance and such data can be misleading. For instance, refractile mineral particles are frequently found in the granulomas of sarcoidosis, and it is quite common to receive consultations suggesting that this process may be some sort of pneumoconiosis. In fact sarcoidosis has no known relation to dust exposure, and the particles are usually calcium oxalate or calcium carbonate, substances produced by macrophages. Visscher et al. (8) reported the presence of such crystals in two-thirds of a large series of cases of nonnecrotizing granulomas of varying etiology, including sarcoid, and Reid and Andersen (9) found an even greater percentage of positive specimens. Another example would be the finding of asbestos bodies in histologic sections of a case of bronchiolitis obliterans organizing pneumonia (BOOP); although this is indeed an "interstitial" lung disease in a worker with asbestos exposure, the correct diagnosis is BOOP, not asbestosis, no matter how many bodies are found (see Chapter 9).

Determination of the source of exposure to a specific substance is usually a medicolegal question, particularly in patients with more than one possible source of exposure. That is, was injury produced by exposure to a product of manufacturer A or manufacturer B or in factory A or B? In some cases demonstration of the presence or absence of a specific mineral, such as different types of asbestos, allow this question to be answered (See Chapter 9).

LIGHT MICROSCOPIC APPROACHES

Histologic examination obviously is the basic routine pathologic tool for classifying occupational lung diseases; the specific microscopic features of each particular disease are discussed and illustrated in the following chapters, and some general features have been summarized in Chapter 2.

Routine microscopy can often provide an indication of the type of dust to which an individual has been exposed and with some caveats, a crude estimate of the lung dust burden. However, not all dust is occupational in origin. Visible dust is present in the lungs of all individuals and is present in greater amounts in cigarette smokers and those living in polluted environments. Dust is typically seen around small airways and blood vessels and in the subpleural and interlobular connective tissue. In those with occupational exposure to dust, fairly large numbers of particles may be observed in these locations, in the alveolar spaces, and in alveolar interstitium. Furthermore, endogenous processes such as normal macrophage metabolism (8, 9), repeated intrapulmonary hemorrhages, and metastatic and dystrophic calcification can produce considerable visible particulate loads (discussed later in this chapter and in Chapter 13).

If dust is present, color and birefringence are useful albeit limited methods of identification (10–14). Table 3.1 provides a short list of these properties. If a dust disease is suspected, tissue should always be examined under polarized light. For routine diagnostic purposes all one needs is an ordinary light microscope and two polarizers; the microscope light must be used at full intensity. This simple system gives useful information about the amount of birefringent dust present and provides data on size and shape (e.g., fiber, plate) of particles. It is again helpful to have some idea of the amount of dust seen by polarization in the general population, since some polarizable dust is always present. But the absence of polarizable dust does not always exclude substantial dust exposure, because some dusts, for example asbestos and tungsten carbide (hard metal), are not birefringent in tissue sections and pure silica (without admixed brightly birefringent silicates) is only weakly birefringent. The finding of numerous large crystals in the interstitium and vessels but not in alveolar spaces should raise the possibility of intravenous (usually drug abuse) origin or endogenous crystal formation (discussed later in this chapter and in Chapter 13.)

TABLE 3.1
Color and Birefringence of Some Common Mineral Dusts in Histologic Sections

DUST	COLOR SHAPE	BIREFRINGENCE
Asbestos	Colorless fibers	–
Barium sulfate	Yellow-white plates	Strong +
Carbon, smoke, lignite Anthracite coal	Black, granular	–
Bituminous coal	Yellow, brown	–
Crystalline silica (e.g., quartz, cristobalite)	Colorless needles and plates	Weak +
Graphite	Black	+
Gypsum (CaSO↓4↑)	White	+
Iron	Red-brown to black, granular	–
Coal fly ash	Usually black, spheres or lacy forms	–
Nonfibrous silicates such as talc, mica, feldspars	Colorless or very pale yellow plates or needles	Strong +
Starch	Colorless or white, round	Strong + Maltese cross
Microcrystalline cellulose	Colorless PAS, Congo red +	+

PAS, periodic acid-Schiff stain.

TABLE 3.2
Types of Ferruginous Bodies

MICROSCOPIC APPEARANCE	NATURE OF MINERAL CORE
Colorless, transparent cores, usually straight, sometimes branched	Asbestos Erionite (only reported from Turkey)
Broad yellow fibers or irregular yellow plates	Sheet silicates such as talc, mica
Black fibers (relatively broad) or plates	Coal, carbon
Fine black fibers	Rutile, silicon carbide, iron (rare)
Black hollow spheres, often with lacy configuration (may also be nonferruginated)	Coal fly ash (mullite)
Small irregular solid black particles	Exogenous iron, ? carbon
Ferruginated fragments of elastin	Elastin fibers in conditions of chronic pulmonary hemorrhage[a]

See Chapter 9 for details.
[a] See Chapter 13.

Specific identification of particulates in tissue sections by measurement of parameters such as refractive index, optical rotation, density, and color with a mineralogic polarizing microscope is theoretically possible (11) but practically difficult, since the particles of interest are rarely cut in the required plane and material is often added to mineral particles by the lung, changing or reducing their birefringence (15). In addition, many particles are at or below the limit of resolution of the light microscope. With a few exceptions, exact identification of individual particles in lung tissue requires an analytic method with a resolution at the electron microscopic level (6).

Ferruginous bodies are mineral particles to which the lung has added an iron protein coat. The asbestos body is a well known example. The ferruginous coating may be linear or beaded, but the key to diagnosis lies in the appearance of the core (Table 3.2). Because relatively few types of minerals are ferruginated and because their golden-yellow or bright blue color on iron stains makes these structures relatively easy to find in sections, their presence can be very helpful in identifying an inhaled dust or making a diagnosis (16). Ferruginous bodies are discussed in detail in Chapter 9 and illustrated in colorplate 1. One word of caution is in order: repeated intrapulmonary hemorrhage can lead to ferrugination of elastic fibers, creating structures that resemble asbestos bodies (see Chapter 13).

One light microscopy approach that is often overlooked is simple chemistry performed on unstained deparaffinized sections to detect any calcium oxalate or calcium carbonate. These particles are, as noted earlier, common in granulomas and in other processes involving abnormal calcification. To detect calcium carbonate 2M acetic acid is applied to the sections and the evolution of gas bubbles observed: a positive reaction indicates calcium carbonate. To detect calcium oxalate, the deparaffinized sections are ashed in a Bunsen burner flame and then concentrated sulfuric acid added. The evolution of gas bubbles is characteristic of calcium carbonate (17). This approach is particularly useful in granulomatous lesions if the question of endogenous versus exogenous material arises.

CHOICE OF SPECIMEN FOR ANALYTIC PROCEDURES

Although in theory any type of lung specimen may be suitable for analytic studies, we believe that as a rule it is unwise to use transbronchial biopsies or histologic sections for *quantitative* procedures. Mineral dust is unevenly distributed in lung, and the unevenness appears to increase as the sample size decreases (18, 19). Hence these small samples can seriously overestimate or underestimate elemental or mineral content. Transbronchial biopsy compounds the distribution problem because it usually samples the peribronchial connective tissues, which, as noted previously, are a common repository for inhaled dust, even in those with no occupational exposure (6).

These types of specimens may be suitable for qualitatively demonstrating that a specific mineral is present (discussed later), and histologic sections can be used for a crude estimation of asbestos body content (effectively none, few, many; see Chapter 9) as well as a similarly crude estimate (none, little, much) of visible colored or polarizable dust. This crude estimate may be all that is required in a given case, but if true quantitative analysis is needed, it should preferably be performed on open lung biopsy samples, resection specimens, or autopsy lungs. Paraffin blocks of open biopsy samples or resection or autopsy specimens are something of an intermediate case: they are certainly better than transbronchial biopsies or paraffin sections but are relatively small samples and are subject to unknown amounts of mineral loss and contamination during tissue embedding and processing. For example, Lee et al. (20) recently reported that paraffin blocks are often contaminated with chrysotile asbestos.

QUANTITATIVE AND QUALITATIVE ANALYTICAL TECHNIQUES

Again, simple observation of light microscopic sections and simple polarization, while not true quantitative methods, provide adequate answers in many cases, and the techniques discussed here are not required in most instances. For example, Chapter 8 illustrates the brightly birefringent particles seen in lungs with exposure to silicates such as talc and mica. Given a suitable history of exposure to talc or mica, pathologic lesions that could be caused by talc or mica, and numerous birefringent plates, a diagnosis of talc or mica pneumoconiosis can be made with confidence.

Table 3.3 lists quantitative methods that have been applied to lung tissue. Most are essentially research procedures that are not widely available. In practice only a few techniques are generally accessible and widely used. Detailed discussion of all the various methods and their limitations and the required methods of tissue preparation is beyond the scope of this book, but reviews are available (6, 14, 21–25). More extensive information on preparative and analytic procedures for beryllium and asbestos is included in Chapters 5 and 9. Figure 3.1 illustrates a schematic approach to the problem of selecting a technique.

Bulk analytic techniques, such as x-ray diffraction, x-ray fluorescence, atomic absorption spectroscopy, and neutron activation analysis, are used to examine the tissue sample as a whole and are excellent for detecting and quantifying individual elements (e.g., beryllium, aluminum). X-ray diffraction can also identify specific minerals and polymorphs, which are chemically identical but structurally different forms of a mineral, for example, quartz, cristobalite, and tridymite, all polymorphs of crystalline silica.

TABLE 3.3
Analytic Methods and Their Applications

METHOD	APPLICATIONS AND LIMITATIONS	EXAMPLES OF ACTUAL OR POTENTIAL USES
Bulk (macroanalytic) techniques	Localization of particle not usually possible; sample generally destroyed	
X-ray diffraction[a]	Qualitative, quantitative; overlapping silicate peaks are a problem; can be used with as little as 100 ng of sample; can identify elements, minerals, and polymorphs of minerals	Identification of quartz polymorphs; sometimes specific identification of silicates
X-ray fluorescence	Qualitative, quantitative	Chemical composition of fly ash
Atomic absorption spectroscopy[a]	Very sensitive for trace elements (down to 0.003 ppm); not all elements identifiable	Analysis of beryllium content
Neutron activation analysis	Relatively high sensitivity (to about 10 ppm) for trace elements; not all elements identifiable; requires on-site nuclear reactor	Largely used for tracers in experimental animal work
Proton-induced x-ray emission spectroscopy	Element detection down to 1 to 10 ppm	
Microanalytic techniques	Identification of specific particle at least theoretically possible; tissue section or digested specimen can be used	
Energy-dispersive x-ray spectroscopy[a]	Equipment available in many labs; very high resolution (depending on electron microscope) and simultaneous analysis of all elements; most systems do not detect elements lighter than sodium	Widely used for analysis of asbestos fibers; also good for identification of other silicates
Wavelength-dispersive x-ray spectroscopy	Good resolution (depending on instrument); can detect all elements; slow	Able to identify light elements such as beryllium
Electron energy loss spectroscopy	Detects light elements in thin sections	Potentially useful for identification of beryllium and other light elements in EM sections
Laser Raman spectroscopy	Detects down to picogram amounts of individual elements; resolution limited to particles several microns and up	Has been used to detect quartz, calcite, rutile in tissue sections
Auger electron spectroscopy	Detects light elements; also good for analysis of materials on particle surfaces	
Secondary ion or laser microprobe mass spectroscopy	Sensitivity for trace elements in ppm range. Resolution 0.5–1 micron	Has been used for in situ beryllium analysis and element mapping
Electron diffraction	Identification of individual crystals of any size; time-consuming and often difficult to interpret	Confirmation of particle identification when chemical composition alone is not sufficient

[a] Commonly available techniques.
EM, electron microscope.

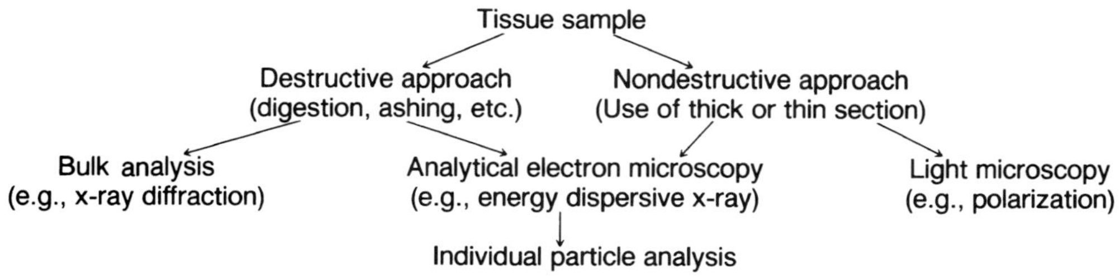

FIGURE 3.1
Schematic approach to analytic techniques.(Modified from Green FHY, Tucker IM, Vallythan V. Occupational diseases of the lung. Lab Med 1983;14:103–111.)

These methods are sensitive and can provide extremely accurate quantitation but have several limitations. They usually necessitate destruction of the sample and thus do not provide a correlation with specific lesions. Except for x-ray diffraction, these techniques cannot identify specific minerals but merely indicate which elements are present. For some purposes, such as beryllium analysis, this is adequate, but both crystalline silica and various silicates are found in every lung (1–6) (see next section), and here the distinction can be vital. Even x-ray diffraction, while providing excellent specificity for relatively pure minerals, may be unable to separate silicate minerals extracted from lung tissue because of overlapping x-ray peaks and other confounding factors.

Microanalytic techniques, such as x-ray energy spectroscopy and electron diffraction using a suitably equipped electron microscope, allow one to examine and identify individual mineral particles in tissue sections or tissue digests. Figure 9.2 illustrates the application of these particular techniques to asbestos fiber identification. Electron energy loss spectroscopy, when available, is useful for identifying light elements in thin sections, as are some of the more esoteric techniques listed in Table 3.3.

In situ microanalytic examination, for example examination of individual particles in light microscopic or electron microscopic tissue sections using an electron microscope equipped with x-ray energy spectrometer, allows direct correlation of mineral dust content with specific lesions, and comparisons can also be made between the lesions and adjacent tissue. An example is identification of a refractile particle seen in the center of a granuloma (26). The x-ray energy spectrometer essentially provides a microchemical analysis, and in many instances this information is adequate to identify the particle. If need be a portion of the paraffin block can be embedded and cut for transmission electron microscopy, or a section can be cut and mounted for scanning electron microscopy. If the paraffin block is not available, the actual light microscopic section can be used on the slide in a scanning electron microscope (26).

This approach is particularly useful when only histologic sections exist, but it is time-consuming, produces qualitative (which may be all that is required) or at best semiquantitative information on particle concentration, and may be misleading because of the inhomogeneous distribution of the agent in question. Indeed, because of their extremely small volume, electron microscope sections may contain no mineral particles even when very substantial pulmonary burdens are present!

Application of a microanalytic technique to tissue digests eliminates many of the problems of inhomogeneity of dust within the lung, provided a sufficiently large sample is used (6). These techniques can be applied to normal lung or to specific lesions; for example, it is possible to analyze the content of dust-induced nodular lesions by cutting the nodules out of the lung and digesting them individually. Because these techniques can eliminate problems of inhomogeneity and because they allow analysis of large numbers of particles, extremely accurate determinations of particle number, type, and size are possible. Many of these methods allow examination of particles well below the level of light microscopic resolution and thus are suitable for very small particles such as asbestos fibers and for much of the background dust seen in human lungs (see next section). Their main drawbacks are that some techniques lack the resolution required to examine individual particles (Table 3.3) and that the requirement for particle-by-particle analysis makes them extremely slow and expensive.

The choice of analytic procedure in a given case depends on instrument availability, sample size, and the exact question being asked. Electron microscopes equipped with energy-dispersive x-ray spectrometers (often called analytic electron microscopes), atomic absorption spectrometers, and x-ray diffraction cameras are available in most academic institutions. Many of the other instruments and methods listed in Table 3.3 can be found only in research laboratories. When selecting a method, it is helpful to know (or to make a good guess) about the minerals and elements likely to be found and to have an idea how concentrations are usually expressed for a given mineral. Silica, for example, is usually analyzed in terms of weight, and quantitative x-ray diffraction is a useful method of measuring silica content. Asbestos, however, is usually quantified in terms of numbers of fibers. Hence an electron microscopic technique that allows counting of fibers is required.

For documenting the pulmonary asbestos burden, simple quantification of asbestos bodies with a light microscope may be adequate, since these structures can easily be extracted from lung tissue, collected on membrane filters, and accurately identified and counted. A detailed procedure is provided in Chapter 9, which also reviews other methods of quantifying pulmonary asbestos burden. Again, some knowledge of the limitations of even simple techniques is required; for example, quantifying asbestos bodies provides some estimate of the lung burden of amphibole asbestos fibers but is a poor indicator of the lung burden of chrysotile asbestos fibers (see Chapter 9).

Sample preparation for bulk and microanalysis depends on the technique to be employed. In situ techniques require only minor modifications of conventional light and electron microscope procedures. For most other types of analysis the tissue must be digested to remove organic matter and concentrate the mineral dust; common digestion procedures include treatment with a strong acid or base, oxidizing agents such as bleach and enzymes, microincineration, and plasma ashing (25). These techniques must not substantially alter the chemistry and/or morphology of a mineral (6), and hence appropriate controls are required. For these reasons it is advisable to check with a laboratory that routinely carries out the type of procedure that one contemplates for a particular patient to determine how material should be fixed (if at all) and what preparatory steps should be undertaken.

LUNG MINERAL DUST IN THE GENERAL POPULATION

The normal human lung contains relatively large numbers of particles inhaled from ambient air and derived from rock and soil weathering as well as from human activity. Three reports on the mineral particle content of human lung parenchyma in the general population are listed in Table 3.4. All of these data were derived by digestion of lung tissue and identification and quantification of particles by analytic electron microscopy. Note the fairly wide range of particle concentrations from person to person and the remarkably high (hundreds of millions of particles per gram of dry lung tissue) level of particles found (1–5). Our own data were derived entirely from lungs that were morphologically unremarkable except for pneumonia, which emphasizes the fact that this particle burden produces no obvious deleterious effects.

Particles are present not only in the parenchyma but also in the airway mucosa (as analyzed, airway mucosa is the tissue between the airway epithelium and the cartilage plates) (4, 5). The airway mucosal particle concentration is also relatively high, albeit lower than the concentration of particles in the parenchyma supplied by a given airway; nonetheless, typical concentrations are in the range of tens of millions of particles per gram of dry tissue. Airway mucosal particle loads increase with increasing airway generation (i.e., distance from the carina). Again, as is true of parenchymal particle loads, there is a quite marked individual variation in airway particle burden, even among persons without occupational dust exposure who lived many years in a similar environment. These differences most likely reflect differences in individual particle clearance rates.

Table 3.5 provides data from our laboratory on the types of particles found in the parenchyma and airway mucosa (4, 5). These two sites show different rel-

TABLE 3.4
Mineral Particle Concentration in the General Population

REPORT	MEDIAN	MEAN	RANGE
Stettler et al. (2)	480	570	110–1610
Churg and Wiggs (1)	340	470	180–1090
Kalliomaki et al. (3)		970	

All values as millions of particles per gram of dry lung.

TABLE 3.5
Types of Particles in Airway versus Parenchyma in Nonsmokers in the General Population

MINERAL TYPE	PARENCHYMA	AIRWAY MUCOSA
Silica	24.4	42.5
Kaolin	23.1	14.5
Mica	20.6	11.9
Feldspars	11.2	15.9
Metals	11.1	8.0
Talc	3.5	2.9
Miscellaneous	6.1	4.3

As mean percent of total particles.

Adapted from Churg A, Wright J, Stevens B. Exogenous mineral particles in the human bronchial mucosa and lung parenchyma: 1. Nonsmokers in the general population. Exp Lung Res 1990;16: 169–175.

ative proportions of the various mineral species, but all are substances commonly found in ambient air. Asbestos was also found in these lungs but is not included in these tables. It is also important to understand that most of this particle load is invisible by ordinary light microscopy. These observations reinforce the idea that analyses of pulmonary particulate loads must document the normal range before attempting to determine whether an abnormally high burden is present (4, 5, 27).

REFERENCES

1. Churg A, Wiggs B. Types, numbers, sizes, and distribution of mineral particles in the lungs of urban male cigarette smokers. Environ Res 1987;42:121–129.
2. Stettler LE, Growth DH, Platek SF, Burg JR. Particulate concentrations in urban lungs. In: Ingram P, Shelburne JD, Roggli VL, eds. Microprobe analysis in medicine. New York: Hemisphere Press, 1989:133–146.
3. Kalliomaki PL, Taikina-aho O, Paakko P, et al. Smoking and the pulmonary mineral particle burden. In: Bignon J, Peto J, Saracci R, eds. Non-occupational exposure to mineral fibres. Lyon: International Agency for Research on Cancer, 1989:323–329.
4. Churg A, Wright J, Stevens B. Exogenous mineral particles in the human bronchial mucosa and lung parenchyma: 1. Nonsmokers in the general population. Exp Lung Res 1990;16:169–175.
5. Churg A, Wright JL, Stevens B, Wiggs B. Exogenous mineral particles in the human bronchial mucosa and lung parenchyma: 2. Smokers without emphysema. Exp Lung Res 1992;18:687–714.
6. Gibbs AR, Pooley FD. Analysis and interpretation of inorganic mineral particles in "lung" tissues. Thorax 1996;31:327–334.
7. Goldbach PD, Mohsenifar Z, Abraham JL, et al. Talcum powder pneumoconiosis: diagnosis by transbronchial biopsy using energy-dispersive x-ray analysis. West J Med 1982;136:439–442.
8. Visscher D, Churg A, Katzenstein ALA. Significance of crystalline inclusions in lung granulomas. Mod Pathol 1988;1:415–419.
9. Reid JD, Andersen ME. Calcium oxalate in sarcoid granulomas. Am J Clin Pathol 1988;90:545–558.
10. Johnson FB. Crystals in pathologic specimens. Pathol Ann 1972;7:321–344.
11. McCrone WC, Delly JG. Particle atlas. 2nd ed. Ann Arbor: Ann Arbor Sciences, 1973.
12. Hartshorne NH, Stuart A. Crystals and the polarizing microscope. 4th ed. London: Arnold, 1970.
13. Heinrich WE. Microscopic identification of minerals. New York: McGraw-Hill, 1965. Vallyathan NV, Green FHY, Craighead JE. Recent advances in the study of mineral pneumoconiosis. Pathol Ann 1980;15(pt 2):77–104.
14. Green FHY, Tucker IM, Vallythan V. Occupational diseases of the lung. Lab Med 1983;14:103–111.
15. Kleinerman J, Green F, Laqueur W, et al. Pathology standards for coal worker's pneumoconiosis. Arch Pathol Lab Med 1979;103:375–430.
16. Crouch E, Churg A. Ferruginous bodies and the histologic evaluation of mineral dust exposure. Am J Surg Pathol 1984;8:109–116.
17. Johnson FB. Identification of graphite in tissue sections. Arch Pathol Lab Med 1980; 104:491–492.
18. Churg A, Wood P. Observations on the distribution of asbestos fibers in lung. Environ Res 1983;31:374–380.
19. Morgan A, Holmes A. Distribution and characteristics of amphibole asbestos fibres, measured with the light microscope, in the left lung of an insulation worker. Br J Ind Med 1963;40:45–30.
20. Lee RJ, Florida RG, Stewart IM. Asbestos contamination in paraffin tissue blocks. Arch Pathol Lab Med 1995;119:528–532.

21. Roggli VL, Ingram P, Linton RW, et al. New techniques for imaging and analyzing lung tissue. Environ Health Perspect 1984;56:163–183.
22. Roggli VL, Mastin JP, Shelburne JD, et al. Inorganic particulates in human lung. In: Lynn WS, ed. Inflammatory cells and lung disease. Boca Raton: CRC Press, 1984.
23. Stika KM, Morrison GH. Analytical methods for the mineral content of human tissues. Fed Proc 1981;40:2115–2119.
24. deMull FF, Buiteveld H, Lankester J, et al. Raman microspectroscopy in human pathology. Hum Pathol 1984;15:1062–1068.
25. Ingram P, Shelburne JD, Roggli VL. Microprobe analysis in medicine. New York: Hemisphere, 1989.
26. Pickett JP, Ingram P, Shelburne JD. Identification of inorganic particulates in a single histologic section using both light microscopy and x-ray microprobe analysis. J Histotech 1980;3:155–158.
27. Churg A. The uptake of mineral particles by pulmonary epithelial cells. Am J Respir Crit Care Med 1996;154:1124–1140.

CHAPTER 4

Diseases Caused by Gases and Fumes

❖ J. L. Wright
❖ Andrew Churg

This chapter covers diseases caused by gases and fumes. Strictly speaking, fumes are metal oxides produced by heating metals (1), but the term is often used for vapors and gases of nonmetallic origin. Fumes are different from dusts, which are solid particles derived from rocks, minerals, metals, or man-made products and dispersed in air by mechanical means such as grinding or crushing (1). In general dust particles are larger than fume particles, and the small size of fume particles tends to promote their passage into distal airspaces. Nonetheless, the distinction between lesions caused by fumes and those caused by metallic dusts (see Chapter 5) may be moot; for example, morphologically similar macules are commonly found in welders, who encounter iron oxide as a fume, and hematite miners, who encounter it as a dust. Alternatively, some agents may have one effect as a dust and another as a fume; for example, nickel salts are principally important in the field of occupational lung disease because of their carcinogenic properties, but nickel oxide fume has occasionally been reported to produce adult respiratory distress syndrome (ARDS). We have therefore made some arbitrary decisions about whether particular agents should be included in this chapter or the subsequent one on effects of metals.

PATHOLOGIC REACTION PATTERNS

The basic design of this chapter is a tabular listing of agents according to pathologic reactions. This format is particularly useful in the area of gases and fumes because the pathologic reactions they produce tend to be monotonously similar, and there is usually nothing in either the clinical features or pathologic picture that specifically identifies the causative agent. Instead one must depend on a detailed history in a given case or general knowledge of the types of exposures likely in various occupations. A brief summary of specific agents and the occupations in which they are encountered is provided in Table 4.1. Further details on occupations and industrial processes associated with risk can be found in ref-

TABLE 4.1
Agents Encountered as Gases and Fumes and Uses and Occupations Associated with Risk

AGENTS	OCCUPATIONS WITH EXPOSURE, USES
Ammonia	Fertilizer manufacture Pharmaceutical production Plastic manufacture Explosive manufacture
Antimony trichloride and antimony pentachloride	Coloring metals Chemical catalysts
Beryllium[a]	Beryllium mining and extraction Beryllium metallurgy and production of beryllium alloys, ceramics (see Chapter 5)
Boranes	Fuels Welding Fungicides
Cadmium[a]	High-friction metal alloys Soldering, welding cadmium alloys Electroplating Paints, ceramics, glass, plastics Refining of other ores (zinc, lead, copper)
Chlorine	Bleach manufacture Chemical manufacture Pulp and paper industries
Chromium[a]	Mining, refining Chrome plating Paints and pigments (as chromates) Welding
Cobalt, hard metal[a]	Hard metal production and use In alloys and steel As paint and china pigment Catalyst in the oil and chemical industry
Hydrogen chloride	Dye, fertilizer, textile, rubber manufacture
Hydrogen sulfide	Dye manufacture Rubber manufacture Sewer cleaners
Nickel[a]	Mining and smelting of nickel ores Stainless steel welding Electroplating
Oxides of nitrogen	Farmers (silo work) Explosive manufacture Welding, electroplating Metal cleaning Diesel exhaust
Ozone	Welding Pulp and paper production
Phosgene	Welding Fire fighting Isocyanate and pesticide production
Sulfur dioxide	Chemical, pulp, and paper manufacture Bleach and fumigation Smelters
Titanium[b]	Manufacture of ceramics, paints Machining titanium metal
Zinc[a]	Welding, metal plating
Zirconium[c]	Mining, refining ores (also exposure to silica) Production of steel Manufacture of refractory ceramics In foundries as sand substitute In enamels and glasses As a polishing and abrasive agent

[a] Reported to cause ARDS when encountered as a fume.
[b] Titanium tetrachloride reported to cause ARDS.
[c] Zirconium chloride reported to cause ARDS.

erences 2–5. Table 4.2 provides a general summary of the types of lesions caused by fumes and gases, and Tables 4.3 to 4.6 indicate the specific agents reported to produce each lesion.

For many of the agents listed in the tables only a handful of case reports exist, and many of these have no or little pathologic documentation. An additional

TABLE 4.2
Diseases Caused by Inhaled Gases and Fumes

Adult respiratory distress syndrome (diffuse alveolar damage)
Necrotizing bronchitis and bronchiolitis
Bronchiolitis obliterans (proliferative bronchiolitis and constrictive bronchiolitis)
BOOP, cryptogenic organizing pneumonia
Bronchiectasis
Occupational asthma
Chronic airflow obstruction
Metal fume fever
Lung cancer (?)

TABLE 4.3
Agents Producing Adult Respiratory Distress Syndrome (Diffuse Alveolar Damage)

AGENT	REFERENCES
Acetaldehyde	5
Acrolein	5
Ammonia	6, 7
Antimony trichloride or pentachloride	8
Beryllium	Chapter 5
Boranes	8
Cadmium and cadmium salts	9, 10–12
Chlorine	8, 12–15
Cobalt metal	5
Fire smoke	3, 16
Hydrogen bromide	17
Hydrogen chloride	5
Hydrogen sulfide	8
Hydrogen selenide	5, 18
Mercury	19, 20
Methyl bromide	21
Methylene chloride (paint remover)	22
Nickel (fume)	23
Nickel carbonyl	16, 24
Nitrogen oxides	25, 26
Ozone	27
Perchloroethylene	This report
Phosgene	8
Phosphorus tribromide	17
Sulfur dioxide	8, 28–30
Sulfuric acid	31
Thionyl chloride	32
Titanium tetrachloride	33, 34
Zinc oxide and chloride	10, 35
Zirconium chloride	8

TABLE 4.4
Agents Producing Bronchiolitis Obliterans

Ammonia
Chlorine
Fire smoke
Hydrogen bromide
Hydrogen selenide
Oxides of nitrogen
Sulfur dioxide
Thionyl chloride

TABLE 4.5
Agents Producing Bronchiectasis

Ammonia
Fire smoke
Kerosene
Nickel carbonyl
Phosgene

TABLE 4.6
Fumes and Gases Generated in Fires

FUME OR GAS	SOURCE
Household Fires	
Sulfuric and nitric acid	Soot
Acrolein, acetaldehyde, formaldehyde	Plastics, acrylates, synthetic fibers, wood, cotton, paper
Cyanide, halogens, benzene	Plastics
Phosgene, chlorine gas, hydrogen chloride	Polyvinylchloride
Ammonia	Plastics, refrigeration materials
Wildland Fires	
Aldehydes, acrolein, formaldehyde	Organic materials

problem arises from the fact that our views of pathologic mechanisms and nomenclature for pulmonary processes have changed considerably over the past 30 years, particularly in the areas of ARDS and interstitial fibrosis. Many of the reports listed have therefore been classified into what appears to be the best modern equivalent (discussed later). In some instances the pathologic descriptions are obscure or lacking and we have included the agents on the basis of clinical features; this is particularly common with the agents producing ARDS. In other reports the descriptions suggest terminal changes (e.g., pneumonia) which are probably not directly related to the original insult. Our compilation is therefore to a certain extent based on extrapolation.

Adult Respiratory Distress Syndrome and Diffuse Alveolar Damage

ARDS is by far the most common serious reaction to gases and fumes. It is likely that any noxious fume or gas, inhaled in sufficient concentration, will produce it (Table 4.3). Diffuse alveolar damage, the pathologic equivalent of ARDS, appears grossly as extremely firm diffusely consolidated lung with effacement of lung markings (Figs. 4.1 and 4.2) and microscopically as hyaline membranes in the alveolar ducts, with variable degrees of interstitial inflammation and/or alveolar collapse (Figs. 4.1 and 4.2). As diffuse alveolar damage organizes, tufts of granulation tissue appear in the alveoli (Fig. 4.2) and are gradually incorporated into the interstitium by overgrowth of the alveolar epithelium.

Many reports of exposure to occupational agents describe processes labeled chemical pneumonia, chemical pneumonitis, noncardiogenic pulmonary edema, or hemorrhagic edema (8, 9, 17, 22, 28). The reported clinical features, particularly the rapid (hours) onset after exposure, the lack of evidence of cardiac failure (indicating that this is low-pressure "edema"), the often severe respiratory compromise with widespread infiltrates on chest radiograph (Fig. 4.1), and the occasional pathologic description are those of ARDS of mild or severe degree. We have included such reports under that category.

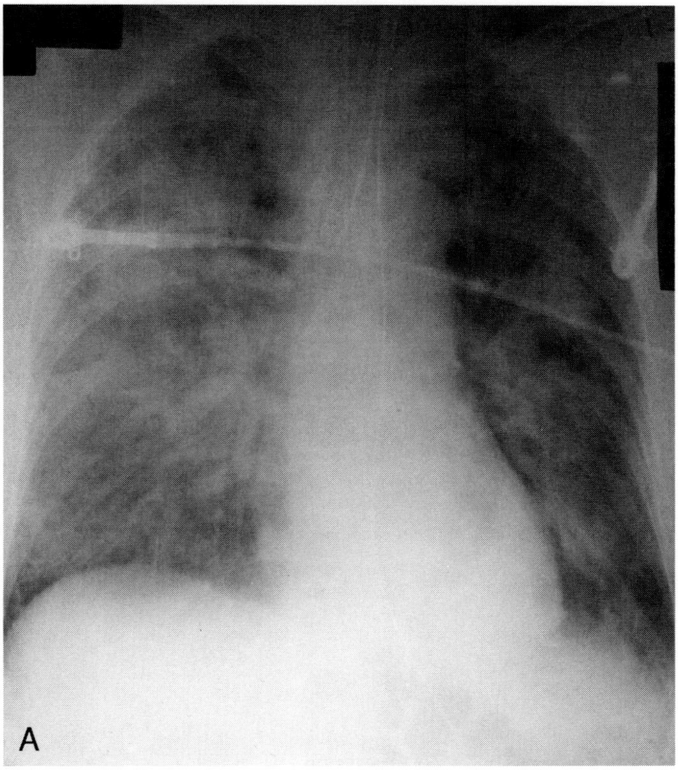

FIGURE 4.1
Diffuse alveolar damage, airway epithelial necrosis, and bronchiolitis obliterans in a patient exposed to smoke and fumes in a gasoline fire. **A.** Chest radiograph on admission approximately 24 hours after exposure. There are widespread diffuse infiltrates in a pattern typical of ARDS. **B.** Gross appearance at autopsy 1 week after exposure. There is extensive consolidation of the parenchyma with obliteration of lung markings, findings typical of diffuse alveolar damage. **C.** Micrograph showing hyaline membranes in alveolar ducts and early foci of organization, findings characteristic of acute diffuse alveolar damage of any cause. As a rule the pathologic features of diffuse alveolar damage provide no information about the nature of the insult, and the complete diagnosis requires historical data. (×64.) **D.** Large bronchiole demonstrating necrosis of the airway epithelium. This lesion can be seen with any noxious fume or gas. (×64.) **E.** Centrilobular area showing tuft of necrotic material in bronchiolar lumen. The epithelium (*arrow*) is growing over this material, and it will become a focus of granulation tissue producing the pattern of bronchiolitis obliterans. The surrounding parenchyma shows hyaline membranes and proliferating fibroblasts and alveolar lining cells, typical of diffuse alveolar damage. (×64.)

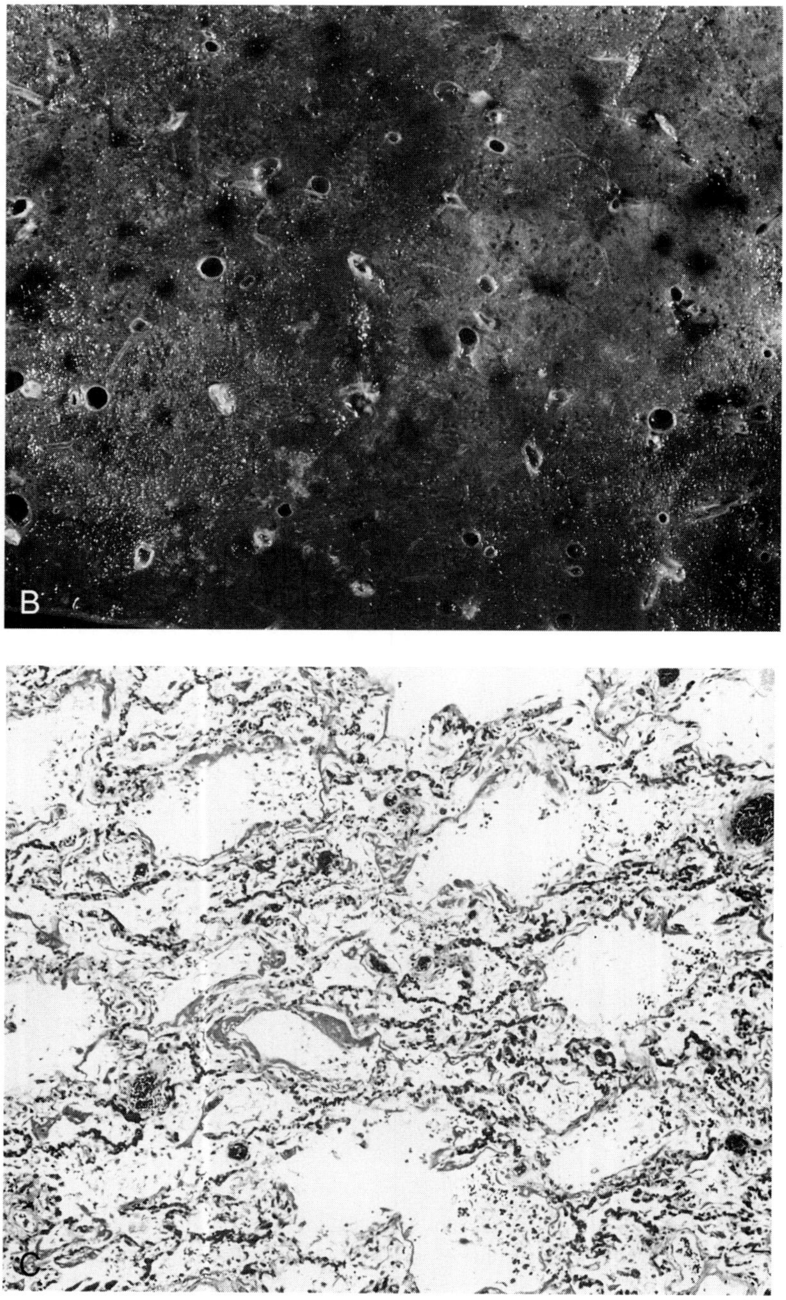

FIGURE 1.10 *(continued)*

The literature frequently confuses organizing diffuse alveolar damage and interstitial fibrosis of the type seen in fibrosing alveolitis or usual interstitial pneumonia (UIP) (10, 11, 19, 35) (see Chapter 5). These two processes are clinically quite different: ARDS is acute, usually related to an obvious episode of exposure, and the fibrosing reaction develops in a matter of days to weeks. UIP usually develops slowly and progresses over months to years.

Pathologic separation of these processes is usually easy. As a rule, organizing

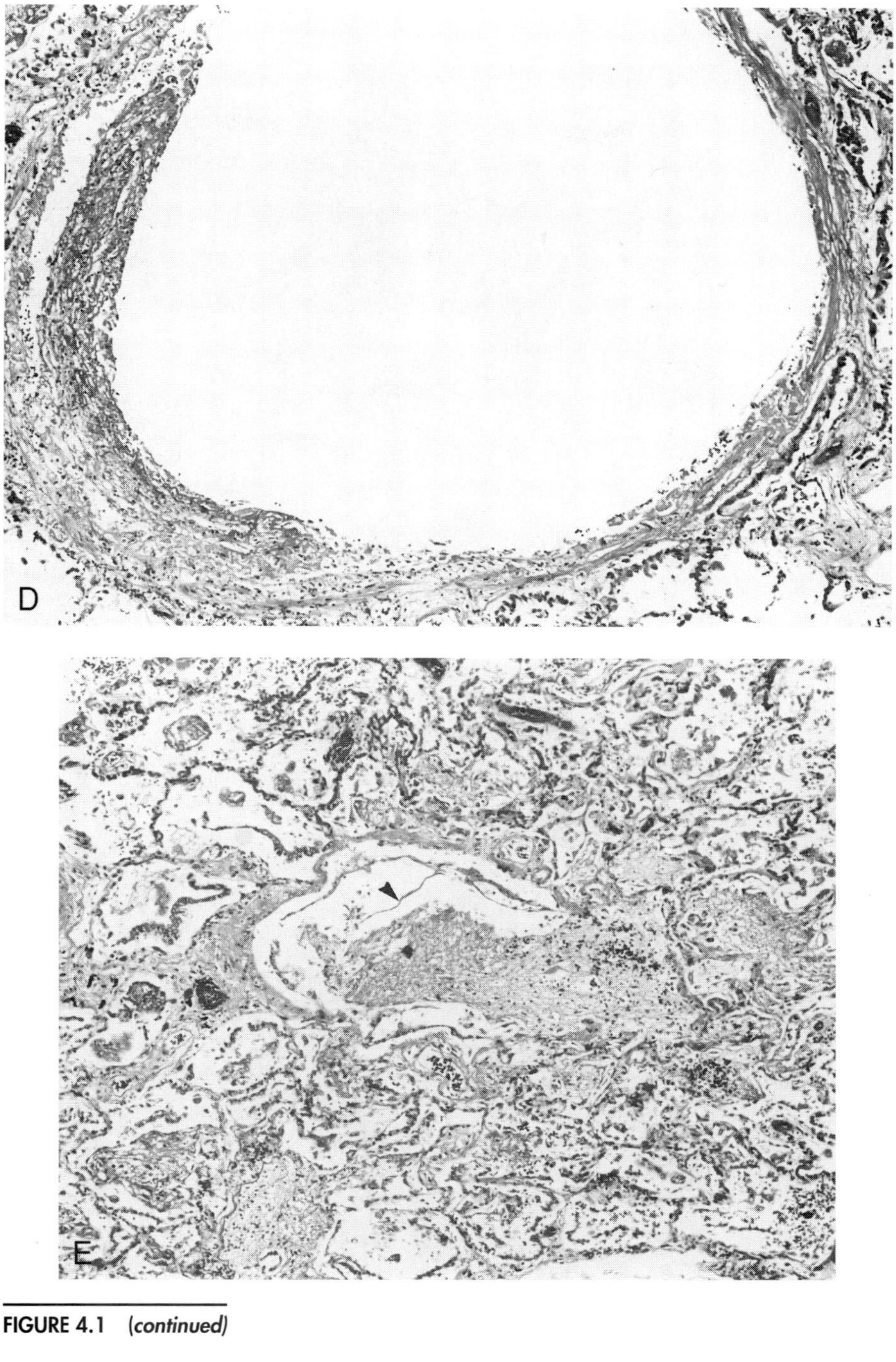

FIGURE 4.1 *(continued)*

diffuse alveolar damage is both grossly and microscopically homogeneous in distribution. Also, it tends to have little true fibrosis but a large component of recently formed granulation tissue in airspaces and numerous proliferating fibroblasts in both airspaces and interstitium (Fig. 4.2). Furthermore, the process appears temporally similar in all affected areas. By contrast, true interstitial fibrosis of the type seen in UIP and some pneumoconioses (see Chapters 5, 9, and 12) appears as old, relatively dense fibrosis, is generally much patchier in distri-

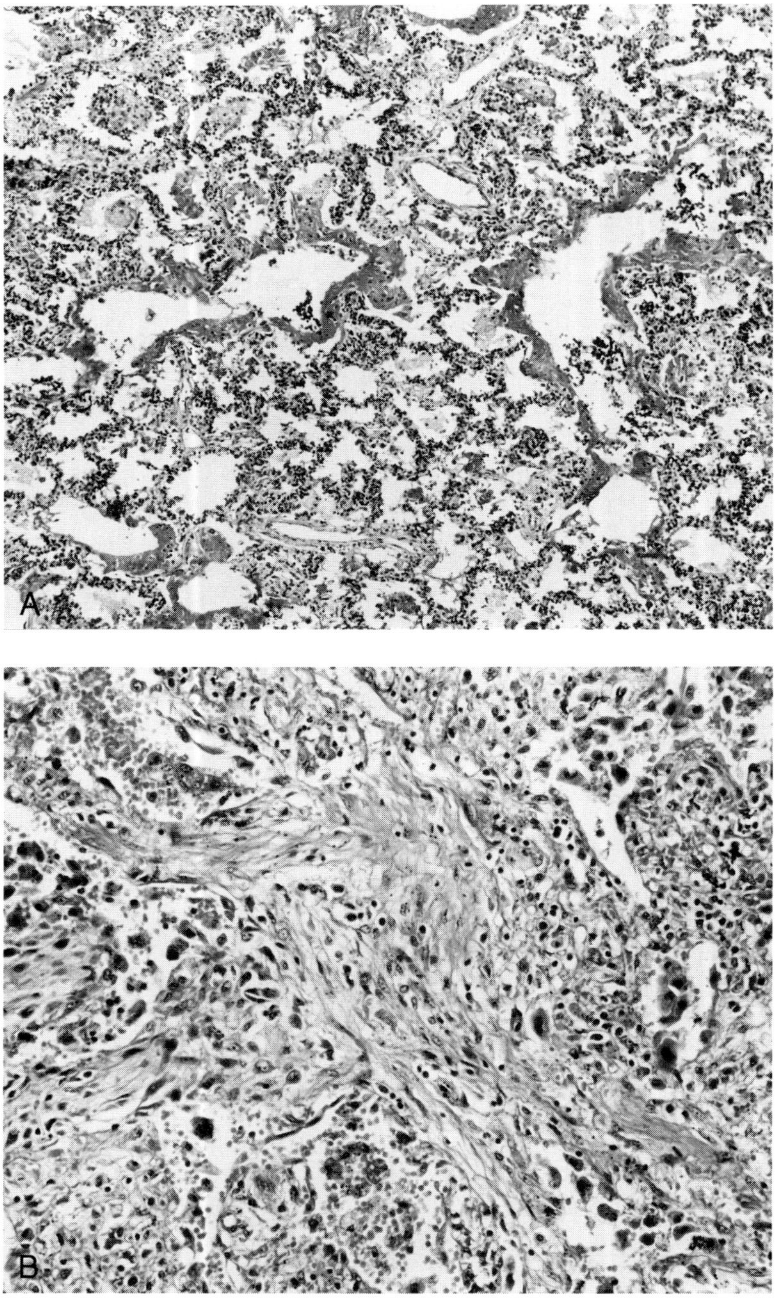

FIGURE 4.2
Diffuse alveolar damage secondary to inhalation of perchloroethylene. **A.** Low-power view showing hyaline membranes in alveolar ducts and interstitial inflammation in alveolar walls. (×40.) **B.** Higher-power view of another area demonstrating proliferating granulation tissue in airspaces. This appearance has been confused in the past with interstitial fibrosis; it really is a form of organization of diffuse alveolar damage. (×160.) (Courtesy Dr. C. Bloor, San Diego.)

bution and severity, has little or no airspace component, and appears to vary in age. However, organized diffuse alveolar damage sometimes develops a pattern of collapsed alveolar parenchyma with dilated respiratory bronchioles and alveolar ducts secondary to use of positive pressure ventilation (see Fig. 13.5) and may resemble a honeycombed lung of the sort seen in UIP. Again, recourse to clinical history usually makes the distinction clear: a story of acute exposure followed by the development of pulmonary edema and then, 1 to several weeks later, "interstitial fibrosis" (11, 19, 24, 35) surely describes ARDS with organization and not true interstitial fibrosis at all.

It is clear from the literature that many patients with relatively mild ARDS (typically reported as chemical pneumonitis) recover rapidly and probably have no residual deficits. The long-term prognosis for those who survive severe acute ARDS of any cause is uncertain, and some patients are left with residual functional deficits (36). However, there is a dearth of information about the prognosis and residual impairment in survivors of severe gas- and fume-induced ARDS.

Necrotizing Bronchitis, Bronchiolitis, and Bronchiolitis Obliterans

The same agents that produce diffuse alveolar damage may also damage airway epithelium. Very severe acute injury appears as necrosis of the airway epithelium in both large and small airways (Fig. 4.1*D*). Necrotizing bronchitis and bronchiolitis is an uncommon lesion that is seen with inhaled gases and fumes and with infections, particularly viral infections, but with little else. We have observed that when epithelial necrosis is a result of exposure to fire smoke, aggregates of black material derived from the smoke mixed with necrotic tissue may be visible (Fig. 4.1*D*), but with other types of inhaled agents no specific features are present.

Inhaled gases and fumes can also produce bronchiolitis obliterans (Table 4.4). Functionally significant bronchiolitis obliterans has been reported after exposure to ammonia, oxides of nitrogen (discussed later), fire smoke, hydrogen selenide, hydrogen bromide, sulfur dioxide, chlorine gas, and thionyl chloride (thionyl chloride generates a combination of hydrogen chloride and sulfur dioxide) (7, 17, 18, 25, 32, 37–44), but it is likely that many more agents can produce this condition. Small airway damage is most common after inhalation of fumes in a closed space where the concentrations are very high and is less frequent after inhalation in the open air (42, 43).

It has been suggested that the degree of damage to the trachea and large airways reflects the solubility of the inhaled agent, with highly soluble agents such as ammonia and sulfur dioxide producing more proximal damage than less soluble agents such as nitrogen dioxide (3, 4). In practice it appears that either site or both sites may be affected to some extent by any noxious gas or fume (25, 37–41); it is likely that both the solubility and the concentration of the agent are important in determining where injury occurs in the individual case. Proximal airway damage in the form of epithelial necrosis, ARDS, and bronchiolitis obliterans may in fact result from the same inhalation event (18, 28–30; Fig. 4.1). In other cases the acute events are less dramatic and bronchiolitis obliterans develops after a matter of weeks (3, 37, 45; Fig. 4.3); the clinical picture is progressive shortness of breath associated with marked degrees of airflow obstruction.

Colby and Carrington (46) propose that what has traditionally been called bronchiolitis obliterans comprises two morphologically and probably prognos-

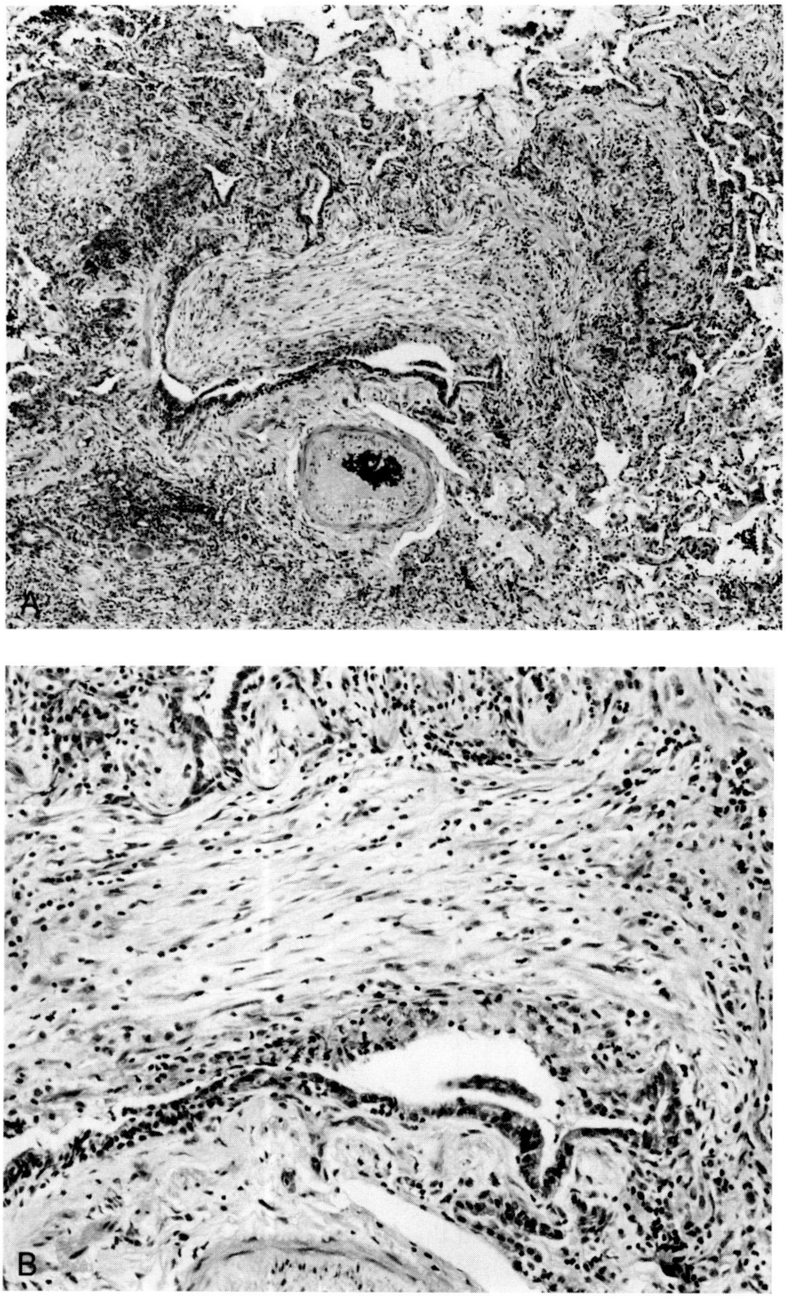

FIGURE 4.3
Bronchiolitis obliterans (proliferative bronchiolitis) secondary to fume inhalation. The patient was exposed to fumes in a nickel-plating plant after a chemical spill. She developed shortness of breath and airflow obstruction several weeks after exposure. From the description the fumes appear to have been NO_2. Low- and high-power views (**A** and **B**, respectively) showing tuft of granulation tissue virtually filling the lumen of a respiratory bronchiole. This is the characteristic lesion of active bronchiolitis obliterans. There is also surrounding inflammation and fibrosis extending for a short distance from the airway, but between airways the parenchyma is for the most part normal. If this process does not resolve, the granulation tissue will become re-epithelialized and the airway lumen reduced, obstructed, or markedly narrowed (Fig. 4.6). (**A**, ×40, **B**, ×160.)

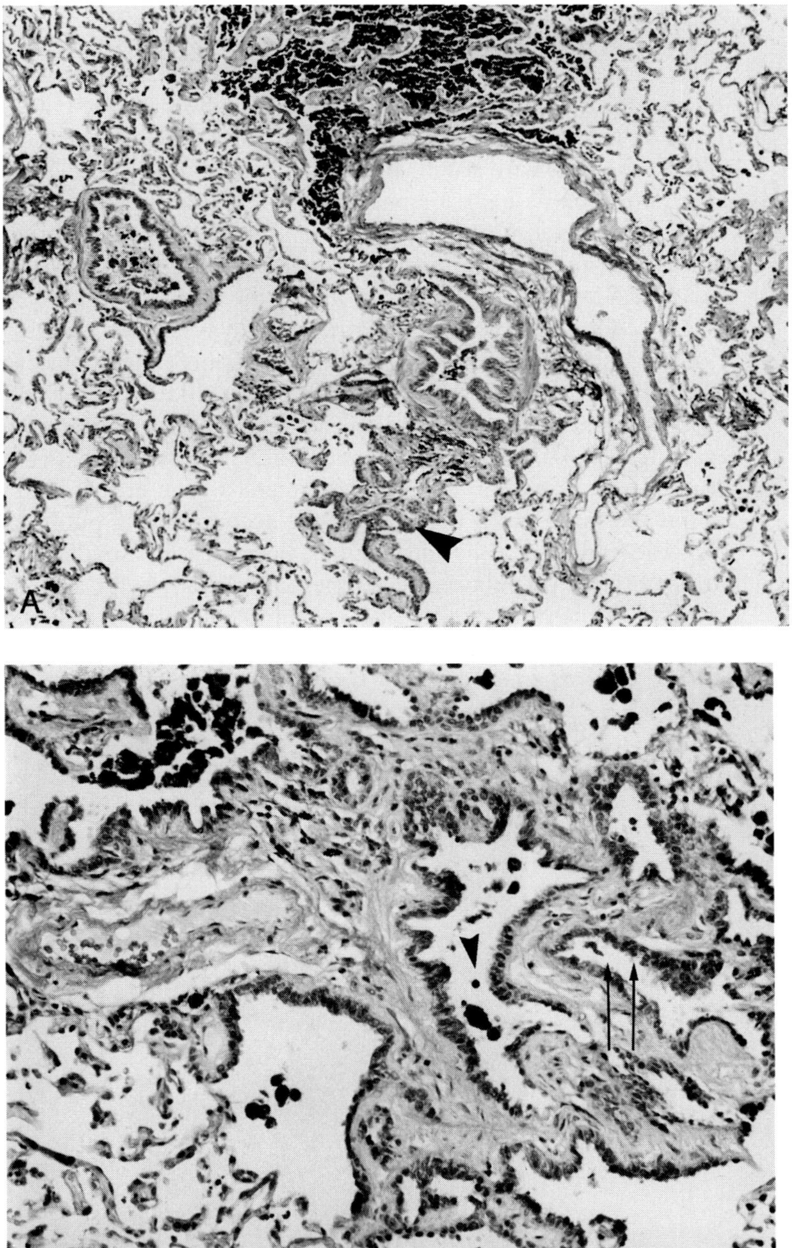

FIGURE 4.4

Old healed bronchiolitis obliterans (constrictive bronchiolitis) in an arc welder. This patient was a man with a history of many years of arc welding who presented with shortness of breath and was found to have severe obstructive lung disease. Open lung biopsy was performed to determine the nature of his pulmonary disease. **A.** Low-power micrograph showing large amounts of iron pigment and deformed and scarred respiratory bronchiole (*arrow*). Intervening parenchyma is essentially normal. (×40.) **B.** Higher-power view of another airway. The airway is abnormally thick-walled, and the central lumen (*arrow*) is deformed and stenotic. Other small luminal channels (*double arrows*) are also present, and irregular tongues of epithelium-covered fibrous tissue extend into the parenchyma. These are characteristic lesions of healed bronchiolitis obliterans, presumably induced in this instance by exposure to welding fumes. (×160.)

tically dissimilar entities. Under this scheme the classical type of bronchiolitis obliterans, which appears as granulation tissue plugs in the lumens of membranous and respiratory bronchioles, is called proliferative bronchiolitis . This is by far the most common type of bronchiolitis obliterans seen after gas and fume inhalation (Fig. 4.1*E*). Occasionally fumes also produce the lesion called bronchiolitis obliterans with patchy organizing pneumonia (BOOP) (46), a combination of granulation tissue in airspaces and interstitial inflammation that morphologically overlaps into abnormalities confined to the small airways. BOOP is not confined to metallic fume inhalations: Moya et al. (47) recently reported an outbreak of BOOP in workers spraying textile dyes.

Less commonly recognized pathologically but probably functionally more significant, is the form of bronchiolitis obliterans called constrictive bronchiolitis (46). Microscopically this appears as narrowed and distorted respiratory bronchioles, usually with obviously thickened, fibrotic, and sometimes inflamed walls (Fig. 4.4). Constrictive bronchiolitis may be subtle and easily overlooked. A good rule of thumb is that the diameter of the bronchiolar lumen should be about the same as the diameter of the accompanying pulmonary artery lumen; thus the finding of either bronchioles that are much smaller than the pulmonary artery branch or pulmonary arteries with nondescript accompanying scars instead of bronchioles should bring to mind constrictive bronchiolitis.

An additional lesion that we have observed in workers with fume and gas exposure consists of respiratory bronchioles that end in multiple small fibrous-

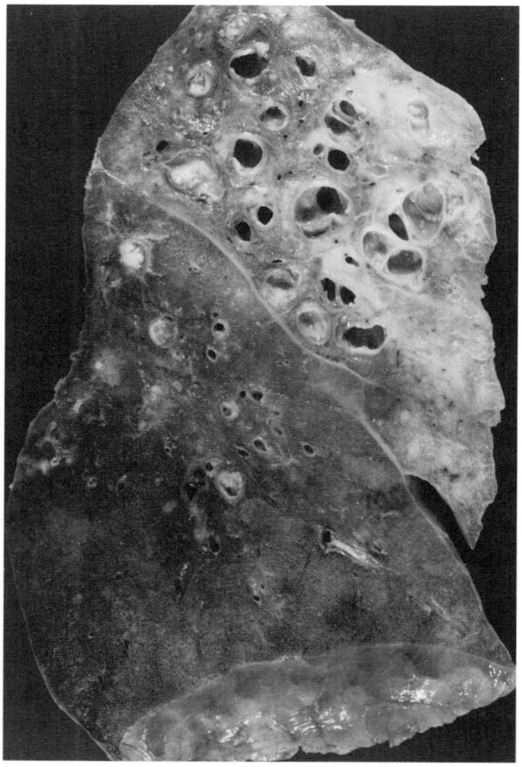

FIGURE 4.5

Severe upper lobe bronchiectasis in a patient who inhaled kerosene as a child and lived to adulthood. (Reprinted with permission from Churg A, Green FHY. Occupational lung disease. In: Thurlbeck WM, Churg A, eds. Pathology of the lung. 2nd ed. New York: Thieme, 1995).

walled channels (Fig. 4.4*B*) rather than opening into thin-walled alveolar ducts in the usual fashion. This appears to be yet another variant of constrictive bronchiolitis.

Many patients who develop bronchiolitis obliterans and acute airflow abnormalities improve over a few weeks to months (15, 29, 44, 48, 49), often in response to steroid therapy (3, 42). However, bronchiolitis obliterans may progress to death from respiratory failure. It is believed (although data correlating pathologic findings and clinical outcome are scanty) that resolution is much more likely when the pathologic findings are those of proliferative bronchiolitis and that constrictive bronchiolitis is likely to result in fixed or worsening airflow obstruction (46).

Emphysema, Bronchiectasis, and Occupational Asthma

Except for the disputed area of cadmium exposure (see Chapter 5), there is no evidence that any of these agents produces emphysema, and older reports that mention emphysema after exposure to fumes, gases, or metals (Chapter 5) appear to describe changes induced by cigarette smoke or the dilated airspaces of honeycomb lung seen in true interstitial fibrosis and some cases of organizing ARDS.

Occupational asthma is seen after exposure to many types of fumes and metals; reported agents are listed in Chapter 12.

Bronchiectasis has been reported in workers inhaling ammonia (7, 40, 50), fire smoke (51, 52), phosgene (4), and possibly nickel carbonyl (16) (Table 4.5). We have seen a case in which upper zone bronchiectasis developed after accidental kerosene aspiration (Fig. 4.5). Typically the lesions develop over years.

DISEASE ASSOCIATED WITH SPECIFIC AGENTS AND OCCUPATIONS

Effects of Welding

Welding is the joining of metal to metal by use of heat and/or pressure. There are several methods of welding. The two main types, which also generate the most fumes and gases, are manual arc and metal inert gas welding. The latter produces approximately 100 times the fume emissions of the former (53). The nature of the fume also depends on whether the electrode is nonconsumable, as in carbon or tungsten arc welding, or consumable. The main fume generated by consumable electrodes is iron oxide. Cadmium, chromium, beryllium, aluminum, titanium, and nickel may also be present. Chromium is most common in stainless steel welding. Inhalable material may also be generated by the electrode coating and flux, producing exposure to acrolein and isocyanate as well as oxides of nitrogen.

By far the most common clinical effect of welding is the appearance of fine nodular lesions on the chest radiograph; these correspond to the pathologic picture of dust macules, that is, collections of dust-laden macrophages surrounding small airways and vessels. Because iron is the principal metallic fume in most types of welding, the dust macules in welders contain largely iron, and the condition is termed siderosis (54). Although dust macules are generally considered radiographic and pathologic findings having no functional significance, there is considerable evidence that in some cases macules progress to fibrotic lesions of the small airways. They may also be associated with the type of focal emphysema commonly seen in coal miners; these pathologic lesions, which are discussed as a general phenomenon in Chapter 5, may be a cause of airflow obstruction (discussed later).

Apart from siderosis, clinical respiratory tract abnormalities in welders are mostly related to effects on large airways but do not appear to reflect the total amount of dust in the lung (55). Hayden et al. (56) found an increased frequency of upper respiratory tract infections in welders, but chronic bronchitis (i.e., increased sputum production) was increased only in welders who smoked. Naslund and Hogstedt (57), using magnetopulmonography to estimate degree of exposure, found that 23% of highly exposed welders had chronic bronchitis regardless of smoking history. Akbarkhanzadeh (58), investigating metal arc welders, showed that the welders with chronic bronchitis had longer exposure histories than welders without. Of course, chronic bronchitis is excessive sputum production and is not by itself associated with airflow obstruction.

The issue of chronic airflow obstruction in welders is confusing, controversial, and complicated by the effects of cigarette smoking. Cross-sectional analyses of mild steel welders and arc welders of all types were performed by Mur et al. (59) and Keimig et al. (60). Neither study showed significant differences in pulmonary function tests between the test and control groups, although the mild steel welders had an overall slightly decreased FEF_{25-75}. Akbarkhanzadeh et al. (58) examined metal arc welders in a shipyard and found a greater deterioration of FEV_1 and FVC with age in welders and lower FEV_1 for both smoking and nonsmoking welders than in controls. Hayden et al. (56) found decreased FEF_{25-75}, but only in the welders who smoked; nonsmokers showed no difference from controls. Kalliomaki et al. (53) compared welders of stainless steel with those primarily welding mild steel. Pulmonary function test impairment was found in the stainless steel welders who used the metal arc but not in those using the inert gas technique. Although the metal arc stainless steel welders had more dust in their lungs (as measured by magnetometry), tests of metal arc mild steel welders showed more small airway disease.

Sferlazza and Beckett (61) extensively reviewed the literature on this subject and came to the following conclusions: (*a*) Most welding, in the absence of an acute inhalation injury, does not appear to lead to clinically apparent lung dysfunction. (*b*) Shipyard welders have more negative effects on lung function than do outdoor welders, a finding attributed to the confined and poorly ventilated areas in which shipyard welders work. (*c*) There appears to be significant interaction between cigarette smoking and welding, resulting in diminution of the mid and late flow rates; these findings are attributed to the hypothesis that both agents are likely to affect the small bronchioles. However, these function decrements are not associated with disability and do not predict accelerated decline in pulmonary function.

These studies suggest that although small airway disease (see Chapter 5) may exist in some welding populations, this phenomenon is not universal, and the degree of impairment is minimal in most workers. However, there is a need for longitudinal analyses with careful control of smoking, welding technique, and welding materials to examine directly the long-term effects of welding. Of course, individual welders may develop lesions such as bronchiolitis obliterans as a result of exposure to welding fumes.

Lung cancer risk in welders is also controversial, with some studies showing no increased risk while others found increased mortality (61, 62). In a review of the world literature Stern (62) found a risk of lung carcinoma approximately 30% above that of the nonwelding population, even after excluding effects for shipyard working and smoking. Beaumont and Weiss (63) examined a large group of welders in Washington state and found a 32% elevated mortality from lung carcinoma. If the group with exposure longer than 20 years was considered, the excess was 74%. Mutagenicity of welding fume, ascribed to chromium, has been described by Hedenstedt et al. (64), who examined metal arc and inert gas fumes. Stainless steel but not mild steel welding fumes were mutagenic, and metal arc fumes were more mutagenic than inert gas fumes. These studies may indicate that welders have an increased risk of developing lung carcinoma; since there is no apparent limitation to or accentuation of the carcinoma risk in stainless steel welders, the risk cannot be entirely attributed to chromium. Thus, although welding fumes are a suspected carcinogen, this must be confirmed by epidemiologic studies devised to distinguish between the welding fume components and the confounding factors of cigarette smoke and possibly asbestos exposure. Furthermore, there is no diagnostic finding that would allow the pathologist to attribute a case of lung cancer in a smoking welder to occupational exposure.

Metal Fume Fever

Metal fume fever is seen most commonly in shipyard welders who are exposed to oxides of zinc, copper, magnesium, and sometimes cadmium (65). A similar symptom complex seen in response to polytetrafluorethylene in the manufacture of Teflon is known as polymer fume fever. The clinical features consist of excessive thirst accompanied by a metallic taste in the mouth that commences 4 to 8 hours after work begins. After 10 to 12 hours flulike symptoms consisting of fever, myalgia, rigors, and weakness occur. The symptoms subside after 24 to 48 hours. During this time peripheral leukocytosis is accompanied by diffuse crepitations in the lung, but with a normal chest radiograph. There is no latent period for sensitization. Workers develop tolerance on repeated exposures, so that over the course of a workweek symptoms disappear, but tolerance is rapidly lost when exposure stops; hence the worst symptoms are seen at the beginning of the workweek ("Monday morning fever"). The disease is thought to be an immunologic reaction to fumes and metal particulates less than 1.5 μm in size (3, 65), but the pathologic changes in metal fume fever are not known.

Effects of Oxides of Nitrogen

Since NO_2 is poorly soluble, its conversion to nitrous acid (HNO_2) and nitric acid (HNO_3) occurs slowly, allowing the gases to reach the distal airways and alveoli; the propensity of high concentrations of NO_2 to produce bronchiolitis obliterans has been attributed to this effect (3, 25) (Fig 4.5). Nitric acid, a source of oxides of nitrogen, is used in the manufacture of various nitrates, jewelry, and leather substitutes; in the cleaning of copper and brass articles; and in conjunction with other acids in stripping steel sheets. Smaller amounts of nitrous fumes are released during detonation of nitro explosives and during welding and brazing. In addition, various oxides of nitrogen are produced in the fermentation of silage, and it is here that probably the majority of massive exposures occur, resulting in silo workers' disease.

The incidence of silo workers' disease is difficult to assess, but data from Horvath et al. (25) suggest that of approximately 164,000 farmers in Wisconsin, 6,700 have encountered potentially dangerous gas concentrations. A retrospective study of farmers in the state of New York identified an incidence of 5 cases per year among 100,000 farm workers exposed to silos(66). In the New York study mortality was 20%; thus there is a substantial population at risk.

In the silo anaerobic fermentation, which begins within a few hours after ensilement, breaks down plant materials by bacterial enzymatic degradation, producing acetic and lactic acid, carbon dioxide, and nitrites. The amount of nitrites produced is positively related to the immaturity of plants, plants grown in drought, and plants given abundant nitrate-based fertilizers. The nitrites react with organic acids to form nitrous acid, which is further converted to NO, N_2O_5, NO_2, and N_2O_4. The last two, the most common gases, are generally present in a ratio of 30:70, although N_2O_4 breaks down rapidly to nitrogen dioxide. A peak concentration of gas is reached in 1 to 5 days; common concentrations are 150 to 1900 ppm, but up to 4000 ppm has been reported.

Since both carbon dioxide and NO_2 are heavier than air, the gases concentrate at the surface and in surface pits of the silage. They may be seen as a yellow–red to orange vapor. The farmer is exposed when he jumps into the silage surface to remove feed. Acute high exposures often result in death from asphyxiation or ARDS; bronchiolitis obliterans usually becomes clinically apparent in 3 to 6 weeks and may or may not be preceded by clinically evident acute disease. In a study of 22 patients with silo workers' disease, five developed persistent airway dysfunction, probably bronchiolitis obliterans (25).

Disease in Firefighters

In the course of fires in houses, apartment buildings, hotels, automobiles, and aircraft, numerous chemicals are released by the hot or burning materials (Table 4.6). Many of these substances are toxic, and they may be present in high concentrations. For example, polyvinyl chloride, when heated to 225 to 475°C, loses approximately 60% of its weight in the form of chlorine gas, phosgene, and hydrochloric acid (67). Exposure to chemicals and fumes is highly variable, depending on what is burning and whether any form of respiratory protection is worn. Fighters of wildland fires are also exposed to fumes and gases, particularly of the aldehyde group (Table 4.6) in addition to high levels of particulates. Unlike fighters of household or industrial fires, these workers rarely if ever wear respiratory protection (68).

Firefighters and individuals caught in fires may acutely develop necrosis of the upper respiratory epithelium, ARDS, or both (Fig. 4.1). Bronchiolitis obliterans developing several weeks after exposure has also been described, as has bronchiectasis (45, 51, 69).

Although transient decreases in flow rates have been found after acute exposures to a single fire (70–72), the question of chronic pulmonary function abnormalities in firefighters is controversial. A long-term study of Boston firefighters initially suggested an increased rate of decline in function (73), but this was not confirmed on a repeat study of the same population (74, 75). Another study (76) found a greater rate of decline of FEV_1 in firefighters than in a control cohort but could not relate this either to symptoms or years of exposure. Further longitudinal studies in both firefighter groups will be required to establish whether firefighting is associated with airflow abnormalities and any morphologic correlates of such abnormalities.

REFERENCES

1. Parkes WR. Aerosols: their deposition and clearance. In: Parkes WR, ed. Occupational Lung Disorders. 3rd ed. London: Butterworth-Heinemann, 1994:35–49.
2. Brooks SM. Lung disorders resulting from the inhalation of metals. Clin Chest Med 1981;2:235–254.
3. Summer W, Haponik E. Inhalation of irritant gases. Clin Chest Med 1981;2:273–287.
4. Weiss SM, Lakshminarayan S. Acute inhalation injury. Clin Chest Med 1994;15:103–116.
5. Waldron HA. Nonneoplastic disorders due to metallic, chemical, and physical agents. In: Parkes WR. Occupational Lung Disorders. 3rd ed. London: Butterworth-Heinemann, 1994:593–643.
6. Walton M. Industrial ammonia gassing. Br J Ind Med 1973;30:78–86.
7. Sobonya R. Fatal anhydrous ammonia inhalation. Hum Pathol 1977;8:293–299.
8. Cordasco EM, Stone FD. Pulmonary edema of occupational origin. Chest 1973;64:182–185.
9. Beton DC, Andrews GS, Davies HJ, et al. Acute cadmium fume poisoning. Br J Ind Med 1966;23:292–301.
10. Anthony JS, Zamel N, Aberman A. Abnormalities in pulmonary function after brief exposure to toxic metal fumes. Can Med Assoc J 1978;119:586–588.
11. Yamamoto K, Ueda M, Kikuchi H, et al. An acute fatal occupational cadmium poisoning by inhalation. Z Rechtsmed 1983;91:139–143.
12. Weston JT, Liebow AA, Dixon MG, Rich TH. Untoward effects of exogenous inhalants on the lung. J Forensic Sci 1972;17:199–279.
13. Beach FXM, Sherwood Jones E, Scarrow GD. Respiratory effects of chlorine gas. Br J Ind Med 1969;26:231–236.
14. Tibbits PA, Milroy WC. Pulmonary edema induced by exposure to cadmium oxide fume: case report. Mil Med 1980;145:435–437.
15. Weill H, George R, Schwarz M, Ziskind M. Late evaluation of pulmonary function after acute exposure to chlorine gas. Am Rev Respir Dis 1969;99:374–379.
16. Jones Williams W. The pathology of the lungs in five nickel workers. Br J Ind Med 1958;15:235–242.
17. Kraut A, Lilis R. Chemical pneumonitis due to exposure to bromine compounds. Chest 1988;94:206–210.
18. Schecter A, Shanske W, Stenszler A, et al. Acute hydrogen selenide inhalation. Chest 1980;77:554–555.
19. Jaeger A, Tempe JD, Haegy JM, et al. Accidental acute mercury vapor poisoning. Vet Hum Toxicol 1979;21(Suppl):62–63.
20. Hallee TJ. Diffuse lung disease caused by inhalation of mercury vapor. Am Rev Respir Dis 1969;99:430–436.
21. Rathus EM, Landy PJ. Methyl bromide poisoning. Br J Ind Med 1961;18:53–57.
22. Synder RW, Mishel HS, Christensen GC. Pulmonary toxicity following exposure to methylene chloride and its combustion product, phosgene. Chest 1992;101:860–861.
23. Rendell RE, Phillips JI, Renton KA. Death following exposure to fine particulate nickel from a metal arc process. Ann Occup Hyg 1994;38:921–930.
24. Sunderman FW, Kincaid JF. Nickel poisoning: 2. Studies on patients suffering from acute exposure to vapors of nickel carbonyl. JAMA 1954;155:889–894.
25. Horvath EP, doPico GA, Barber RA, Dickie HA. Nitrogen-dioxide induced pulmonary disease. J Occup Med 1978;20:103–110.
26. Suzuki K, Tachibana A, Hatakeyama S, Okano H. Five cases of acute pulmonary failure associated with nitrogen dioxide inhalation. Jpn J Thorac Dis 1993;31:517–522.
27. Stockinger HE. Ozone toxicology: a review of research and industrial experience, 1954–1964. Arch Environ Health 1965;10:719–731.

28. Charan NB, Myers CG, Lakshminarayan S, Spencer TM. Pulmonary injuries associated with acute sulfur dioxide inhalation. Am Rev Respir Dis 1979;119:555–560.
29. Chester EH, Kaimal PJ, Payne CB, Kohn PM. Pulmonary injury following exposure to chlorine gas: possible beneficial effects of steroid treatment. Chest 1977;72: 247–250.
30. Woodford DM, Coutu RE, Gaensler EA. Obstructive lung disease from acute sulfur dioxide exposure. Respiration 1979;38:238–245.
31. Knapp MJ, Bunn WB, Stave GM. Adult respiratory distress syndrome from sulfuric acid fume inhalation. South Med J 1991;1031–1033.
32. Konchezky S, Schattner A, Ezri T, et al. Thionyl chloride-induced lung injury and bronchiolitis obliterans. Chest 1993;104:971–973.
33. Lawson JJ. The toxicity of titanium tetrachloride. J Occup Med 1961;3:7–12.
34. Park T, DiBenedetto R, Morgan K, et al. Diffuse endobronchial polyposis following a titanium tetrachloride inhalation injury. Am Rev Respir Dis 1984;130:315–317.
35. Millikan JA, Waugh AD, Kadish ME. Acute interstitial pulmonary fibrosis caused by a smoke bomb. Can Med Assoc J 1963;88:36–39.
36. Ghio AJ, Elliott CG, Crapo RO, et al. Impairment after adult respiratory distress syndrome. Am Rev Respir Dis 1989;139:1158–1162.
37. Murphy DMF, Fairman RP, Lapp NL, Morgan WKC. Severe airway disease due to inhalation of fumes from cleansing agents. Chest 1976;69:372–373.
38. Woodford DM, Coutu RE, Gaensler EA. Obstructive lung disease from acute sulfur dioxide exposure. Respiration 1979;38:238–245.
39. Seggev JS, Mason UG 3rd, Worthen S, et al. Bronchiolitis obliterans. Chest 1983;83: 169–174.
40. Close LG, Catlin FI, Cohn AM. Acute and chronic effects of ammonia burns of the respiratory tract. Arch Otolaryngol 1980;106:151–158.
41. Morgenroth K. Morphological alterations to the bronchial mucosa in high-dosage long-term exposure to sulfur dioxide. Respiration 1980;39:39–48.
42. Arora NS, Aldrich TK. The use of steroids in bronchiolitis obliterans after smoke inhalation. Crit Care Med 1981;9:72.
43. Darke CS, Warrack AJN. Bronchiolitis from nitrous fumes. Thorax 1958;13: 327–333.
44. Ploysongsang Y, Beach BC, DeLisio RE. Pulmonary function changes after acute inhalation of chlorine gas. South Med J 1982;75:23–26.
45. Aurora NS, Aldrich TK. Bronchiolitis obliterans from a burning automobile. South Med J 1980;73:507–510.
46. Colby TV, Carrington CB. Interstitial lung disease. In: Thurlbeck WM, Churg A, eds. Pathology of the lung. 2nd ed. New York: Thieme, 1995:589–738.
47. Moya C, Anto JM, Taylor AJN. Outbreak of organising pneumonia in textile printing sprayers. Lancet 1994;343:498–502.
48. Barret L, Faure J. Chlorine poisoning. Lancet 1984;1:561–562.
49. Hasan FM, Gehshan A, Fuleihan FJD. Resolution of pulmonary dysfunction following acute chlorine exposure. Arch Environ Health 1983;38:76–80.
50. Hoeffler HB, Schweppe HI, Greenberg SD. Bronchiectasis following pulmonary ammonia burn. Arch Pathol Lab Med 1982;106:686–687.
51. Perez-Guerra F, Walsh RE, Sagel SS. Bronchiolitis obliterans and tracheal stenosis: late complications of inhalation burn. JAMA 1971;218:1568–1570.
52. Slutzker AD, Kinn R, Said SI. Bronchiectasis and progressive respiratory failure following smoke inhalation. Chest 1989;95:1349–1350.
53. Kalliomaki PL, Kalliomaki K, Korhonen O, et al. Respiratory status of stainless steel and mild steel welders. Scand J Work Environ Health 1982;8:117–121.
54. Morgan WKC, Kerr HD. Pathologic and physiologic studies of welder's siderosis. Ann Intern Med 1963;58:293–304.
55. Kalliomaki PL, Alanko K, Korhonen O, et al. Amount and distribution of welding fume lung contaminants among arc welders. Scand J Work Environ Health 1978;4: 122–130.

56. Hayden SP, Pincock AC, Hayden J, et al. Respiratory symptoms and pulmonary function of welders in the engineering industry. Thorax 1984;39:442–447.
57. Naslund PE, Hogstedt P. Welding and bronchitis. Eur J Respir Dis 1982;118:69–72.
58. Akbarkhanzadeh F. Long-term effects of welding fumes upon respiratory symptoms and pulmonary function. J Occup Med 1980;22:337–341.
59. Mur JM, Cavelier C, Meyer-Bisch C, et al. Étude de la fonction pulmonaire de soudeurs à l'arc. Respiration 1983;44:50–57.
60. Keimig DG, Pomrehn, Burmeister LF. Respiratory symptoms and pulmonary function in welders of mild steel: a cross-sectional study. Am J Ind Med 1983;4:489–499.
61. Sferlazza SJ, Beckett WS. The respiratory health of welders. Am Rev Respir Dis 1991; 143:1134–1148
62. Stern RM. Assessment of lung cancer risk for welders. Arch Environ Health 1983; 38:148–155.
63. Beaumont JJ, Weiss NS. Lung cancer among welders. J Occup Med 1981;23: 839–844.
64. Hedenstedt A, Jenssen D, Lidesten BM, et al. Mutagenicity of fume particles from stainless steel welding. Scand J Work Environ Health 1977;203–211.
65. Johnson JS, Kilburn KH. Cadmium induced metal fume fever: results of inhalation challenge. Am J Ind Med 1983;4:533–540.
66. Zwemer FL, Pratt DS, May JJ. Silo filler's disease in New York state. Am Res Respir Dis 1002;146:650–653.
67. Dyer RF, Esch VH. Polyvinyl chloride toxicity in fires. JAMA 1976;235:393–397.
68. Liu D, Tager IB, Balmes JR, Harrison RJ. The effect of smoke inhalation on lung function and airway responsiveness in wildland fire fighters. Am Rev Respir Dis 1992;146:1469–1473.
69. Loke J, Farmer W, Matthay RA, et al. Acute and chronic effects of fire fighting on pulmonary function. Chest 1980;77:369–374.
70. Musk AW, Smith TJ, Peters JM, McLaughlin E. Pulmonary function in firefighters: acute changes in ventilatory capacity and their correlates. Br J Ind Med 1979;36: 29–34
71. Large AA, Owens GR, Hoffman LA. The short term effects of smoke exposure on the pulmonary function of firefighters. Chest 1990;97:806–809.
72. Sheppard D, Distefano S, Morse L, Becker C. Acute effects of routine firefighting on lung function. Am J Ind Med 1986;9:333–340.
73. Peters JM, Theriault GP, Fine LJ, Wegman DH. Chronic effect of fire fighting on pulmonary function. N Engl J Med 1974;291:1320–1322.
74. Musk AW, Peters JM, Wegman DH. Lung function in fire fighters: 1. A three year follow-up of active subjects. Am J Public Health 1977;67:626–629.
75. Musk AW, Peters JM, Wegman DH. Lung function in fire fighters: 2. A five year follow-up of retirees. Am J Public Health. 1977; 67:630–633
76. Sparrow D, Bosse R, Rosner B, Weiss ST. The effect of occupational exposure on pulmonary function. Am Rev Respir Dis 1982;125:319–322.

CHAPTER 5

Diseases Caused by Metals and Related Compounds

❖ Andrew Churg
❖ Thomas V. Colby

Chapter 4 discussed lesions produced by gases and fumes, including effects of metals and metal compounds commonly encountered as fumes (see Chapter 4 for definitions of fumes and dusts). This chapter discusses diseases caused by metals and metal compounds generally encountered as dusts rather than fumes, although, as noted in Chapter 4, this distinction is sometimes difficult, since dusts and fumes can produce similar lesions, such as macules. Specific causative agents and occupations associated with risk are shown in Table 5.1, (1–4) and the general types of lesions produced are listed in Table 5.2.

PATHOLOGIC REACTIONS

Dust Macules, Small Airway Fibrosis, Emphysema, and Their Relation to Chronic Airflow Obstruction

A dust macule is a nonpalpable and (theoretically) nonfibrotic collection of pigmented dust and dust-laden macrophages around small airways and vessels in the center of the pulmonary lobule (1). Most metals, metal oxides, and metal salts can produce dust macules, and in fact many produce no other lesions (Table 5.3). Other types of dust, such as coal, silica, and some silicates, also produce macules.

Because the dusts making up the macules are radiodense, on chest radiographs these lesions appear as fine nodules that are generally more prominent in the upper zones (Fig. 5.1). Thus by definition they constitute a simple pneumoconiosis (see definitions and illustrations in Chapter 1). When the macules are caused by very radiodense metals, such as tin or barium, the chest radiograph may be spectacular (1). Such radiographs may also show Kerley B lines; these are manifestations of dust collected along interlobular septa. When macules are found by pathologic examination or fine nodules consistent with simple pneumoconiosis show up on radiographic examination, specific names related to the

TABLE 5.1
Metals and Related Compounds, Uses, and Occupations Associated with Risk

AGENTS	OCCUPATIONS WITH EXPOSURE; USES
Aluminum and aluminum oxide	Mining bauxite Aluminum smelting Production of aluminum metal or specific product (numerous) Aluminum grinding, polishing, welding
Antimony	Mining, processing, and smelting antimony ores Production and use of antimony alloys In paints, glass Linotype setting
Antimony trichloride and antimony pentachloride	Coloring metals Chemical catalysts
Arsenic	Smelting of copper, aluminum, and other ores
Barium	Mining, refining ores Glass manufacture Filler for paints, papers, tectiles Sandblasting Medical contrast agent
Beryllium	Beryllium mining and extraction Beryllium metallurgy and production of beryllium alloys, ceramics (see Table 5.6)
Cadmium	High-friction metal alloys Soldering and welding cadmium alloys Electroplating Paints, ceramics, glass, plastics Refining of other ores (zinc, lead, copper)
Chromium	Mining and refining Chrome plating Paints and pigments (as chromates) Welding
Cobalt, hard metal	Hard metal production and use In alloys and steel As paint and china pigment Catalyst in the oil and chemical industry
Copper	Mining and refining ores (also produces exposure t silica, arsenic, cadmium) Vineyard spraying Welding
Iron	Iron and steel millwork Steel grinding and cleaning Welding Foundry work Boiler scaling Mining hematite, magnetite, limonite, siderite Mining or processing emery Mining iron containing clays

TABLE 5.1
(continued)

AGENTS	OCCUPATIONS WITH EXPOSURE; USES
Lanthanum and rare earths	Mining and refining ores (also produces exposure to silica) Polishing glass (cerium) Glass manufacture High-temperature ceramics and alloys In carbon arc lamps
Nickel and nickel salts	Mining and smelting of nickel ores Stainless steel welding Electroplating
Silicon carbide	Carborundum abrasives
Tin	Tin mining (also produces exposure to silica) Refining of tin ore Tinplating and soldering In fungicides and pesticides
Titanium	Manufacture of ceramics, paints Machining titanium metal
Zinc oxide and zinc chloride	Welding
Zirconium	Mining and refining ores (also produces exposure to silica) Production of steel Manufacture of refractory ceramics In foundries as sand substitute In enamels and glasses As a polishing and abrasive agent

TABLE 5.2
Lesions Produced by Metals and Metal Compounds

ARDS (from fume exposure)
Dust macules
Small airways fibrosis
Emphysema (?)
Diffuse interstitial fibrosis
Lung cancer
Alveolar proteinosis
Giant-cell interstitial pneumonia (hard metal disease)
Granulomas (berylliosis, ?other agents)

TABLE 5.3
Agents Usually Producing Only Dust Macules

Antimony
Barium
Chromium ore
Iron
Rare earths
Tin
Titanium
Tungsten

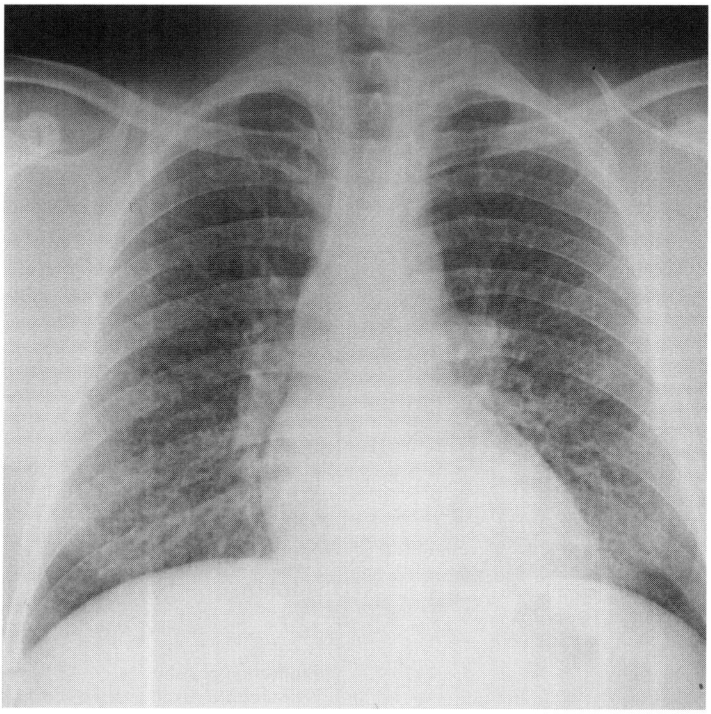

FIGURE 5.1
Chest radiograph showing so-called arc welders' pneumoconiosis (siderosis). This appearance is nonspecific and can be seen with a wide variety of mineral dusts.

dust, for example siderosis from iron inhalation or stannosis from tin inhalation, are often applied.

Grossly dust macules appear as colored spots in the centers of the lobules. Similar collections of dust frequently extend along the interlobular septa (routes of lymphatic drainage) and pleural lymphatics (Fig. 5.2). The exact color of the macule depends on the nature of the dust: the most common macule is the collection of black pigment, largely carbon, seen in the centers of lobules in cigarette smokers and many city dwellers. Macules in hematite (iron ore) miners are red-brown (Fig. 5.2); those in coal miners are black (see Chapter 6); macules caused by tin are gray; and macules produced by the paint pigment titanium dioxide are white.

The dust macule was originally defined to separate these lesions, which were thought to be nonfibrotic blemishes of little functional significance, from the heavily collagenized nodules of silicosis (1), a disease thought to produce major functional impairment. From this separation arose the concept that dusts producing only macules were inert (1). However, it now appears that although macules may initially have little associated fibrosis (compare Figs. 5.3 and 5.4), with time and/or continued dust accumulation, considerable fibrosis can occur. Whether this is true of every dust remains uncertain, but it is likely that with sufficient exposure no dust is truly inert.

We have proposed elsewhere that the fibrotic lesion of the small airways that appears to evolve from true nonfibrotic dust macules be called mineral dust–induced small airway disease (5–9). In its simplest form this small airway lesion consists of linear accumulations of collagen and pigment that extend down the

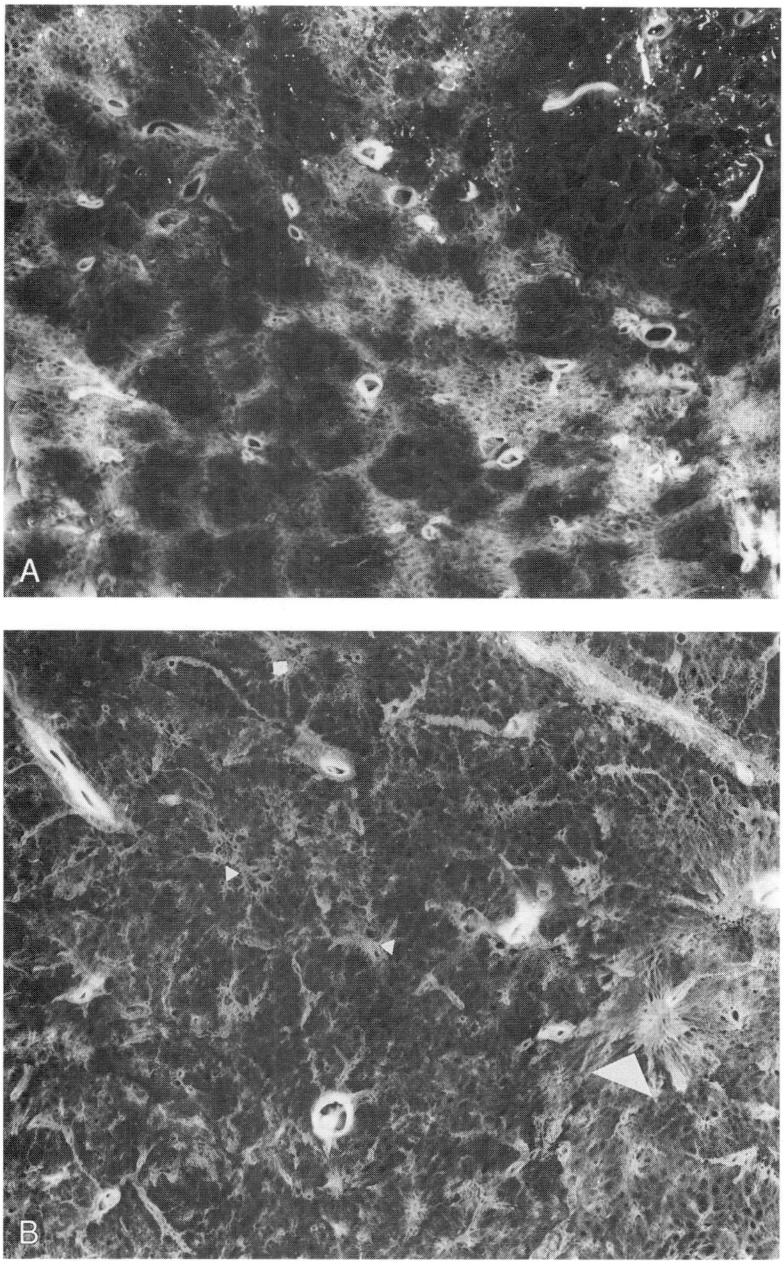

FIGURE 5.2
Gross appearances of the effects of a prototypical so-called inert dust, iron. **A.** Gross appearance of the lung of a hematite miner showing macular lesions superimposed on centrilobular emphysema. These red-brown lesions consist of pigmented but nonpalpable foci. The intervening parenchyma is unremarkable. **B.** Lung from another hematite miner showing a variety of lesions. Nodules (*large arrowhead*) of a medusa head configuration are palpable and raised. Macules (*small arrowheads*) are less well defined in the absence of emphysema but consist of pigment deposited around vessels and small airways. Interlobular septa are also prominent because of the accumulation of iron pigment. Nodules, macules, and septa are bright red in the original.

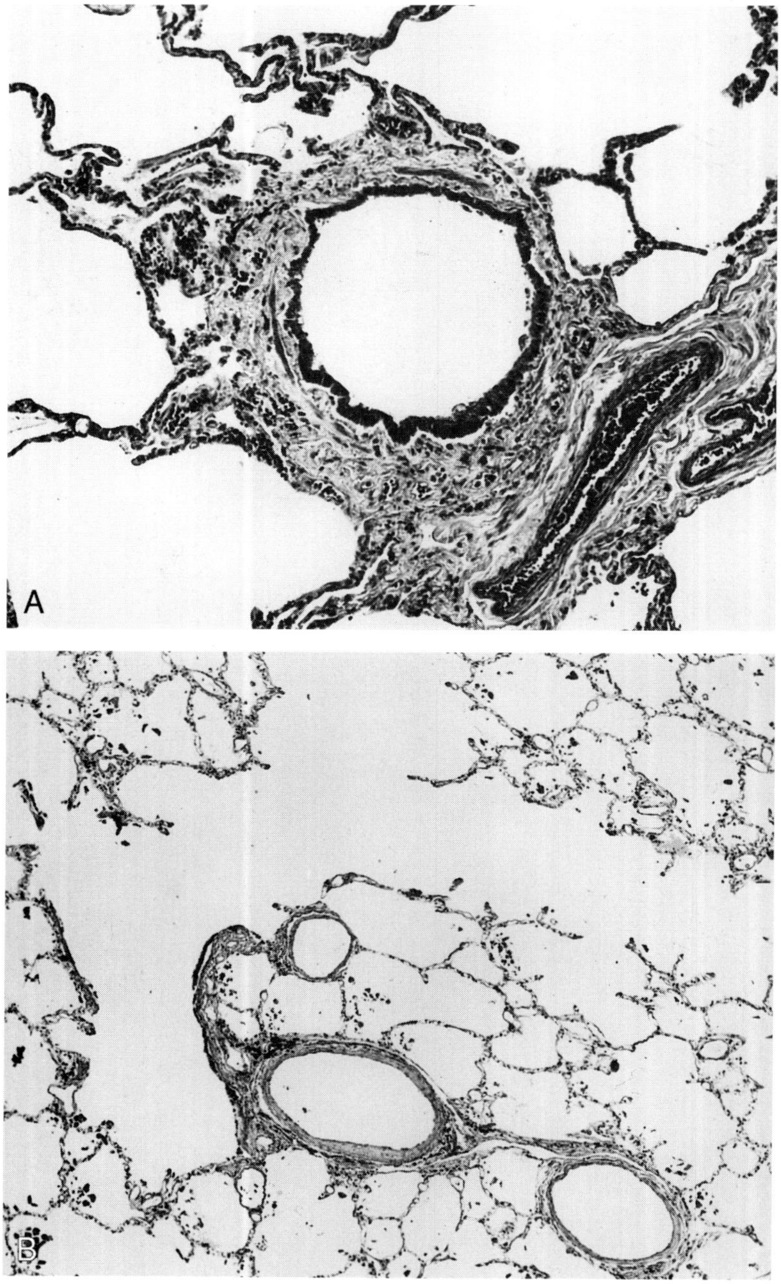

FIGURE 5.3
Typical small airways in cigarette smokers without dust exposure. **A.** Membranous bronchiole from a cigarette smoker. This airway is defined by a noncartilaginous continuous wall of muscle and fibrous tissue. Inflammation and fibrosis produced by cigarette smoking are found in many lungs. A membranous bronchiole from a nonsmoker has a thinner wall and little inflammation or fibrosis. **B.** Normal respiratory bronchiole and alveolar ducts. This is the typical appearance of the distal portion of the airways in a cigarette smoker or a nonsmoker. The respiratory bronchiole has a partly muscular and partly alveolated wall, and the alveolar ducts have completely alveolated walls. Note how thin the walls are in this example. (**A** reprinted with permission from Churg A, Wright JL. Small airways disease and mineral dust exposure. Pathol Ann 1983;18:233–251. **B** reprinted with permission from Wright JL, Churg A. Morphology of small-airway lesions in patients with asbestos exposure. Hum Pathol 1984;15:68–74.)

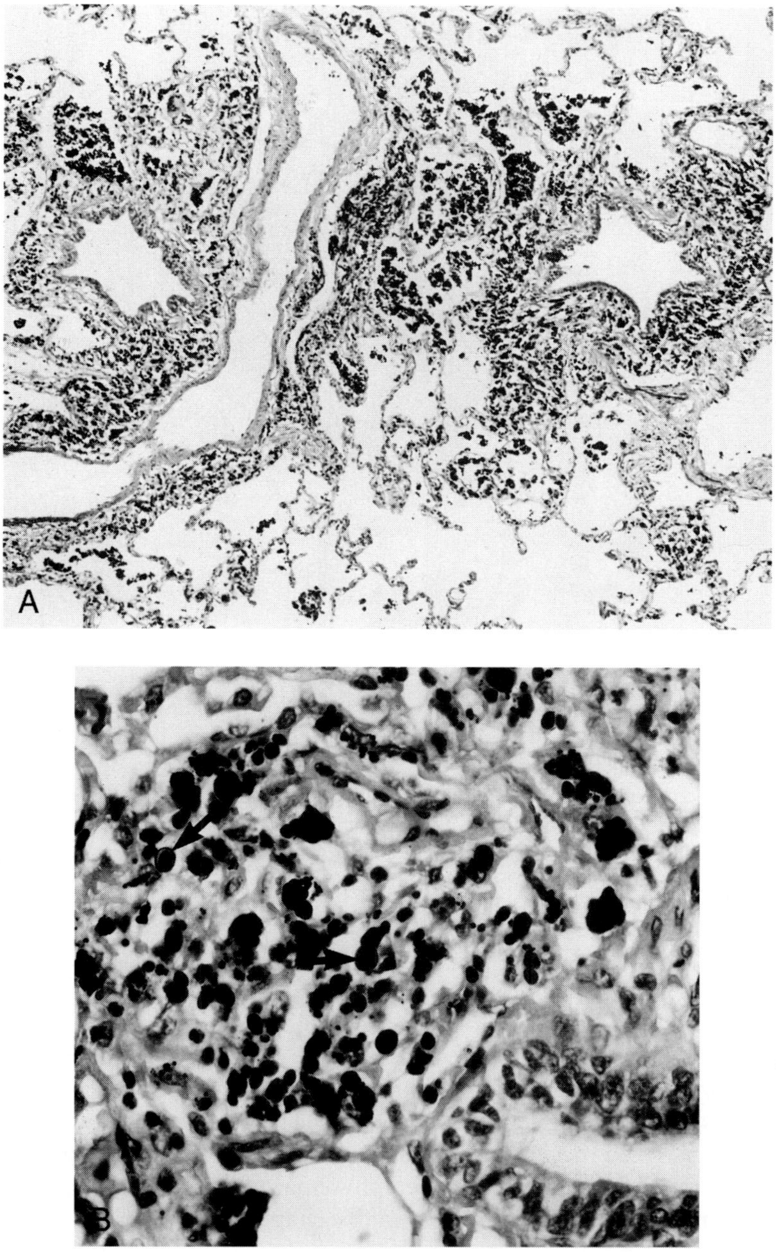

FIGURE 5.4
Microscopic appearance of classical nonfibrotic dust macules. **A.** Dust macule from the lung of an arc welder. The lesions consist of iron pigment associated with some degree of fibrous tissue around small vessels and airways. **B.** Higher-power view of another macule from this patient. Note the round ferruginous bodies (*arrows*) formed on particles of inhaled iron. It is probably the ferruginous coating that gives a positive iron stain in these cases.

walls of membranous and respiratory bronchioles and often into alveolar ducts (Figs. 5.5 and 9.11). As the lesion becomes more severe, the airway walls gradually become quite thick and fibrotic and the airway quite distorted (Figs. 5.6 and 9.11). In its most marked form the lesion consists of a central collagenized

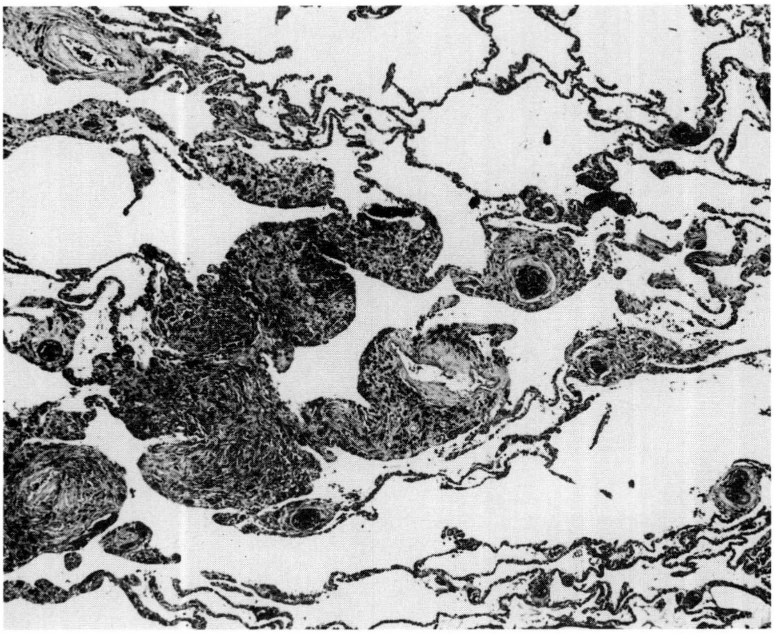

FIGURE 5.5
Appearance of mineral dust–induced small airway disease (progressively fibrotic dust macules with the contour of the airway still readily discernible). The respiratory bronchiole in this example, which is from the lung of a hard rock miner, has a greatly thickened and distorted wall and distorted lumen. Analysis of the lung revealed largely silica, mica, and kaolinite. Compare Figure 9.11*A*, which shows a very similar lesion in an asbestos worker. (Reprinted with permission from Wright JL, Cagle P, Churg A, et al. State of the art: disease of the small airways. Am Rev Respir Dis 1992;146:240–262.)

scar with surrounding enlarged air spaces in which the relation to an underlying airway is difficult to discern (Fig. 5.6, *C* and *D*).

The whole issue of the dust macule and its relation to fibrosis of the small airways is confounded by terminology. For some specific pneumoconioses, notably coal workers' pneumonoconiosis, the type of distorted and quite fibrotic airway illustrated in Figure 5.6 is still by definition a macule and the surrounding enlarged airspaces are focal emphysema, which is simply a form of centrilobular emphysema (discussed later in this chapter; also see Chapter 6). Many would use similar nomenclature for the same morphologic lesions in workers with other types of dust exposure. But whatever name one applies, it appears that these morphologic changes are common stereotypical reactions to a wide variety of mineral dusts, including coal, asbestos, and many nonasbestos silicates, as well as metals such as iron (5–9).

We have recently reviewed the pathogenesis of these lesions (9). Airway wall fibrosis probably is a direct effect of high dust loads derived from direct deposition of particles in the small airways, from proximal drainage of particles phagocytized by macrophages, or from both; the long-standing inflammatory response that these dusts evoke within the airway wall presumably leads to the elaboration of fibrogenic cytokines, fibroblast proliferation, and increased collagen production. We have also shown in laboratory animals that after simple intratracheal instillation of dusts such as silica and even titanium dioxide, both

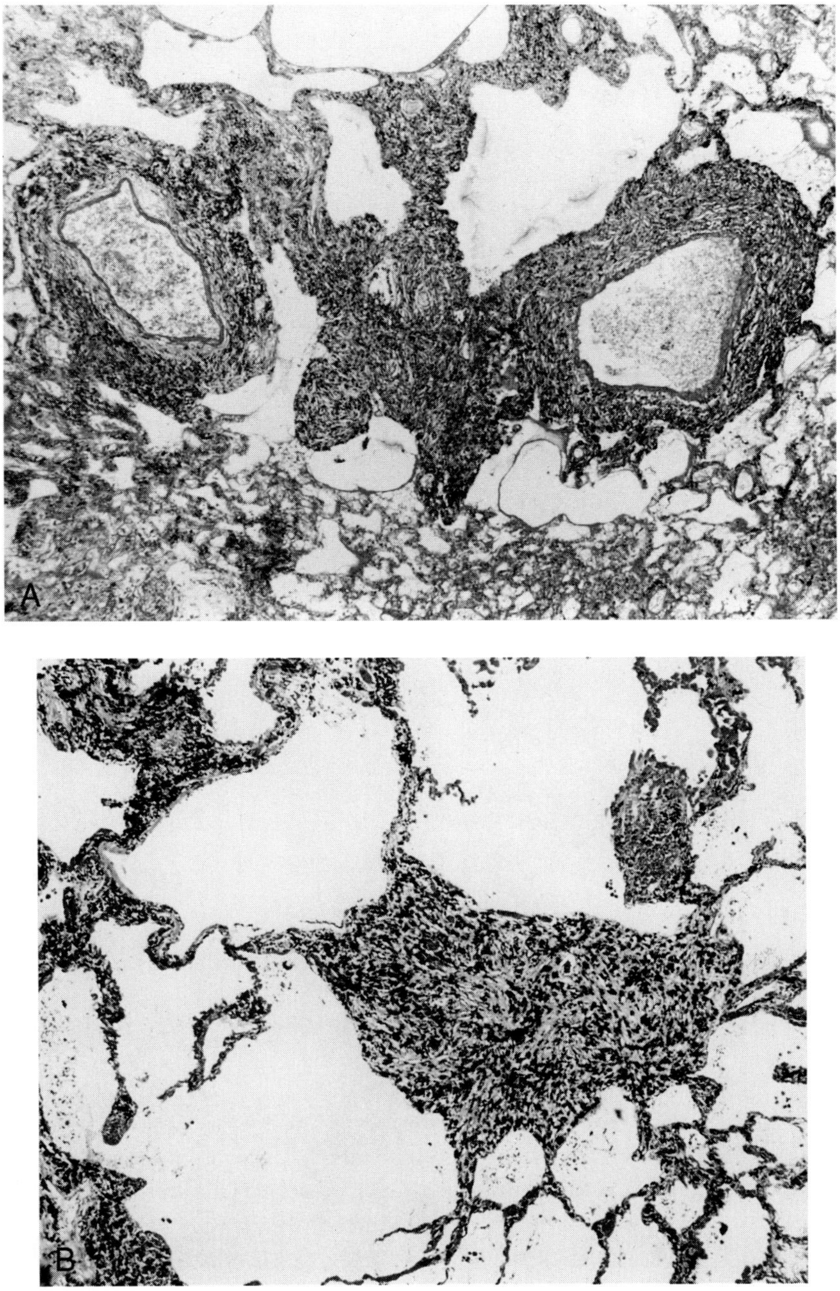

FIGURE 5.6
Progressively fibrotic small airway lesions. **A.** Distorted but still recognizable small airways from the lung of an arc welder ((120). **B.** A lesion in which part of the residual airway wall (respiratory bronchiolar wall) appears almost nodular. From the lung of a hematite miner. **C.** Low-power view of another area from the lung of a hematite miner showing marked distortion and barely recognizable respiratory bronchioles with surrounding focal emphysema. Note the similarity of this image to that shown in Figure 9.11*B* from the lung of an asbestos worker. **D.** Higher-power view of a similar lesion to show marked fibrosis of the distorted airway wall. (**B** Courtesy of Dr. A. Katzenstein, Syracuse, NY.)

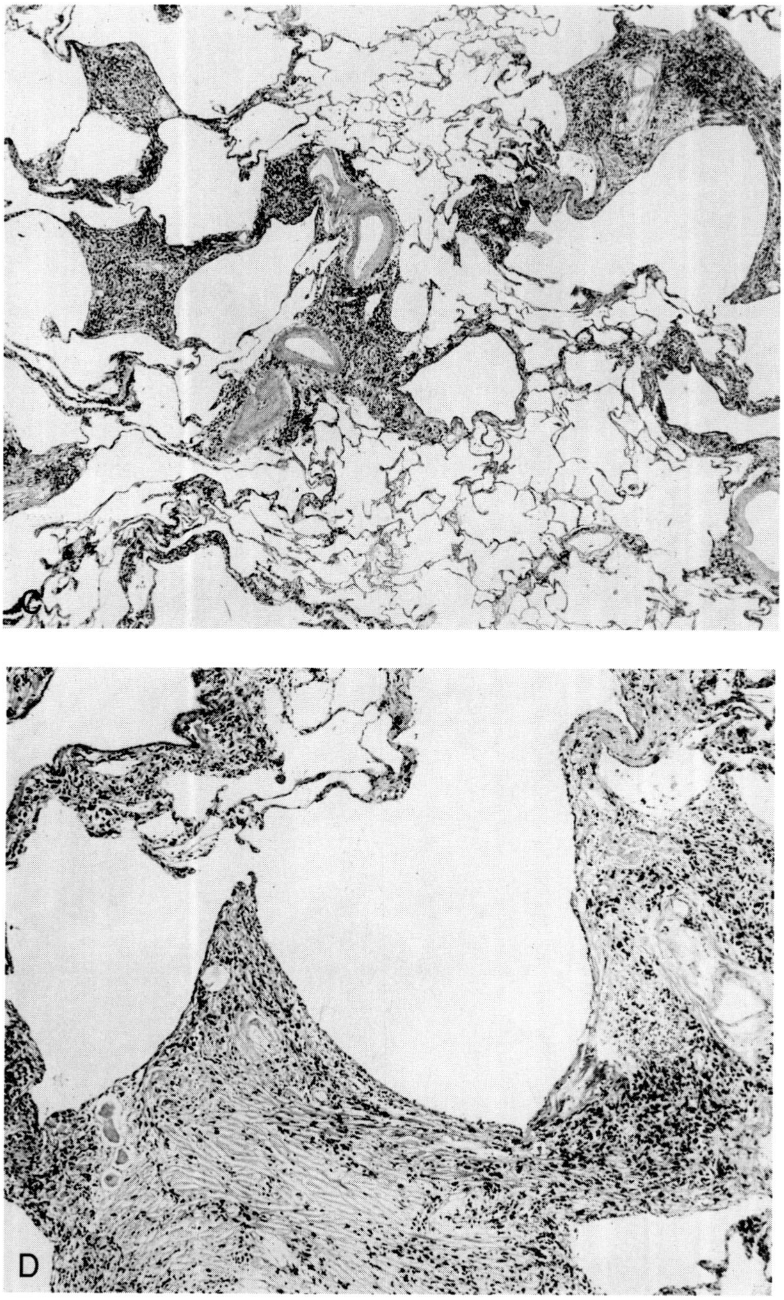

FIGURE 5.6 *(continued)*

desmosine, a marker of elastin breakdown, and hydroxyproline, a marker of collagen breakdown, can be found in lavage fluid (10); the degree and time course of connective tissue breakdown appears to parallel the magnitude of the polymorphonuclear leukocyte response. These findings suggest that dust-induced inflammation in the airspaces surrounding the small airways leads to emphysema because of persisting inflammatory cell recruitment and excess local release of proteolytic enzymes from these cells in much the same fashion as is believed to be true of cigarette smoke (9). Thus mineral dusts appear to produce the same two pathologic lesions, namely small airway inflammation with fibrosis and emphysema, that are responsible for airflow obstruction in cigarette smokers (9). The distribution of cigarette smoke–induced small airway disease is more proximal than that of mineral dust–induced small airway disease (6, 7). While the lesions in the membranous bronchioles are essentially identical with both agents, cigarette smoke rarely produces severe fibrosis of the respiratory bronchioles and never causes fibrotic lesions in the alveolar ducts. Thus it is usually possible to determine by simple visual inspection whether dust-induced rather than cigarette smoke–induced lesions are present (Figs. 5.3–5.6).

The recognition that mineral dusts can cause small airway fibrosis and a form of centrilobular emphysema occurred at the same time as epidemiologic studies demonstrated the association of mineral dust exposure and chronic airflow limitation (11–14). The association was again first recognized in coal miners, but there is now extensive evidence of chronic airflow obstruction in hard-rock miners and other workers with silica exposure (11–18) and more controversial data in workers with asbestos exposure (9–14, 19–24). In some studies the degree of airflow obstruction appears to be closely related to total dust exposure and in others to radiographically visible pneumoconiosis (11–18).

Even in workers with exposures accepted as causing airflow obstruction, the exact frequency and clinical significance of dust-induced abnormalities require further elucidation. Longitudinal studies based on large cohorts of workers suggest that the effects of high-level prolonged dust exposure on functional decline can be as great as the effects of cigarette smoke, and the two agents may in fact be synergistic (11–14). Nevertheless, accelerated rates of functional loss measured in a large cohort do not indicate that everyone in the cohort has either measurable impairment or clinical disease; rather the implication of the longitudinal epidemiologic surveys is that some workers develop significant airflow obstruction because of dust exposure and some show few or no effects.

The possible association of cadmium exposure with emphysema is discussed in the section on cadmium.

Interstitial Fibrosis

The clinical and pathologic differences between organizing acute respiratory distress syndrome (ARDS) and true diffuse interstitial fibrosis described in Chapter 4 have only recently been clearly explained in the occupational lung disease literature, and, as a result the number of agents reported to produce fibrosis is probably exaggerated. While chronic interstitial fibrosis certainly does occur after exposure to metals and metal compounds (Table 5.4), it is relatively uncommon. Some of the forms of diffuse fibrosis associated with these agents have distinctive features: both beryllium- and aluminum-induced fibrosis, for example, are often upper zonal, as opposed to the lower zonal distribution of fibrosis induced by silicates such as asbestos and talc. Hard metal (cobalt) disease appears to be associated with a desquamative or giant cell interstitial pneumonia.

As a rule metals do not induce nodular fibrosis of the silicotic type, and the appearance of fibrotic nodules suggests that exposure to silica, perhaps mixed with the dust in question, has occurred. An example is the mixed-dust fibrosis sometimes seen in hematite miners. Beryllium is an exception; it produces a granulomatous response that may evolve into either fibrotic nodules composed of coalesced granulomas or a pattern of diffuse fibrosis.

TABLE 5.4
Agents Producing Interstitial Fibrosis

Iron (usually mild)
Aluminum
Hard metal (cobalt)
Copper (vineyard sprayer's lung)
Rare earths
?Brass, steel, lead
Beryllium (but granulomas and nodules more common)
Silicon carbide
Dental technician's pneumoconiosis (agent uncertain)

TABLE 5.5
Occupationally Encountered Agents Producing Carcinoma of the Lung

Definite or probable carcinogens
Asbestos (with asbestosis)
Arsenic
Beryllium
Cadmium
Chloromethyl ether
Foundry work
Hexavalent chromium compounds
Nickel (?nickel monoxide, nickel subsulfide)
Radon and radon daughters
Smelting (probably arsenic)
Possible carcinogens/exposures
Antimony trioxide
Crystalline silica
Iron mining (probably radon)
Welding (?chromium)

Lung Cancer

Table 5.5 lists a number of metals, metal salts, gases, and other substances that have been associated, with varying degrees of certainty, with the development of lung cancer (25–46). However, the issue of an increased risk of lung cancer and occupational exposures is complicated. Even when the substance in question is clearly associated with lung cancer, there may be marked differences in carcinogenicity among different forms of the mineral or metal. For example, chrysotile asbestos appears to be a much weaker mesothelial carcinogen than is amphibole asbestos (see Chapter 10), and the carcinogenicity of chromium compounds is probably limited to hexavalent chromium (28, 29).

In some instances the carcinogenic agent appears to be not the compound nominally handled but a contaminant or another substance related to the industrial process. For example, smelting of copper, zinc, and aluminum has been associated with an increased cancer risk (30–33) that is commonly attributed to the arsenic in the ores being smelted; analysis of lung tissue from such workers has shown relatively high levels of arsenic (34). Another good example is iron ore mining, in which the apparently increased risk is probably associated with exposure to radon daughters in the mines; this is likely true of other types of metal mining as well (28–30, 35–37). In some occupational settings, such as foundries, a variety of organic carcinogens may also be present (33, 38, 39).

A further complication is that the exact salts or compounds of a metal that are the true carcinogens may be difficult to discern, often because of lack of detailed information on exposure. Nickel, which in a generic sense is clearly carcinogenic (26, 28, 29), is an excellent example: workers are exposed to many nickel compounds, but the ones that are actually human lung carcinogens (possibly nickel monoxide, nickel subsulfide) remain uncertain.

For some substances the proximate cause of lung cancer may not be the agent itself but the underlying fibrosing process caused by the agent. The best example is asbestos exposure; lung cancer appears to be associated with asbestosis (diffuse interstitial fibrosis) rather than with exposure itself (see Chapter 10). The relation between crystalline silica and lung cancer is much less certain, but here again the strongest evidence specifically links silicosis rather than just silica exposure with cancer (40).

Last, studies of occupational lung cancer must by definition deal with confounding by cigarette smoke, but in many studies such information is not available, and for some exposures, notably asbestos (see Chapter 10) and radon (41), cigarette smoke appears to act synergistically.

The establishment of an association between a given agent and the development of lung cancer is primarily an epidemiologic task, and detailed discussion is beyond the scope of this book. The major question for the pathologist is whether any pathologic features allow ascription of cause in a given case. Some authors believe that histologic type of cancer can be used for this purpose for most agents (42). Others conclude that for some very specific substances, for example chloromethyl ether, with which small-cell carcinomas appear to occur in nonsmokers (43, 44), and uranium mining, with which very high level radiation exposure may be associated with an increased frequency of small-cell carcinoma (44, 45), cell type can be helpful in establishing cause. However, in most instances there are either insufficient data or no real evidence to associate a specific cell type with a specific occupational agent (44, 46). Rather, as a general rule no pathologic features allow the pathologist to conclude that an occupational exposure caused a particular tumor (carcinoma developing in the presence of asbestosis is an exception to this rule: see Chapter 10).

Specific Agents

Iron. Iron is probably the metal most commonly encountered in the occupational setting; it has been estimated that some 4 million workers in the United States are exposed (2). Inhalation of iron alone produces the disease called siderosis; when free silica is also present, the resulting condition is labeled silicosiderosis, a form of mixed-dust fibrosis.

Exposure to iron is encountered in mining hematite, magnetite, limonite, and siderite. It also occurs in mining and milling of emery (aluminum oxide), which is used for grinding, and crocus, a finely powdered form of iron oxide used for polishing (1, 2). A variety of iron-containing ores, including hematite, limonite, ocher, and umber, are mined for use in paint pigments. In most of these occupations there may be considerable exposure to crystalline silica as well as iron.

Extensive iron exposure is also common in steel mills, foundries, welding, silver and steel grinding and polishing, boiler scaling, and production and refining of many metal alloys. Some of these occupations, for example foundry work, may entail considerable quartz exposure, and many of them, particularly foundry work and welding, also expose the worker to a wide variety of other metals and to fumes, all of which may be irritant, toxic, and/or carcinogenic.

Exposure to iron in and of itself is generally said to produce no clinical disease (1, 47, 48), and functional abnormalities in such workers have usually been ascribed to smoking (1); however, as is demonstrated in Figure 5.6, sufficiently high-level exposure to iron alone can produce small airway abnormalities and probably emphysema, which may result in airflow obstruction (discussed later in the chapter and in the earlier section on macules). As well, other agents encountered in foundries and welding can cause asthma and possibly irreversible airflow changes as well (49–51; see Chapter 4).

On radiography workers with long-term exposure typically show fine nodules measuring up to about 2 mm (1) (Fig. 5.1); the distribution of the nodules is similar to that seen in silicosis, but they tend to be more radiodense; indeed, early authors were at pains to point out the distinction between such "benign pneumoconioses" and silicosis (52, 53). Kerley B lines are occasionally found as well; presumably they represent accumulations of dust along interlobular septa (Fig 5.2*B*). In a study of 661 welders, Attfield and Ross (54) found a 7% prevalence of grade 0/1 or greater rounded opacities. Freedman et al. (55) and Kalliomaki et al. (56), using magnetic measurements of retained iron in welders, showed that there was a correlation between radiographic changes and measured amounts of dust and that total dust burden increased from an average of 7 mg iron for those with 2 years' exposure to 200 to 700 mg for those with 18 years' exposure (56). Occasionally much larger amounts are found without obvious deleterious effects. For example, Kalliomaki et al. (57) measured a total lung burden of 10 g of iron in one stainless steel welder. Iron is slowly cleared from the lungs after cessation of exposure (56), and radiographic abnormalities also regress, in contrast to the situation in silicosis and coal workers' pneumoconiosis (58).

Macroscopically lungs from workers with iron exposure typically show macules that vary from brick red in hematite miners (Fig. 5.2, *A* and *B*) to degrees of reddish brown, gray, or black (59). Linear dust collections may be seen along interlobular septa (Fig. 5.2*B*). Microscopically brown to black particles of iron are found scattered throughout the lung but tend to collect around bronchioles and small vessels (60), forming the microscopic picture of macules (Fig. 5.4, *A* and *B*). Many of the particles appear as rounded ferruginous bodies with round or polygonal black cores (Fig. 5.4*B* and colorplate 2). Although exogenous iron does not stain with Prussian blue (1), almost all particles in such lungs do stain, most likely because the exogenous particles have become ferruginated. The extent of this process can be appreciated from the data of Kalliomaki et al. (61), who showed that only about 10% of the total iron in the typical welder's lung is actually of exogenous origin; the other 90% is presumably the endogenous iron forming the ferruginous body coatings.

Although iron is typically described as inert, there is no doubt that with sufficient exposure some degree of fibrosis occurs in the macules (Fig. 5.6) or other sites where the dust collects; this is true of both workers mining iron ores and welders (47, 59). The macular lesions in some instances progress to typical quite fibrotic mineral dust airway disease, sometimes associated with a process identical to focal emphysema, at least in smokers (Fig. 5.6, *C* and *D*); whether focal emphysema occurs in this setting in nonsmokers is unknown. The functional consequences of these lesions are discussed at the beginning of this chapter.

Dense nodular fibrosis (Fig. 5.7), even in welders, has been commonly ascribed to the concomitant presence of silica (59, 60, 62, 63) and some modern studies examining the location of particles within the tissue lent support to this notion (64). However, Hicks et al. (65) and Hewitt and Hicks (66) showed experimentally that nodular fibrosis could be produced with instillation of very large amounts of welding fume. Most likely this was a reaction to the iron itself, although other components of the welding fume, such as chromium, nickel, and manganese, also accumulate in the lung in such experimental animals (67) and in humans (68). We have microdissected and analyzed a number of such nodules from hematite miners' lungs and found that many contained little or no silica, again suggesting that iron can produce nodular fibrosis (Katzenstein ALA and Churg A, unpublished data). Furthermore, diffuse interstitial fibrosis sufficient to produce cor pulmonale is seen in patients with long-standing idiopathic hemosiderosis and is presumably caused by iron (69). The implication of these observations is that iron can occasionally produce significant amounts of fibrosis, either simply from the presence of large numbers of particles evoking a fibrogenic inflammatory response or less probably because of the concomitant presence of other types of particle.

Microscopically the macular and mineral dust–induced small airway lesions in welders appear to be identical to those of iron ore miners (70–74). Effects of welding are considered in Chapter 4.

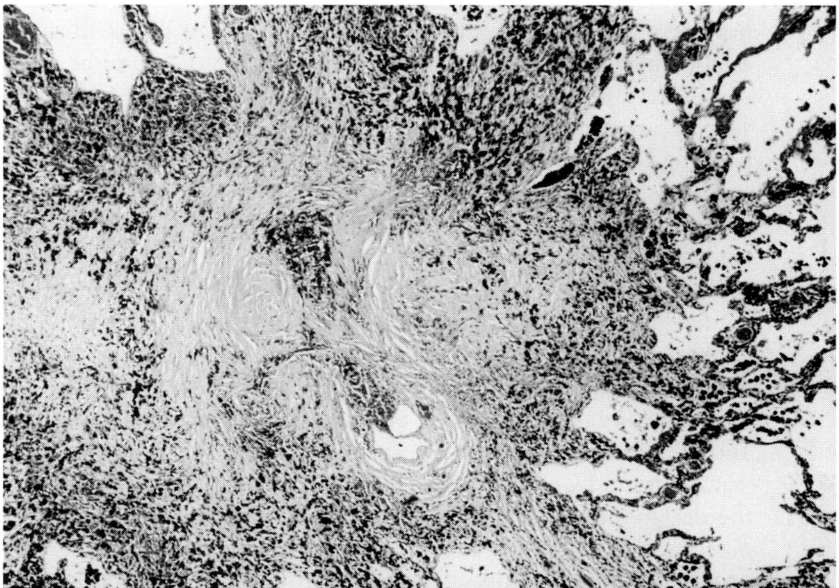

FIGURE 5.7
Nodular lesion from the hematite miners' lung shown in Figure 5.2*B*. This palpable lesion has a medusa head configuration and whorled collagenous center. It is unclear whether the lesion is a result of exposure to quartz along with the iron oxide or is produced by iron oxide alone. (Courtesy of Dr. A. Katzenstein, Syracuse, NY.)

Other "Inert" Metals. Tin, barium, antimony, zirconium, chromium ore, and titanium also produce so-called benign pneumoconioses, characterized radiographically by very dense nodules and often Kerley B lines (2). These agents have a wide range of commercial uses (Table 5.1), and in some instances a surprisingly large number of workers are at risk. For example, the National Institute for Occupational Safety and Health (NIOSH) has estimated that some 1.4 million workers in the United States are exposed to antimony and 1.3 million to zirconium (2). In some industries radiographic changes are common; for example, Robertson and Whittaker (cited in reference 2) found abnormal chest radiographs in 121 of 215 tin refinery workers. Similarly, Doig (75) found radiographic evidence of pneumoconiosis in the majority of workers at a small factory processing barium ores.

Pathologic descriptions are scanty, but it appears that these agents generally produce only macular lesions. Those caused by tin (stannosis) are gray–black (76), and titanium dioxide (rutile) produces white lesions (77). Histology includes dust accumulation around small vessels and airways in the centers of the pulmonary lobules and along interlobular septa (76). The presence of fibrosis is again disputed, although some reports do mention or illustrate slight fibrosis around airways (77–79), and presumably any of these dusts can produce at least minor degrees of fibrosis. The amount of dust that can be tolerated in the lung is large: Robertson et al. (76) found up to 3 g of tin oxide in their patients. Barium salts, tin oxide, and titanium oxide are birefringent in tissue section, and barium sulfate often has a greenish tinge in sections stained with hematoxin and eosin.

In general these pneumoconioses are said to produce no significant functional impairment (the issue of chronic airflow obstruction has for practical purposes not been examined), but occasional cases of more severe fibrotic disease associated with some of these agents have been reported, and some animal studies have produced abnormalities where none commonly appears in man (80). Whether such changes are actually caused by the reputed agent or are induced by accompanying substances such as silica, for example the case reported by Pendergrass and Greening (81), is unclear.

Aluminum. Aluminum has numerous uses (1, 2) (Table 5.1), and large numbers of workers are exposed to various forms of it: NIOSH estimates that in the United States 1.8 million persons encounter alumina ($A1_2O_3$) and 1.6 million encounter coated aluminum metal (discussed later) in an occupational setting; an additional half a million deal directly with the bare metal (2).

Aluminum is derived from bauxite, an ore that consists of alumina with iron and other minerals. The alumina is extracted from the ore and reduced to metallic aluminum by electrolysis (82). This process is carried out in large pots (hence the designation pot room) that can hold 10 tons of mixture. The pot room atmosphere contains not only alumina dust but a variety of gases, including hydrogen fluoride and sulfur dioxide; metal fumes; cyanide; ozone; and aromatic hydrocarbons (1, 2, 33, 82).

Exposure to aluminum, alumina, and pot room fumes has been putatively associated with a variety of pathologic reactions, including acute asthma, chronic airflow obstruction, diffuse interstitial fibrosis, and lung cancer (33), although almost all are a matter of dispute.

The earliest reaction described was pulmonary fibrosis resulting from exposure to aluminum metal powder, first seen in Germany before World War II and with increasing frequency during World War II. Mitchell (83) gives a brief historical review. Goralewski (cited in 83) found a 26% incidence of radiographic pneumoconiosis in the German cases. However, a variety of studies from England and the United States failed to demonstrate any risk until the reports by Mitchell et al. (83, 84) showing pulmonary fibrosis in 6 of 27 workers making a very fine aluminum powder. A scattering of subsequent case reports document the same phenomenon (85, 86). Fibrosis in aluminum pot room workers was described by Shaver and Riddell (87), who found definite pulmonary fibrosis in 35 of 344 patients and probable disease in 13 others, with 7 fatalities.

Aluminum-associated pulmonary fibrosis appears to be associated with a high frequency of spontaneous pneumothorax (83). Radiographically the noteworthy feature is fibrosis in the upper and mid lung zones (83–87) (Fig. 5.8*A*). This observation was confirmed pathologically by Riddell (88), who described the process as central scarring with peripheral emphysema. Whether the latter is a form of scar emphysema or merely honeycombing with extensive cysts is unclear from the published reports.

Microscopic descriptions and illustrations show both interstitial fibrosis of the type seen in usual interstitial pneumonia (Fig. 5.8*B*) and a more nodular process associated with aggregates of dust (83–86, 88). By transmitted light the dust appears black. Extraordinarily large particles (some measuring 25 (m) have been observed histologically (83); their size is such as to suggest that the material may aggregate after inhalation. If enough dust is present, the lung may have a slate gray color on gross examination (86, 88).

The exact agent responsible for the fibrosing process is uncertain. Powdered aluminum is coated with stearin or mineral oil to prevent oxidation and aggregation of the particles, and it has been suggested that the mineral oil actually causes the fibrosis. However, Corrin (89) showed that stearin-coated, mineral oil–coated, and bare aluminum metal powder were all equally effective in producing fibrosis in experimental animals. The patient with fibrosis reported by McLaughlin et al. (86) was also exposed to a stearin-coated material. Corrin did observe, however, that a granular aluminum powder failed to cause fibrosis; he speculated that fibrosis was produced by dissolved aluminum from the lipid-coated or bare metal, whereas the granular powder had acquired a coating of aluminum oxide and was not soluble in lung tissue fluid (89, 90). Gilks and Churg (91) analyzed the lungs from a pot room worker with predominantly upper zone fibrosis and reported an approximately thousandfold increase in aluminum particles over background. The presence of relatively large numbers of fine aluminum fibers was notable; it was suggested that fibers might in fact be the agent of aluminum-induced fibrosis.

Results from animal studies are also confused by species and route of administration. Gross et al. (92) found fibrosis of both parenchyma and airway walls after intratracheal instillation of large amounts of metallic aluminum powder to rats, but not after inhalation. This result may indicate that heavy exposure is required to develop fibrosis. However, Tian-Xi et al. (93) found only minimal fibrosis in rats given comparable amounts of bare metal powder by intratracheal instillation. Even here aggregates of dust were associated with greater degrees of fibrosis. Tian-Xi et al. (93) also observed severe diffuse fibrosis in dogs given stearin-coated powder by inhalation.

It has been proposed that the agent responsible for fibrosis is not aluminum but silica, especially cristobalite, encountered as a contaminant, particularly in the pot room (1). This does not explain the disease in workers exposed to alu-

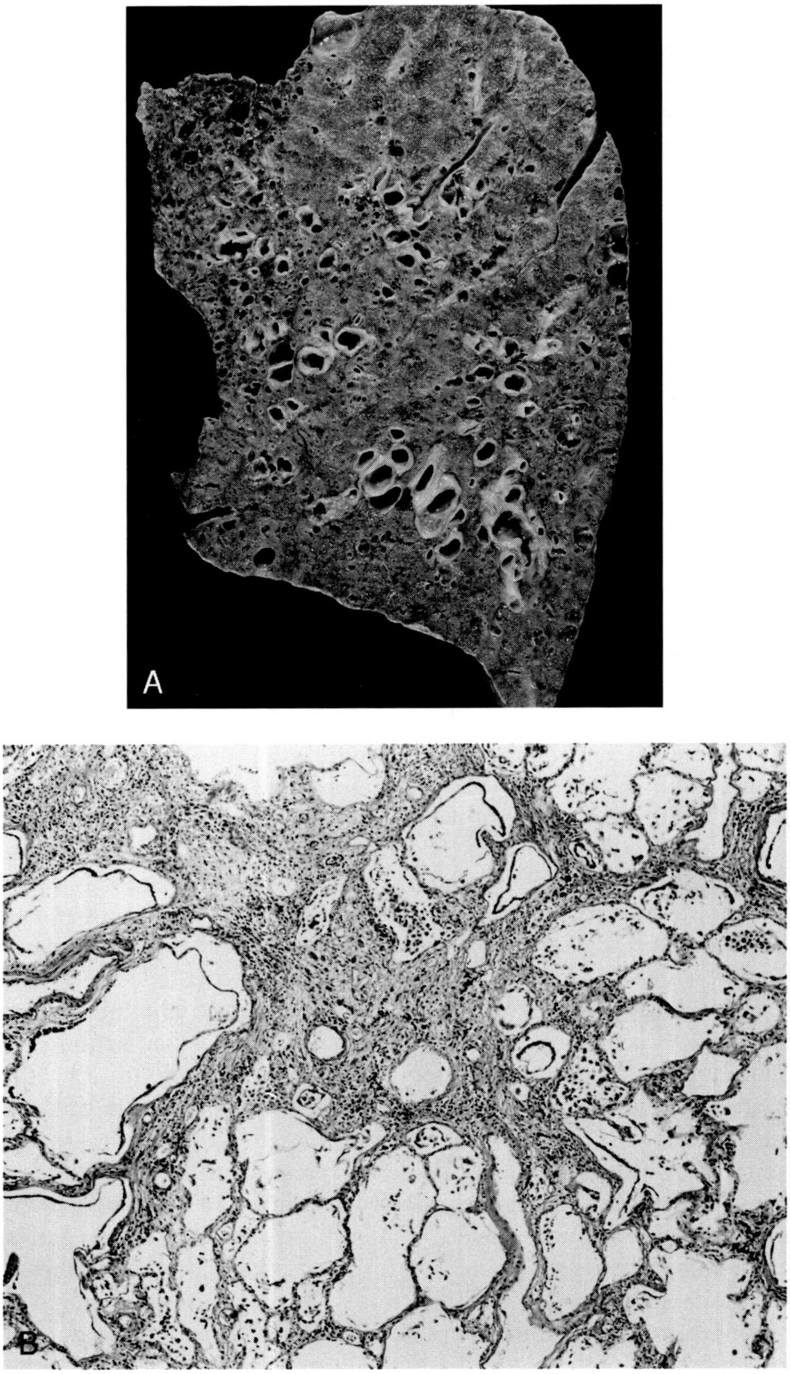

FIGURE 5.8
Interstitial fibrosis in a worker employed for many years in an aluminum pot room. Chest radiograph showed diffuse interstitial fibrosis with some tendency to upper zone distribution. Pulmonary function tests revealed a restrictive impairment with decreased diffusing capacity. Patient died of respiratory failure. **A.** Gross lung showing marked honeycombing and fibrosis with suggestion of more severe disease in the upper zones. **B.** Microscopic view shows diffuse interstitial fibrosis. Analysis of this specimen revealed large numbers of aluminum particles, and the combination of history, distribution of fibrosis, and mineral analysis suggests that aluminum work produced the lung disease.

minum powder, and the fibrosing process is pathologically very different from silicosis. Another hypothesis is that the causative factor is gamma aluminum oxide evolved in the pot fumes; it has been claimed that the gamma form of alumina is fibrogenic in experimental animals and the ordinary alpha form is not (94). However, gamma aluminum oxide should be destroyed at the working temperature of the pots (1).

The issue of aluminum-induced fibrosis thus remains unresolved, and given the large population at risk, it is clearly not a common disease; in fact a recent review of disease in aluminum smelter workers concludes that smelter work is not associated with interstitial fibrosis (33). However, the peculiar distribution of fibrosis, the association with specific exposures, and the animal data all suggest that either aluminum or some substance related to the processing of aluminum can, albeit infrequently, produce fibrosis.

Diffuse interstitial fibrosis has also been reported in workers making aluminum oxide (alumina) abrasives. Jederlinic et al. (95) described 9 cases of interstitial disease in 1000 workers from a plant producing alumina grinding wheels and alumina-tipped tools. Analysis of lung particle content in 3 cases showed large numbers of aluminum particles but also very substantial numbers of asbestos fibers in one subject. Although the incidence of interstitial fibrosis in these workers was clearly increased over background, the potential for confounding by asbestos exposure remains a problem. Bellot et al. (96) published a report of interstitial fibrosis in a worker engaged in crushing bauxite ore; aluminum oxide was present in large amounts in the lung.

A variety of other pathologic reactions have been seen in workers exposed to aluminum. Miller et al. (97) reported a case of alveolar proteinosis in an aluminum rail grinder (Fig. 5.9). Corrin (98) and Gross et al. (92) have shown experimentally that large doses of finely divided aluminum powder can produce proteinosis in animals, and the lung of the patient reported by Miller et al. (97) contained large numbers of aluminum spheres, almost all of them smaller than 1 μm in diameter.

Interstitial fibrosis has been reported in aluminum arc welders by Vallyathan et al. (99) and Herbert et al. (100). The lung tissue from the latter case contained fine aluminum spheres of the type reported by Miller et al. (97). Welders are, of course, exposed to a variety of substances, and ascription of the lesions to aluminum alone is difficult. Chen et al. (101) reported a case of granulomatous lung disease in a welder in the aircraft construction industry. Aluminum particles were demonstrated in the granulomas, but whether this process was a reaction to aluminum or some other condition, especially sarcoidosis, is uncertain. A very similar patient was reported by De Vuyst et al. (102); this case is noteworthy because the patient's peripheral blood lymphocytes showed blast transformation after exposure to soluble aluminum compounds, an observation that provides more support for an aluminum origin. De Vuyst et al. (103) also reported diffuse interstitial fibrosis in a worker who polished aluminum with unspecified abrasives. Given a lack of epidemiologic support, all of these cases are difficult to interpret.

The data on the relation of aluminum smelting work to both asthma and chronic airflow obstruction have recently been reviewed by Abramson et al. (33). These authors concluded that pot room workers do develop an asthmalike syndrome, although it is unclear whether the reaction is an allergic or irritant one. They also concluded that aluminum smelter workers develop chronic airflow obstruction, although it is uncertain whether this is ever disabling.

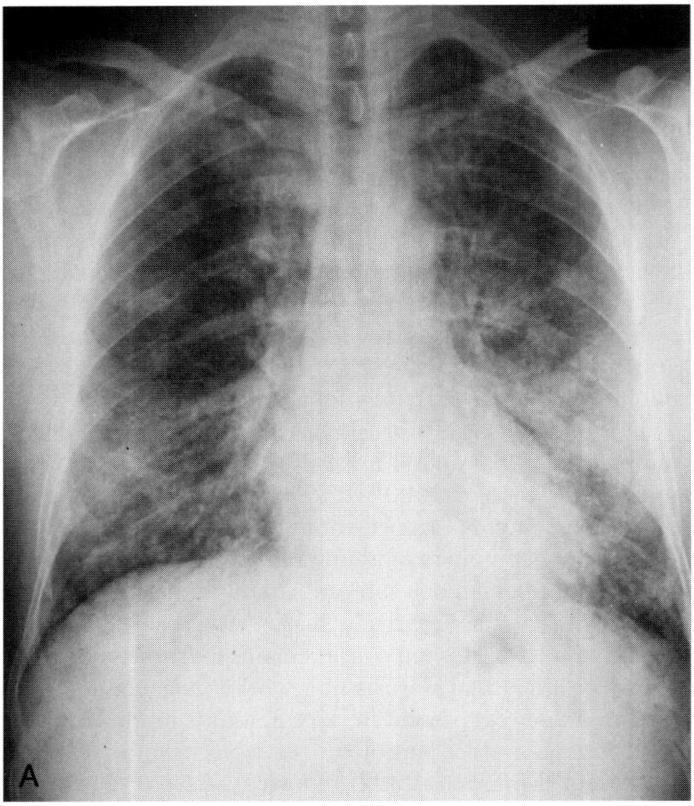

FIGURE 5.9
Alveolar proteinosis in a worker exposed to high dust levels grinding aluminum rails. The patient had shortness of breath and weight loss. Pulmonary function tests showed a restrictive pattern. **A.** Chest radiograph showing bilateral diffuse alveolar and interstitial infiltrates. **B.** Micrograph showing filling of alveoli by granular material. Notice typical clefts and dense bodies of alveolar proteinosis. **C.** High-power view of periodic acid-Schiff stain section showing positive staining of the intra-alveolar material. **D.** Metal spheres extracted from lung by digestion. Analysis by energy-dispersive x-ray spectroscopy showed that they were composed of pure aluminum (×20, 000). (Reprinted with permission from Miller R, Churg AM, Hutcheon M, Lam S. Pulmonary alveolar proteinosis and aluminum dust exposure. Am Rev Respir Dis 1984;130: 312–315.).

The relation of aluminum smelting, particularly pot room work, to lung cancer is also problematic. Although some studies have demonstrated increased relative risks, others have not, and the magnitude of the increases have generally been small. Moreover, confounding by cigarette smoking has usually not been controlled for (33). Given the large variety of irritating, sensitizing, and potentially carcinogenic compounds in the pot room atmosphere, the role of aluminum itself, if any, in lung cancer, asthma, and chronic airflow obstruction remains to be established.

Hard Metal (Cobalt) Disease. Hard metal (cemented tungsten carbide with cobalt) is a synthetic compound that approaches the hardness of diamond. It is used in applications that require strength and rigidity even at high operating

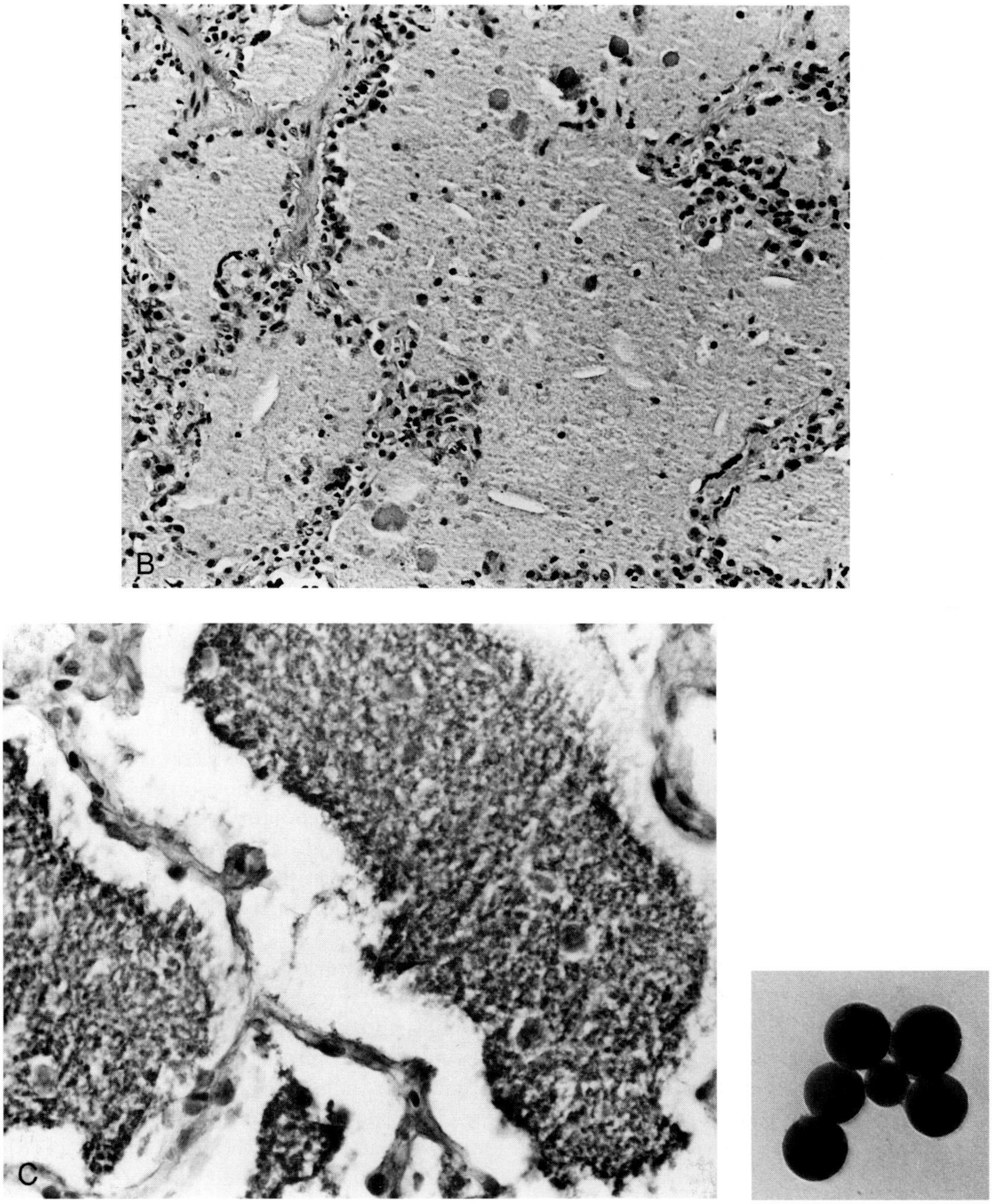

FIGURE 5.9 *(continued)*

temperatures. It is particularly valuable for cutting edges on tools; drills of all types, including those used in mining; and high-temperature bearings (104–105). Hard metal is prepared by first heating finely divided tungsten and carbon to form tungsten carbide. Then cobalt and sometimes titanium, tantalum, or chromium carbide are added, and the mixture fused at high temperature to form the final product. The whole process generates very fine dust, mean particle size less than 2 μm (104, 105). NIOSH estimates some 30,000 workers are exposed to hard metal in the United States (2), but the number of workers exposed to cobalt, which is probably the causative agent of hard metal disease (discussed later), is considerably greater (106).

Hard metal exposure can produce interstitial fibrosis, occupational asthma, and sometimes a syndrome resembling extrinsic allergic alveolitis, as well as contact dermatitis. The history of hard metal disease is briefly reviewed by Bech et al. (105). First reported in Germany, radiographic evidence of disease was seen in as many as 20% of workers. Lower incidences have generally been found in other countries, although the proportion of affected workers varies considerably from report to report. Coates and Watson (104) observed only 9 cases of interstitial fibrosis in an industry employing 1500 workers. Sprince et al. (107) reviewed pulmonary function tests and chest radiographs in 1039 production workers at 22 facilities and found work-related wheeze in 10.9% and a radiographic interstitial infiltrate read as 1/1 or greater with accompanying restrictive changes in 0.7%. Meyer-Bisch et al. (108) reported a 12.8% prevalence of 0/1 or 1/1 chest radiographs in 425 production workers.

There is fairly strong evidence to suggest that the actual causative agent of hard metal disease is cobalt rather than tungsten or tungsten carbide. A process clinically and histologically identical to hard metal asthma and hard metal interstitial lung disease occurs in diamond polishers who use polish containing cobalt but not hard metal (109, 110). Cobalt alone also provokes asthmatic attacks in some patients with the hard metal occupational asthma syndrome (106, 111). Shirakawa et al. (112) have demonstrated anticobalt antibodies in the sera of patients with hard metal–induced asthma. Analysis of hair and nails shows that cobalt accumulates in body tissues (113). Hard metal grinding and saw blade sharpening, activities in which a coolant is used as the metal is worked, appear to be particularly associated with disease, and this phenomenon probably reflects leaching of cobalt from the metal into the coolant and inhalation of the evaporated coolant (107, 114, 115). Kennedy et al. (114) reported hard metal disease in tungsten carbide blade sharpeners in British Columbia sawmills, emphasizing the idea that toxic exposures are not confined to hard metal production workers.

The interstitial process is generally either lower or mid zonal in chest radiographs (104). Histologically it appears to be characterized by a tendency to more severe fibrosis in the centers of the lobules and a desquamative interstitial pneumonia–like picture with numerous alveolar macrophages and at least sometimes alveolar giant cells that appear to originate from both macrophage and alveolar lining (104, 105, 111, 116, 117) (Fig. 5.10). The combination of giant cells and a desquamative interstitial pneumonia–like pattern was labeled by Liebow (118) giant-cell interstitial pneumonia (GIP). It has been suggested that most cases of GIP actually are hard metal disease (116, 117, 119). However, we have seen cases of GIP in which there was no historical or analytic (discussed later) evidence of hard metal exposure, and the reaction pattern should be regarded as suggestive rather than specific.

Black particulate material, some of it birefringent, can be found in macrophages and giant cells, although in the cases we have seen, particulate matter was not abundant. Analysis by energy-dispersive x-ray spectroscopy has revealed largely tungsten particles. Particulate cobalt has been seen in some (110, 111, 116, 120) but not all instances, which is not surprising, since cobalt is soluble in lung tissue fluid (121, 122). Elevated levels of cobalt in lung tissue have been also shown by atomic absorption spectroscopy (121, 122).

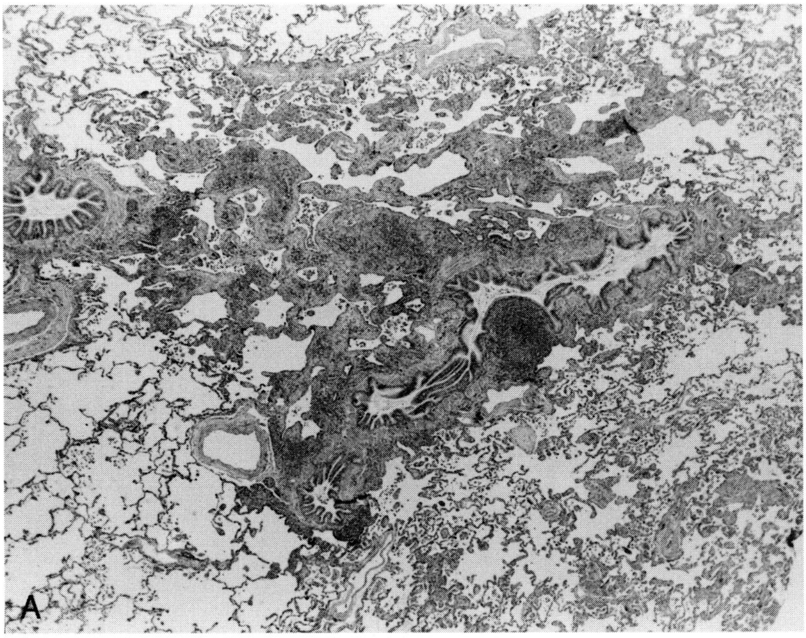

FIGURE 5.10

Hard metal disease. **A.** Low-power view of the lung of a worker exposed to hard metal in a sawmill. Note the typical airway-centered pattern of interstitial inflammation and fibrosis. **B.** High-power view showing bizarre giant cells along with interstitial inflammation and fibrosis. This particular example shows a relatively small number of alveolar macrophages in the airspaces. **C.** Low-power micrograph from the lung of a worker in the hard metal industry showing marked fibrosis in the region of a respiratory bronchiole. Remaining nonfibrotic parenchyma is obscured by an infiltrate of alveolar macrophages filling airspaces. **D.** An area slightly away from the centrilobular zone showing a pattern very much like that of a desquamative interstitial pneumonia. Giant cells are also present; the combination of giant cells and macrophages with an interstitial infiltrate (so-called giant cell interstitial pneumonia) is characteristic of hard metal disease. Particles of tungsten were demonstrated in this case by energy dispersive x-ray spectroscopy. (**C** and **D** courtesy Dr. B. Corrin. London, UK.)

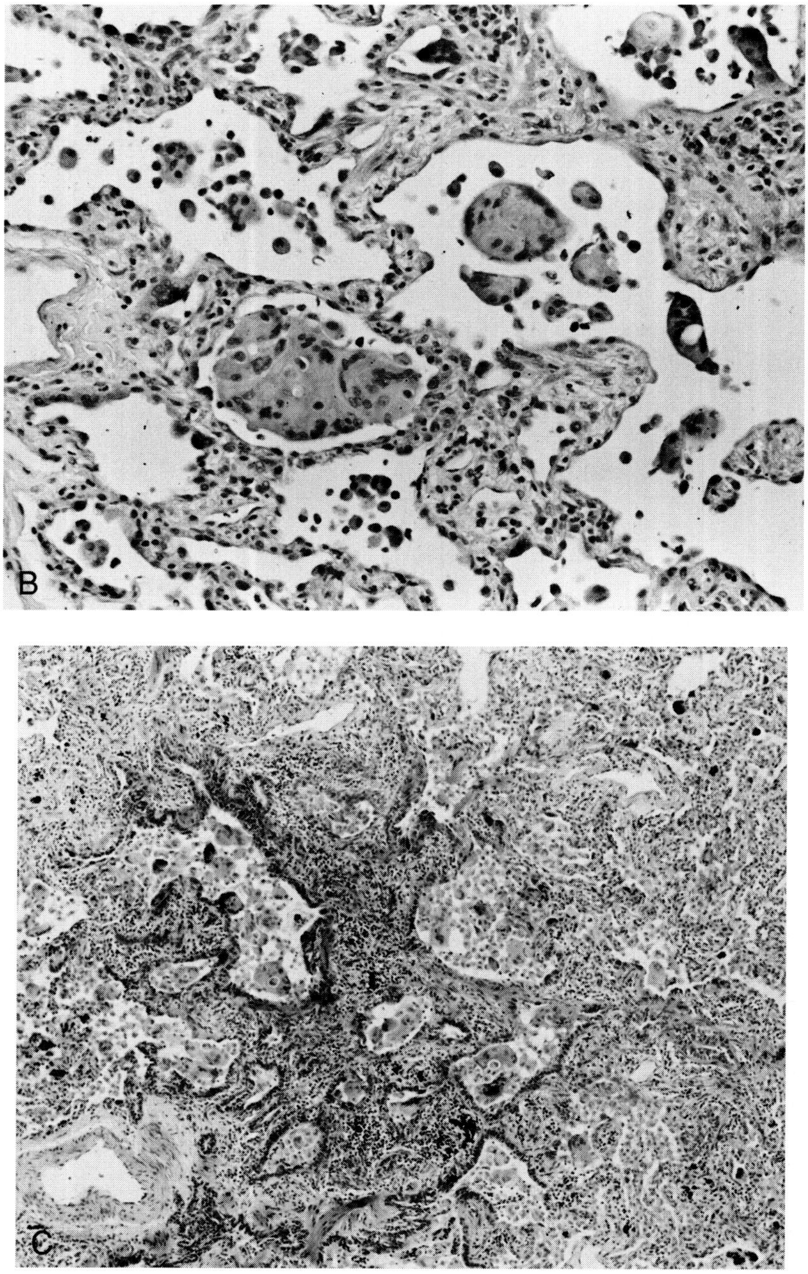

FIGURE 5.10 *(continued)*

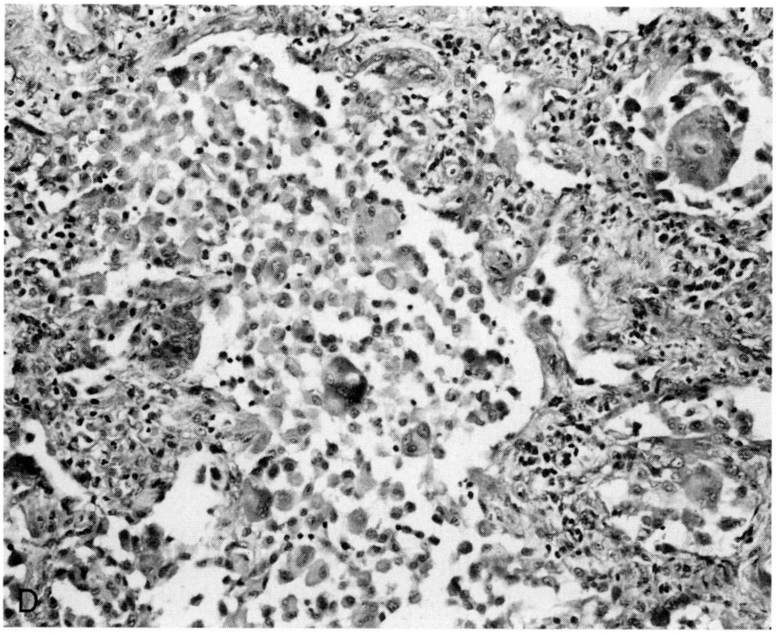

FIGURE 5.10 *(continued)*

From the point of view of practical diagnosis, if there is historical or histologic evidence of hard metal disease and if analysis of lung tissue by analytical electron microscopy (usually energy-dispersive x-ray spectroscopy) shows tungsten, tantalum, or cobalt particles, metals that are not found in the lungs of the general population (Churg, unpublished data), the diagnosis can be considered established. However, in our experience these metals sometimes cannot be found by electron microscopy, even in patients with unequivocal histories of exposure and a typical picture of GIP, and their absence in this situation does not detract from the diagnosis.

Not all reports have described a histologic pattern suggesting desquamative interstitial pneumonia or GIP (123, 124), and it is possible that some hard metal disease resembles usual interstitial pneumonia pathologically. In this setting analytic electron microscopy can have particular benefit. The three patients reported by Sjogren et al. (115) to have interstitial infiltrates also showed decreases in airflow after exposure, and the authors suggested that the process clinically resembled extrinsic allergic alveolitis; in their patients, signs and symptoms disappeared after removal from exposure and reappeared, somewhat worse each time, on re-exposure. One of their patients finally failed to clear radiographically, leading the authors to propose that the disease starts as reversible allergic alveolitis and proceeds to irreversible fibrosis. However, a classic histologic picture of allergic alveolitis does not appear to have been reported in hard metal workers.

Hard metal (cobalt) disease is one of the few forms of occupational interstitial fibrosis that often responds to steroids and/or removal from exposure (104, 111, 109, 115, 125. Thus accurate clinical and histologic diagnosis is crucial to patient management. However, steroids are not always effective, and death from respiratory failure may result (105, 106, 121, 126).

Silicon Carbide. Silicon carbide (carborundum) is a widely used synthetic abrasive. It is produced by heating crystalline silica and carbon at high temperature. The finished product consists of compact particles and at least in some instances, silicon carbide fibers.

Infranterivard et al. (127) surveyed 585 Québec silicon carbide production workers and found an increased risk of nonmalignant interstitial respiratory disease. Funahashi et al. (128) reported a peculiar pattern of slightly nodular aggregates of dust and fibrosis in 2 workers in a factory making silicon carbide; radiographically this appeared as a reticulonodular infiltrate. By x-ray diffraction the total quartz content of the lungs was low and silicon carbide was the major dust. Masse et al. (129) examined lung tissue from 3 workers whose chest radiographs showed finely nodular or reticulonodular infiltrates. Pathologically there was both diffuse interstitial fibrosis and nodular disease that appeared to be silicosis or a mixed-dust pneumonoconiosis. Various types of particulate, including carbon, silica, and silicon carbide fibers, were observed; ferruginous bodies with a black fibrous silicon carbide core were also present. Bégin et al. (130) administered silicon carbide fibers and compact silicon carbide particles to sheep and produced fibrotic lesions with the fibers but not the particles. These studies suggest that silicon carbide production work can be associated with interstitial lung disease, most likely because of the presence of silicon carbide fibers.

Other Causes of Interstitial Fibrosis. A recent epidemiologic study (131) of cases labeled as cryptogenic fibrosing alveolitis (usual interstitial pneumonia) suggests an association between interstitial fibrosis and exposure to steel, brass, and lead, as well as wood dusts. However, as the authors note, it is unclear whether these specific substances are the causative agents or there is an associated exposure in the workplace.

As a rule, exposure to rare earths such as cerium oxide appears to produce only macular lesions, but cases of interstitial fibrosis have been reported in workers exposed to rare earth–containing dusts from carbon arcs (132, 133).

Fibrosis of a more nodular type has been reported in workers exposed to a mixture of copper sulfate and hydrated lime used to prevent mildew in grapes; it is called vineyard sprayers' lung (134, 135). Radiographically the lesions resemble those of silicosis, with upper zonal fine nodules and in some instances massive fibrosislike changes (134). Microscopically the earliest lesions appear to be interstitial collections of dust and macrophages forming ill-defined granulomas; these scar to nodules that very much resemble silicotic nodules. The mass lesions are green–blue to dark blue and may cavitate. They included dust stains as copper (135).

Dental technicians' pneumoconiosis is a somewhat ill-defined condition seen in workers who make dental protheses. The prostheses contain a variety of metals, including chromium, cobalt, molybdenum, beryllium, and nickel. In addition, silica sandblasting may be used in preparing the prosthesis (136). Chest radiographs have shown reticulonodular infiltrates, and the clinical and histologic patterns have been interpreted variously as those of berylliosis, hard metal disease, and silicosis (136–138). Morgenroth et al. (139) examined 30 lung biopsies from patients believed to have dental technicians' pneumoconiosis. A variety of linear and nodular fibrotic changes, along with considerable dust in macrophages, were observed. Some of the nodular lesions appeared to be silicotic. Chromium, cobalt, copper, zinc, silica, and large quantities of iron were identified by energy-dispersive x-ray spectroscopy. Kotloff et al. (140) reported a patient who had in vitro proliferation of lavaged lung lymphocytes exposed to beryllium salts. Although it does appear that some dental technicians develop pneumoconiosis, it remains uncertain whether this process is histologically specific.

The development of interstitial infiltrates in a dental student who inhaled acrylic resin vapors has also been described (141); histologic and ultrastructural examination revealed numerous acrylic particles in macrophages. The radiographic lesions gradually resolved after cessation of exposure.

Cadmium. Acute high-level exposure to cadmium produces ARDS as well as possibly renal impairment (1, 142–144). The evidence for development of lung disease with chronic exposure to cadmium is controversial. A number of older studies reported emphysema in workers exposed to cadmium (145, 146) but these reports are flawed by a lack of information on smoking status. Furthermore, the descriptions and illustrations in these studies are those of ordinary centrilobular emphysema, despite the authors' claims that the process is morphologically unusual.

A recent report by Davison et al. (147), examining lung function and chest radiographs of 101 men who worked in a plant manufacturing a copper–cadmium alloy, is more convincing. Compared with a referent group with comparable age, sex, and smoking status, the cadmium-exposed workers showed a statistical excess of airflow obstruction and radiographic emphysema. Unfortunately, it appears that no morphologic data were available to document the type of emphysema present.

Animals acutely exposed to cadmium fume show early pulmonary edema or ARDS, much like that appearing in acute human exposure, followed by an interstitial infiltrate of monocytes and fibroblasts, with return toward normal in 10 days to 2 weeks (148, 149). Snider et al. (150) induced emphysema in animals by exposure to $CdCl_2$ aerosol, but this process was pathologically different from ordinary cigarette smoke–induced emphysema in man or animals in that there was no loss of elastin and there was a quite distinct increase in fibrous tissue. Snider et al. (150) postulated that airspace enlargement ("emphysema") in this model reflected focal distention of the airspaces secondary to fibrosis rather than an imbalance of proteolysis and antiproteolysis of the type thought to occur with cigarette smoke and dusts such as coal and silica (see section on macules).

Cadmium is classified by the International Agency for Research on Cancer (IARC) as a definite human carcinogen, although this classification has been disputed (27, 28).

Beryllium

Chemistry and Mineralogy. Beryllium is an extremely light metal with excellent thermal and electrical conductivity and a modulus of elasticity that is one-third greater than that of steel; it is an excellent sound conductor and has the highest heat of fusion of all metals (151). It is an excellent moderator and reflector of neutrons, is translucent to x-rays, and is not magnetic (152).

Beryllium is found in a variety of minerals, most commonly beryl ($3BeOAl_2O_36SiO_2$), (151), which occurs in granite pegmatite formations, from which it is mined. Beryllium is extracted from beryl at high temperatures by sulfate or fluoride techniques (152, 153). Beryllium hydroxide is produced and converted to beryllium oxide (beryllia) or any of a number of salts: fluoride, chloride, nitrate, and sulfate. Synthetic beryllium silicates are also produced.

Beryllium oxide is widely used because of its high thermal conductivity; it is prepared by high-fired (1600°C) or low-fired (500 to 1000°C) techniques (152). The low-fired technique has been more often associated with human disease (152). Beryllium is commonly alloyed with copper (4% or less beryllium), from which other alloys are made with nickel, aluminum, manganese, and zinc (152, 154). Beryllium alloys have a high resistance to fatigue (155). Beryllium phosphors were formerly used in the fluorescent light bulb industry but were abandoned because of the high association with beryllium-induced lung disease (152). Beryllium and compounds that contain it are all toxic to humans, although beryl itself is relatively safe (152).

Industrial Uses and Occupational Exposures. Because of its exceptional physicochemical properties, beryllium is widely used in many industries. Before strict controls were instituted, beryllium disease was relatively common in individuals exposed during extraction of the metal from the ore, especially associated with the fluoride moiety, and in industries that used its compounds and alloys (155). In the late 1940s and early 1950s strict exposure limits were imposed, and the number of cases of beryllium disease have greatly decreased since then (154). Nevertheless, estimates of individuals now at risk vary from 30,000 to 870,000 (156), and since chronic berylliosis may be caused by relatively low levels of exposure, new cases will continue to be identified.

Beryllium disease has been seen in a wide variety of settings (Table 5.6) (152–171). Workers who produced fluorescent lamps that incorporated beryllium phosphors were one of the earliest risk groups identified, and exposure from breakage or during disposal of such lamps is still possible. A variety of metal workers, including those engaged in recovery of scrap metals and in construction of switchboards, aircraft engines, precision tools, plastic molds, and marine propellers, are exposed to beryllium. Beryllium oxide is used in the ceramics industry. Beryllium alloys are important in the manufacture of transistors, tubes, and computers. Aerospace workers may be exposed to both the metal and beryllium alloys, which are incorporated in gyroscopes, nuclear reactors, missile guidance systems, neutron deflectors, space vehicles, space mirrors, and satellite antennae; beryllium is also a potential component of rocket fuel. Workers who extract beryllium from beryl are also at risk for exposure, as are experimental chemists and physicists who work with beryllium and its com-

TABLE 5.6
Workers, Occupations, and Sources of Beryllium Exposure

Extraction of beryllium from beryl
Fluorescent lamp manufacture (beryllium phosphors)
Metal workers (beryllium metal and alloys)
Ceramic manufacturing (beryllium oxide)
Electronics industry (beryllium alloys)
Rockets and space industry (beryllium metal and alloys)
Dental technicians (beryllium alloys)
Experimental chemists and physicists working with beryllium
Employees in beryllium processing plants not directly exposed to the products
Individuals living in the vicinity of factories using beryllium
Individuals exposed while handling the clothing of beryllium workers

pounds. Beryllium is used in some dental prostheses, and some cases of dental technicians' pneumoconiosis may be beryllium disease (164).

Several recent studies have confirmed that cases of chronic beryllium disease continue to be recognized, affecting approximately 2% of exposed individuals (171). Recent cases of berylliosis have been identified in epidemiologic studies of metal refineries, (165) nuclear workers (168), and ceramic workers (169). Some of these studies show that the risk of developing chronic beryllium disease increases with the level of exposure (168, 169).

A number of cases of berylliosis have been reported in people without direct exposure (152, 156, 168, 169, 172, 173). Many of these cases were recognized before strict control measures. They included factory employees such as secretaries who were not directly exposed to beryllium but worked in the same building, people living in the vicinity of factories using beryllium, and individuals exposed while handling the clothing of beryllium workers. Among neighbors of factories higher incidence of disease was associated with living closer to the plants (most patients within a mile). Recent studies have reconfirmed that bystander cases of chronic beryllium disease continue to be recognized (168, 169, 172), and in one study a case developed in a dust disturber who worked in a plant in which beryllia production had stopped eight years earlier (169). Four cases of berylliosis without air-identified exposure source were reported to the Beryllium Case Registry from 1973 to 1980 (156).

Beryllium-Induced Human Disease. Recent reviews of pulmonary toxicity of beryllium attest to the continued identification of cases of the human disease primarily chronic beryllium disease (174–176). Historically beryllium-induced human disease has been divided into acute and chronic syndromes.

Acute Beryllium Disease. The incidence of acute beryllium disease has dramatically decreased with the reduction in permitted levels of beryllium exposure, since most cases of acute berylliosis were associated with high levels of exposure (154). At present acute pneumonitis from beryllium is virtually limited to large accidental exposures (152), and skin and mucosa beryllium lesions have historical interest only. The acute lesions induced by beryllium are shown in Table 5.7.

Beryllium-induced dermatitis (177) is a pruritic papulovesicular eruption on exposed parts of the body that is usually associated with conjunctivitis. A contact dermatitis, it subsides with termination of exposure. Beryllium ulcer (177) is a local necrotizing ulceration caused by physical implantation of beryllium or beryllium-containing compound in the skin. The ulcer festers until the material is removed. Beryllium-induced nasopharyngitis and tracheobronchitis usually follow exposure to large amounts of beryllium dusts, fumes, or mists and precede acute beryllium pneumonitis (177). The inflammation subsides a few weeks after cessation of exposure.

TABLE 5.7
Patterns of Acute Beryllium Disease

Dermatitis, conjunctivitis
Beryllium ulcer
Nasopharyngitis, tracheobronchitis
Acute beryllium pneumonitis
Fulminant (2–3 days after exposure)
Subacute (weeks after exposure)

Acute beryllium pneumonitis can be divided into two categories (177). One is a fulminant illness that evolves in 2 to 3 days following massive exposure; the other is a more insidious process that is heralded by dry cough and progressive dyspnea over a few weeks. Both ultimately progress to an illness resembling ARDS. Historically, the latter form of the disease has been more common; however, since most current acute disease results from accidental exposure to very high levels of beryllium, the fulminant form may be encountered.

Mortality of 10% is reported for historical cases of acute beryllium pneumonitis (152, 177). Most patients recover 1 to 6 months after development of symptoms, with or without steroid therapy. Approximately 10% subsequently develop chronic beryllium disease (177). Some of these patients have radiographic abnormalities that never resolve, and there appears to be a direct and continuous transition from acute to chronic disease (177, 178). The acute pneumonitis may recur with repeated exposure (161).

Chronic Beryllium Disease. Chronic berylliosis is a multisystem disease caused by hypersensitivity to beryllium; it has a marked similarity to sarcoidosis in clinical, functional, radiographic, and pathologic respects (152, 154, 155, 165, 166, 171–176, 179, 180). The amount of beryllium to which affected individuals have been exposed and their tissue levels of beryllium may be quite low, and there is a latency period, sometimes lasting many years, before symptoms become manifest. The risk of developing the disease rises with levels of exposure (168, 169, 171).

Because of the latency period and the often low levels of exposure, eliciting an exposure history in a patient with chronic beryllium disease may require considerable detective work. In historical series nearly half the patients developed symptoms while on the job, and another third developed symptoms within 5 years of last exposure (177). Nevertheless, latency periods of 40 years or more are known (162). Chronic berylliosis accounts for all the bystander cases of neighborhood and paraoccupational berylliosis.

The disease continues to be identified among active employees as well as ex-employees of industries where exposure occurs (165, 168–171). One recent series identified patients who were sensitized to beryllium and without evidence of disease yet who developed pulmonary granulomas on lung biopsy during the following 2 years (168).

Most symptomatic patients present with progressive dyspnea and cough (152, 153). Some are asymptomatic and are recognized with beryllium sensitization testing or on radiography or have their disease unmasked by pneumothorax, respiratory infection, or re-exposure to beryllium (152, 153). Skin lesions that are clinically and histologically identical to sarcoid disease may be found.

Chest radiographic findings in chronic berylliosis are nonspecific (152, 153). Miliary small (granular) opacities, larger nodules with or without line shadows, and small, contracted lungs are usually described. The upper lung zones may be more severely affected. Hilar adenopathy may be present and rarely is the only abnormality on the chest radiograph. Thin-section CT scans are more sensitive than routine chest radiography, but not all cases are recognized, and the CT appearances of chronic beryllium disease are not specific (181, 182).

Pulmonary function abnormalities—decreased total lung capacity, vital capacity, residual volume with arterial denaturation, diffusing capacity, and compliance—may be identical to those in sarcoid and other forms of fibrosing lung disease (152, 153, 170, 183). Serial diffusing capacity may be used to document the course and progression of the disease. Slightly more than half of surveillance-identified patients in the study of Pappas and Newman (170) were found to have functional abnormalities. These patients were identified on the basis of beryllium sensitization, not clinical complaints.

Pathologic Features of Acute Beryllium Pneumonitis. Acute beryllium pneumonitis is a chemical pneumonitis with histologic features of acute lung injury (diffuse alveolar damage) (184–187). As such, the findings depend on the elapsed time since the onset of the disease and on the fact that only severe cases are encountered histologically. Early cases show alveolar hemorrhage, edema, and hyaline membranes. Later, type II pneumocyte hyperplasia, increased alveolar macrophages, and organization within airspaces are seen along with an interstitial infiltrate of lymphocytes and plasma cells (Fig. 5.11). Occasional giant cells may be seen, but granulomas are not found, and neutrophils are generally scant. Presumably, mild cases show less severe pathologic changes.

Although approximately 10% of patients with acute disease develop chronic disease, the histologic sequence from one to the other is not clear; the lung is usually not examined until chronic berylliosis is present. Individuals who have recovered from acute berylliosis may have a slight but recognizable increase in connective tissue in their lungs (188).

Pathologic Features of Chronic Beryllium Pneumonitis. The pathology of chronic berylliosis has been the subject of a number of reports (187–191). There is a chronic interstitial pneumonia with interstitial cellular infiltrates of lymphocytes and plasma cells, progressive interstitial fibrosis, and usually a prominent accompanying granulomatous reaction (Figs. 5.12–5.17). Some patients have confluent masses of well-formed granulomas distributed along the lymphatic routes with relatively little interstitial infiltrate. These cases are indistinguishable from sarcoid disease. In other cases the granulomas are relatively small, poorly formed, and randomly scattered throughout the parenchyma. None of the histologic changes are pathognomonic, and as shown in Figure 5.16, granulomas may be lost over time, leaving nonspecific honeycombing. Laminated calcospherites (Schaumann bodies) are usually prominent in the giant cells in alveolar spaces or amid the interstitial fibrous tissue. Schaumann bodies are nonspecific, and when granulomas are sparse or absent, they represent a fossilized remnant of the earlier granulomatous inflammation. Asteroid bodies and cholesterol clefts within giant cells are another common nonspecific feature.

Large hyalinized fibrotic nodules are seen in 40% of cases of chronic berylliosis, and 15% of these show evidence of amorphous central degeneration or necrosis (189). Similar nodules may be seen in the lymph nodes. Dystrophic calcification and even ossification may occur in the nodules. The nodules resemble silicotic nodules, but they have less fibrous whorling and lack a cuff of dust-filled macrophages.

Interstitial fibrosis accompanies the interstitial inflammatory infiltrate and the granulomas. The granulomas are progressively replaced by a hyalinized connective tissue. Scarring and destruction of lung parenchyma lead to progressive architectural distortion and honeycombing, which varies in extent and severity. Granulomas may be lacking in some cases of chronic berylliosis (189).

Extranodal granulomatous infiltrates identical to sarcoidosis may be found in the skin, nodes, liver, spleen, pancreas, kidneys, adrenal glands, marrow, muscle, central nervous system, and rarely the myocardium (152).

Analysis of Human Tissue for Beryllium. Beryllium in human tissues and urine may be detected and measured by a number of techniques. The conventional techniques are spectrographic or fluorometric (192, 193), among which

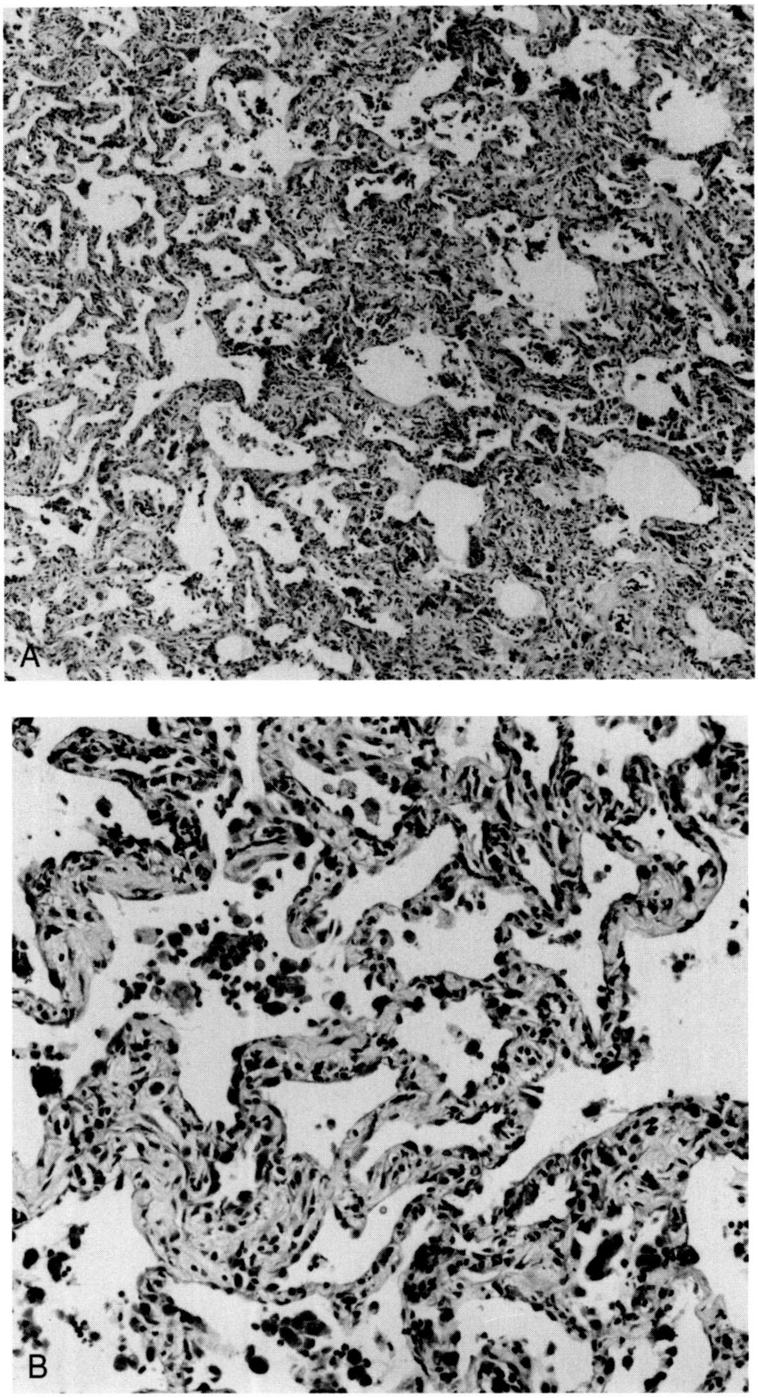

FIGURE 5.11

A. Acute berylliosis showing organizing acute diffuse alveolar damage. The alveolar walls are edematous and widened, and they contain a sparse mononuclear infiltrate. **B.** A proliferation of type II pneumocytes lines most of the alveolar walls. (Courtesy of Joel Green, MD, Salt Lake City.)

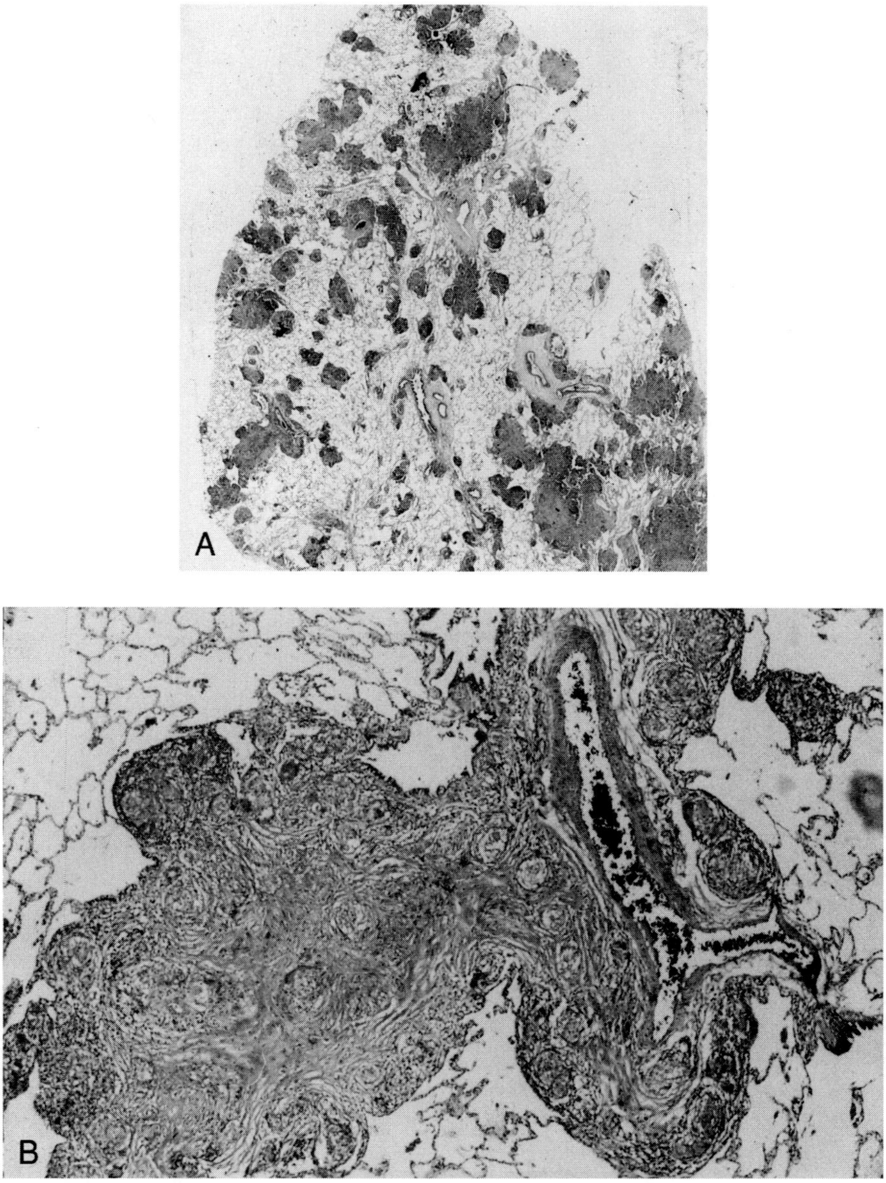

FIGURE 5.12

A. Chronic berylliosis histologically identical to sarcoidosis. **B.** Confluent well-formed noncaseating granulomas distributed along lymphatic routes in the pleura, septa, and along airways and vessels. (Courtesy of E. A. Gaensler, MD, Boston.)

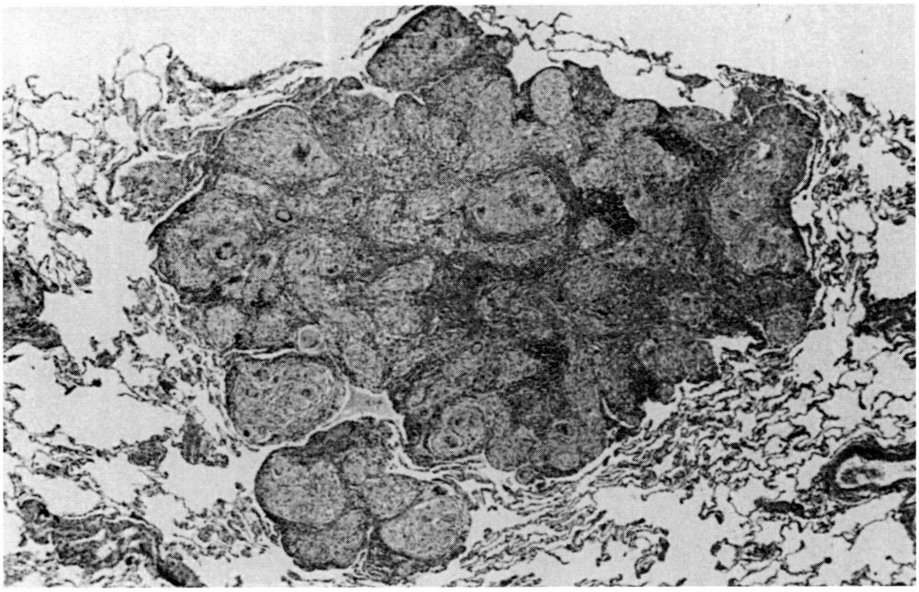

FIGURE 5.13
Chronic berylliosis with a nodular mass of sarcoidlike granulomas. Such a lesion may also be seen in sarcoidosis and granulomatous infections. (Courtesy of E. A. Gaensler, MD, Boston.)

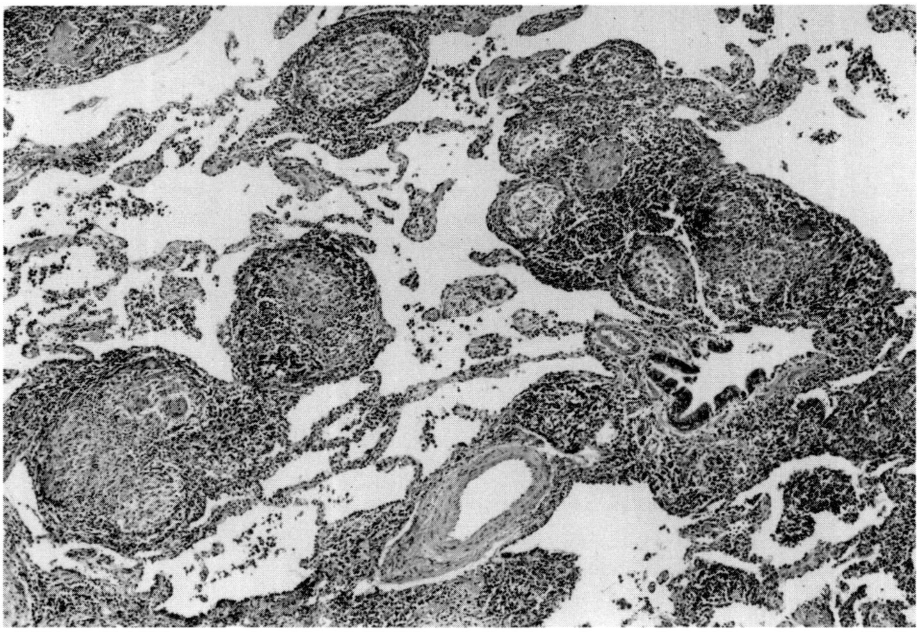

FIGURE 5.14
Chronic berylliosis that shows discrete granulomas and a prominent associated chronic inflammatory infiltrate. Sarcoidosis could produce an identical picture. (Courtesy of E. A. Gaensler, MD, Boston.)

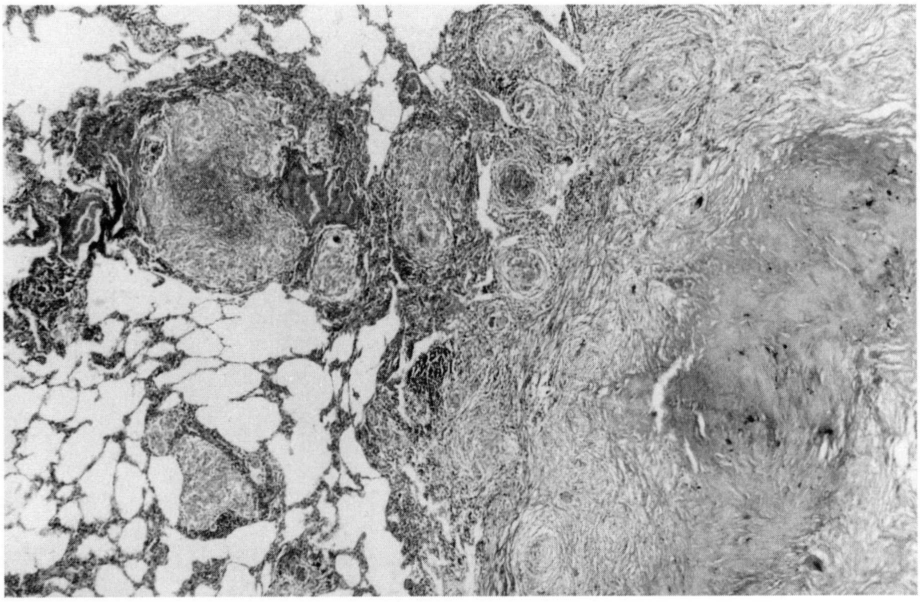

FIGURE 5.15
Chronic berylliosis with coalescent sarcoidlike granulomas associated with central hyaline sclerotic degenerative change. Hyaline nodule formation is unusual in sarcoidosis. (Courtesy of E. A. Gaensler, MD, Boston.)

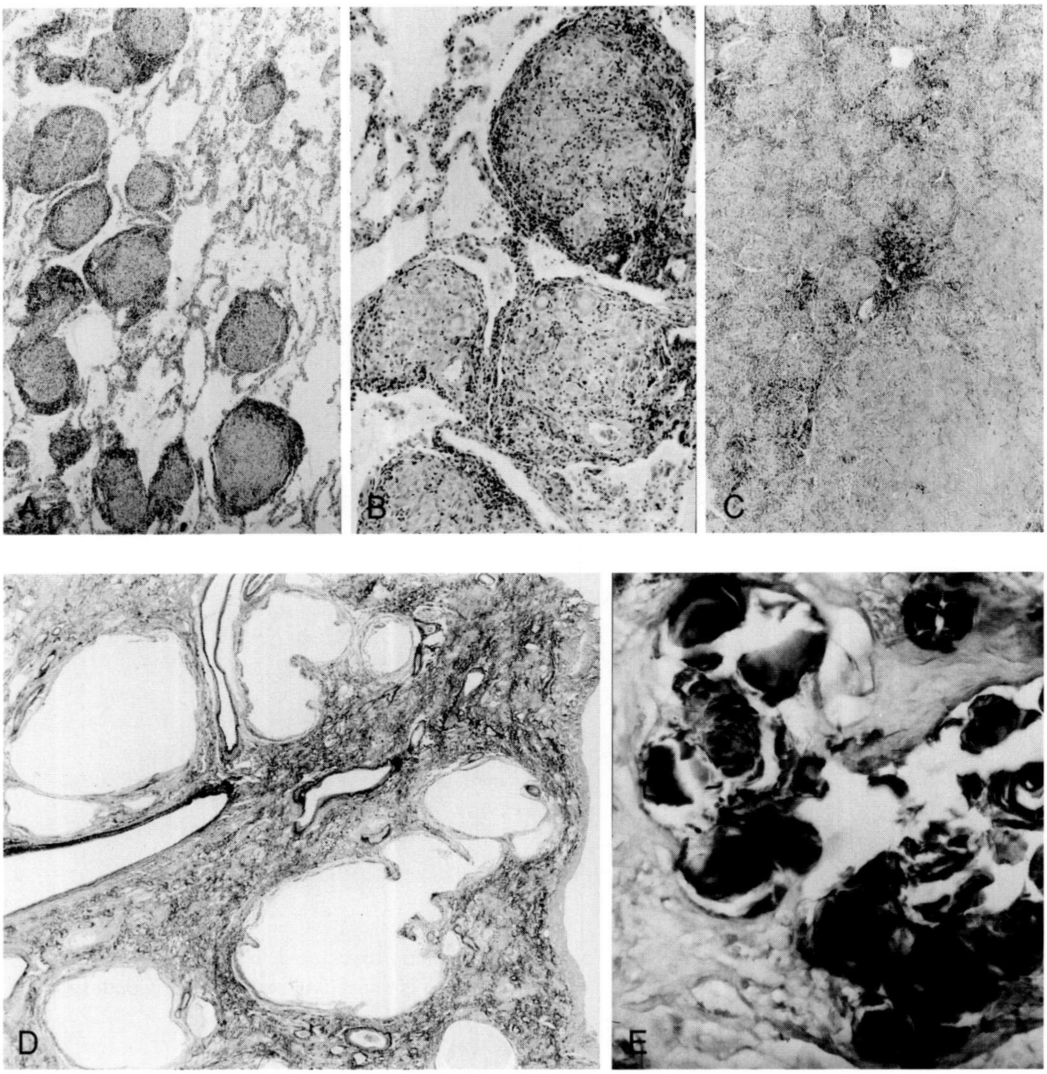

FIGURE 5.16

Chronic berylliosis progressing to nonspecific honeycombing. Lung (**A** and **B**) and hilar lymph node (**C**) biopsy specimens 29 years before death show randomly distributed sarcoidlike granulomas with hyaline nodule formation in the lymph node (*lower right*). At autopsy there is chronic pulmonary fibrosis with honeycombing (**D**). No granulomas remain, but they have left a record of their presence in the form of numerous laminated Schaumann bodies (**E**) embedded in the fibrous tissue. (Courtesy of E. A. Gaensler MD, Boston.)

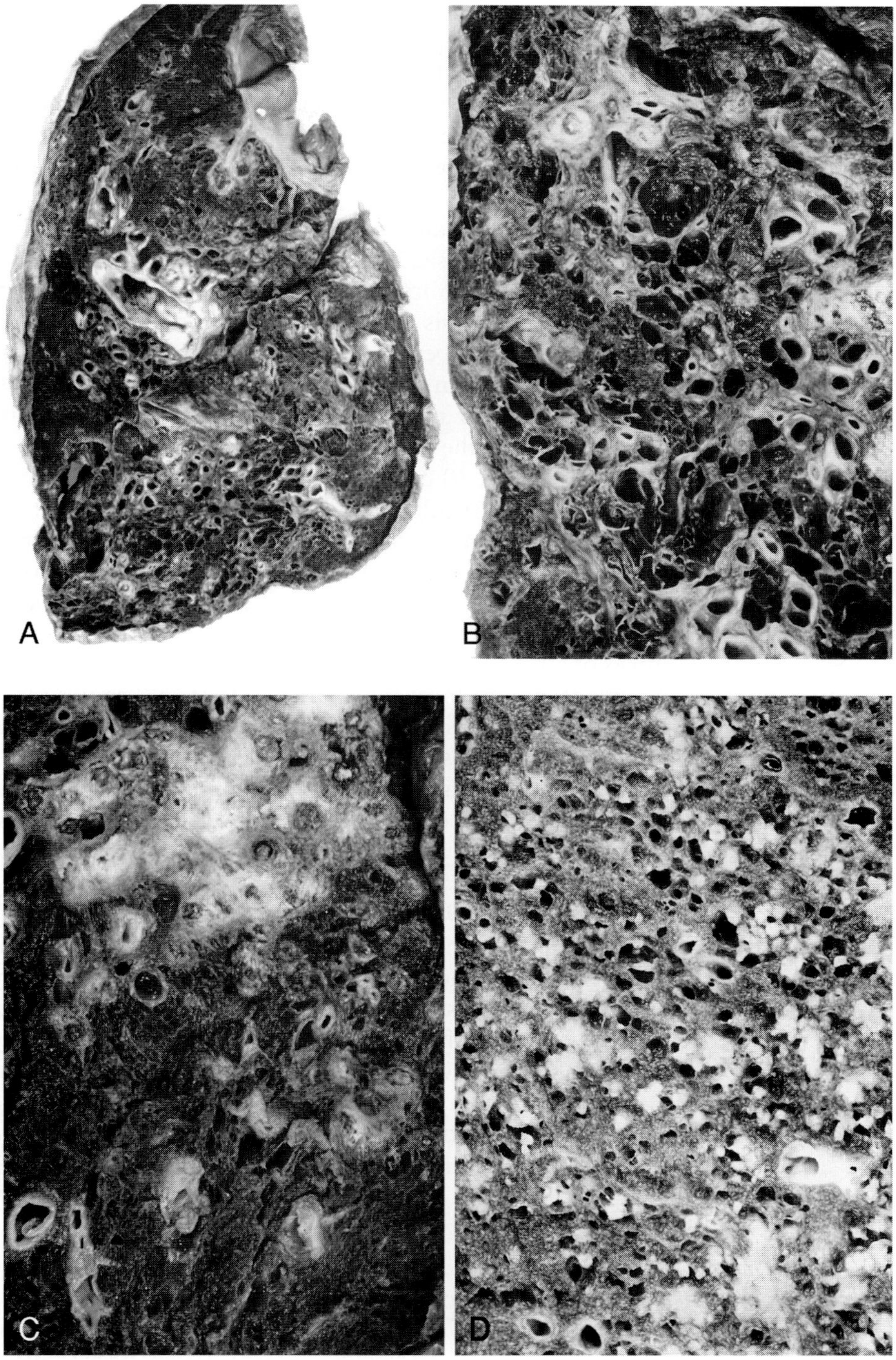

FIGURE 5.17.
Gross features of chronic berylliosis at autopsy. Both cases shown had a long history of berylliosis, and neither patient died directly of the effects of the lung disease. **A–C,** Fibrotic nodules with some coalescence (**C**) with intervening patchy honeycombing and emphysema. The large nodules represent coalescent granulomas with central fibrosis and degenerative change. **D.** Small nodules that were calcified and were composed entirely of Schaumann bodies embedded in dense fibrosis. The intervening parenchyma shows mild emphysematous change, probably a manifestation of pericicatricial emphysema.

atomic absorption spectroscopy is the most widely available. The results are quantifiable, and the sensitivity depends on the size of the sample studied. Although small samples (as small as 1 g of tissue or 50 mL of urine) may be analyzed, the results are more reliable with much larger samples (approximately 50 g or more of tissue, 500 mL or more of urine). For practical purposes with biopsy material, 1 to 2 g is probably sufficient (152). Levels are measured in micrograms per gram of dry weight.

Microemission spectrochemical analysis of 50-μm tissue sections with frozen or formalin-fixed tissues may be used to detect beryllium semiquantitatively in specific histologic structures recognized on paired hematoxylin and eosin sections (194). Ion microprobe analysis in conjunction with scanning electron microscopy has been used to identify beryllium in conventional, routinely prepared light microscope sections of human lung tissue (195–197). Jones Williams and Wallach (197) showed with laser microprobe mass spectrometry analysis that beryllium could be identified in the granulomas of all 33 cases of chronic beryllium disease and was absent in 30 comparison cases of sarcoidosis. However, these analyses are technically difficult and available in only a few centers.

Background levels of beryllium are found in the ambient environment and in tissues of people without any known exposure to beryllium. Small amounts of beryllium are found in the air, soil, and atmosphere, particularly where soft coal is burned (192). Cholak (192) found a range of 0.0001 to 0.003 $\mu g/m^3$ among 933 random samples of air. Background levels of beryllium have been quantified in unexposed individuals and in those with sarcoid. Table 5.8 shows results of analysis for beryllium in unexposed control individuals. The recent NIOSH recommendation for workplace exposure limits are 0.5 $\mu g/m^3$ (198).

Tissue analysis for beryllium has in the past been part of the pathologic examination in suspected cases of berylliosis. The data from Dutra and a series from the Beryllium Case Registry are representative of cases of berylliosis that have been analyzed (Table 5.9).

The data in Tables 5.8 and 5.9 and from the study of Freiman et al. (189) point out several features. Patients with acute berylliosis generally have about four times as much beryllium in their lungs as do patients with chronic berylliosis. Patients with chronic berylliosis who were suspected of having prior acute beryllium pneumonitis had levels intermediate between those of acute berylliosis and those in whom only chronic berylliosis was recognized (189). Of course, a significant quantity of beryllium in the lung indicates exposure only, and acceptable clinical and histologic patterns of abnormalities must be present before disease can be ascribed to beryllium (discussed later). There is a wide variation

TABLE 5.8
Beryllium Levels in Individuals without Occupational Exposure

TISSUE SAMPLE	CHOLAK (192)	SPRINCE ET AL. (193)
Lung	0–0.198 μg/g (average 0.0033) (70 cases)	0.003–0.01 μg/g (average 0.005) (6 cases)
Lymph nodes	—	0.006–0.019 μg/g (average 0.011) (7 cases)
Lung (patients with sarcoid)	—	0.002–0.019 μg/g (average 0.008) (5 cases)

TABLE 5.9
Beryllium Levels in Individuals with Beryllium Disease

TISSUE SAMPLE	DUTRA[187]	SPRINCE[193]
Acute beryllium pneumonitis	0.09–0.22 μg/g (average 0.78) (5 cases)	—
Chronic beryllium pneumonitis	0.00–0.78 μg/g (average 0.19) (5 cases)	0.004–45.7 μg/g (average 1.19) (66 cases)
Mediastinal lymph nodes in chronic berylliosis	—	0.05–8.50 μg/g (average 3.41) (5 cases)
Peripheral lymph nodes in chronic berylliosis	—	0.002–0.49 μg/g (average 0.11) (5 cases)

in the amount of beryllium in the lung in both acute and chronic berylliosis, especially the latter, and the apparent absence of beryllium may not exclude cases otherwise acceptable as chronic berylliosis (see diagnostic criteria later in the chapter). Conversely, beryllium may be found at low background levels in the lungs of people without known exposure and without recognizable lung disease. Lymph nodes that directly drain the lung are more likely to have beryllium than peripheral lymph nodes. When sampling tissue for analysis, mediastinal lymph nodes as well as lung tissue should be sampled. Beryllium in urine indicates exposure to beryllium (152, 199). As shown by Stoeckle et al. (199), beryllium excretion in the urine may be found as long as 15 years after exposure, but lack of measurable beryllium in the urine less than a year from last exposure does not exclude chronic berylliosis.

Immunologic Features of Berylliosis. Chronic berylliosis has an immunologic basis as a delayed hypersensitivity reaction. Over the years a number of clinical tests assaying sensitivity to beryllium have been developed. In addition, recent evidence suggests that exposed individuals with certain major histocompatibility antigen subtypes (specifically HLA-DPβ-1) are at increased risk for developing chronic beryllium disease (175).

Beryllium Patch Test. In a positive patch test there is an erythematous skin reaction 48 to 72 hours after cutaneous application of a solution of beryllium sulfate (152). Granulomas develop in 3 to 4 weeks. Patients may have a positive reaction without evidence of disease, and a negative reaction may be seen in patients with chronic berylliosis. The test itself may induce hypersensitivity to beryllium and may exacerbate existing beryllium-induced diseases, so it is no longer used. Patients with chronic berylliosis usually have a negative Kveim test (152, 153).

Studies of Lymphocyte Blast Transformation and Macrophage Migration Inhibition. In the 1970s in vitro tests were developed to assess peripheral blood lymphocyte reactivity to beryllium, usually beryllium sulfate (152, 200–202). These include lymphocyte blast transformation and guinea pig macrophage migration tests. In the former, peripheral blood lymphocytes are incubated with a beryllium-containing compound, and the number of lymphocytes that transform to lymphoblasts is assessed morphologically or by uptake of tritiated thymidine. In the latter, lymphocytes are incubated with beryllium, and macrophages are exposed to the supernatant. The degree of inhibition of macrophage migration is then assessed. Positive lymphocyte blast transformation tests and macrophage migration inhibition tests are seen in most patients who are sensitive to beryllium; however, a positive test is not always associated with clinical disease (152, 171, 201). The lymphocyte blast transformation test appears to be the more sensitive of the two, and unlike the macrophage inhibition test, it is not suppressed by steroid therapy (202).

Bronchoalveolar lavage (BAL) has also been used as a means of harvesting lymphocytes for the study of sensitivity to beryllium (203–206). Epstein et al. (203) showed that the response of lymphocytes from BAL fluid was greater than in those derived from the peripheral blood. They concluded that BAL may be more useful in the diagnosis of chronic berylliosis. BAL also has been useful harvesting cells for a variety of studies of lymphocyte subsets (204).

Rom et al. (205) have shown that sensitization to beryllium as assessed by BAL-derived lymphocytes may be reversible and that reversibility may correlate with a reduction in exposure levels. Such a finding may be analogous to the reversible radiographic and pulmonary function defects noted by Sprince et al. (207).

Newman (171) and Kreiss et al. (175) in Denver have extensively studied chronic beryllium disease and the usefulness of beryllium sensitivity testing. Their current preferred term is beryllium lymphocyte proliferation testing (BLPT). This can be performed on both blood and BAL lymphocytes. BLPT on BAL lymphocytes may be more sensitive, although BLPT on peripheral blood lymphocytes was capable of identifying more than 94% of the patients who had an abnormal BLPT on BAL and was easier to perform. The ease and reliability of BLPT make it likely to replace tissue analysis in the diagnosis of chronic beryllium disease, as evidenced by recent suggested changes in the diagnostic criteria for this condition (discussed later).

While not all beryllium-sensitized individuals have clinically recognized disease, it may ultimately develop in individuals who have been identified solely on the basis of a positive BLPT (170). In patients who have clinical and pathologic changes consistent with chronic beryllium disease, a positive BLPT is significant and may confirm the diagnosis.

Diagnosis of Berylliosis. The diagnosis of acute beryllium disease in most cases rests on an obvious exposure and pulmonary disease developing shortly thereafter; the histologic features are nonspecific. Appreciable quantities of beryllium can be found with tissue analysis if it can be performed. Criteria for diagnosing chronic berylliosis have varied somewhat (152, 153, 160, 193) but historically have included most or all of the following:

1. Significant history of exposure to beryllium
2. Clinical, functional, and radiographic evidence of pulmonary disease consistent with chronic berylliosis, including chest radiograph with interstitial fibronodular disease and restrictive or obstructive functional deficit with decreased diffusing capacity
3. Histologic changes consistent with berylliosis, especially granulomatous inflammation
4. Detection of beryllium in tissue and/or urine
5. Evidence of sensitivity to beryllium
6. Exclusion of other granulomatous diseases
7. Negative Kveim test

The mere existence of such a list testifies to the difficulty in confirming the diagnosis of chronic berylliosis, and not all cases accepted as such fulfill all of these criteria (193). From the clinical perspective the main problem in differential diagnosis is sarcoid, and cases may masquerade as sarcoidosis (172). A confident diagnosis may require compilation of many clinical, radiographic, biochemical, and histologic parameters and the results of tissue analysis and BLPT (152, 172, 193).

The Beryllium Case Registry in a 1984 review required at least four of the following six criteria to establish a diagnosis of chronic beryllium disease (156):

1. Documented exposure, preferably including air samples in the workplace
2. Objective evidence of lower respiratory disease and clinical course consistent with berylliosis
3. Chest radiograph showing interstitial fibronodular disease
4. Functional evidence of restriction, obstruction, or decreased diffusing capacity
5. Pathology consistent with berylliosis in lung or thoracic lymph nodes
6. Beryllium in lung, lymph nodes, or urine

Although granulomas are characteristic of chronic beryllium disease, the series of Freiman confirms that granulomas may be absent in a significant number of cases (189), and the case illustrated in Figure 5.16 shows that granulomas may disappear with time.

The use of BLPT is a significant diagnostic aid in the identification of patients with sensitivity to beryllium and of chronic beryllium disease and has been incorporated into the diagnostic criteria recently proposed by Newman et al. (171) (Table 5.10). From the point of feasibility, it is clear that BLPT is preferable to tissue analysis in diagnosing chronic beryllium disease.

Diagnostic Considerations for the Pathologist. The pathologic spectrum of beryllium pneumonitis is wide, and no one feature or constellation of features is pathognomonic (189). Acute berylliosis is indistinguishable from diffuse alve-

TABLE 5.10

Proposed Criteria for the Diagnosis of Chronic Beryllium Lung Disease, Subclinical Beryllium Lung Disease, and Beryllium Sensitization

History of exposure to beryllium
Beryllium-specific immune response; positive blood or BAL BLPT
Lung biopsy histopathology consistent with chronic beryllium disease (granulomas and/or mononuclear cell infiltrates)
Constellation of clinical findings that may include any of the following:
Respiratory symptoms or signs
Reticulonodular infiltrates on chest imaging
Altered pulmonary physiology with restrictive and/or obstructive changes
Decreased diffusing capacity, ventilatory impairment, or altered gas exchange on exercise testing

Diagnosis of chronic beryllium disease requires all four criteria.
Diagnosis of subclinical beryllium disease requires criteria 1–3.
Diagnosis of beryllium sensitization requires criteria 1 and 2.
Modified from Kreiss K, Mroz MM, Zhen B, et al. Epidemiology of beryllium sensitization and disease in nuclear workers. Am Rev Respir Dis 1993;148:985–991.

TABLE 5.11
Histologic Differential Diagnosis of Chronic Berylliosis

Sarcoidosis	Tendency to confluent masses of granulomas that follow lymphatic routines along bronchovascular bundles, pulmonary veins and in the septa and pleura; hyalinized nodules usually absent; sarcoid often histologically indistinguishable from chronic berylliosis
Extrinsic allergic alveolitis	Small, randomly scattered noncaseating granulomas that may only manifest as tiny nodules of epithelioid histiocytes or a small cluster of giant cells; cellular infiltrate along airways and in the interstitium usually prominent
Lymphocytic interstitial pneumonia	Marked prominence of the interstitial infiltrate relative to the granulomas and lack of hyalinization in the granulomas
Usual interstitial pneumonia and lesions associated with this pattern (such as drug reactions and collagen diseases)	Absence of granulomas and Schaumann bodies in the interstitial fibrous tissue; berylliosis may assume this pattern
Asbestosis	Asbestos bodies identified histologically; fibrosing pleural lesions usually prominent
Granulomatous infections, active or healed	Schaumann bodies generally not conspicuous; active granulomatous infections usually not a problem because of necrosis and demonstration of organisms; differentiation may be difficult in the absence of these features
Silicosis	No epithelioid granulomas; silicotic nodules often show birefringent crystals and often more fibrous whorling of the nodules than in berylliosis

olar damage (acute interstitial pneumonia). The diagnosis rests on a confirmed history of exposure and is further supported by demonstration of beryllium in the tissues or urine. A diagnosis of chronic berylliosis based on histologic features alone is also not possible (153). Table 5.11 shows the lesions that should be included in the differential diagnosis along with their distinguishing features.

Table 5.12 lists histologic features that should at least raise the question of chronic berylliosis in a case of undiagnosed granulomatous and/or fibrotic pulmonary disease. The hyalinized nodules, though not specific, are probably the feature that most helps to separate chronic berylliosis from other granulomatous lung diseases (189). Although the features listed may be helpful in statistical separation of large groups of cases, most investigators agree that in individual cases berylliosis and sarcoidosis cannot be distinguished histologically, and some cases may be extremely difficult to distinguish from allergic alveolitis (189, 191). The histologic findings are only one of the several clinicopathologic findings that are assessed to confirm or exclude a diagnosis of berylliosis.

Treatment and Prognosis of Beryllium Disease. Historically, acute berylliosis has relatively low mortality, and most patients recover within a few months with or without steroid therapy and supportive care (177). However, acute berylliosis is now rare, and most cases are the result of accidental exposure, which can be massive. Thus the 10% mortality figure in historical se-

TABLE 5.12
Histologic Features That Raise the Possibility of Berylliosis

Nonnecrotizing granulomas with a prominent interstitial infiltrate
Nonnecrotizing sarcoidlike granulomas
Tendency of granulomas to form round hyalinized nodules with or without central degenerative, necrotic changes in nonsilicotic lung or lymph nodes
Large and numerous clusters of Schaumann bodies embedded in the connective tissue in a fibrotic lung with or without associated granulomas

TABLE 5.13
Prognosis of Chronic Berylliosis as a Function of Histologic Features

	MEAN DURATION OF ILLNESS	PERCENT ALIVE
Group IA	8 years	15
Group IB	8 years	40
Group II	11 years	95

ries may be misleading, since the prognosis is worse with larger exposures (162, 184).

Steroids ameliorate symptoms in chronic berylliosis, but the long-term effect on prognosis is unproved in controlled trials (152, 176, 183, 208). Apparent resolutions or long-term remissions may occur with or without steroid therapy. Among the patients of Andrews et al. (208), 75% of whom had follow-up of 10 years or more, 30% died. The authors identified a spectrum of pulmonary function abnormalities in 41 patients with chronic berylliosis. They divided their series into three groups: one with abnormal diffusing capacity and normal lung volumes (interstitial group); a second with normal FEV_1 but decreased total lung capacity, vital capacity, and diffusing capacity (restrictive group); and a third with parameters of obstruction (obstructive group) that could not be fully explained by other factors (e.g., smoking). The latter two groups had more disabling disease.

Sprince et al. (207) reported that a decrease in the concentration of beryllium in a beryllium plant was associated with improvement in radiographic changes and pulmonary functions in a subset of abnormal patients identified at the initial screening.

Freiman et al. (189) divided cases of chronic berylliosis into three histologic categories based on the presence and degree of interstitial infiltrate and the character of the granulomas: group I, moderate to marked interstitial cellular infiltrate with no or poorly formed granulomas (group IA) or well-formed granulomas (group IB); and group II, numerous well-formed granulomas with little interstitial infiltrate. Group IA fared the worst and group II the best (Table 5.13).

The major complication and cause of mortality in chronic berylliosis is cor pulmonale due to extensive pulmonary fibrosis; other complications include spontaneous pneumothoraces (approximately 15% of patients), myocarditis (giant cell and/or granulomatous), renal calculi due to hypercalcemia, and gout due to hyperuricemia (152).

Beryllium Exposure and Lung Cancer. The issue of an increased incidence of lung cancer in individuals exposed to beryllium has been controversial. The weight of clinical and experimental evidence supports the presumption that beryllium is carcinogenic in humans (209–212). An IARC working group meeting reported in 1993, "The overall evaluation of the working group is that beryllium and beryllium compounds are carcinogenic to humans . . ." (212). Reviewing cases from the Beryllium Case Registry, Steenland and Ward (211) concluded that there was a lung cancer excess among cases in the registry with standard mortality that varied from 1.57 for chronic beryllium disease to 2.32 for acute beryllium disease. These findings notwithstanding, MacMahon (213) concluded that the case for increased lung cancer risk was unproved and that the excess risk of death from lung cancer in two post-1987 studies, including that of Steenland and Ward, was "compatible with a number of explanations other than that they are attributable to occupational exposure to beryllium."

REFERENCES

General

1. Parkes WR. Occupational Lung Disorders, 3rd ed. London: Butterworth-Heinemann, 1994.
2. Brooks SM. Lung disorders resulting from the inhalation of metals. Clin Chest Med 1981;2:235–254.
3. Summer W, Haponik E. Inhalation of irritant gases. Clin Chest Med 1981;2:273–287.
4. Weiss SM, Lakshminarayan S. Acute inhalation injury. Clin Chest Med 1994;15:103–116.

Macules, Small Airway Disease, and Emphysema

5. Churg A, Wright JL. Small airways disease and mineral dust exposure. Pathol Ann 1983;18:233–251.
6. Churg A, Wright JL. Small-airway lesions in patients exposed to nonasbestos mineral dusts. Hum Pathol 1983;14:688–693.
7. Wright JL, Churg A. Morphology of small-airway lesions in patients with asbestos exposure. Hum Pathol 1984;15:68–74.
8. Churg A, Wright JL, Wiggs B, et al. Small airways disease and mineral dust exposure. Am Rev Respir Dis 1985;131:139–143.
9. Wright JL, Cagle P, Churg A, et al. State of the art: disease of the small airways. Am Rev Respir Dis 1992;146:240–262.
10. Li K, Keeling B, Churg A. Mineral dusts cause collagen and elastin breakdown in the rat lung: a potential mechanism of dust-induced emphysema. Am J Respir Crit Care Med 1996;153:644–649.
11. Becklake MR. Chronic airflow limitation: its relationship to work in dusty occupations. Chest 1985;88:608–617.
12. Becklake MR. Occupational exposures: evidence for a causal association with chronic obstructive pulmonary disease. Am Rev Respir Dis 1989;140:S85–S91.
13. Becklake MR. Occupational pollution. Chest 1989;96:372S–378S.
14. Oxman AD, Muir DCF, Shannon HS, et al. Occupational dust exposure and chronic obstructive pulmonary disease: a systematic overview of the evidence. Am Rev Respir Dis 1993;148:38–48.
15. Becklake MR, Irwig L, Kielkowski D, et al. The predictors of emphysema in South African gold miners. Am Rev Respir Dis 1987;135:1234–1241.
16. Hnizdo E, Sluis-Cremer K, Abramowitz J. Emphysema type in relation to silica dust exposure in South African gold miners. Am Rev Respir Dis 1991;143:1241–1247.
17. Bégin R, Filion R, Ostiguy G. Emphysema in silica and asbestos exposed workers

seeking compensation: a CT scan study. Chest 1995;108:647–55.
18. Hnizdo E, Sluis-Cremer GK, Baskind E, Murray J. Emphysema and airway obstruction in nonsmoking South African gold miners with long exposure to silica dust. Occup Environ Med 1994;51:557–563.
19. Bégin R, Cantin A, Berthiaume Y, et al. Airway function in lifetime-nonsmoking older asbestos workers. Am J Med 1983;75:631–638.
20. Bégin R, Boileau R, Peloquin S. Asbestos exposure, cigarette smoking, and airflow limitation in long-term Canadian chrysotile miners and millers. Am J Ind Med 1987;11:55–66.
21. Jodoin G, Gibbs GW, Macklem PT, et al. Early effects of asbestos exposure on lung function. Am Rev Respir Dis 1971;104:525–535.
22. Harless KW, Watanabe S, Renzetti AD. The acute effects of chrysotile asbestos exposure on lung function. Environ Res 1978;16:360–372.
23. Rodriquez-Roisin R, Merchant JA, Cochrane GE, et al. Maximal expiratory flow volume curves in workers exposed to asbestos. Respiration 1980;39:158–165.
24. Secker-Walker RH, Ho JE. Regional lung function in asbestos workers. Respiration 1982;43:8–22.

Lung Cancer

25. International Agency for Research on Cancer. Monograph on the evaluation of carcinogenic risks to humans, vol 43: Man-made mineral fibres and radon. Lyon: International Agency for Research on Cancer, 1988.
26. International Agency for Research on Cancer. Monograph on the evaluation of carcinogenic risks to humans, vol 49: Chromium, nickel, and welding. Lyon: IARC, 1990.
27. International Agency for Research on Cancer. Monograph on the evaluation of carcinogenic risks to humans, volume 58: Beryllium, cadmium, mercury, and exposures in the glass manufacturing industry. Lyon: IARC, 1993.
28. Harington JM. Problems encountered in determining metal carcinogenesis through epidemiological studies. In: JM Duffus, ed. International Symposium on Assessment of Carcinogenic Risk from Occupational Exposure to Inorganic Substances. Cambridge, UK: Royal Society of Chemistry (in press).
29. Bernard A. Overview of epidemiologic studies on the carcinogenicity of metals. In: JM Duffus, ed. International Symposium on Assessment of Carcinogenic Risk from Occupational Exposure to Inorganic Substances. Cambridge, England, Royal Society of Chemistry (in press).0
30. Weiss W. Lung cancer and occupational lung disease. Clin Chest Med 1981;2: 289–300.
31. Enterline PE, Marsh GM. Mortality studies of smelter workers. Am J Ind Med 1980;1:251–259.
32. Welch K, Higgins I, Oh M, Burchfiel C. Arsenic exposure, smoking, and respiratory cancer in copper smelter workers. Arch Environ Health 1982;37:325–335.
33. Abramson MJ, Wlodarczyk JH, Saunders NA, Hensley MJ. Does aluminum smelting cause lung disease? Am Rev Respir dis 1989;139:1042–1057.
34. Wester PO, Brune D, Nordberg G. Arsenic and selenium in lung, liver and kidney tissue from dead smelter workers. Br J Ind Med 1981;38:179–184.
35. Stokinger HE. A review of world literature finds iron oxides noncarcinogenic. Am Ind Hyg Assoc J 1984;45:127–133.
36. Fox AJ, Goldblatt P, Kinlen LJ. A study of the mortality of Cornish tin miners. Br J Ind Med 1981;38:378–380.
37. Radford EP, Renard KGS. Lung cancer in Swedish iron miners exposed to low doses of radon daughters. New Engl J Med 1984;310:1485–1494.
38. Palmer WG, Scott WD. Lung cancer in ferrous foundry workers: a review. Am Ind Hyg Assoc J 1981;42:329–340.
39. Gibson ES, McCalla DR, Kaiser-Farrell CK, et al. Lung cancer in a steel foundry: a search for causation. J Occup Med 1983;25:573–578.

40. Weill H, McDonald JC. Exposure to crystalline silica and risk of lung cancer: the epidemiological evidence. Thorax 1996;51:97–103.
41. Samet JM. Radon and lung cancer. J Natl Cancer Inst 1989;81:745–757.
42. Morton WE, Treyve EL. Histologic differences in occupational risks of lung cancer incidence. Am J Ind Med 1982;3:441–457.
43. Weiss W, Moser RL, Auerbach O. Lung cancer in chloromethyl ether workers. Am Rev Respir Dis 1979;120:1031–1037.
44. Churg A. Lung cancer cell type and occupational exposure. In: Samet JM, ed. Epidemiology of lung cancer. New York: Marcel Dekker. 1994:413–436.
45. Saccomanno G, Archer VE, Auerbach O, et al. Histologic types of lung cancer among uranium miners. Cancer 1971;27:515–523.
46. Ives JC, Buffler PA, Greenberg SD. Environmental associations and histopathologic patterns of carcinoma of the lung. Am Rev Respir Dis 1983;128:195–209.

Iron

47. Morgan WKC, Kerr HD. Pathologic and physiologic studies of welder's siderosis. Ann Intern Med 1963;58:293–304.
48. Morgan WK. Magnetite pneumoconiosis. J Occup Med 1978;20:762–763.
49. Johnson A, Chan-Yeung M, Maclean L, et al. Respiratory abnormalities among workers in an iron and steel foundry. Br J Ind Med 1985;42:94–100.
50. Low I, Mitchell C. Respiratory disease in foundry workers. Br J Ind Med 1985;42: 101–105.
51. Sferlazza SJ, Beckett WS. The respiratory health of welders. Am Rev Respir Dis 1991;143:1134–1148.
52. Doig AT, McLaughlin AIG. X-ray appearances of the lungs of electric arc welders. Lancet 1936;1:771–772.
53. Pendergrass EP, Leopold SS. Benign pneumoconiosis. JAMA 1945;127:701–705.
54. Attfield MD, Ross DS. Radiological abnormalities in electric-arc welders. Br J Ind Med 1978;35:117–122.
55. Freedman AP, Robinson SE, O'Leary K, et al. Noninvasive magnetopneumographic determination of lung dust loads in steel arc welders. Br J Ind Med 1981;38: 384–388.
56. Kalliomaki PL, Alanko K, Korhonen O, et al. Amount and distribution of welding fume lung contaminants among arc welders. Scand J Work Environ Health 1978;4: 122–130.
57. Kalliomaki PL, Kalliomaki KK, Aittonieme K, Korhonen OS. Lungco measurement of particles retained in the lungs. Scand J Work Environ Health 1983;9:219–222.
58. Marek K, Kujawska A. Evolution of functional respiratory disorders in different types of pneumoconiosis. Bull Physiopathol Respir 1975;11:597–610.
59. Stewart MJ, Faulds JS. The pulmonary fibrosis of haematite miners. J Pathol Bacteriol 1934;39:233–253.
60. Heath D, Mooi W, Smith P. The pulmonary vasculature in haematite lung. Br J Dis Chest 1978;72:88–94.
61. Kalliomaki PL, Sutinen S, Kelha V, et al. Amount and distribution of fume contaminants in the lungs of an arc welder post mortem. Br J Ind Med 1979;36: 224–230.
62. Meyer EC, Kratzinger SF, Miller WH. Pulmonary fibrosis in an arc welder. Arch Environ Health 1967;15:462–469.
63. Faulds JS, Nagelschmidt GS. The dust in the lungs of haematite miners from Cumberland. Ann Occup Hyg 1962;4:225–263.
64. Guidotti TL, DeNee PB, Abraham JL, Smith JR. Arc welder's pneumoconiosis: application of advanced scanning electron microscopy. Arch Environ Health 1978;33: 117–124.
65. Hicks R, Al-Shamma KJ, Lam HF, Hewitt PJ. An investigation of fibrogenic and other toxic effects of arc-welding fume particles deposited in the rat lung. J Appl Toxicol 1983;3:297–306.

66. Hewitt PJ, Hicks R. An investigation of the effects of inhaled welding fume in the rat. Ann Occup Hyg 1983;16:213–221.
67. Kalliomaki PL, Tuomisaari M, Lakomaa EL, et al. Retention and clearance of stainless steel shield gas welding fumes in rat lungs. Am Ind Hyg Assoc J 1983;44: 649–654.
68. Stettler LE, Groth DH, MacKay GR. Identification of stainless steel welding fume particulates in human lung and environmental samples using electron probe microanalysis. Am Ind Hyg Assoc J 1977;38:76–82.
69. Leatherman JW, Davies SF, Hoidal JR. Alveolar hemorrhage syndromes. Medicine 1984;63:343–361.
70. Charr R. Pulmonary changes in welders: a report of three cases. Ann Intern Med 1956;44:806–812.
71. Charr R. Respiratory disorders among welders. Am Rev Tuber 1955;71:877–884.
72. Angervall L, Hansson G, Rockert H. Pulmonary siderosis in electrical welder: a note on pathological appearances. Acta Pathol Microbiol Scand 1960;49:373–380.
73. Mann BT, Lecutier ER. Arc-welder's lung. BMJ 1957;2:921–922.
74. Harding HE, McLaughlin AIG, Doig AT. Clinical, radiographic, and pathological studies of the lungs of electric-arc and oxyacetylene welders. Lancet 1958;2: 394–398.

Miscellaneous Inert Dusts

75. Doig AT. Baritosis: a benign pneumoconiosis. Thorax 1976;31:30–39.
76. Robertson AJ, Rivers D, Nagelschmidt G, Duncumb P. Stannosis: benign pneumoconiosis due to tin dioxide. Lancet 1961;1:1089–1093.
77. Rode LE, Ophus EM, Gylseth B. Massive pulmonary deposition of rutile after titanium dioxide exposure. Acta Path Micro Scand (A) 1981;89:455–461.
78. Maatta K, Arstila AU. Pulmonary deposits of titanium dioxide in cytologic and lung biopsy specimens: light and electron microscopic x-ray analysis. Lab Invest 1975; 33:342–346.
79. Dundon CC, Hughes JP. Stannic oxide pneumoconiosis. Am J Roentgenol 1950;63: 797–812.
80. Dernehl CU, Nau CA, Sweets HH. Animal studies on the toxicity of inhaled antimony trioxide. J Ind Hyg Toxicol 1945;27:256–262.
81. Pendergrass EP, Greening RR. Baritosis: AMA Archives of Ind Hyg Occup Med 1953;7:44–48.

Aluminum

82. Jephcott CM. Fume exposure in the manufacture of alumina abrasives. J Occup Med 1948;5:701–709.
83. Mitchell J, Manning GB, Molyneux M, Lane RE. Pulmonary fibrosis in workers exposed to finely powdered aluminum. Br J Ind Med 1961;18:10–20.
84. Mitchell J. Pulmonary fibrosis in an aluminum worker. Br J Ind Med 1959;16: 123–125.
85. Jordan JW. Pulmonary fibrosis in a worker using an aluminum powder. Br J Ind Med 1961;18:21–23.
86. McLaughlin AIG, Kazantzis G, King E, et al. Pulmonary fibrosis and encephalopathy associated with the inhalation of aluminum dust. Br J Ind Med 1962;19: 253–263.
87. Shaver CG, Riddell AR. Lung changes associated with the manufacture of alumina abrasives. J Ind Hyg Toxicol 1947;29:145–157.
88. Riddell AR. Pulmonary changes encountered in employees engaged in the manufacture of alumina abrasives. J Occup Med 1948;5:710–717.
89. Corrin B. Aluminum pneumoconiosis: 2. Effect on the rat lung of intratracheal injections of stamped aluminum powders containing different lubricating agents and of a granular aluminum powder. Br J Ind Med 1963;20:268–276.

90. Corrin B. Aluminum pneumoconiosis: 1. In vitro comparison of stamped aluminum powders containing different lubricating agents and a granular aluminum powder. Br J Ind Med 1963;20:264–267.
91. Gilks C, Churg A. Aluminum-induced pulmonary fibrosis: do fibers play a role? Am Rev Respir Dis 1987;136:176–179.
92. Gross P, Harley RA, deTreville RTP. Pulmonary reaction to metallic aluminum powders. Arch Environ Health 1973;26:227–236.
93. Tian-Xi H, Jun-shan L, Bao-kui T, et al. The fibrogenic effect of metallic aluminum powder in the lungs of rats and dogs. Am Rev Respir Dis 1983;127(Part 2):174.
94. Stacy BD, King EJ, Harrison CV, et al. Tissue changes in rat lungs caused by hydroxides and phosphates of aluminum and iron. J Pathol Bacteriol 1959;77: 417–426.
95. Jederlinic PJ, Abraham JL, Churg A, et al. Pulmonary fibrosis in aluminum oxide workers. Am Rev Respir Dis 1990;142:1179–1184.
96. Bellot SM, van Westrum JAFMS, Wagenvoort CA, Meijer AEFH. Deposition of bauxite dust and pulmonary fibrosis. Pathol Res Pract 1984;179:225–229.
97. Miller R, Churg AM, Hutcheon M, Lam S. Pulmonary alveolar proteinosis and aluminum dust exposure. Am Rev Respir Dis 1984;130:312–315.
98. Corrin B, King E. Pathogenesis of experimental pulmonary alveolar proteinosis. Thorax 1970;25:230–236.
99. Vallyathan V, Bergeron WN, Robichaux PA, Craighead JE. Pulmonary fibrosis in an aluminum arc welder. Chest 1982;81:372–374.
100. Herbert A, Sterling G, Abraham J, Corrin B. Desquamative interstitial pneumonia in an aluminum welder. Hum Pathol 1982;13:694–699.
101. Chen W, Monnat RJ, Chen M, Mottet NK. Aluminum induced pulmonary granulomatosis. Hum Pathol 1978;6:705–77l.
102. De Vuyst P, Dumortier P, Schandene L, et al. Sarcoidlike lung granulomatosis induced by aluminum dusts. Am Rev Respir Dis 1987;135:493–497.
103. De Vuyst P, Dumortier P, Rickaert F, et al. Occupational lung fibrosis in an aluminum polisher. Eur J Respir Dis 1986;68:131–140.

Hard Metal

104. Coates EO, Watson JHL. Diffuse interstitial lung disease in tungsten carbide workers. Ann Intern Med 1971;75:709–716.
105. Bech AO, Kipling MD, Heather JC. Hard metal disease. Br J Ind Med 1962;19: 239–252.
106. Demedts M, Ceuppens JL. Respiratory disease from hard metal or cobalt exposure: solving the enigma. Chest 1989;95:2–3.
107. Sprince NL, Oliver LC, Eisen EA, Greene RE, Chamberlin RI. Cobalt exposure and lung disease in tungsten carbide production. Am Rev Respir Dis 1988;138: 1220–1226.
108. Meyer-Bisch C, Pham QT, Mur JM, et al. Respiratory hazards in hard metal workers: a cross-sectional study. Br J Ind Med 1989;46:302–309.
109. Demedts M, Gheysens B, Nagels J, et al. Cobalt lung in diamond polishers. Am Rev Respir Dis 1984;130:130–135.
110. Nemery B, Nagels J, Verbeken E, . Rapidly fatal progression of cobalt lung in a diamond polisher. Am Rev Respir Dis 1990;141:1373–1378.
111. Davison AG, Haslam PL, Corrin B, et al. Interstitial lung disease and asthma in hard-metal workers: bronchoalveolar lavage, ultrastructural, and analytical findings, and results of bronchial provocation tests. Thorax 1983;38:119–128.
112. Shirakawa T, Kusaka Y, Fujimura N, . Occupational asthma from cobalt sensitivity in workers exposed to hard metal dust. Chest 1990;95:29–36.
113. Stebbins AI, Horstman SW, Daniell WE, Atallah R. Cobalt exposure in a carbide tip grinding process. Am Ind Hyg Assoc J 1992;53:186–192.
114. Kennedy SM, Chan-Yeung M, Marion S, et al. Maintenance of Stellite and tungsten carbide saw tips. Occup Environ Med 1995;52:185–191.
115. Sjogren I, Hillerdal G, Andersson A, Zetterstrom O. Hard metal lung disease: importance of cobalt in coolants. Thorax 1980;35:653–659.

116. Anttila S, Sutinen S, Paananen M, et al. Hard metal lung disease: a clinical, histological, ultrastructural and x-ray microanalytical study. Eur J Respir Dis 1986;69: 83–94.
117. Ohori NP, Sciurba FC, Owens GR, et al. Giant cell interstitial pneumonia and hard-metal pneumoconiosis. Am J Surg Pathol 1989;13:581–587.
118. Liebow AA. New concepts and entities in pulmonary disease. In: Liebow AA and Smith DD, eds. The lung. Baltimore: Williams & Wilkins, 1968:332–365.
119. Abraham JL, Hertzberg MA. Exposure to hard metal. Chest 1985;87:554 (letter).
120. Stettler LE, Groth DH, Platek SF. Automated characterization of particles extracted from human lungs: three cases of tungsten carbide exposure. Scanning Electron Microscopy 1983;(Part 1):439–448.
121. Kitamura H, Kitamura H, Tozawa T, Kimula Y. Cemented tungsten carbide pneumoconiosis. Acta Pathol Jpn 1978;28:921–935.
122. Hartung M, Schaller KH, Brand E. On the question of the pathogenetic importance of cobalt for hard metal fibrosis of the lung. Int Arch Occup Environ Health 1982; 50:53–57.
123. Hartung M, Valentin H. Lungenfibrosen durch Hartmetallstaube. Zen Bak Mikro Hyg (B) 1983;177:237–250.
124. Baudouin J, Jobard P, Moline J, et al. Fibrose pulmonaire interstitiele diffuse: responsabilité des métaux durs. Nouv Presse Med 1975;4:1353–1355.
125. Pelletier A, Leroy MJ, Oswald T, et al. Pneumopathie interstititelle diffuse liee au carbue de tungstene confirmes par lavage broncho-alveolaire, regressive sous corticotherapie. Rev Pneumol Clin 1984;40:131–134.
126. Scherrer M, Paramkbadathumalail A, Burki H, et al. Drei Falle von Hardmetallstaublunge. Schweiz Med Wschr 1970;100:2251–2255.

Silicon Carbide

127. Infranterivard C, Dusfresne A, Armstrong B, et al. Cohort study of silicon carbide production workers. Am J Epidemiol 1994;140:1009–1015.
128. Funahashi A, Schlueter DP, Pintar K, et al. Pneumoconiosis in workers exposed to silicon carbide. Am Rev Respir Dis 1984;129:635–640.
129. Masse S, Begin R, Cantin A. Pathology of silicon carbide pneumoconiosis. Mod Pathol 1988;1:104–108.
130. Bégin R, Dufresne A, Cantin A, et al. Carborundum pneumoconiosis: fibers in the mineral activate macrophages to produce fibroblast growth factors and sustain the chronic inflammatory disease. Chest 1989;95:842–849.

Miscellandous Causes of Interstitial Fibrosis

131. Hubbard R, Lewis S, Richards K, et al. Occupational exposure to metal or wood dust and aetiology of cryptogenic fibrosing alveolitis. Lancet 1996;347:284–289.
132. Kappenberger L, Buhlmann AA. Lungenveranderungen durch "Seltene Erden." Schweiz Med Woch 1975;105:1799–1801.
133. Vocaturo G, Colombo F, Zanoni M, et al. Human exposure to heavy metals: rare earth pneumoconiosis in occupational workers. Chest 1983;83:780–782.
134. Villar T. Vineyard sprayer's lung: clinical aspects. Am Rev Respir Dis 1974;110: 545–555.
135. Pimental JC, Marques F. 'Vineyard sprayer's lung': A new occupational disease. Thorax 1969;24:678–688.
136. Rom WN, Lockey JE, Lee JS, et al. Pneumoconiosis and exposures of dental laboratory technicians. Am J Public Health 1984;74:1252–1257.
137. Kronenberger H, Morgenroth K, Tuengerthal S. Pneumoconiosis in dental technicians: clinical, physiological, radiological, and histological findings. Am Rev Respir Dis 1981;123:127.
138. Carles P, Fabre J, Pujol M, et al. Pneumoconioses complexes chez les prothésistes dentaires. Poumon Coeur 1978;34:189–192.
139. Morgenroth K, Kroneneberg H, Michalke G, Schnabel R. Morphology and patho-

genesis of pneumoconiosis in dental technicians. Pathol Res Pract 1985;179: 528–536.
140. Kotloff RM, Richman PS, Greenacre JK, Rossman MD. Chronic beryllium disease in a dental laboratory technician. Am Rev Respir Dis 1993;147:205–207.
141. Barrett TE, Pietra GG, Maycock RL, et al. Acrylic resin pneumoconiosis: report of a case in a dental student. Am Rev Respir Dis 1989;139:841–843.

Cadmium

142. Beton DC, Andrews GS, Davies HJ, et al. Acute cadmium fume poisoning. Br J Ind Med 1966;23:292–301.
143. Anthony JS, Zamel N, Aberman A. Abnormalities in pulmonary function after brief exposure to toxic metal fumes. Can Med Assoc J 1978;119:586–588.
144. Yamamoto K, Ueda M, Kikuchi H, et al. An acute fatal occupational cadmium poisoning by inhalation. Z Rechtsmed 1983;91:139–143.
145. Bonnell JA. Emphysema and proteinuria in men casting copper cadmium alloys. Br J Ind Med 1955;12:181–195.
146. Lane RE, Campbell ACP. Fatal emphysema in two men making a copper cadmium alloy. Br J Ind Med 1954;11:118–125.
147. Davison AG, Newman-Taylor AJ, Darbyshire J, et al. Cadmium fume inhalation and emphysema. Lancet 1988;663–667.
148. Bus JS, Vinegar A, Brooks SM. Biochemical and physiologic changes in lungs of rats exposed to a cadmium chloride aerosol. Am Rev Respir Dis 1978;118:573–580.
149. Dervan PA, Hayes JA. Peribronchiolar fibrosis following acute experimental lung damage by cadmium aerosol. J Pathol 1979;128:143–149.
150. Snider GL, Lucey EC, Faris B, Jet al. Cadmium-chloride-induced air-space enlargement with interstitial pulmonary fibrosis is not associated with destruction of lung elastin. Am Rev Respir Dis 1988;137:918–923.

Beryllium

151. Krejci LE, Scheel LD. The chemistry of beryllium. In: Stokinger HE, ed. Beryllium: its industrial hygiene aspects. New York: Academic Press, 1966:45–131.
152. Parkes WR. Occupational lung disorders. 2nd ed. Boston: Butterworths, 1982: 333–358.
153. Jones William W. Beryllium disease. In: Parkes WR. Occupational lung disorders. 3rd ed. Boston: Butterworth-Heinemann, 1994:571–592.
154. Eisenbud M. Commentary and update: chemical pneumonia in workers extracting beryllium oxide. Cleve Clin Q 1984;51:441–447.
155. Reeves AL. Beryllium in the environment. Clin Toxicol 1977;10:37–48.
156. Sprince NL, Kazemi H. Beryllium disease In: Rom WN, ed. Environmental and occupational medicine. Boston: Little, Brown, 1984:481–490.
157. Sprince NL, Kazemi H. U.S. beryllium case registry through 1977. Environ Res 1980:21:44–47.
158. Hassan FM, Kazemi H. Chronic beryllium disease: a continuing epidemiologic hazard. Chest 1974;65:289–293.
159. Izumi T, Kobara Y, Inui S, et al. The first seven cases of chronic beryllium disease in ceramic factory workers in Japan. Ann N Y Acad Sci 1976;278:636–653.
160. Jones William W. Beryllium disease: pathology and diagnosis. J Soc Occup Med 1977;27:93–96.
161. Constantinidis K. Acute and chronic beryllium disease. Br J Clin Pract 1978;32: 127–136.
162. Eisenbud M, Lisson J. Epidemiological aspects of beryllium-induced nonmalignant lung disease: a 30-year update. J Occup Med 1983;25:196–202.
163. Beryllium disease among workers in a spacecraft-manufacturing plant: California morbidity and mortality weekly report. Bethesda, MD: U.S. Department of Health and Human Services: 419–425, 1983.
164. Rom WN, Lockey JE, Lee JS, et al. Pneumoconiosis and exposures of dental laboratory technicians. Am J Public Health 1984;74:1252–1257.

165. Cullen MR, Kominsky JR, Rossman MD, et al. Chronic beryllium disease in a precious metal refinery. Am Rev Respir Dis 1987;135:201–208.
166. Newman LS, Kreiss K, King TE Jr, et al. Pathology and immunologic alterations in early stages of beryllium disease. Am Rev Respir Dis 1989;139:1479–1486.
167. Kotloff RM, Richman PS, Greenacre JK, et al. Chronic beryllium disease in a dental laboratory technician. Am Rev Respir Dis 1993;147:205–207.
168. Kreiss K, Mroz MM, Zhen B, et al. Epidemiology of beryllium sensitization and disease in nuclear workers. Am Rev Respir Dis 1993;148:985–991.
169. Kreiss K, Wasserman S, Mroz MM, et al. Beryllium disease screening in the ceramics industry. J Occup Med 1993;35:267.
170. Pappas GP, Newman LS. Early pulmonary physiologic abnormalities in beryllium disease. Am Rev Respir Dis 1993;148:661–666.
171. Newman LS. Immunology, genetics, and epidemiology of beryllium disease. Chest 1996;109:40s-44s.
172. Newman LS, Kreiss K. Nonoccupational beryllium disease masquerading as sarcoidosis: identification of blood lymphocyte proliferative response to beryllium. Am Rev Respir Dis 1992;145:1212–1214.
173. Eisenbud M, Wanta RC, Dustan C, et al. Nonoccupational berylliosis. J Ind Hyg Toxicol 1949;31:282–294.
174. Kriebel D, Brian JD, Sprince NL, et al. The pulmonary toxicity of beryllium. Am Rev Respir Dis 1988;137:464–473.
175. Kreiss K, Miller F, Newman LS, et al. Chronic beryllium disease: from the workplace to cellular immunology, molecular immunogenetics, and back. Clin Immunol Immunopathol 1994;71:123–129.
176. Meyer KC. Beryllium and lung disease. Chest 1994;106:942–946.
177. Tepper LB, Hardy HL, Chamberlain RI. Toxicity of beryllium compounds. New York: Elsevier, 1961:1–107.
178. Rees PJ. Unusual course of beryllium lung disease. Br J Dis Chest 1979;73:192–194.
179. Newman LS. Beryllium disease and sarcoidosis: clinical and laboratory links. Sarcoidosis 1995;12:7–19.
180. Deodhar SD, Barna BP. Immune mechanisms in beryllium lung disease. Cleve Clin J Med 1991;Mar–Apr:157.
181. Newman LS, Buschman DL, Newell JD Jr, et al. Beryllium disease: assessment with CT. Radiology 1994;190:835–840.
182. McConnochie KMH, Adams H. The computed tomographic appearances in chronic berylliosis. Clin Radiol 1993;47:26–31.
183. Gaensler EA, Verstraeten JM, Weil WB, et al. Respiratory pathophysiology in chronic beryllium disease. Arch Ind Health 1959;19:132–145.
184. Hazard JB. Pathologic changes of beryllium disease. Arch Ind Health 1959;19: 179–183.
185. Katzenstein ALA, Askin FB. Surgical pathology of nonneoplastic lung disease. Philadelphia: WB Saunders, 1982.
186. Van Ordstrand HS. Acute beryllium poisoning. In: Vorwald AJ, ed. Sixth Saranac Symposium (1947). Pneumoconiosis: beryllium bauxite fumes, compensation. New York: PB Hoeber, 1950:65–81.
187. Dutra FR. The pneumonitis and granulomatosis peculiar to beryllium workers. Am J Pathol 1948;24:1137–1152.
188. Vorwald AJ. Medical aspects of beryllium disease. In: Stokinger HE, ed. Beryllium: its industrial hygiene aspects. New York: Academic Press, 1966:167–200.
189. Freiman DG, Hardy HL. Beryllium disease: the relation of pulmonary pathology to clinical course and prognosis based on a study of 130 cases from the U.S. Beryllium Case Registry. Hum Pathol 1970;1:25–44.
190. Jones Williams W. A histological study of the lungs in 52 cases of chronic beryllium disease. Br J Ind Med 1958;15:84–91.
191. Carrington CB, Gaensler EA, Mikus JP, et al. Structure and function in sarcoidosis. Ann N Y Acad Sci 1976;278:265–283.
192. Cholak J. The analysis of traces of beryllium. Arch Ind Health 1959;19:205–210.

193. Sprince NL, Kazemi H, Hardy HL. Current (1975) problem of differentiating between beryllium disease and sarcoidosis. Ann N Y Acad Sci 1976;654–664.
194. Robinson FR, Brokeshoulder SF, Thomas AA, Cholak J. Microemission spectrochemical analysis of human lungs for beryllium. Am J Clin Pathol 1968;49: 821–825.
195. Abraham JL, Rossi R, Marques N, Wagner RM. Ion microprobe mass analysis of beryllium in situ in human lung: preliminary results. Scanning electron microscopy 1976 (part 3), Proceedings of the workshop on techniques for particulate matter studies in SEM. ITT Research Institute, Chicago, April 1976:501–506.
196. Abraham JL. Recent advances in pneumoconiosis: the pathologist's role in etiologic diagnosis. In: Thurlbeck WM, ed. The lung: structure, function and disease. Baltimore: Williams & Wilkins, 1978:96–137.
197. Jones Williams W, Wallach ER. Laser microprobe mass spectrometry (LAMMS) analysis of beryllium, sarcoidosis, and other granulomatous diseases. Sarcoidosis 1989;6:111–117.
198. NIOSH recommendation for occupational safety and health standards. Morbidity and mortality weekly report (Suppl). Bethesda, MD: U.S. Department of Health and Human Services publication 35–315, 1985.
199. Stoeckle JD, Hardly HL, Weber AL. Chronic beryllium disease. Am J Med 1969; 46:545–561.
200. Deodhar SD, Barna B, Van Ordstrand HS. A study of the immunologic aspects of chronic berylliosis. Chest 1973;63:309–313.
201. Reeves AL. Berylliosis as an auto-immune disorder. Ann Clin Lab Sci 1976;6: 256–262.
202. Williams WR, Jones William W. Comparison of lymphocyte transformation and macrophage migration inhibition tests in the detection of beryllium hypersensitivity. J Clin Pathol 1982;35:684–687.
203. Epstein PE, Dauber JH, Rossman MD, Daniele RP. Bronchoalveolar lavage in a patient with chronic berylliosis: evidence for hypersensitivity pneumonitis. Ann Intern Med 1982;97:213–216.
204. Kern JA, Rossman MD, Daniele RP. Blood and lung T lymphocyte surface antigen expression in chronic berylliosis. Am Rev Respir Dis 1985;13 (suppl):A17 (abstract).
205. Rom WN, Lockey JE, Bank KM, et al. Reversible beryllium sensitization in a prospective study of beryllium workers. Arch Environ Health 1983;38:302–307.
206. Daniele RA, Elias JA, Epstein PE, Rossman MD. Bronchoalveolar lavage: role in the pathogenesis, diagnosis and management of interstitial lung disease. Ann Intern Med 1985;102:93–108.
207. Sprince NL, Kanarek DJ, Weber AL, et al. Reversible respiratory disease in beryllium workers. Am Rev Respir Dis 1978;117:1011–1017.
208. Andrews JL, Kazemi H, Hardy HL. Patterns of lung dysfunction in chronic beryllium disease. Am Rev Respir Dis 1969;100:791–800.
209. Kuschner M. The carcinogenicity of beryllium. Environ Health Perspect 1981;40: 101–105.
210. Aller AJ. The clinical significance of beryllium. J Trace Elem Electrolytes Health Dis 1990;4:1–6.
211. Steenland K, Ward E. Lung cancer incidence among patients with beryllium disease: a cohort mortality study. J Natl Cancer Inst 1991;83:1380–1385.
212. Meeting of the International Agency for Research on Cancer working group on beryllium, cadmium, mercury and exposures in the glass manufacturing industry. Scand J Work Environ Health 1993;19:360–363.
213. MacMahon B. The epidemiological evidence on the carcinogenicity of beryllium in humans. J Occup Med 1994;36:15.

CHAPTER 6

Coal Workers' Pneumoconiosis and Pneumoconiosis Due to Other Carbonaceous Dusts

❖ Francis H. Y. Green
❖ Val Vallyathan

The earliest morphologic description of coal workers' pneumoconiosis (CWP) is in a report by Gregory in 1831 (1) that describes black fibrotic lesions with cavitation in the lungs of British coal miners. In subsequent years conditions improved in the British mines and occupational mortality statistics published by the registrar general indicated declining mortality for coal miners. These statistics reinforced the generally held opinion that coal dust was innocuous and might even exert a beneficial effect on the lungs (2, 3). Pulmonary disease in miners was considered to be due to crystalline silica exposure. It was not until 1928 that this view was challenged by Collis and Gilchrist (4),who reported pneumoconiotic changes in the lungs of 426 coal trimmers exposed to coal dust that had been washed relatively free of silica. These findings were confirmed by Gough et al. (5) and reinforced by a series of reports published by the Medical Research Council of Great Britain showing that surface coal workers and coal trimmers developed pneumoconiosis despite low exposure to silica.

The emphasis on silica as a sole cause of pneumoconiosis was even more deeply entrenched in the United States. This was partly due to reports from the anthracite coal fields in eastern Pennsylvania, where both the prevalence of pneumoconiosis and the silica exposures were high and partly because CWP and silicosis were indistinguishable on the chest radiograph. However, in 1957 Levine and Hunter (6) demonstrated a high rate of pneumoconiosis in Ohio bituminous miners exposed to relatively low levels of silica.

Today there is general acceptance that CWP can be distinguished pathologically from silicosis. This distinction is reinforced by the observation that workers in the graphite and carbon electrode industries who are exposed to carbonaceous dusts free of silica develop pulmonary lesions morphologically identical to simple CWP (7–9). This view does not preclude a role of silica in the pathogenesis and progression of CWP, nor is it meant to imply that silica is not an important respiratory hazard in the coal mines. Indeed, approximately 12% of cases submitted to the United States National Coal Workers' Autopsy Study (NCWAS) demonstrate the pathologic lesions of silicosis (10).

This chapter is primarily concerned with the diagnosis of CWP by the pathologist. However, the pathologist is frequently required to answer complex questions regarding impairment, disability, or cause of death; therefore, reference to the mineralogic, epidemiologic, radiologic, and clinical aspects have been included so that the pathologist can place the pathologic features in perspective.

CWP is not synonymous with black lung. Black lung is a legal term (see Chapter 14) that includes, in addition to the medical condition CWP, other chronic lung conditions, notably chronic bronchitis, that are also causally related to employment in the coal mines.

COAL FORMATION AND COMPOSITION

Coal is derived from compressed organic material in sedimentary strata. Source materials, which may be recognizable in coal, include wood, bark, roots, leaves, spores, and seeds. Accumulation of these materials in swampy areas produces peat; burial of peat and the effects of heat and pressure over geologic time produce coal. The younger coals, such as lignite, are soft and closely resemble peat. Older coals, such as anthracite, are hard and glistening and contain little or no recognizable plant remains. Coal is classified according to its type, grade, and rank. Type describes the plant materials from which the coal originated; grade describes the amount of impurities (ash and sulfur) in the coal; and rank describes the degree of metamorphosis of the coal. Rank includes factors such as geologic age, percent of fixed carbon, volatile matter, moisture content, agglomerating indices, and caloric value. The four major ranks from highest to lowest are anthracite, bituminous, subbituminous, and lignite. The characteristics of these ranks are shown in Table 6.1. In the United States anthracite accounts for 1.1% of reserves and is found only in northeastern Pennsylvania. Bituminous and subbituminous coals, which account for 43% and 28% of United

TABLE 6.1
Distinctive Features of Coals of Varying Rank

RANK	PHYSICAL CHARACTERISTICS	FIXED CARBON	OXYGEN	MOISTURE CONTENT	CALORIC VALUE	GEOLOGIC AGE
Lignite	Brown to brownish black; soft; plant residues obvious	Low	High	High	Low	Young
Subbituminous	Black; dull or waxy luster; weathers easily; plant residues apparent	↓	↑	↑	↓	↓
Bituminous	Black, dense, brittle; moderately resistant to weathering; plant structure visible with microscope; burns with short blue flame					
Anthracite	Black; hard; glassy luster; brittle; resistant to weathering; usually no plant residues; burns with almost no smoke	High	Low	Low	High	Old

Adapted with permission from Meyers RA. Coal handbook. New York: Marcel Dekker, 1981:1–17.

TABLE 6.2
Major Mineral Inclusions in Coal

MINERAL CLASS	SPECIFIC MINERAL	CHEMICAL FORMULA
Alumino silicate (clay)	Illite	$(OH)_4K_2(SiAl_2)Al_4O_{20}$
	Kaolinite	$(OH)_8SiAl_4O_{10}$
Sulphide	Pyrite	FeS_2
Carbonates	Dolomite	$CaCo_3MgCo_3$
	Ankerite	$2CaCo_3MgCo_3FeCo_3$
	Calcite	$CaCo_3$
Silica	Quartz	SiO_2
Feldspars	Albite	$Na(Si_3Al)O_8$

Adapted from Meyers RA. Coal handbook. New York: Marcel Dekker, 1981: 1–17.

States reserves, respectively, are found in Appalachia and in the mid and far west. Lignite is found principally in the Dakotas, with small deposits in Texas.

When coal burns, a mineral residue, ash, is left. The ash derives from clays and sand washed into the peat swamp, inorganic materials in the plant residue, and elements derived from infiltrating groundwater. The elements in groundwater may undergo ion exchange with clays or organic matter and precipitate as minerals.

Thus coal may contain any element in the earth's crust. The most common inorganic elements in coal are silicon (1 to 4%), aluminum, iron (0.3 to 2.5%), calcium (0.1 to 2.5%), sulphur (0 to 2%), magnesium, titanium, sodium, and potassium (0 to 2%) (11). Eight trace elements, boron, mercury, lead, molybdenum, arsenic, cadmium, antimony, and selenium, are selectively enriched in coal. Many of these are cytotoxic and/or carcinogenic in low concentration. The radioactive nuclides uranium-238, uranium-235, and thorium-232 are present in trace amounts in coal deposits, usually in concentrations of a few parts per million, but relatively high concentrations are found in coal deposits in Missouri and southern Iowa and in lignite deposits in South Dakota (12). The South Dakota deposits were at one time exploited commercially for uranium.

The major mineral inclusions are shown in Table 6.2. Other minerals that occur less frequently but that may be important locally include calcium sulphate, siderite, magnetite, and mica (11, 13). The mineral matter is closely admixed within the organic matrix and so may not be biologically available.

Organic compounds are important components of coal. Benzene, cyclohexane, cyclohexanone, methylene, naphthalene, phenol, phenyl ether, polymethylene, phenanthrene, and dihydroaromatics are all present in significant amounts (14).

COAL RESOURCES AND PRODUCTION

Coal is the world's most abundant fossil fuel. The largest reserves exist in the former Soviet Union and the United States. In the United States these amount to approximately 3.6 trillion metric tons and underlie 14% of the contiguous land area. Approximately 396 billion metric tons of U.S. reserves can be mined economically for several centuries at current rates of production. Figures 6.1 and

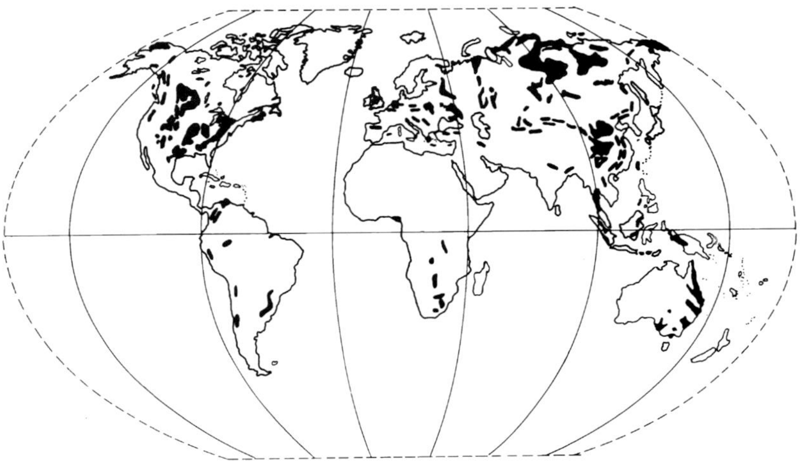

FIGURE 6.1
Distribution of coal deposits worldwide. (Reprinted with permission from Fettweiss E, Gunter B. World coal resources, methods of assessment and results: developments in economic geology, vol 10. New York: Elsevier, 1979.)

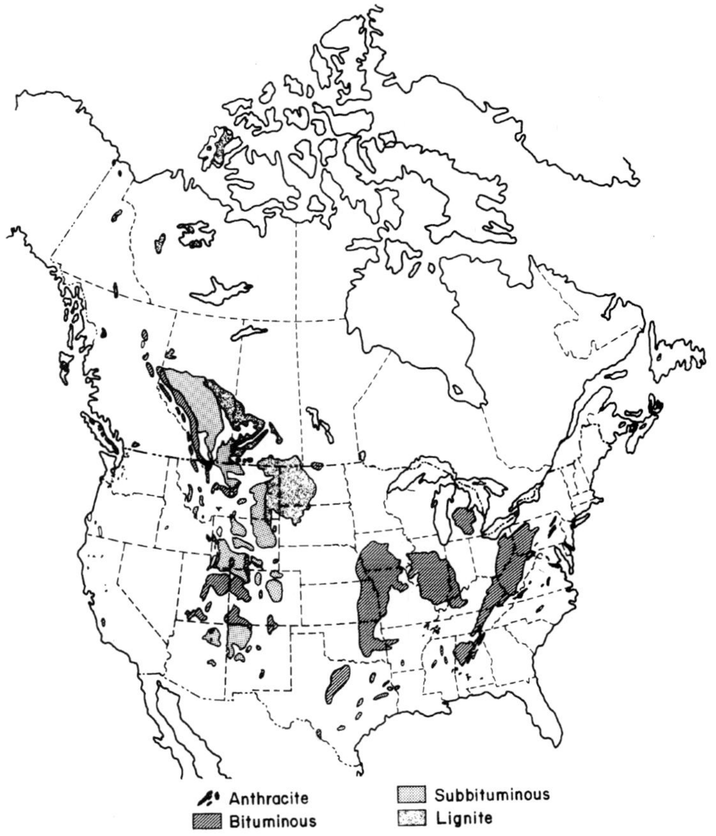

FIGURE 6.2
North American coal deposits by rank.

6.2 show the major coal deposits worldwide and in North America, respectively. China, Germany, the United Kingdom, Canada, Poland, South Africa, and Australia each have more than 60 billion metric tons of reserves. Coal seams range in thickness from a few inches to 100 feet. Those less than 2 feet thick are rarely exploited commercially.

The workforce necessary to sustain production has declined in recent decades because of mechanization and increased productivity. In 1992 an estimated 118,733 miners were employed in U.S. underground and surface coal mines (15). This contrasts with a historic high of 441,000 in 1949 (16). Since 1950, when large-scale mechanization occurred in the U.S. mines, productivity has increased fivefold (Fig. 6.3).

In developed countries coal mining is almost entirely mechanized. Two methods of coal extraction are commonly used in underground mines,. The first, called *room and pillar mining*, involves cutting a series of parallel tunnels into the coal seam and linking them by crosscuts. The cutting machine, called a *continuous miner*, can advance only several feet before the roof must be supported. This task is performed by a roof bolter, who is exposed to free silica from the overburden. The second method, *long-wall mining*, uses a system of cutting machines and hydraulic jacks that advance along a continuous face several hundred feet long. The coal is removed by a conveyer system that runs parallel to the face. As the cutting machine advances, the roof behind collapses. This method is more efficient than room and pillar mining but causes considerable subsidence. It is increasingly popular in the United States.

When the coal is close to the surface, strip or open cast mining is the most efficient method. The thickness of overburden removed at surface coal mines

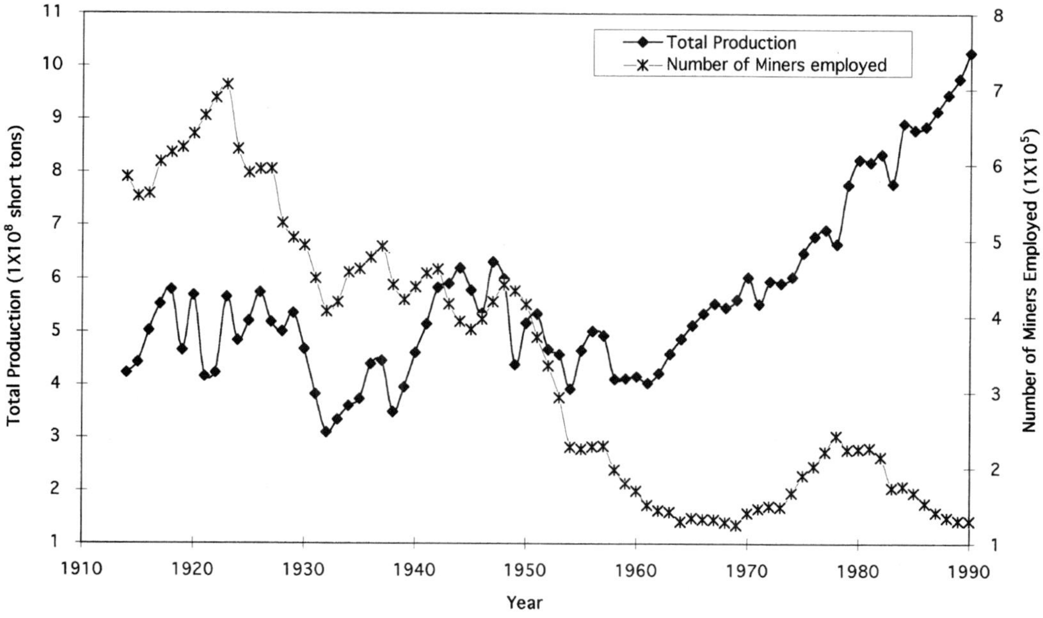

FIGURE 6.3

Number of miners employed and production of bituminous coal for U.S. mines from 1910 to 1990. (Adapted from National Institute for Occupational Safety and Health. Criteria for a recommended standard occupational exposure to respirable coal mine dust. National Institute for Occupational Safety and Health, Education and Information Division, Cincinnati, OH. Department of Health and Human Services (National Institute for Occupational Safety and Health) publication 95–106, September 1995:1–336.)

ranges from 30 to 60 feet. Many of the coal seams in the western United States are suited to strip mining, and in 1987 two-thirds of U.S. coal production was mined this way (17).

The type of mine and the specific occupation of the miner in large measure determine the health hazard. Dust exposure is generally low in surface mines, and this is reflected in a low prevalence of pneumoconiosis (18). In underground mining the greatest concentrations of respirable dust are found at the face. Workers in transportation, maintenance, and surface work are exposed to lower concentrations of dust and are thus at less risk for pneumoconiosis. Certain occupations within underground mines, such as construction, roof bolting, locomotive operation, and tunneling (19), along with overburden drilling at surface coal mines (20), are associated with increased exposure to crystalline silica. Miners employed in these jobs may develop classic silicosis (10). The risk of accidental death is also strongly linked to work within the mines. Workers with high rates of traumatic death include roof bolters and foremen. Coal loaders and electricians have relatively low rates (21).

COAL MINE DUST

The underground mining environment contains a complex mixture of suspended particulates of various shapes and sizes derived from the coal seam, adjacent rock strata, and rock dust used to dampen explosions. This mixture, which constitutes the coal mine dust, may differ in composition from the parent seam. The type of coal, the inclination of the seam, and the mining methods affect the composition of the coal mine dust (19). In addition, the relative proportions of min-

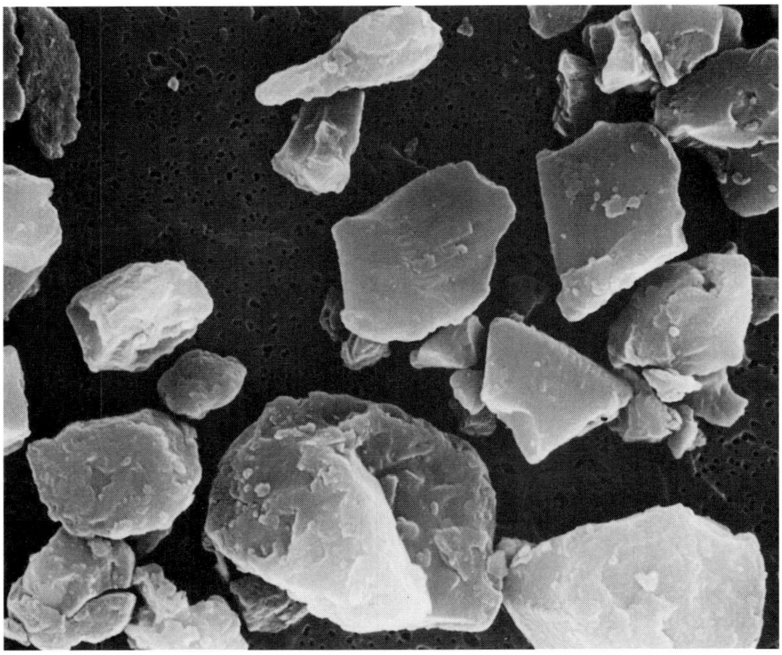

FIGURE 6.4
Scanning electron micrograph of coal dust particles. Most of the particles are within the respirable range ($< 5\mu$).

erals may vary according to particle size (22). Coal mine dust usually has a higher mineral (ash) and silica content than the parent seam (19). Dust derived from high-rank coal has more surface free radicals (23), more respirable silica (24),and a greater surface area for a given particle size (25) than lower-ranked coals. These factors have all been implicated in the pathogenesis of CWP and may account for the higher prevalence of disease in anthracite miners (10, 26).

The airborne dust within a mine is classified by its aerodynamic size into respirable, thoracic, and inhalable mass fractions. The respirable fraction (smaller than 10 μm) contains the smallest particles that can penetrate to the alveolar region of the lung (Fig. 6.4). The thoracic dust and inhalable dust fractions include larger particles that can impinge the conducting airways and nasal passages, respectively. The proportion of thoracic dust may be up to seven times greater than the respirable fraction (27).

OTHER RESPIRATORY HAZARDS IN UNDERGROUND COAL MINES

Coal mine dust is not the only respiratory hazard in mines. Diesel-powered haulage equipment has been used extensively in underground mines, though its use in underground coal mines in the United States is relatively recent. Diesel exhaust contains a large number of toxic and potentially toxic compounds, many of which have yet to be characterized. These include smoke particulates, oxides of nitrogen, sulphur dioxide, carbon dioxide, carbon monoxide, aldehydes, and hydrocarbons (28, 29). The particulate fraction of diesel exhaust is entirely within the respirable range, consisting of particles 0.01 to 0.08 μm in mass median diameter (28). For this reason diesel particulates may account for 27 to 62% of the measured respirable dust fraction in underground mines using diesel equipment (29). Hydrocarbons and gases are readily absorbed by the diesel exhaust particulates, and many of these are mutagenic and genotoxic in bioassay systems (30, 31). Animal inhalation studies designed to compare the toxicities of diesel exhaust and coal dust using levels of respirable particulate permissible in U.S. underground coal mines indicate that diesel exhaust is more toxic to the lung than coal dust (32–34). Synergism between coal dust and diesel emissions has not been demonstrated.

Very few epidemiologic studies have been conducted. A morbidity study reported by Ames et al. (35) on approximately 1000 underground coal miners working in diesel-equipped mines indicated only minor acute respiratory effects of diesel emissions on airway function. Reger et al. (36) found that the prevalence of cough and phlegm was higher among 1,646 U.S. underground miners in diesel mines than in control subjects from nondiesel mines matched for age, height, and years worked underground. Lung volumes and forced expiratory flow at 75% of forced vital capacity (FEF_{75}) were also reduced in the diesel exposed miners, indicating small airway disease. The carcinogenic potential of diesel emissions in underground coal mines has yet to be evaluated.

Other respiratory hazards in underground coal mines include toxic fumes released from electrical fires, welding and/or brazing operations, and oxides of nitrogen produced during shot firing. Small quantities of radon daughters are released from the rock strata and during the fracture of coal. These are not usually sufficiently concentrated to pose a significant health hazard (12).

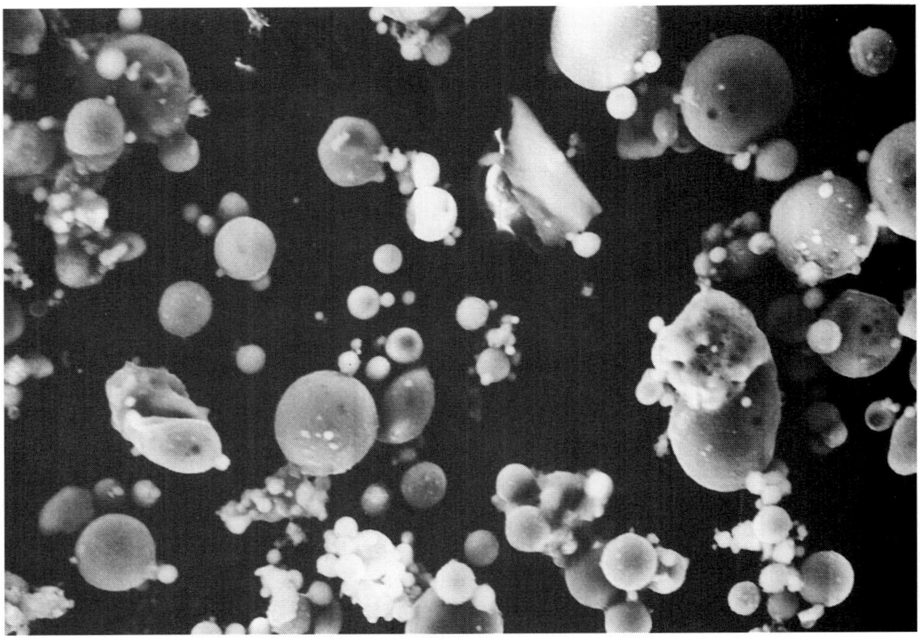

FIGURE 6.5
Scanning electron micrograph of fly ash particles.

PRODUCTS OF COAL COMBUSTION

When coal is burned in power-generating plants, the mineral inclusions fuse to form glassy, sometimes hollow aluminosilicate spheres (fly ash) (Fig. 6.5). In addition, oxides of aluminum, titanium, iron, calcium, magnesium, sodium, and potassium are formed (37). The health effects of these highly respirable particles have not been adequately characterized. Fly ash may be carcinogenic (38) but appears only weakly fibrogenic according to radiologic surveys among exposed power plant workers (39).

The mineral slags produced in certain types of coal-fired electric utility boilers are used as abrasive blasting materials. The molten slag produced from burning powdered coal is allowed to drop into water, where it frits into small, hard, sharp particles. Slags with similar properties are also formed during the smelting of copper and chromium (40). These slags contain less than 1% free silica and are being promoted as substitutes for the highly fibrogenic silica sand traditionally used in abrasive blasting. Animal studies indicate that they are considerably less fibrogenic than quartz (40).

MANDATORY DUST STANDARDS

In the United States the federal Coal Mine Health and Safety Act of 1969 (41) established permissible levels of respirable dust in underground coal mines at 2 mg/m^3, with a quartz content in the dust not to exceed 0.1 mg/m^3. The 2-mg/m^3 respirable dust standard was based on chest radiograph studies of British coal miners (42). Epidemiologic studies since 1972 have shown that miners have an elevated risk of simple and complicated CWP and chronic obstructive pulmonary disease (COPD) when exposed to respirable coal mine dust over a working lifetime at the current Mine Safety and Health Administration (MSHA) permissible exposure limit. Consequently the National Institute for Occupational Safety and Health (NIOSH) recommends that exposures to respirable coal mine dust be limited to 1 mg/m^3 as a time-weighted average (17). NIOSH estimates that the prevalence of simple CWP and progressive massive fibrosis (PMF) over a working lifetime would be reduced by 66% if the new standard were adopted. Allowable exposures in other countries are generally higher than those in the United States; the United Kingdom currently has a 3.8 mg/m^3 standard; Australia, 3 mg/m^3; and the Federal Republic of Germany a 4 mg/m^3. However, measurements in the United States and other countries may not directly correspond because of differences in sampling techniques and adjustments for silica content (17, 43).

Historically dust levels were much higher; prior to 1970, during the period of large-scale mechanization, average levels exceeded 6 mg/m^3 (3, 44). Because the latency for CWP is long, these exposures are still contributing to disease in the older population.

Respirable dust exposures are lower in surface mining facilities (17, 45), and this probably accounts for the lower prevalence of pneumoconiosis detectable in workers at these sites (18).

EPIDEMIOLOGIC STUDIES OF COAL MINERS

Mortality

Some of the best epidemiologic studies have been conducted on coal workers. Excellent reviews of these studies can be found in the writings of Merchant et al. (46), Seaton (43), Parkes (47) and NIOSH (17). Coal mining is an arduous task; hence those who enter the industry are likely to be healthier and fitter on average than individuals in the general population. This selection bias, which may influence the outcome of mortality studies, is often called the healthy worker effect. The earliest mortality studies showed an overall excess mortality in coal workers that was due as much to specific occupational factors as to the poor socioeconomic conditions prevailing at the time (48). Today the life expectancy of a coal miner is approximately that of the general population (49). Excess deaths are seen for specific causes, including nonmalignant respiratory disease, accidents, and stomach cancer (50–58). Approximately 4% of coal miner deaths are directly attributable to pneumoconiosis (10, 56). The excess mortality from pneumoconiosis is primarily associated with PMF (51, 55–57). Death from pneumoconiosis, chronic bronchitis, and emphysema has been related to cumulative dust exposure (51, 58). Excess deaths from these causes are counterbalanced by decreased mortalities from lung cancer (59) and ischemic heart disease (49, 60).

Prevalence

Epidemiologic studies involving large populations of miners in Britain and the United States have shown that the most important factor determining risk and progression of simple CWP is cumulative exposure to respirable dust (17, 42, 61, 62). In recent decades the prevalence of CWP has been declining in western industrial countries because of the institution and enforcement of strict dust controls (63). Results of the most recent NIOSH coal workers' x-ray surveillance

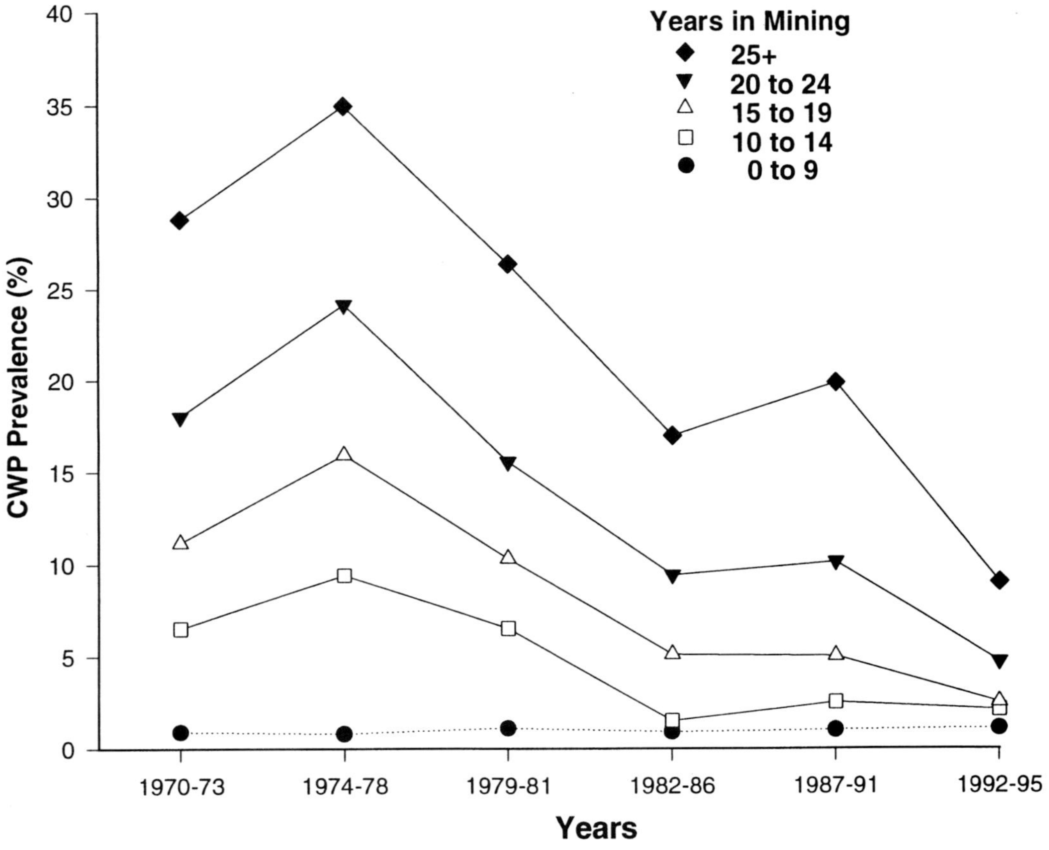

FIGURE 6.6
Declining prevalence of pneumoconiosis in U.S. coal mines from 1970 to 1995. (Adapted from National Institute for Occupational Safety and Health. Criteria for a recommended standard occupational exposure to respirable coal mine dust. National Institute for Occupational Safety and Health, Education and Information Division, Cincinnati, OH. Department of Health and Human Services (National Institute for Occupational Safety and Health) publication 95–106, September 1995:1–336.)

program (1970–1995) involving more than 100,000 American miners show that the prevalence of CWP has decreased from 21.2% in 1970 to approximately 3% in 1995 (17). Risk of both simple CWP and PMF increases with length of employment underground but is rare in those with fewer than 10 years of mining experience (Fig. 6.6). Studies of active miners include a predominance of young miners. Ex-miners who leave the workforce for health-related reasons have a higher prevalence of CWP (64). Autopsy populations are likely to be older, have had greater dust exposures, and include more miners who have retired for health reasons and therefore have a greater prevalence of disease.

The prevalence of CWP is also affected by regional factors. In the United States the prevalence of disease decreases progressively from east to west (46). Similarly, miners from southern Wales develop more severe pneumoconiosis than miners in Scotland (65). These differences, which are noted at equivalent exposure levels, suggest that coal mine dusts vary in their toxicity. Although cigarette smoking impairs clearance of particles deposited in the lungs (66), there is no evidence that cigarette smoking affects the attack rate of CWP (67, 68).

Other host factors may play a role in the pathogenesis of the disease (17, 48, 69–71).

CLINICAL FEATURES OF COAL WORKERS' PNEUMOCONIOSIS

CWP is defined as parenchymal lung disease resulting from a host response to coal dust in the lung. Simple CWP is usually diagnosed on an abnormal chest radiograph. The severity of the disease is classified according to the number, size, and shape of small opacities on the chest radiograph using a system of standard reference films developed by the International Labour Office (ILO) (72) (see Chapter 1). The most common radiologic abnormality in simple CWP is multiple, small rounded opacities (p-, q-, or r-size) that predominate in the upper zones of the lungs (43, 46, 47). Approximately 6% of working U.S. coal miners show small irregular opacities, either alone or with rounded opacities (73). Unlike PMF, radiographic progression of simple CWP is unusual after cessation of exposure (43, 47, 70).

Most miners with simple CWP have no symptoms or physical signs. A proportion of miners develop chronic cough and produce sputum that may be tinged black. This condition, known as *industrial bronchitis*, is thought to be a reaction of the airways to the larger dust particles and is seen in miners with and without radiographic evidence of CWP (74). It is nonspecific, occurring in workers in other dusty trades (75). Dyspnea, while not a feature of simple CWP, may be seen in miners with COPD. Carefully controlled studies of miners with simple CWP have demonstrated several minor abnormalities of pulmonary function. These include minimal reductions of ventilatory capacity and small increases in residual volume. Diffusing capacity may be slightly reduced in miners with p-size (small) opacities (76). Minor abnormalities of ventilation and perfusion may be seen, and the arterial oxygen pressure may be slightly low at rest (43). These abnormalities are most noticeable in miners with higher categories of simple CWP and are also found in nonsmoking miners (77). They are not usually associated with clinical symptoms. The specific basis of these abnormalities and their significance have been recently reviewed by Lapp and Parker (78).

Complicated CWP or PMF, by contrast, is associated with pulmonary disability and premature death (70, 71). It usually develops from a background of severe simple CWP, categories 2 and 3. Although category A PMF may produce no symptoms, categories B and C are associated with severe airway obstruction, restrictive defects, uneven ventilation and perfusion, reduced diffusing capacity, and low arterial oxygen pressure leading eventually to pulmonary hypertension and cor pulmonale (78). The most common initial symptoms are shortness of breath, cough, and sputum. Later stages are likely to be dominated by the signs and symptoms of congestive cardiac failure. The disease progresses even in the absence of further dust exposure (43, 47, 70, 71, 78).

PMF may be confused with carcinoma, tuberculosis, and mycotic infections. All of these conditions produce large radiographic opacities with a tendency to cavitate. PMF is usually bilateral and occurs against a background of nodular simple CWP; these features are useful in distinguishing it from carcinoma. Tuberculosis and other mycobacterial infections may be found in association with PMF. Clinical and bacteriologic testing should be conducted on all patients with PMF to exclude these conditions. Open lung biopsy may be required to establish the diagnosis of PMF but is rarely if ever indicated in simple CWP.

PATHOLOGIC FEATURES OF COAL WORKERS' PNEUMOCONIOSIS

The first accurate descriptions of the pathologic anatomy of CWP were made by Heppleston (79) and Gough et al. (5). Prior to this it was generally thought that CWP was diffuse. It is now generally accepted that the lesions of CWP are focal and specific, occurring in coal workers exposed to coal mine dust irrespective of geographic location of the mine.

The pneumoconiosis of coal workers is radiologically categorized into simple and complicated forms. Simple CWP corresponds to the macular and nodular lesions, and complicated CWP corresponds to PMF and the lesions of rheumatoid pneumoconiosis (Caplan's syndrome). In addition, coal miners are at increased risk for silicosis and COPD.

Although numerous epidemiologic studies have been conducted to determine the prevalence of CWP in active mining populations, very few autopsy prevalence studies have been reported. Data derived from autopsied populations are likely to indicate higher prevalences of disease than are reported in active miners for two reasons. First, autopsy populations are likely to be older and hence have longer latencies and job tenures and to have received their exposures dur-

TABLE 6.3
Demographic Characteristics of the U.S. National Coal Workers Autopsy Study

Number	3,365
Race/sex	94% white males
Mean age (years) at death	63 ± 12 (SD)
Cigarette smokers (ever)	74%
Average pack year consumption for smokers	24 ± 20
Average years worked in underground mines	26 ± 14 (SD)

Adapted from Green FHY, Althouse R, Weber KC. Prevalence of silicosis at death in underground coal mines. Am J Ind Med 1989;16:605–616.

TABLE 6.4
Prevalence of Pneumoconiosis in the U.S. National Coal Workers' Autopsy Study, 1971–1980

TYPE OF LESION	PERCENT SHOWING LESION
Macules	45.6
Macules with focal emphysema	35.8
Nodules (CWP type)	18.9
PMF	5.5
Silicotic nodules	
Lung parenchyma	12.6
Tracheobronchial lymph nodes	52.9

Adapted from Green FHY, Althouse R, Weber KC. Prevalence of silicosis at death in underground coal mines. Am J Ind Med 1989;16:605–616.

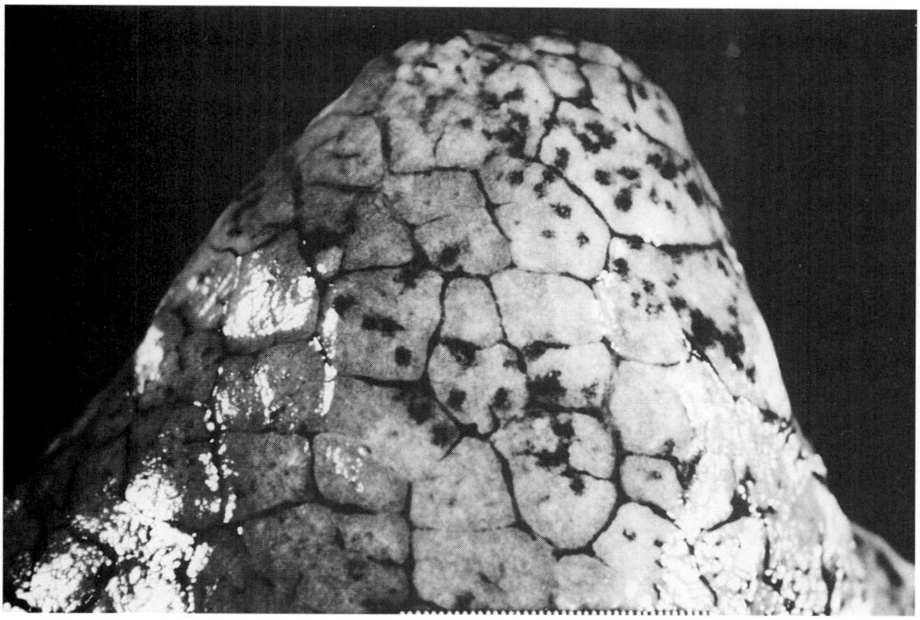

FIGURE 6.7.
Apical pleural surface of coal miner's lung. The black pigment outlines the pleural lymphatic vessels at junctions of lobular septa with the pleura. The focal pigmented areas correspond to accumulations of pigmented macrophages in the subpleural connective tissue and adjacent alveoli.

ing periods when dust levels were high. Second, pathologic techniques are more sensitive than radiology in detecting less severe categories of disease (80–83). The prevalence of various types of pneumoconiotic lesions in cases submitted to the NCWAS (Table 6.3) are shown in Table 6.4. The NCWAS is a voluntary program covering an estimated 10% of coal workers who die. Like all autopsy programs, it suffers from selection biases; however, the population appears fairly representative of all miners, as it is similar demographically to active miners in the United States (10). Although the prevalence of pneumoconiosis is high in this population, deaths from CWP are relatively infrequent, accounting for only 4.1% of all deaths (10). The NCWAS population has mortality rates for CWP similar to those reported in epidemiologic mortality studies (54).

Pleural and Lymphatic Changes

The pleural surfaces of a coal worker's lung show an irregular pattern of bluish-black pigmentation that corresponds to the junctional sites of septal lymphatic vessels and the pleura (Fig. 6.7). These changes are not specific and similar, but less marked pigment is seen in city dwellers and cigarette smokers. The pleura is not usually appreciably thickened unless subpleural nodules or PMF is present. Similar to those seen in silicosis, subpleural nodules are easily palpable and have pale raised centers surrounded by a rim of black pigment (see Chapter 7). Subpleural and intrapulmonary lymph nodes may grossly mimic nodules but are easily distinguished by histologic examination.

Peribronchial, hilar, paratracheal, and occasionally abdominal lymph nodes are enlarged, black, and firm. Microscopically the lymph nodes show large num-

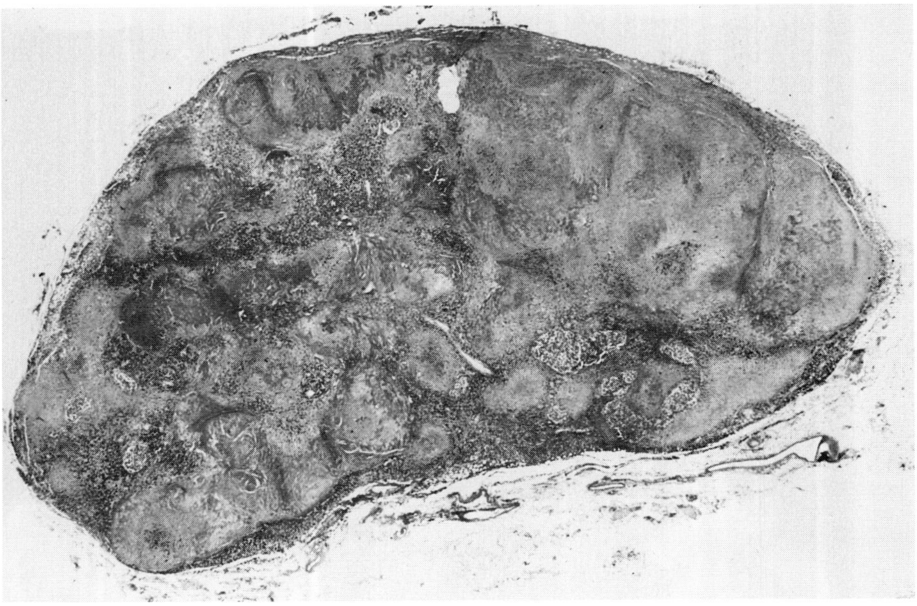

FIGURE 6.8
Section of hilar lymph node from 72-year-old Pennsylvania miner who was employed for 38 years underground, principally as a pipe man. Discrete and confluent silicotic nodules are visible throughout the node. Silicotic lesions were not seen in the lungs.

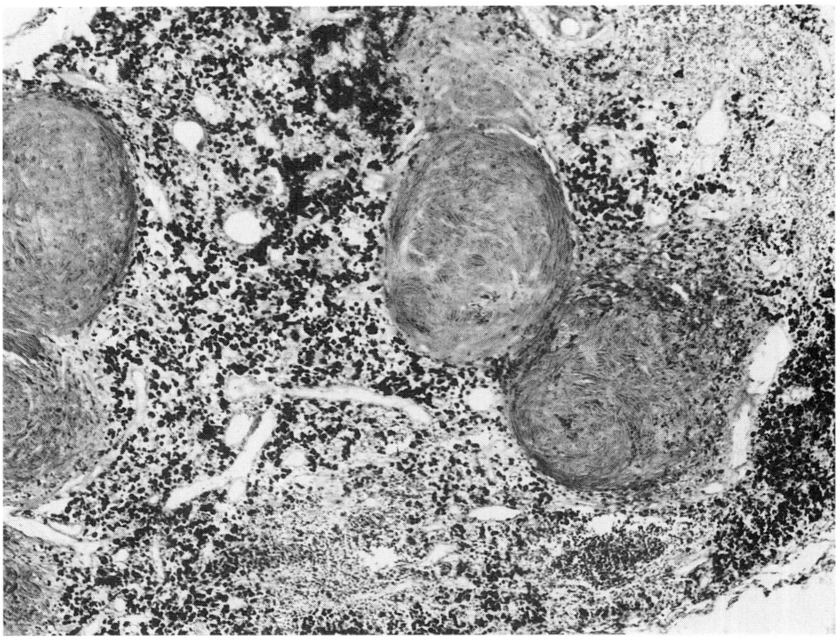

FIGURE 6.9
Silicotic nodules in tracheobronchial lymph node of coal miner. The nodules are histologically identical to those seen in the parenchyma.

bers of pigmented histiocytes and variable degrees of fibrosis. Silicotic nodules are frequently observed in the tracheobronchial lymph nodes of coal workers, usually in the absence of silicotic lesions in the pulmonary parenchyma (Table 6.4) (Figs. 6.8 and 6.9). This phenomenon is due to selective enrichment of quartz in pulmonary lymph nodes (84, 85). Black pigment is also seen in sections of spleen and liver from miners (86), and silicotic nodules are occasionally observed in the spleen.

Coal Dust Macules

On cut section an inflated lung shows numerous uniformly distributed focal areas of black pigmentation (Figs. 6.10 to 6.12). These coal macules may number up to six in each secondary lobule. The density of the lesions is greatest in the upper lobes and upper portions of the middle and lower lobes. The macules range in size from 0.5 to 6 mm in diameter and have irregular borders. The macules are not firm to palpation, and this feature can be used to distinguish them from nodular lesions. The airspaces around the macule are usually enlarged (focal emphysema) (Fig. 6.12).

Microscopically the macule is composed of coal dust–laden macrophages within the walls of the respiratory bronchioles and adjacent alveoli (Figs. 6.13 and 6.14). A fine network of reticulin and collagen runs between the closely packed macrophages. The amount of collagen is variable, probably reflecting the proportion of fibrogenic mineral in the inhaled coal mine dust (87). The lungs of active or recently retired miners also show accumulations of black macrophages in the alveoli adjacent to the respiratory bronchioles (Figs. 6.15 and 6.16). The walls of the affected alveoli are closely opposed to these cells. Incorporation of these aggregates into the walls of respiratory bronchioles may be the mechanism whereby macules evolve (88). For a more detailed discussion of the pathogenesis of macules see Chapter 2.

Macules are also observed in association with exposure to lignite (Fig. 6.17), other carbonaceous dusts (8, 89, 90) (Fig. 6.18), some silicate minerals (see Chapter 8) and some metals (see Chapter 4). Coal dust–containing macrophages are also seen in the connective tissue sheaths of the small pulmonary arteries, bronchi, and veins and in the subpleural and paraseptal connective tissues. This dust distribution is associated with paraseptal emphysema.

Heavy cigarette smokers and residents of polluted urban areas may also develop macules (91). These are frequently labeled anthracosis. This term is best avoided, as it has a specific meaning under black lung legislation in the United States (see Chapter 14). Centriacinar accumulations of black pigment in coal miners can be adequately described without resort to the term *anthracosis*, and the specific nature of the pigment or pigments can be reliably ascertained by microscopic examination. Particles of bituminous coal, when viewed under intense illumination at high magnification, appear as translucent brown or golden brown particles with angular borders (92) (Fig. 6.16). Combustion products of cigarettes and fossil fuels are smaller, opaque, and black, and they have rounder borders.

Focal Emphysema

A zone of enlarged airspaces within and around the coal dust macule, called focal emphysema, is sufficiently common to be considered an integral part of the

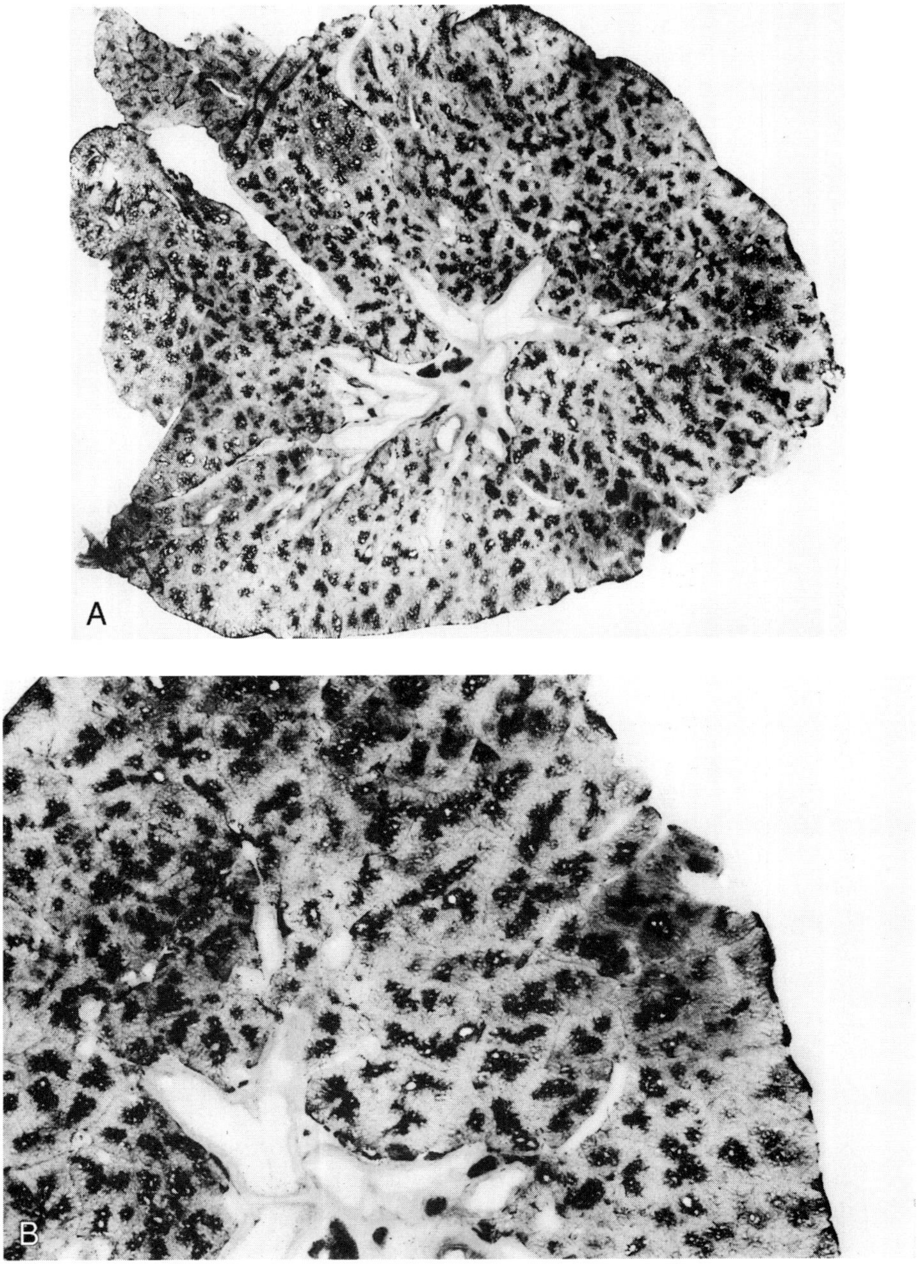

FIGURE 6.10

A. Whole lung section from coal worker showing characteristic lobular distribution of coal dust macules. The miner was 48 years old and had worked underground for 18 years. **B.** Close-up of same patient showing the centriacinar distribution of dust. Focal emphysema is minimal. (Reprinted with permission from Green FHY, Laqueur WA. Coal workers' pneumoconiosis. Pathol Ann 1980;15:333–409.)

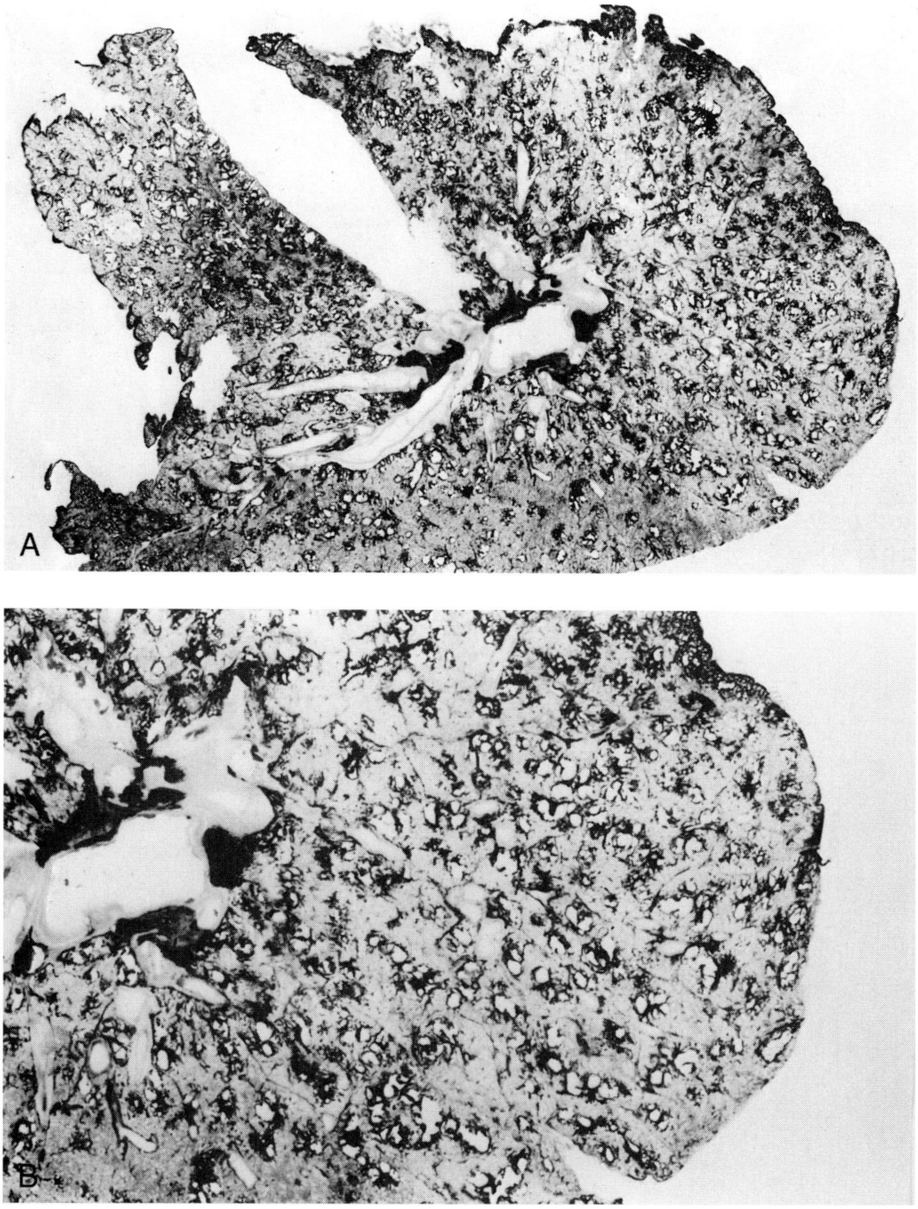

FIGURE 6.11
A. Whole lung section from 80-year-old coal miner from West Virginia whose principal job was loader and machine man. The lung shows coal dust macules with focal emphysema. The miner was a nonsmoker. **B.** Close-up showing relationship of macule to the focal emphysema.

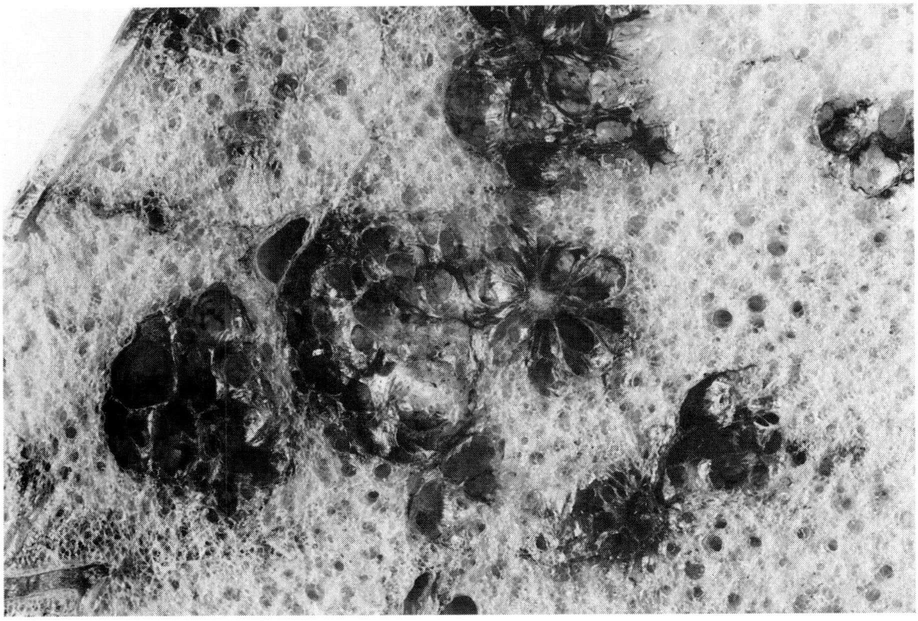

FIGURE 6.12
Cut surface of inflated and freeze-dried coal miner's lung showing coal dust macules with focal emphysema; the lesion at center may be a micronodule. Note the relationship between pigment and emphysema.

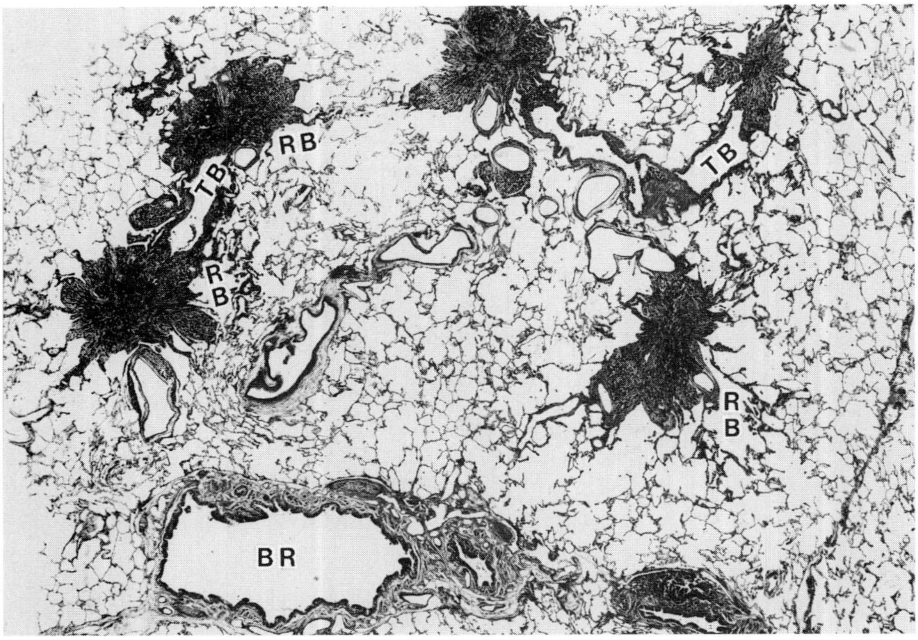

FIGURE 6.13
Section of lung from 59-year-old Pennsylvania coal miner, a cigarette smoker, employed 25 years underground, principally as continuous mining machine operator. The section shows several typical coal dust macules with focal emphysema. Note the centriacinar distribution of the macules. BR, bronchus; TB, terminal bronchiole; RB, respiratory bronchiole.

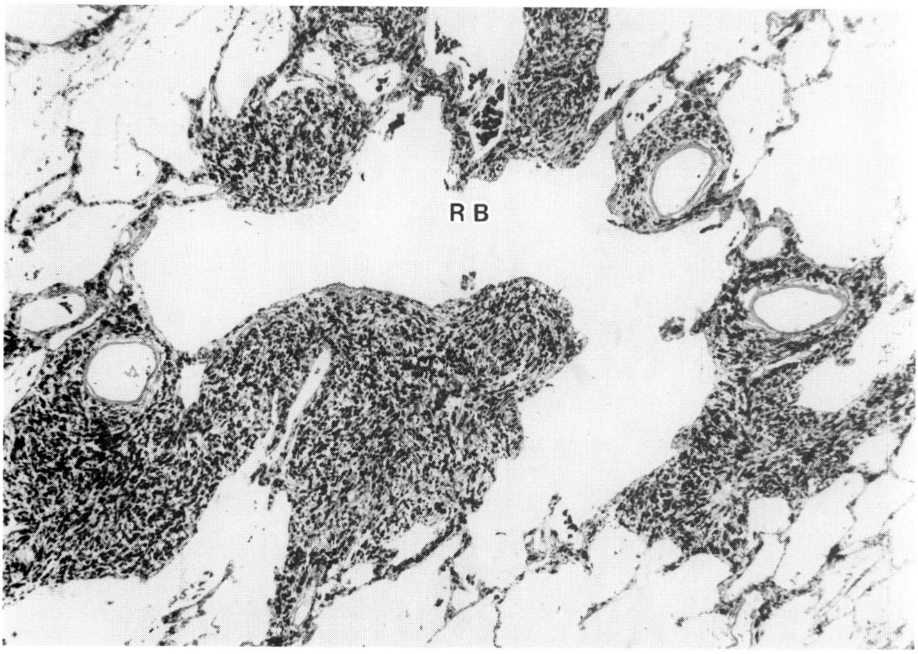

FIGURE 6.14
Same patient as **FIGURE 6.13**. Longitudinal section of coal dust macule showing its relationship to a respiratory bronchiole (RB). Very little collagen is seen in this lesion.

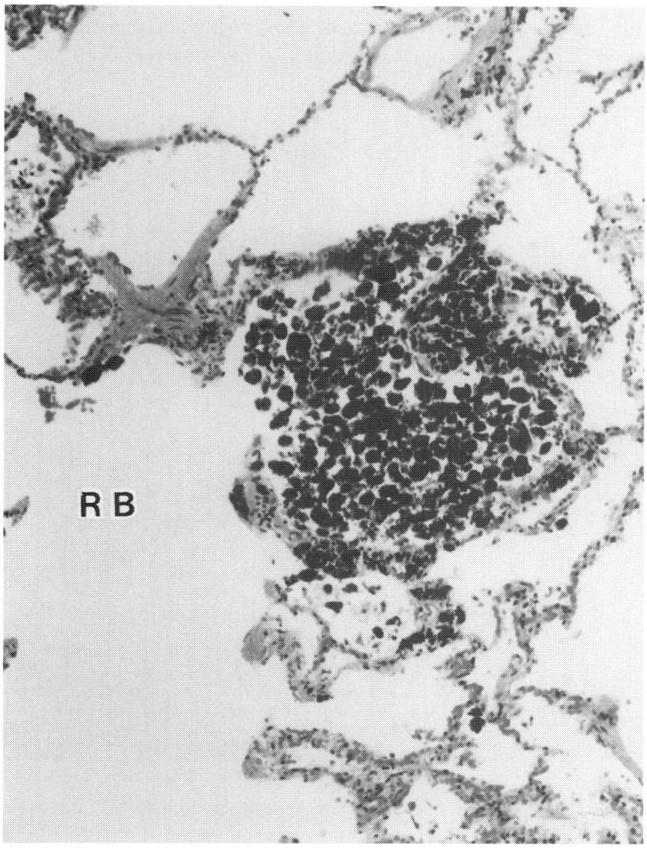

FIGURE 6.15
Section of lung from a 31-year-old coal miner killed in an underground explosion. Clusters of pigmented macrophages pack an alveolus adjacent to a respiratory bronchiole (RB).

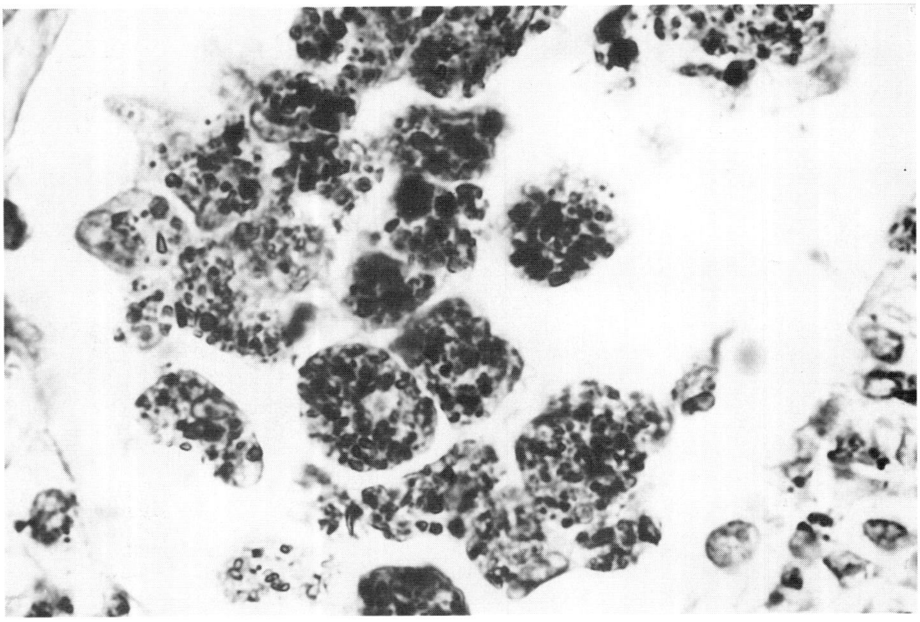

FIGURE 6.16
High-power view of coal dust particles within alveolar macrophages. The intracytoplasmic coal dust particles have a mean diameter of approximately 0.7 mm and angular borders. The latter feature distinguishes them from carbonaceous combustion products. Although each macrophage contains several hundred dust particles, they remain viable.

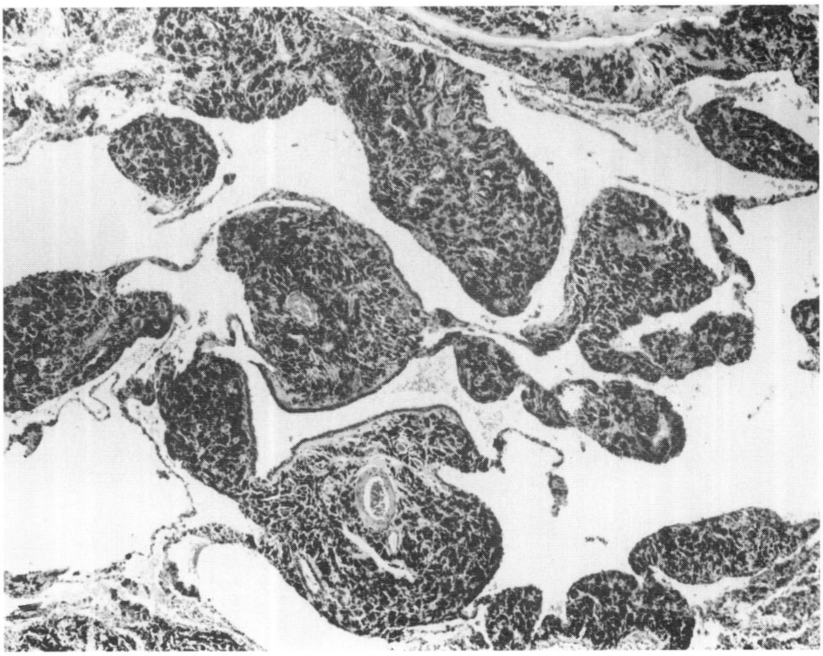

FIGURE 6.17
Macule in a lignite worker. The lesion shows marked focal emphysema. (Courtesy of Drs. E. E. Buckner, C. F. Campbell, and T. L. Rankin.)

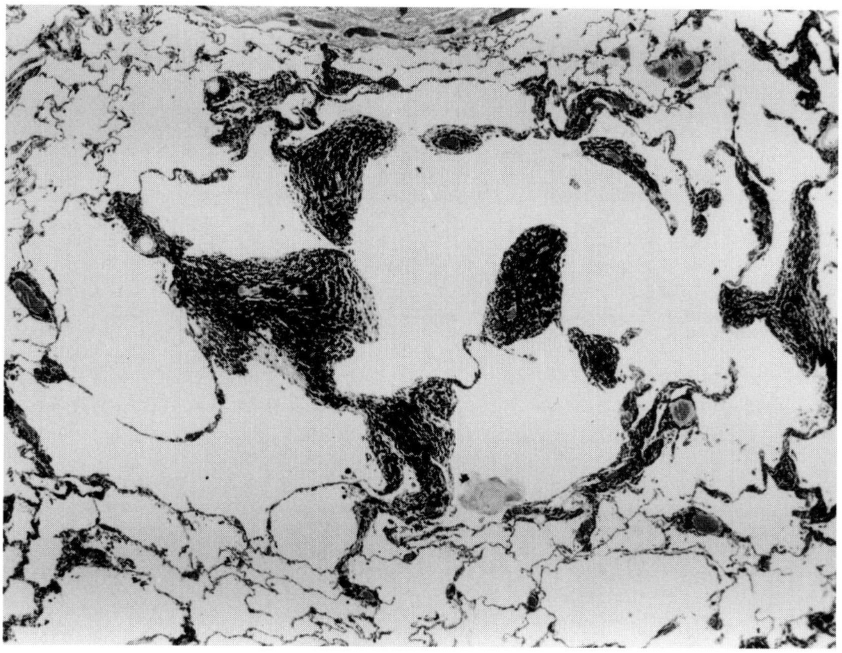

FIGURE 6.18
Lung section from reclusive man who lived in a confined cabin for 40 years. The only source of light and heat was an open kerosene lamp. The section shows a characteristic carbon macule with associated focal emphysema.

lesion of simple CWP and is a necessary criterion for its diagnosis (91). Focal emphysema is a form of centriacinar emphysema. Both involve the proximal acinus and are characterized by airspace dilation and tissue destruction. Thus they can be distinguished only by the presence of coal dust within the walls of the respiratory bronchiole. Focal emphysema occurs in miners who have never smoked (93).

The pathogenesis of focal emphysema is thought to involve secretion of proteolytic enzymes by coal dust–activated macrophages resulting in the inactivation of ${}_1$-antitrypsin and consequent destruction of alveolar and respiratory bronchiolar walls (94). Altered mechanical forces in the region of the macule may also be involved (95). It appears to follow the formation of the macule, as younger miners killed in accidents rarely show the lesion.

Microscopically the initial stages of focal emphysema are characterized by dilation of the respiratory bronchioles at the sites of maximum dust deposition (Figs. 6.18 and 6.19). As the lesion progresses, bronchiolar smooth muscle atrophies (95), and this is succeeded by destructive changes common to all forms of emphysema (abnormal fenestrations, fragmentation of elastic fibers, and loss of septal capillaries). The latter features are more severe in coal miners who are also heavy cigarette smokers. Except in very severe cases the distal portion of the acinus remains unaffected.

Focal emphysema may account for the increases in residual volume and slight decreases in elastic recoil that have been demonstrated in both smoking and nonsmoking miners with simple CWP (96, 97).

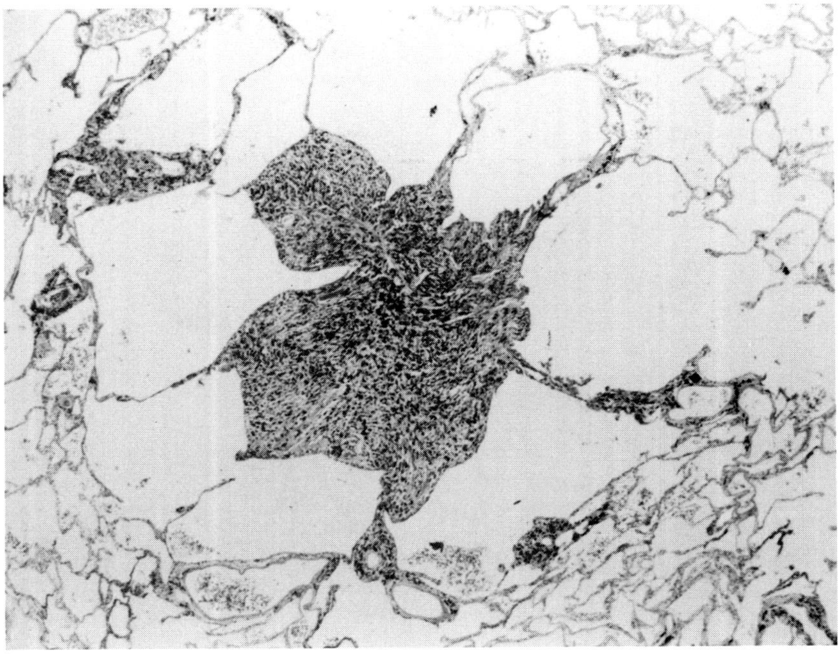

FIGURE 6.19
Section of lung from a retired coal miner showing a coal dust macule and associated focal emphysema. The dust in the alveoli but not in the interstitium has cleared since he left the mines.

Coal Nodules

The nodular lesions of CWP are a form of mixed-dust pneumoconiosis that result from exposure to silica in combination with less fibrogenic dusts, including coal, iron oxides, and silicates (98) (see Chapters 7 and 8). They are classified as micronodules or macronodules (91). Nodules may be the only lesions in the lung but are more commonly seen against a background of macules. Like macules, they are more numerous in the upper zones. Unlike macules, they are not confined to the respiratory bronchioles but are also seen in the subpleural and peribronchial connective tissues. Nodules are firm on palpation and have round, irregular, or serpiginous borders and may be surrounded by enlarged airspaces (Fig. 6.20). There is a tendency for nodules to cluster (Fig. 6.21) and eventually coalesce to produce PMF (Fig. 6.22). Nodules with pale or calcified centers usually demonstrate a silicotic component on microscopy.

Nodules consist of dust-laden macrophages in a fibrotic stroma composed of collagen and reticulin (Figs. 6.23–6.29). The collagen fibers characteristically lack orientation and are arranged in interlacing bundles. A tendency of the collagen to be arranged concentrically (Fig. 6.23) indicates high quartz exposure (87). Nodules centered on respiratory bronchioles probably develop through progressive enlargement and collagenization of pre-existing macules. This type of nodule usually shows a zone of enlarged airspaces at its periphery (Figs. 6.25, 6.26). Degenerative changes commonly observed in the nodular lesions include calcification, cholesterol clefts, and cavitation (Figs. 6.28 and 6.29). Destructive vascular changes similar to those seen in PMF are frequently found in the larger nodules.

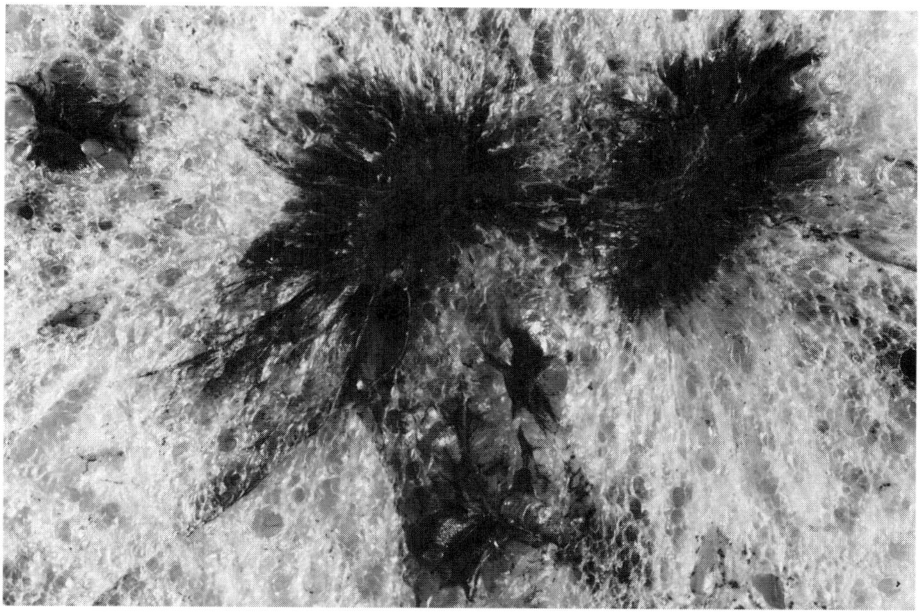

FIGURE 6.20
Same patient as FIGURE 6.12 showing two 0.5-cm-diameter micronodules. The perivascular location is characteristic. There is mild airspace enlargement adjacent to the nodules (scar emphysema).

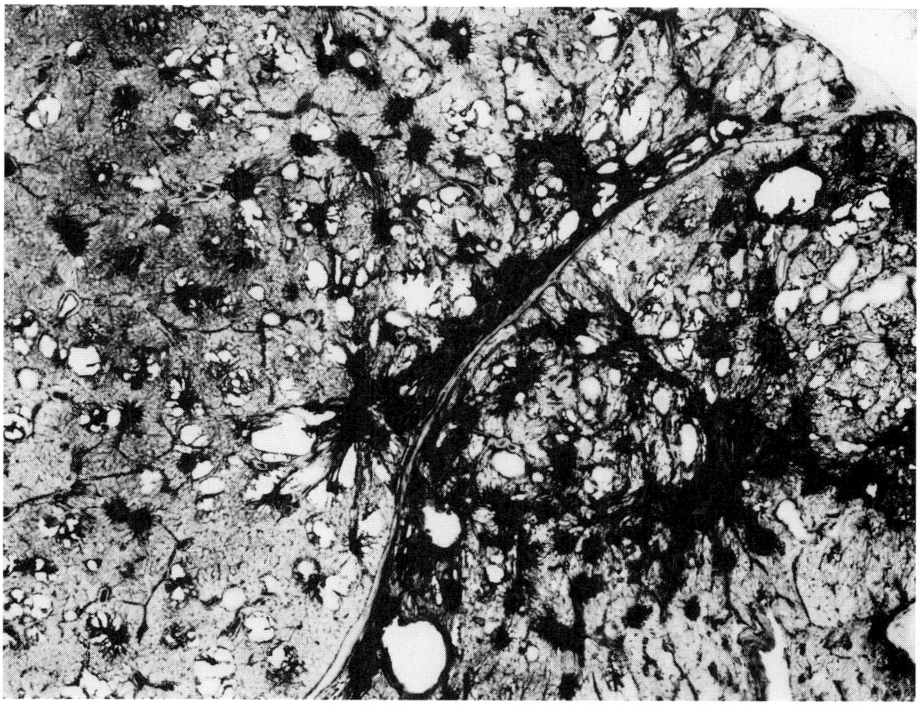

FIGURE 6.21
Close-up of whole lung section showing micronodules and macronodules that are becoming confluent adjacent to the lobar fissure. Macules with focal emphysema are seen at left. From an 80-year-old coal miner and cigarette smoker with 22 years' work in underground mines.

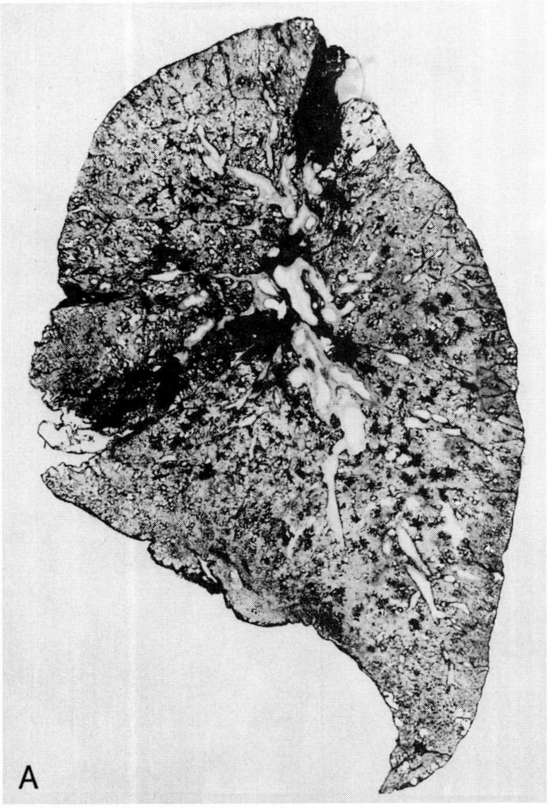

FIGURE 6.22

A. Whole lung section from coal miner showing small PMF lesion at apex set against a background of severe nodular and macular simple CWP. The miner was 90 years old and had worked underground for 43 years. He retired 25 years before death. This case illustrates the slow rate of clearance of dust from the lungs. **B.** Chest radiograph from same patient. ILO-80 classification of this radiograph was category 2/3 profusion small opacities; size/shape q/t; all zones affected. Category A large opacities (PMF) and diffuse pleural thickening.

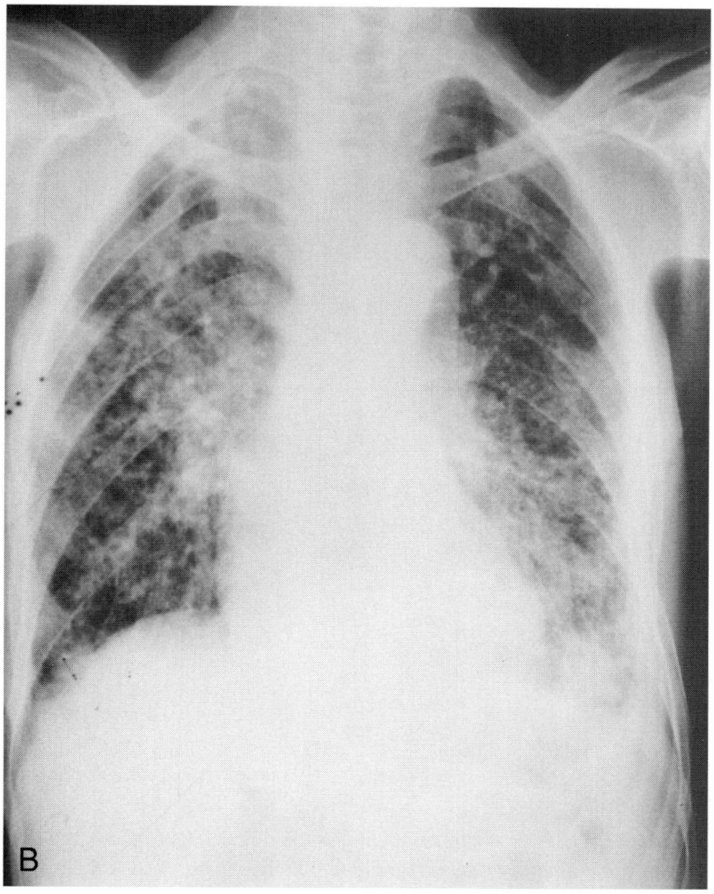

FIGURE 6.22 *(continued)*

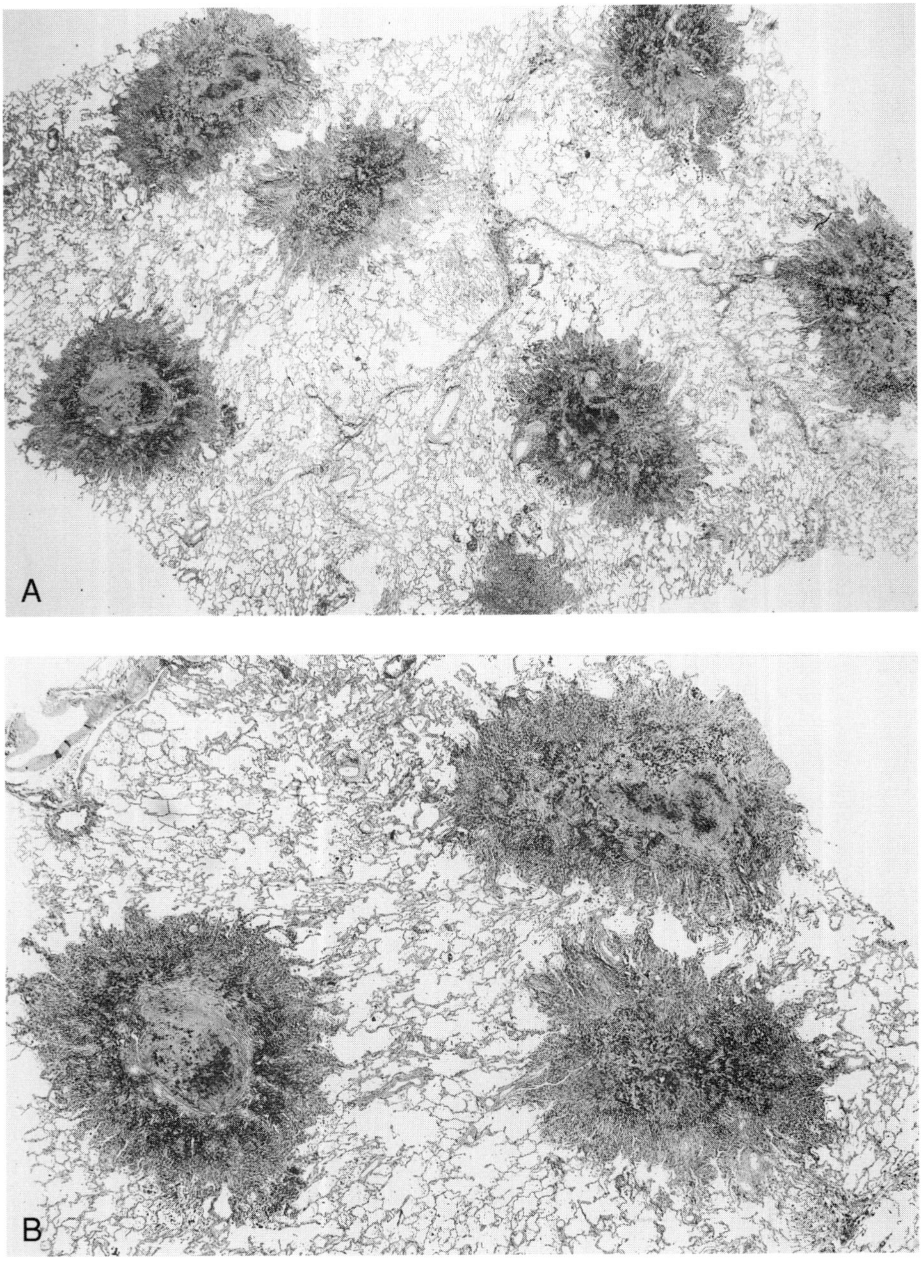

FIGURE 6.23

A. Micronodules. The centriacinar distribution of the nodules suggests origin in the walls of respiratory bronchioles. Microscopic section from the lung of a 59-year-old Pennsylvania coal miner who worked 35 years underground, principally as a continuous mining machine operator. Former cigarette smoker. **B.** Close-up of three nodules from case illustrated in **A**. The nodules show varying amounts of collagen; the concentric arrangement of the collagen in the nodule at left indicates high silica content.

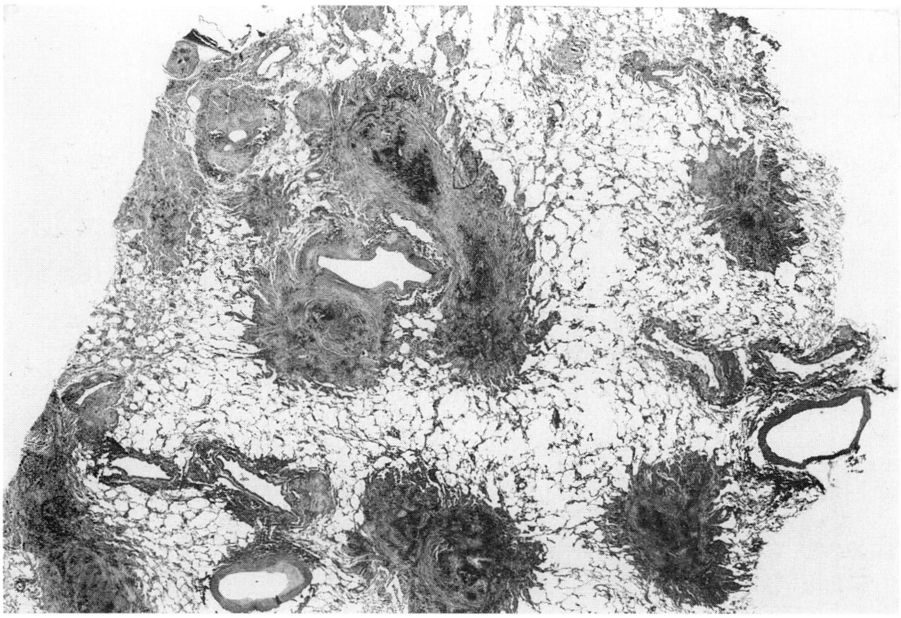

FIGURE 6.24
Micronodules showing central hyalinization of collagen. The perivascular location and tendency to coalesce seen at center are characteristic. From a 59-year-old Pennsylvania coal miner and former smoker, employed 40 years underground, principally as a continuous mining machine operator.

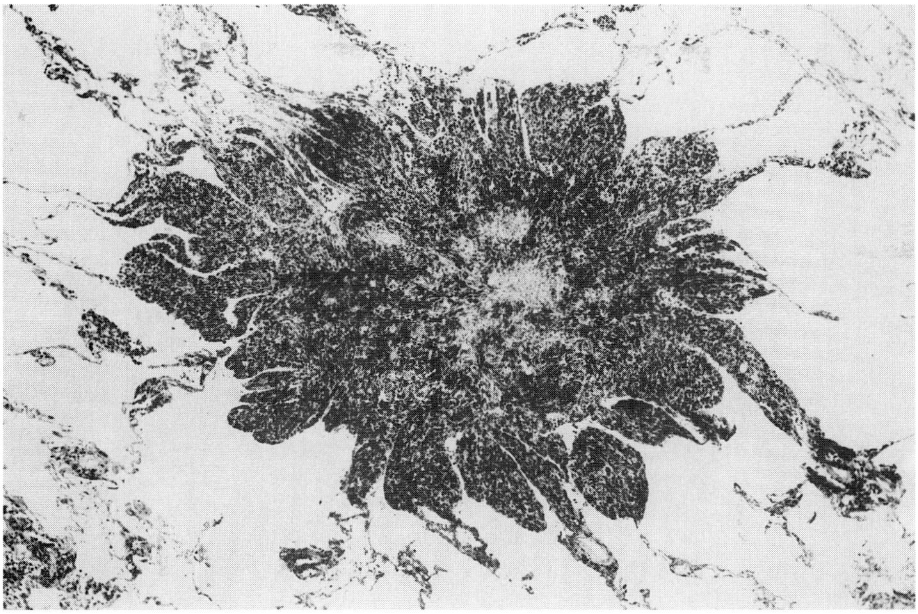

FIGURE 6.25
Micronodule composed of pigmented macrophages in a reticulin and collagen stroma. There is adjacent mild airspace enlargement. From a 59-year-old Pennsylvania coal miner, current smoker with one pack of cigarettes per day for 42 years smoking history, employed 40 years underground, mainly as coal loader.

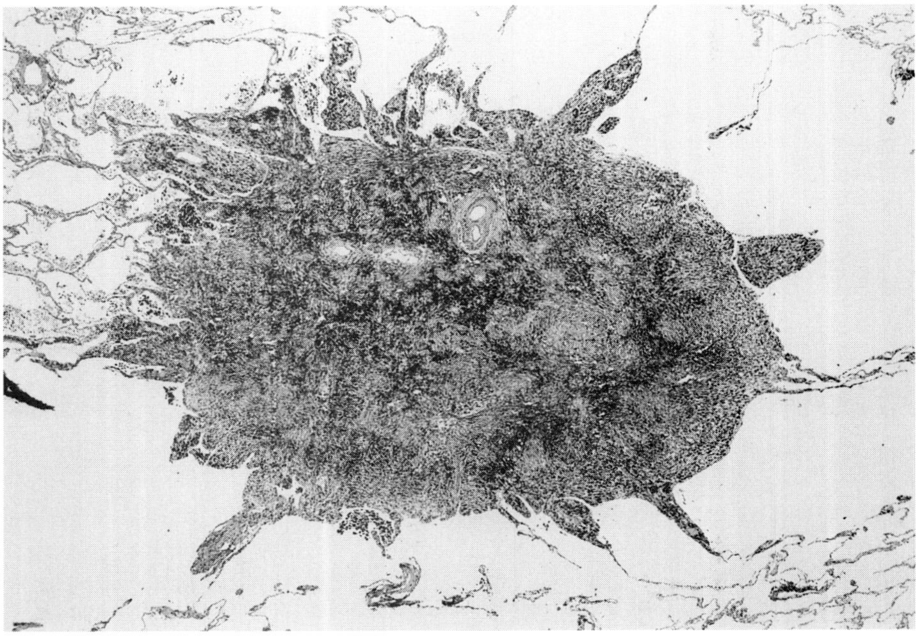

FIGURE 6.26
Micronodule (0.5 cm). The pigment and connective tissue elements are uniformLy distributed throughout the lesion. The connective tissues are arranged randomly. Airspace enlargement is seen adjacent. From a 62-year-old underground coal miner, former smoker with 25 pack-year smoking history.

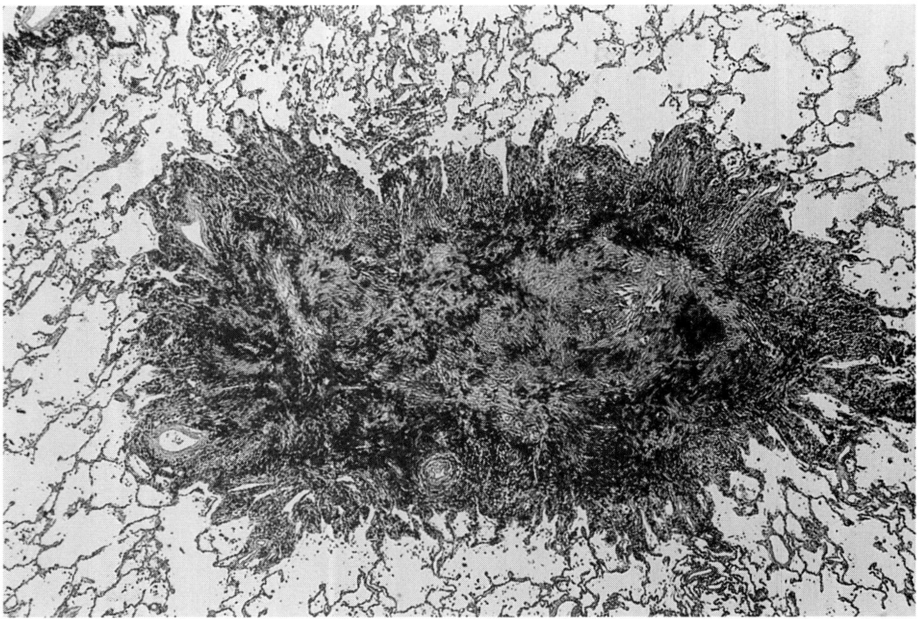

FIGURE 6.27
Micronodule (0.4 cm). The lesion is composed of pigmented macrophages, collagen at center and a peripheral zone of reticulin and dust. The connective tissue fibers are arranged haphazardly. From a 59-year-old Pennsylvania coal miner, former smoker with 35 years of employment underground, principally as continuous mining machine operator.

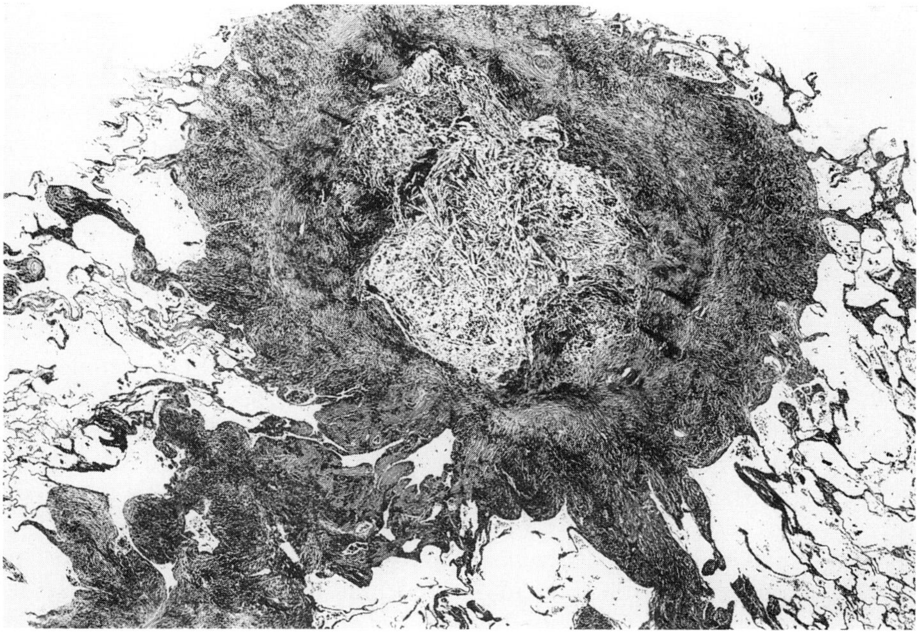

FIGURE 6.28
Macronodule (0.8 cm) with central cavitation and cholesterol clefts. From a 75-year-old West Virginia coal miner, former cigarette smoker with 5 pack-year smoking history, employed 42 years in underground mines, principally as continuous mining machine operator.

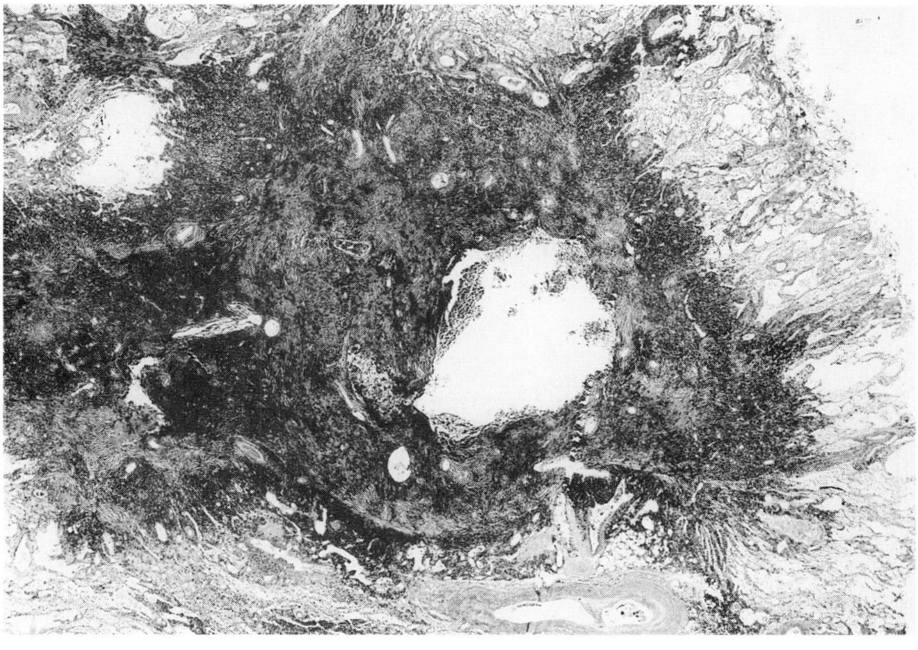

FIGURE 6.29
Macronodule or early PMF (1.1 cm). The lesion shows central cavitation. From a 66-year-old coal miner from Kentucky, cigarette smoker with 50 pack-year smoking history. Employed 16 years underground in transportation activities.

Coal dust nodules must be distinguished from silicotic nodules, rheumatoid nodules, and pigmented (healed) infectious granulomata. Histoplasmosis is particularly troublesome, as it is relatively common in Appalachian coal mining states. Healed infectious granulomata, in contrast to coal dust nodules, are more likely to be calcified, contain less pigment, and have a random, sparse distribution in the lung parenchyma. Moreover, coal dust nodules are usually seen in conjunction with the macular lesions of CWP.

Progressive Massive Fibrosis

The factor or factors responsible for the progression of simple CWP to the more aggressive form, progressive massive fibrosis (PMF), sometimes called complicated CWP, are not fully understood (69, 92). Several factors are associated with the development of PMF: cumulative dust exposure (65, 69), impaired clearance (99), quartz (100–102), immunologic factors (103), and infectious agents (104, 105). There is no association between smoking and the development or progression of PMF (71). In recent decades tuberculosis has become less important, and immunologic factors are known to be directly involved only in the relatively rare cases of rheumatoid pneumoconiosis. Quartz exposure may be an important factor in the development of PMF in a coal miner with a short exposure history (17). Cumulative dust exposure is probably the most important factor in the pathogenesis of PMF. The risk of PMF increases with increasing category of simple CWP (106, 107). In a study of more than 100,000 working British coal miners, the attack rate of PMF over an 8-year period for miners with simple CWP categories 0, 1, 2, and 3 were 0, 1, 11, and 21%, respectively (65).

The attack rate of PMF is also related to the burden of dust in the lungs (99). Lung dust measurements from autopsied British coal miners showed that miners with 5 mg of retained dust per gram of lung showed macules with minimal fibrosis, but 15 mg dust per gram of lung was associated with PMF (Table 6.5). Furthermore, the increases in lung dust burden were disproportionately greater at higher exposure levels, indicating that dust clearance mechanisms had been overwhelmed (see Chapter 2).

PMF may also arise in coal miners with no evidence of simple CWP on the chest radiograph (106), indicating that unidentified host factors are also impor-

TABLE 6.5
Cumulative Exposure, Retained Dust Levels, and Disease in British Coal Miners

NUMBER OF MINERS	MEAN CUMULATIVE EXPOSURE (GH/M^3)[a]	MEAN DUST RETAINED IN LUNGS (MG/G LUNG)	PATHOLOGY
31	136.9	5.4	Macules
26	192.1	5.8	Macules
26	140.6	7.0	Macules
43	194.6	11.3	+Nodules
41	184.8	15.0	PMF

[a] In U.S. coal miners estimates of cumulative exposure to respirable coal mine dust range from 122 to 180 gh/m^3 (i.e., 35 years of exposure at 2 mg/m^3 and 1740 hours per year equals 122 gh/m^3; or 45 years of exposure at 2 mg/m^3 and 200 hours per year equals 180 gh/m^3).

Adapted from Douglas AN, Robertson A, Chapman J, Ruckley VA. Dust exposure, dust recovered from the lung and associated pathology in a group of British coal miners. Br J Md Med 1986;43: 795–801.

tant in the pathogenesis of PMF. Once established, the disease tends to progress with or without further exposure (69). The younger the patient at onset, the more rapid the progression (71).

Pathologic and radiologic definitions of PMF are based on size. The ILO-1980 radiographic classification of the pneumoconioses (see Chapter 1), black lung legislation in the United States (see Chapter 14), and criteria used by British pathologists (99) define PMF as an opacity or fibrotic pneumoconiotic lesion 1 cm in diameter or greater. Size criteria based on lesions 2 cm (91) or 3 cm (104) in greatest dimension have been proposed but have not been generally accepted. In view of the medicolegal significance of a diagnosis of PMF, it is important on gross examination to accurately measure and record the dimensions of all pneumoconiotic lesions 1 cm or greater in diameter. Because PMF usually occurs against a background of severe simple CWP and is usually bilateral, solitary pigmented fibrotic lesions in lungs with mild or absent simple CWP should be interpreted cautiously, as they may be old scars (infectious or otherwise) that have become pigmented.

The lesions of PMF occur in all areas of the lung but have a predilection for the upper and posterior portions. The more advanced categories of disease are almost always bilateral. Smaller lesions are more often unilateral and may appear radiologically as primary neoplasms. They are thus more likely to be sampled for biopsy. The distribution of PMF was studied in 108 autopsied British coal miners who had radiographic categories B and C PMF during life (108). Slightly more right lung zones were affected (57%) than left lung zones (47%), and the upper zones (77%) were involved more often than the middle (43%) or lower zones (31%). Of miners with category C pneumoconiosis, 98% had bilateral lesions, and 67% of miners with category B PMF had bilateral lesions.

Macroscopically PMF lesions appear as black fibrotic masses that may be round, oval, or irregular (Figs. 6.30 to 6.32 and colorplate 1). They are usually well demarcated from the surrounding lung but are not encapsulated. Satellite nodules are usually seen in the adjacent lung (Fig. 6.32). Peripheral lesions are usually firmly tethered to the parietal pleura, and more central lesions tend to contract toward the hilum. In either case the lung and bronchovascular rays become markedly distorted, and this may be apparent on the chest radiograph (Fig. 6.32). A characteristic feature of PMF is the tendency of the lesion to transgress normal anatomic boundaries, with fissures, bronchi, and vessels becoming obliterated as the lesion progresses (Fig. 6.30).

The cut surface of a typical lesion has a rubbery texture and is black. Central necrosis is associated with softening and cavitation. The contents of these may scintillate because of the content of cholesterol crystals (47). The fluid is usually sterile. However, complicating mycobacterial or fungal infection cannot be ruled out by gross examination. Empty cavities with irregular shaggy borders are commonly seen. Other lesions may be harder and have a gritty texture because of calcification. If the cut surface shows multiple ill-defined conglomerate nodules with pale centers, the lesion probably originated from the confluence of silicotic nodules.

Microscopically the lesions are composed of bundles of haphazardly arranged hyalinized collagen fibers and/or reticulin fibers and coal dust (Fig. 6.33). Dust particles near the periphery of the lesion are mainly within macrophages; in the center the dust tends to lie free in clefts and cavities (Fig. 6.34). Areas of liquefactive necrosis containing fragments of degenerating collagen and cholesterol crystals are frequently observed. A giant cell reaction may be seen in association

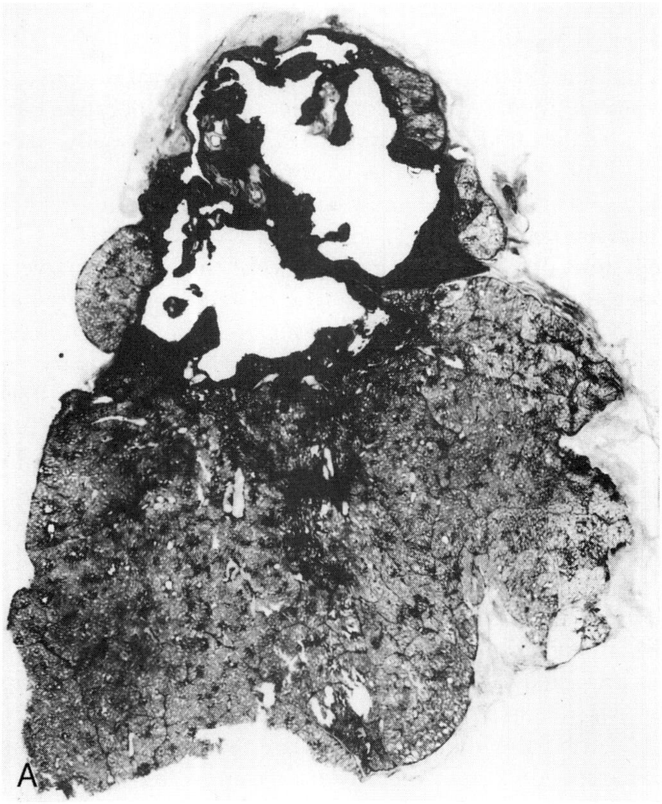

FIGURE 6.30

A. PMF. Whole lung section shows cavitating PMF set against a background of macular and nodular simple CWP. The lesion has transgressed the lobar fissure. There is minimal emphysema. From a 62-year-old miner with 10 years' work underground as a loader and 24 years above ground checking and weighing. **B.** Chest radiograph from same patient showing massive opacities with cavitation. There is marked distortion of the bronchovascular markings. The ILO U/C reading was category B PMF with category 2r round and 2u irregular small opacities. (Reprinted with permission from Green FHY, Laqueur WA. Coal workers' pneumoconiosis. Pathol Ann 1980;15:333–409.)

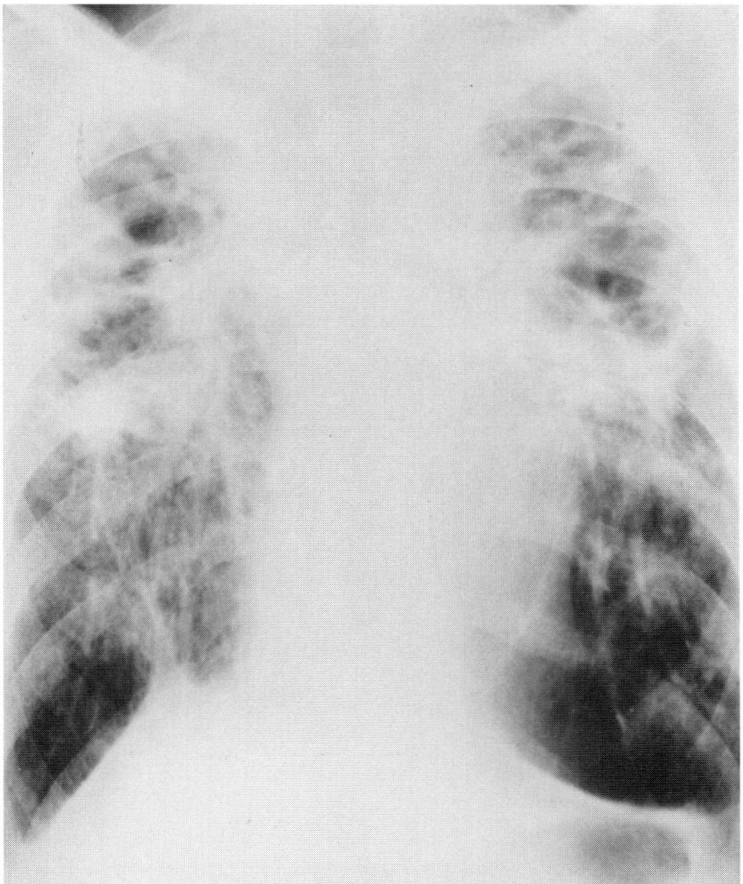
B

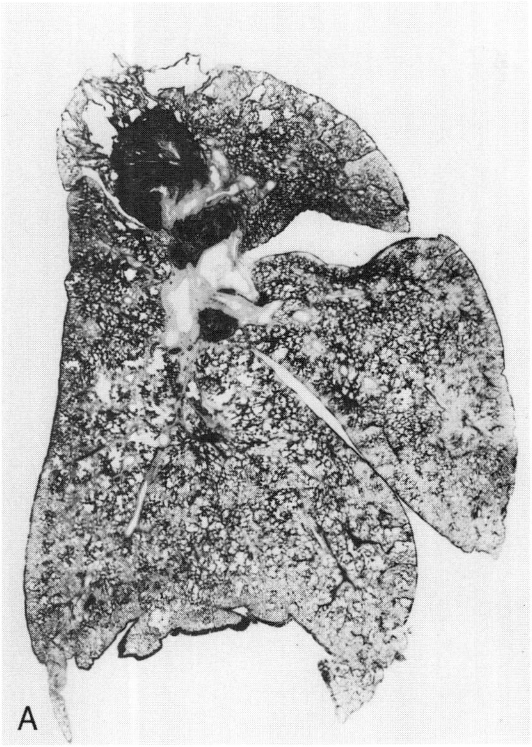

FIGURE 6.31

A. Progressive massive fibrosis. There is macular and diffuse pigmentation with moderate centriacinar and bullous emphysema. From a 74-year-old coal miner with 40 pack-year smoking history who worked 28 years in underground coal mines, principally as a loader. **B.** Chest radiograph from same patient. ILO-80 reading for this radiograph was film quality 1; category 2/2 profusions small opacities, size and shape q/t; category B large opacities (PMF).

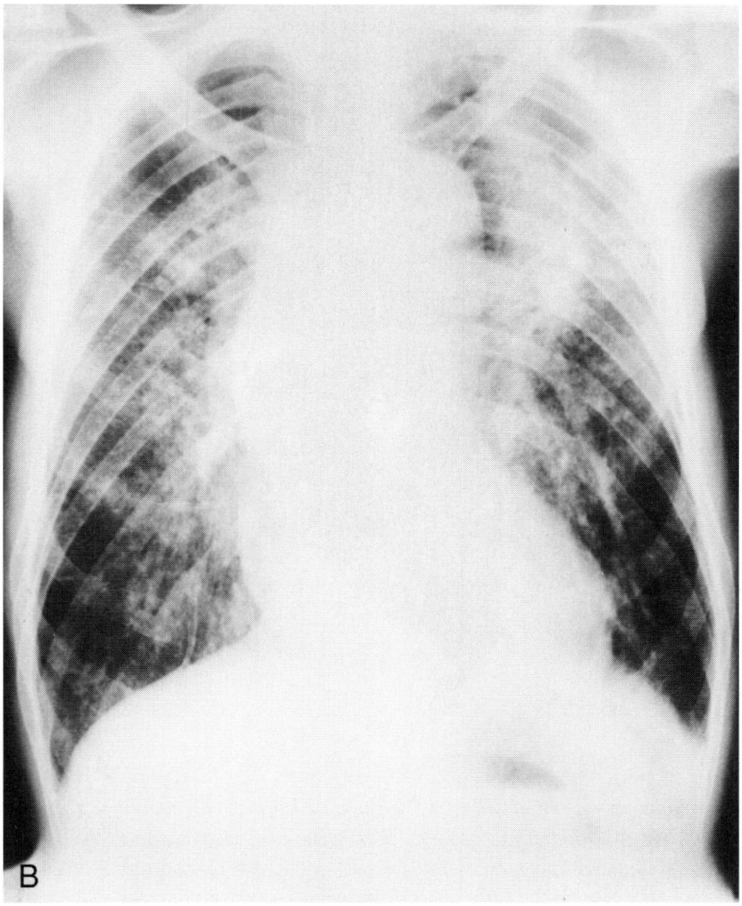

FIGURE 6.31 (*continued*)

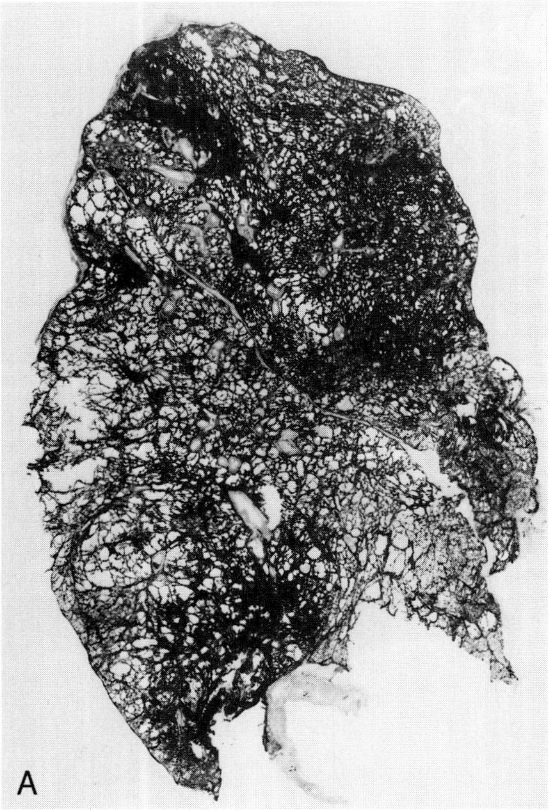

FIGURE 6.32

A. PMF with severe panacinar emphysema. From a 64-year-old miner with 45 pack-year smoking history; worked 40 years underground, principally as a coal loader. Microscopy showed diffuse dust deposition, emphysema, and fibrosis. **B.** Chest radiograph from same patient. There is marked distortion of the right bronchovascular markings associated with several large opacities in the right upper lobe. The hypolucency of the lower lung fields and flattening of the diaphragm indicate emphysema. ILO-80 reading of the radiograph was film quality 2; category 2/1 profusion small opacities; size/shape t/s (upper and middle zones) category B larger opacities (PMF).

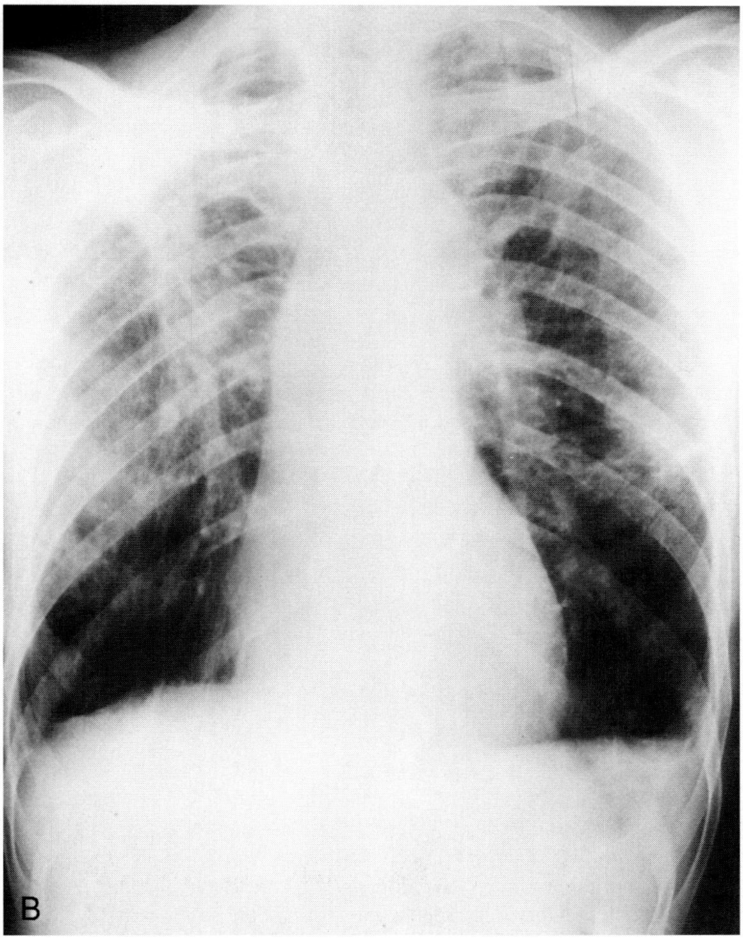

FIGURE 6.32 ***(continued)***

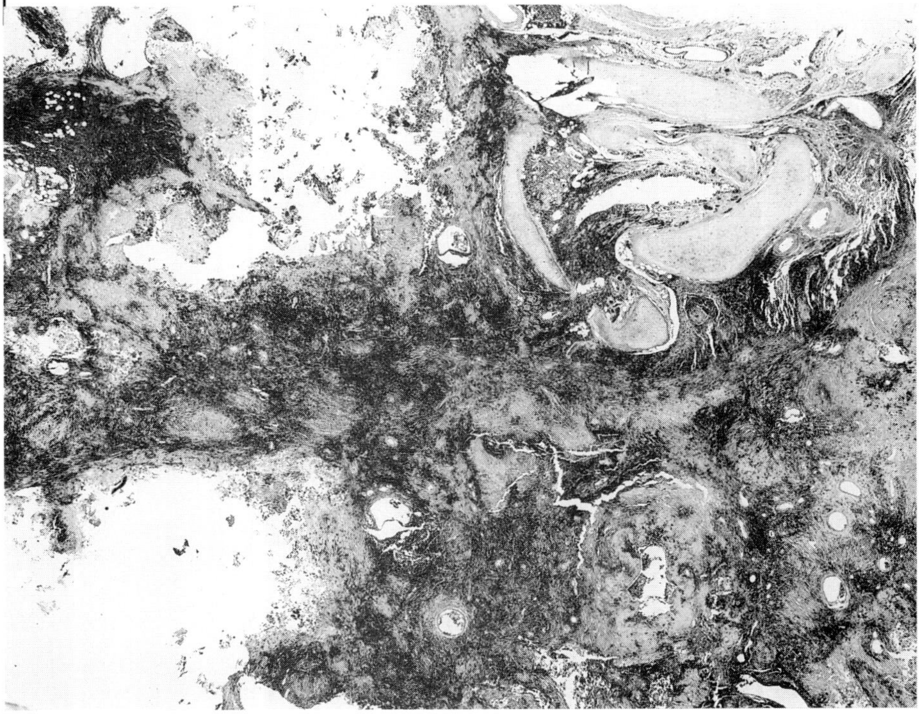

FIGURE 6.33

PMF. Advanced lesion showing cavitation, compression and distortion of a bronchus, and obliteration of blood vessels. From a 64-year-old formerly cigarette-smoking coal miner employed for 29 years underground in Pennsylvania coal mines as motorman and brakeman.

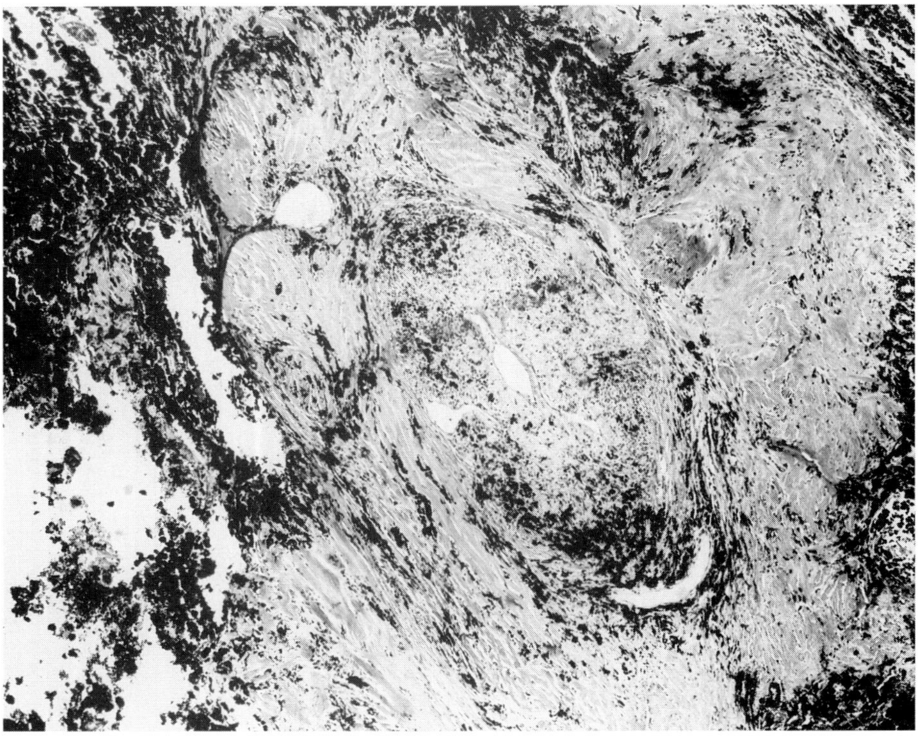

FIGURE 6.34

PMF. The lesion is composed of macrophages, dust, and bundles of hyalinized collagen. Cavitation is seen at left. The cavity contains free dust and degenerating pigmented macrophages. A vessel (center) is almost totally obliterated; the wall is replaced by fibrous tissue and is extensively infiltrated by pigmented macrophages.

with the necrotic collagen (Fig. 6.35). Lymphocytes and plasma cells are few in number. Special stains and culture are necessary to exclude caseation due to mycobacterial or mycotic organisms, as these agents may be present without classic histologic features of infection.

Some PMF lesions contain the conglomerated outlines of nodules with whorled centers indicative of silicosis (Figs. 6.36 and 6.37). Other PMF lesions appear to arise from the enlargement of single nodules (Fig. 6.38). PMF is a destructive process, and the remains of obliterated vessels and airways are apparent in the centers of the lesions (Fig. 6.34). Other airways show marked distortion with displacement of cartilaginous plates and luminal narrowing (Figs. 6.33, 6.39).

Vascular degenerative changes, seen in almost all PMF lesions, affect bronchial and pulmonary arteries, veins, and lymphatic vessels. The affected vessels are infiltrated by dust-containing macrophages and lymphocytes that penetrate to the intimal surface (Fig. 6.40). There is progressive sclerosis of the vessel wall associated with endarteritis obliterans and thrombosis. Immunoglobulins have been demonstrated in some affected vessels (103).

Histologic changes identical to those of PMF may be seen in the peribronchial lymph nodes. The affected lymph node may attain a size greater than 1 cm in diameter. This reaction should not be diagnosed as PMF unless there is also substantial involvement of adjacent lung parenchyma.

Chemical extraction of dusts and other substances in massive lesions reveals 20–50% coal, up to 30% collagen, and lesser amounts of calcium phosphate, silica, silicates, fibrinogen, and immunoglobulins IgA and IgG (109).

The degree and extent of emphysema in the lungs of miners with PMF varies considerably (Figs. 6.30–6.32). Systematic studies conducted on autopsied coal

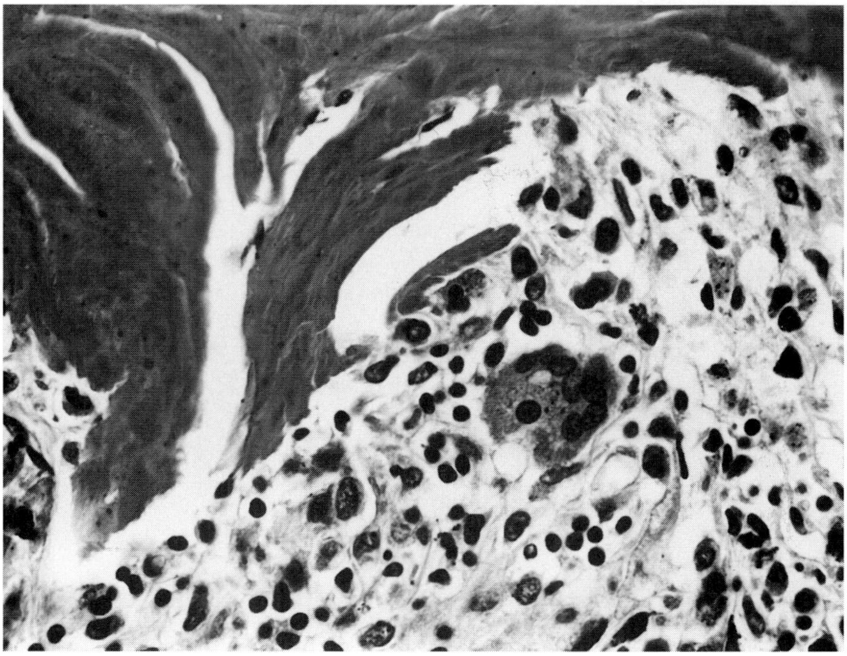

FIGURE 6.35
PMF. A macrophagic and giant cell reaction to necrotic collagen is visible at the center of the lesion.

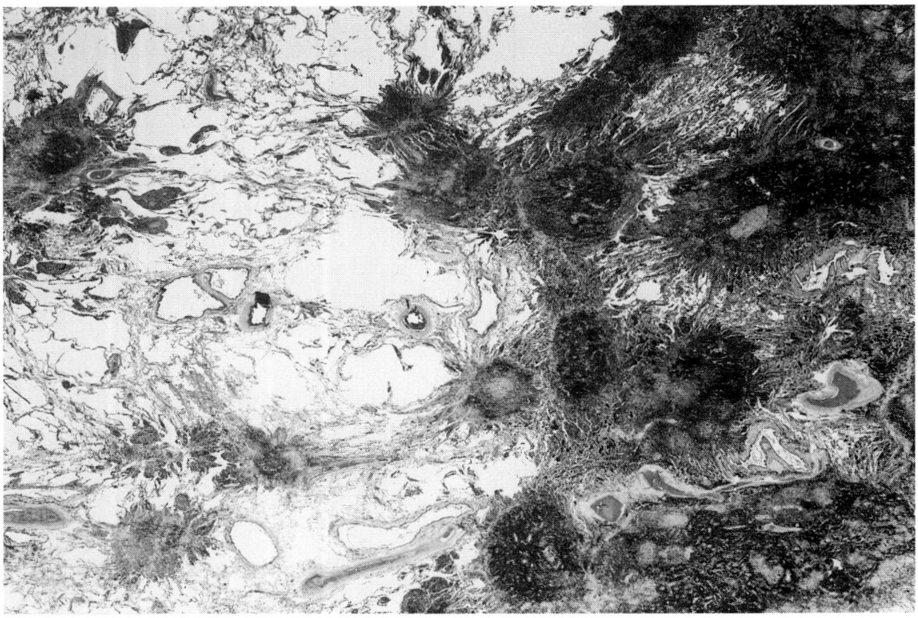

FIGURE 6.36
PMF. Edge of lesion shows confluence of nodules. Irregular emphysema is seen around the nodules.

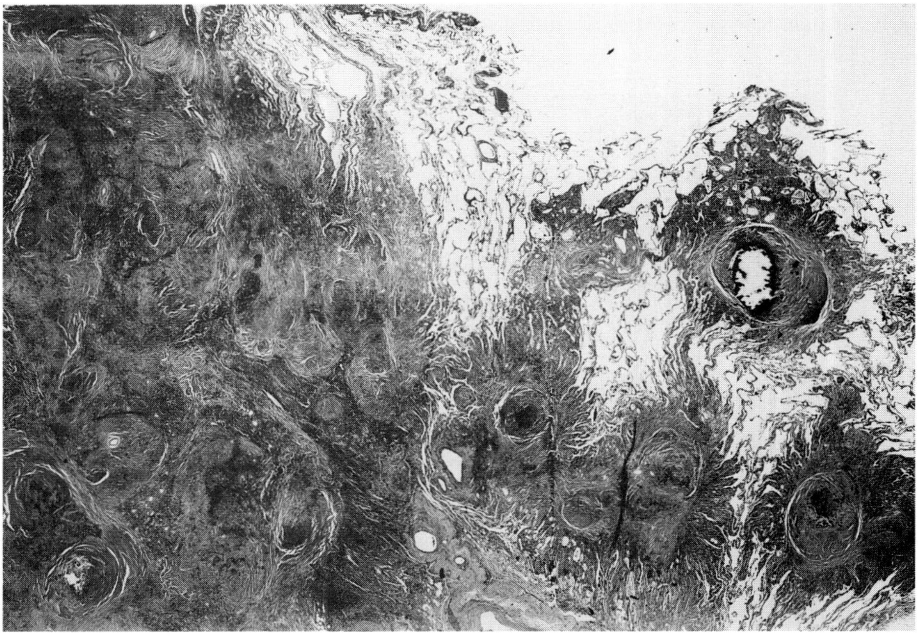

FIGURE 6.37
PMF. The lesion is composed of conglomerated nodules. The central portions of the nodules show whorling of collagen fibers indicative of silicosis. The nodules have stellate borders. From a 76-year-old Pennsylvania coal miner employed 50 years underground in face work.

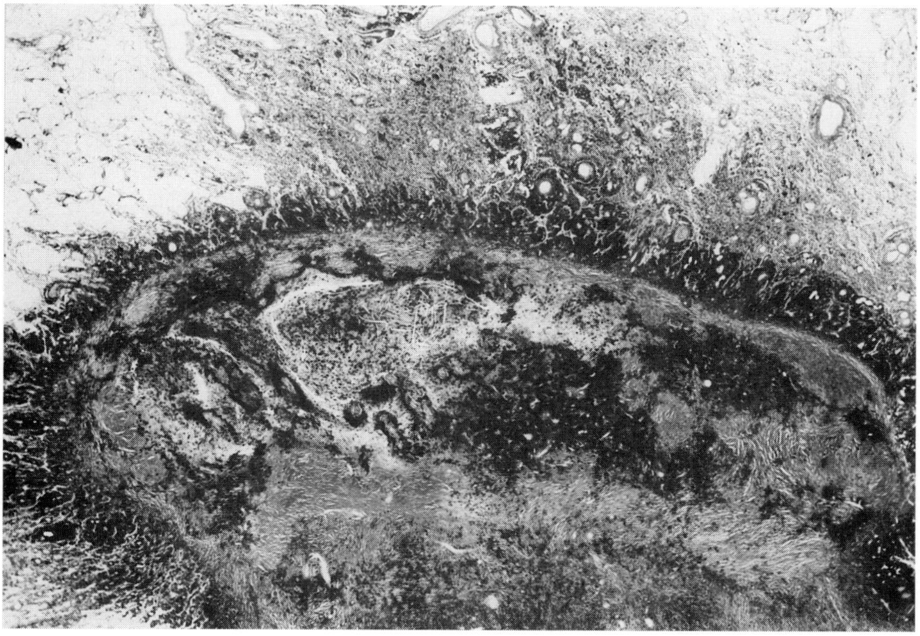

FIGURE 6.38
PMF. This lesion appears to have originated in a single large nodule. It is composed of hyalinized collagen, dust, and cholesterol clefts. It shows an active cellular border. From a 61-year-old coal miner, former smoker, employed 36 years underground in face work.

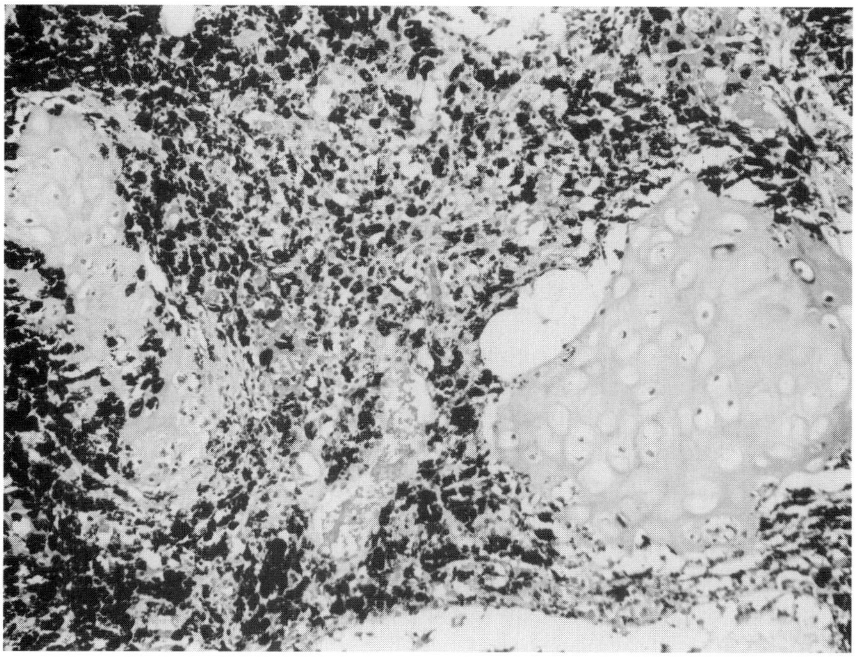

FIGURE 6.39
PMF. Fragments of bronchial cartilage are being eroded and infiltrated by pigmented macrophages.

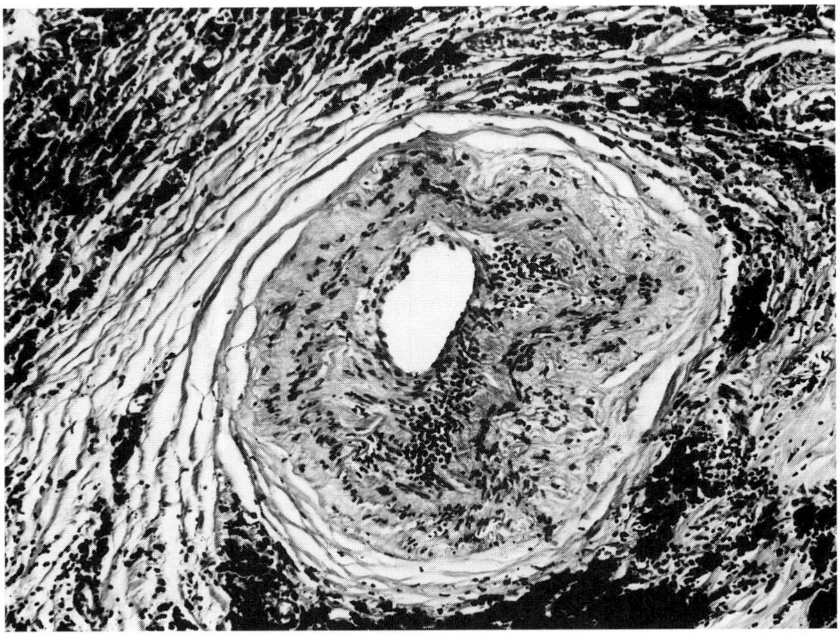

FIGURE 6.40
Muscular pulmonary artery in PMF lesion. The vessel shows fibrosis of the wall and is infiltrated by pigmented macrophages and lymphocytes.

miners have shown that miners with PMF have more severe emphysema than do those with less severe categories of CWP. All types may be observed, but centriacinar emphysema is reported to predominate (108, 110). The study of Lyons and Campbell (108) showed that PMF and emphysema usually make independent contributions to impairment of ventilation in proportion to their size and extent.

Rheumatoid Pneumoconiosis (Caplan's Syndrome)

In 1953 Caplan described a severe form of pneumoconiosis in Welsh coal miners with rheumatoid arthritis (111). Originally called Caplan's syndrome, the condition is now more commonly called rheumatoid pneumoconiosis because it is also known to occur in coal miners with circulating rheumatoid factor but without arthritis (112) and in individuals exposed to silica (113) (see Chapter 7) and nonfibrous silicates (see Chapter 8). It occurs worldwide but for unknown reasons is more common in Europe than in North America (114). Rheumatoid pneumoconiosis occurs in miners of all ages, both active and retired, and may run a rapidly fatal fulminant course. Its epidemiology has been extensively studied. Although some studies have shown an increased prevalence of rheumatoid arthritis or circulating rheumatoid factor in miners with more severe categories of CWP (115), there is no evidence that coal mining predisposes to rheumatoid arthritis (116, 117). The characteristic radiographic feature is rapidly enlarging, evenly distributed, circumscribed nodules ranging in size from 0.3 to 5 cm in diameter, occurring in lungs that otherwise show little evidence of pneumoconiosis. The nodules are likely to cavitate and undergo calcification. Pleural effusion has also been reported (43).

The pathologic features were originally described by Gough et al. (118) in 16 coal miners with rheumatoid arthritis. Of these 8 showed characteristic radiologic opacities. Gross examination shows the lesions to be distributed throughout both lungs and to range in size and shape from small round nodules to large confluent masses several centimeters in diameter (Fig. 6.41). Lesions of classic CWP, usually of mild degree, are observed adjacent to the rheumatoid nodules. The nodules are pale yellow and show a variable number of concentric dark bands. They may show central cavitation and calcification. Superficially they resemble silicotic nodules, but they are softer unless calcified and can be distinguished by histologic examination.

Microscopically the active lesions are similar in many ways to subcutaneous rheumatoid nodules and to rheumatoid nodules in the lungs of non–occupationally exposed individuals. The typical lesion is composed of a central zone of eosinophilic granular necrotic tissue containing nuclear debris and fragments of collagen and elastic fibers (Fig. 6.42). Cholesterol clefts and calcification may be present. The necrotic material is abruptly demarcated from the surrounding tissues by a layer of fibroblasts and macrophages. Giant cells are occasionally seen

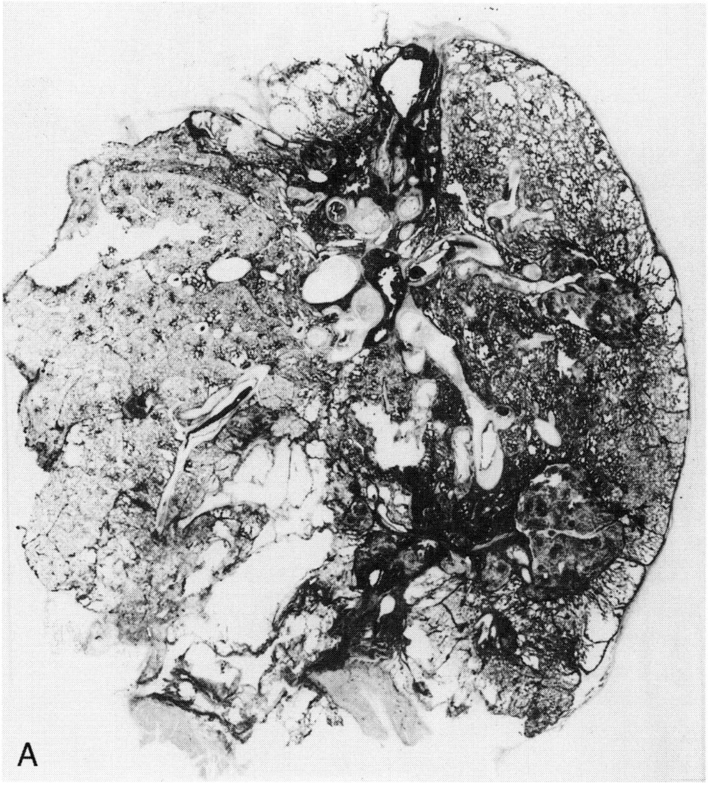

FIGURE 6.41

A. Rheumatoid pneumoconiosis. Whole lung section from 63-year-old underground coal miner with active rheumatoid arthritis. He worked 24 years underground as a machine operator. There is minimal simple macular pneumoconiosis in the upper lobe. Several large, well-circumscribed pale nodules are seen throughout all lung fields. **B.** Close-up of rheumatoid nodule showing a pale center with dust banding. **C.** Chest radiograph shows numerous large round opacities typical of rheumatoid pneumoconiosis. (Reprinted with permission from Green FHY, Laqueur WA. Coal workers' pneumoconiosis. Pathol Ann 1980;15:333–409.)

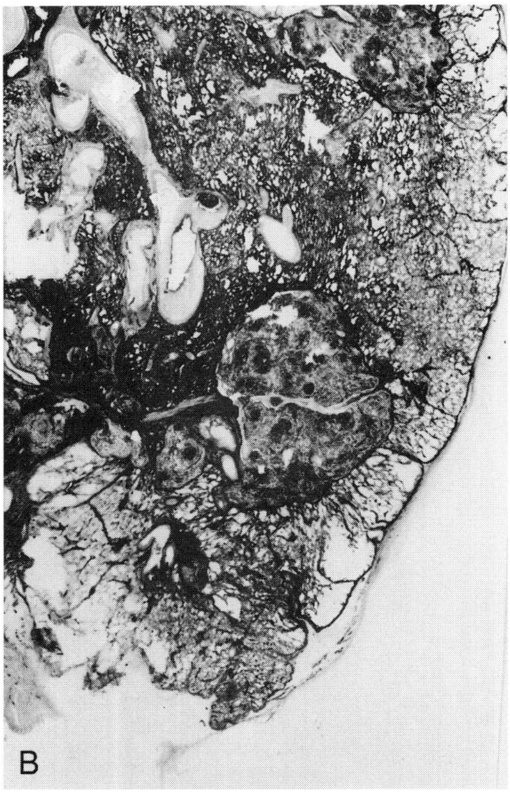

FIGURE 6.41 *(continued)*

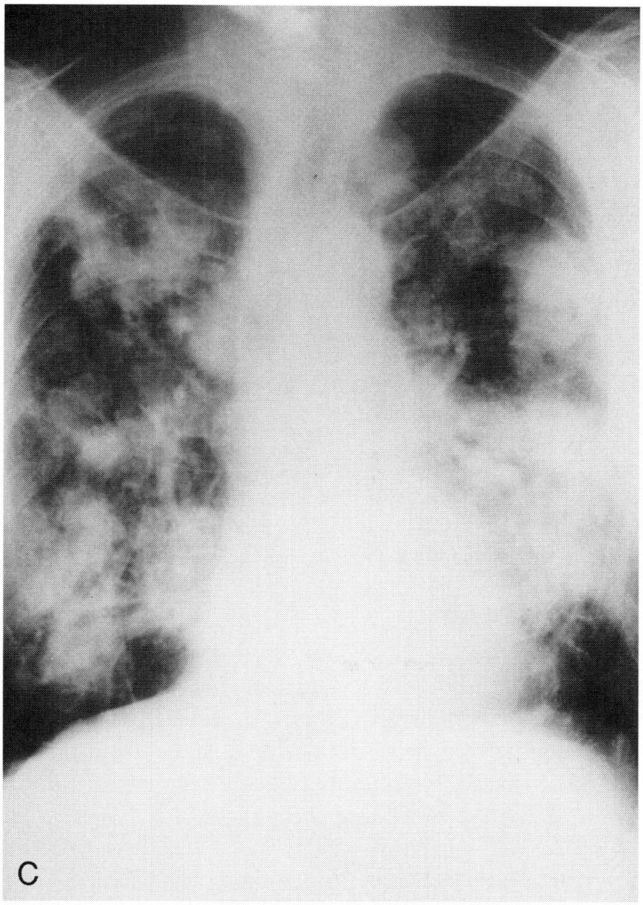

FIGURE 6.41 *(continued)*

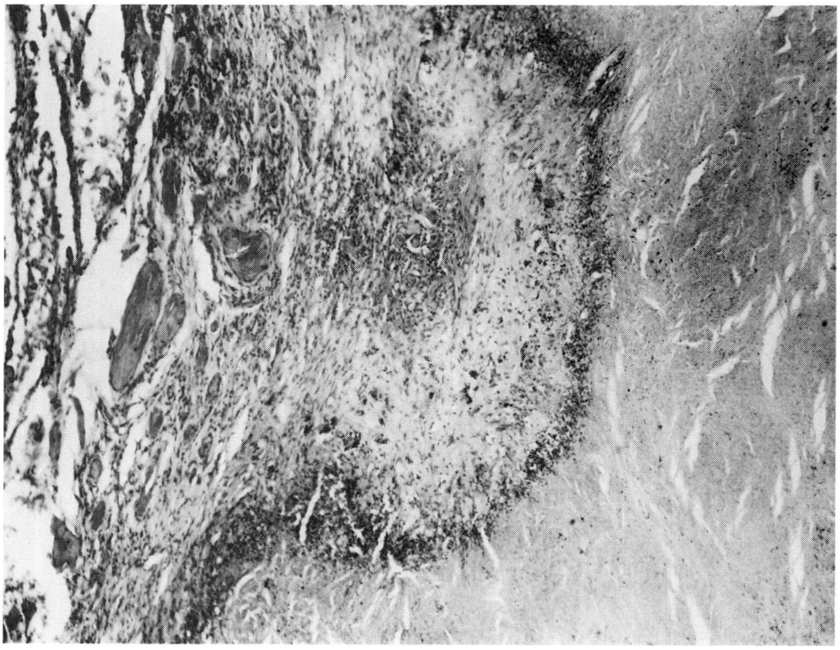

FIGURE 6.42
Rheumatoid pneumoconiosis. The nodule shows central amorphous necrosis surrounded by a band of dust, chronic inflammatory cells, and fibrous tissue. The amount of dust in the surrounding lung is slight.

but are less common than in infective granulomas. Palisading of fibroblasts is characteristic but not seen in every case (Fig. 6.43). The likelihood of finding this feature can be increased by examining multiple sections. The laminations noted grossly are composed of coal dust pigment, both free and within macrophages. The periphery of the lesion is composed of concentrically arranged collagen fibers with variable numbers of lymphocytes, plasma cells, and macrophages. Immunoglobulins, including rheumatoid factor, have been demonstrated immunohistochemically in the plasma cells of rheumatoid pneumoconiosis of coal workers (103). Polymorphonuclear cells are seen in the more active lesions. The older lesions are collagenized and show more closely spaced bands of dust with central calcification. Vasculitis is common in the vessels within and adjacent to the nodules of rheumatoid pneumoconiosis. The major finding is endarteritis obliterans with lymphocyte and plasma cell infiltration of the wall.

It is necessary to distinguish the lesions of rheumatoid pneumoconiosis from those of tuberculosis and other infective granulomata such as histoplasmosis. Tuberculosis and rheumatoid pneumoconiosis have many features in common: both may show central necrosis, dust rings, and giant cells (Figs. 6.42 and 6.44). Plasma cells and palisading of fibroblasts may be prominent in the lesions of rheumatoid pneumoconiosis but are rare in tuberculosis and other infectious granulomata. The dust rings in rheumatoid pneumoconiosis are usually more pronounced. In practice differentiation can be made only by special stains for organisms and culture of the fresh lesion. Gough et al. (118) found histologic or other evidence of tuberculosis in 40% of their cases, and they postulated that rheumatoid pneumoconiosis was a modified form of infective pneumoconiosis. No evidence has been forthcoming in this regard, and it seems more likely that

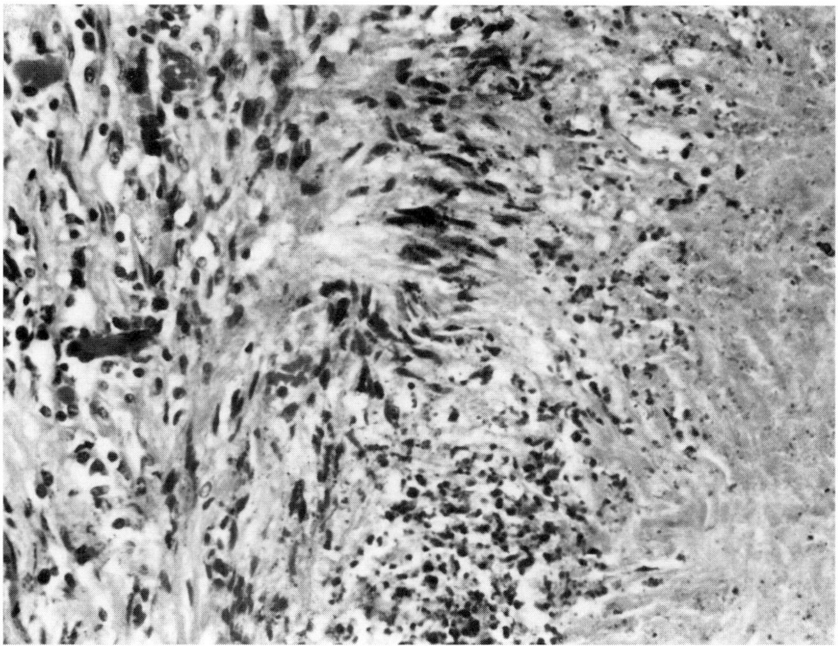

FIGURE 6.43
Rheumatoid pneumoconiosis. Edge of lesion in FIGURE 6.42 showing palisading of fibroblasts adjacent to area of necrosis.

rheumatoid pneumoconiosis is a local hypersensitivity triggered by some component of mineral dust. The term *rheumatoid pneumoconiosis* should be restricted to cases that have characteristic histologic features and in whom infectious disease has been excluded. When an infectious agent is identified in an otherwise typical lesion, the diagnosis should reflect this, bearing in mind that the histologic features may be modified by coexistent pneumoconiosis and immunologic abnormalities.

Silicosis in Coal Workers

The role of silica in causing CWP has been hotly debated for more than a century. The early conviction that CWP was due to quartz alone was seriously undermined by the observation in 1928 that miners exposed to coal dust containing negligible quartz developed classic radiologic signs of CWP (4). Subsequent large prospective epidemiologic studies of coal miners exposed to coal mine dust containing varying amounts of quartz have shown that risk and progression of pneumoconiosis are primarily related to cumulative exposure to total dust and not to quartz content (62, 119). The results of autopsy studies and experiments conducted on animals exposed to coal dust containing varying concentrations of quartz indicate that other minerals in coal, such as aluminosilicate clays and iron oxides, are capable of reducing the fibrogenic effect of quartz (120–123). The mechanism whereby this occurs is not fully understood but may involve an alteration in the surface chemistry of the quartz particles (124).

Studies from the British coal fields show that high quartz exposure is an important factor affecting risk and progression of PMF for some miners (102, 125).

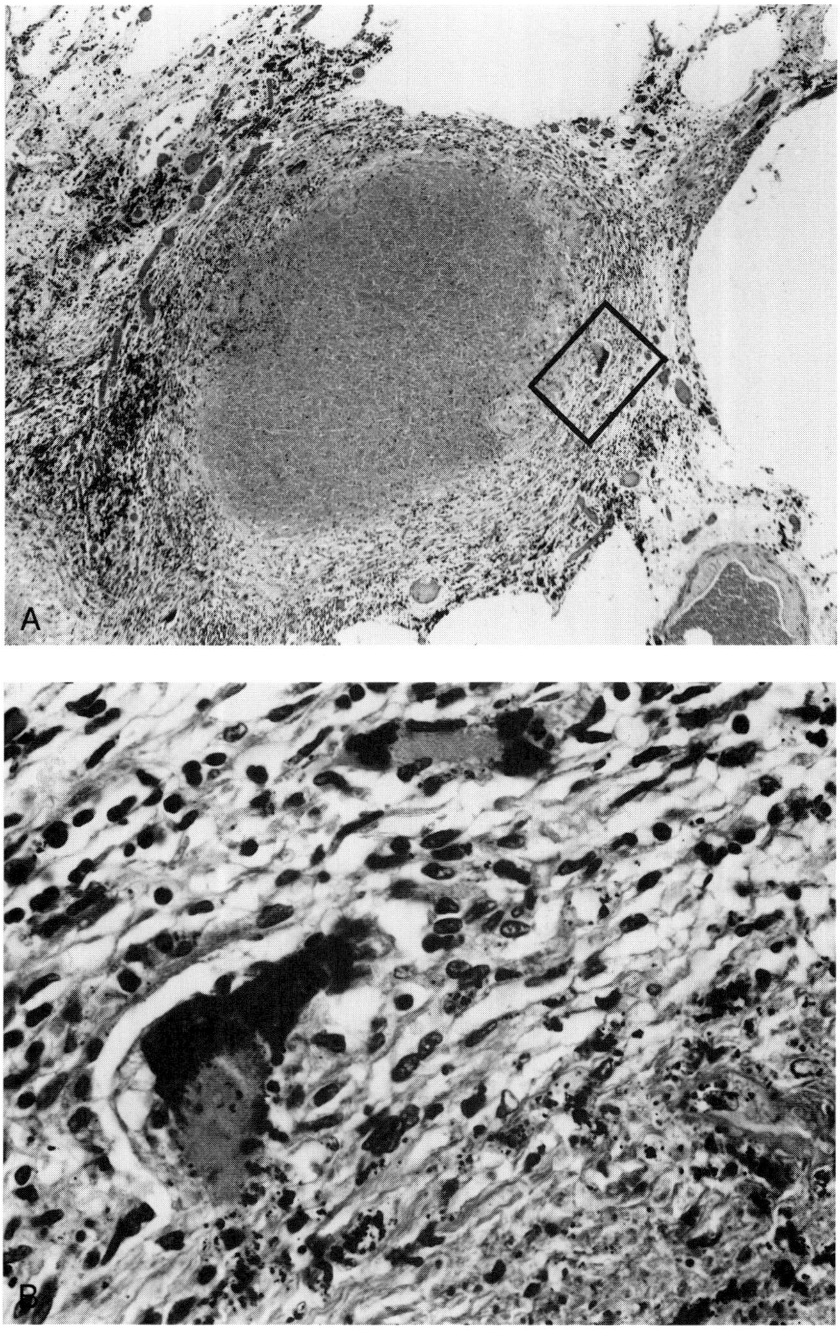

FIGURE 6.44
A. Tuberculosis in a coal worker. Tuberculous granuloma shows central caseous necrosis. Dust is present at periphery, but laminations are not seen in this lesion. **B.** Inset shows giant cells and dust at periphery of necrosis. Stains for acid-fast bacilli were positive.

It is also well recognized that risk of silicosis is related to specific jobs within the mine. High-risk jobs include tunnel drilling, roof bolting, and transportation (10). Transportation workers are at increased risk for silicosis because of the use of sand as a traction material.

A difficulty encountered in clinical and epidemiologic studies of coal workers is the inability of the chest radiograph to distinguish between silicosis and CWP. The radiographic sign of eggshell calcification, although indicative of silica exposure, is nondiagnostic, as silicotic nodules are frequently observed in hilar lymph nodes in the absence of parenchymal disease. Consequently the prevalence of silicosis in coal workers can be reliably determined only at autopsy. Laqueur found silicosis in 13% of a series of autopsied coal miners from southern West Virginia (126). This is similar to the 12.5% prevalence recorded in the NCWAS (10) (Table 6.4), which demonstrated a consistent relation between length of underground mining with prevalence and severity of silicosis, indicating a dose–response effect. The study also showed that job category (Table 6.6) and geographic location of the mine were important determinants of silicosis prevalence and that silicosis was strongly associated with higher categories of CWP.

Silicosis is very rarely an isolated form of pneumoconiosis in coal workers; it usually occurs against a background of simple nodular and macular CWP. Macroscopically silicotic nodules appear more uniform in size and have smoother borders and paler centers than the nodules of CWP (Fig. 6.45). They have a similar distribution to the coal dust nodules. They are most common in the upper lung zones and can be found in interstitial, peribronchial, and subpleural locations. Involvement of the hilar lymph nodes is invariably present, and these may be calcified. Coalescence of silicotic nodules to produce conglomerate silicosis (PMF) is common (Figs. 6.46 and 6.47). The outlines of individual nodules can still be seen in the largest of these lesions.

Microscopically the mature silicotic nodule resembles that observed in non–coal workers (see Chapter 7). It is composed of laminated bundles of mature collagen surrounding a hyalinized or partially necrotic and calcified center. The nodule is usually surrounded by an irregular mantle of black histiocytes in a reticulin stroma (Fig. 6.48). Polarized light microscopy may reveal numerous weakly birefringent and sharply angular particles in the centers of the nodules. The peripheral mantle of coal dust and reticulin usually contains large numbers of brightly birefringent silicate minerals that can be recognized by their intense birefringence and needlelike or platelike morphologies (see Chapter 3). Subpleural and conglomerate silicotic nodules are shown in Figures 6.49 and 6.50, respectively. Immature nodules in which histiocytes predominate and the concentricity of the collagen is less pronounced may also be observed; some of these appear to originate within alveoli (Fig. 6.51).

TABLE 6.6
Silicosis Prevalence by Major Job Classification in NCWAS (1971–1980)

JOB GROUPING	TOTAL NO. IN JOB GROUP	PERCENT SILICOSIS IN JOB GROUP
Transportation	821	24.2
Face activities	1,490	12.5
Miscellaneous (foremen, section boss)	410	12.2
Maintenance	439	8.4
Surface activities (at underground mines)	249	6.4

Reprinted with permission from Green FHY, Althouse R, Weber KC. Prevalence of silicosis at death in underground coal miners. Am J Ind Med 1989;16:605–616.

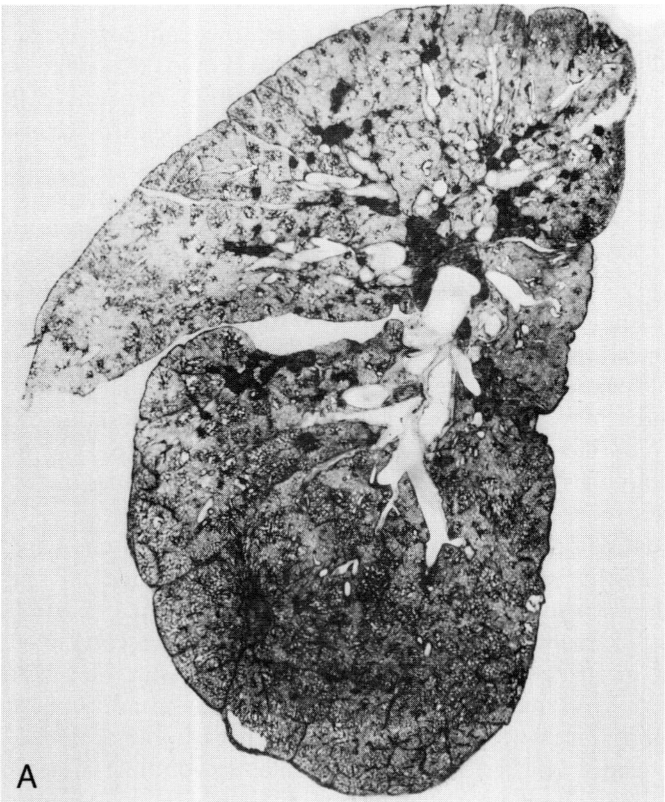

FIGURE 6.45

A. Silicosis in a coal miner. Whole lung section shows numerous round nodular lesions with pale centers that are more numerous in the upper lobe. **B.** Chest film shows bilateral category B PMF against a background of category 3r small round opacities. There is calcification of the hilar lymph nodes, indicating silicosis. The 60-year-old miner worked for 30 years underground as a brakeman and motorman, jobs that are associated with a high prevalence of silicosis. (Reprinted with permission from Green FHY, Laqueur WA. Coal workers' pneumoconiosis. Pathol Ann 1980;15:333–409.)

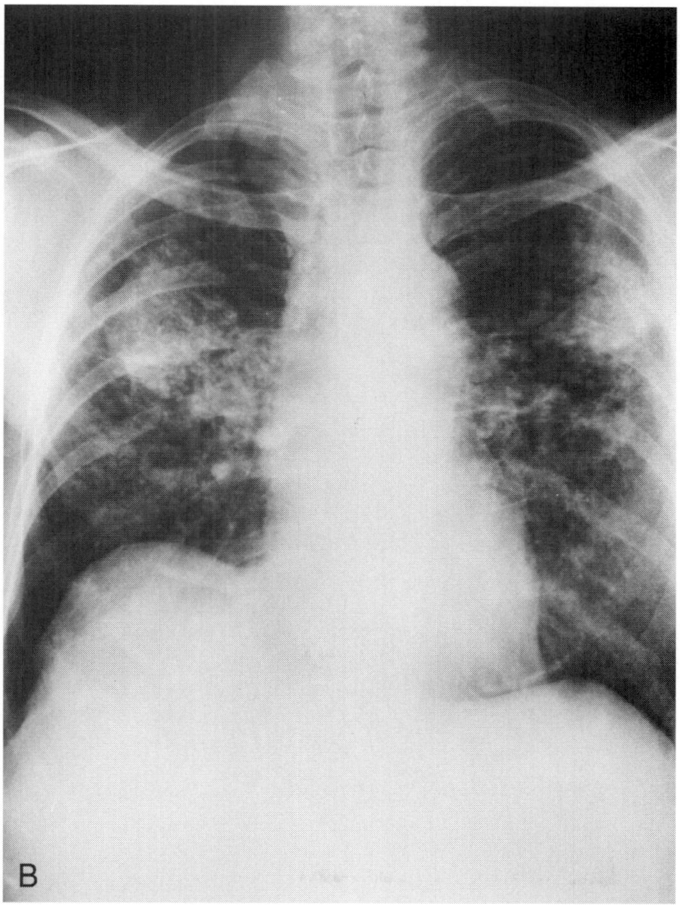

FIGURE 6.45 *(continued)*

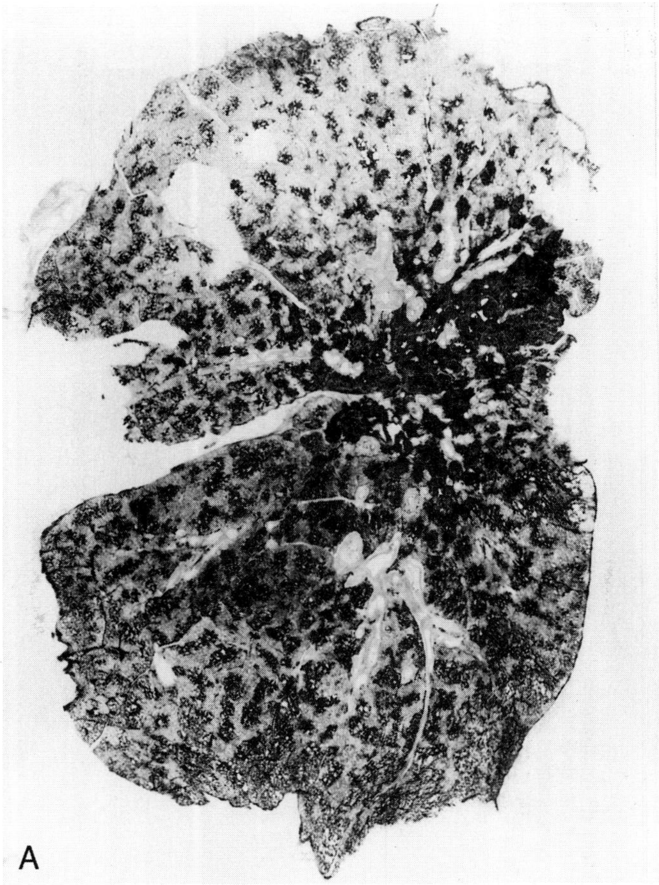

FIGURE 6.46
A. Whole lung section shows conglomerate silicosis in a coal worker. The peripheral portions of the lung show macular simple CWP. **B.** In a close-up the silicotic nodules show characteristic pale centers.

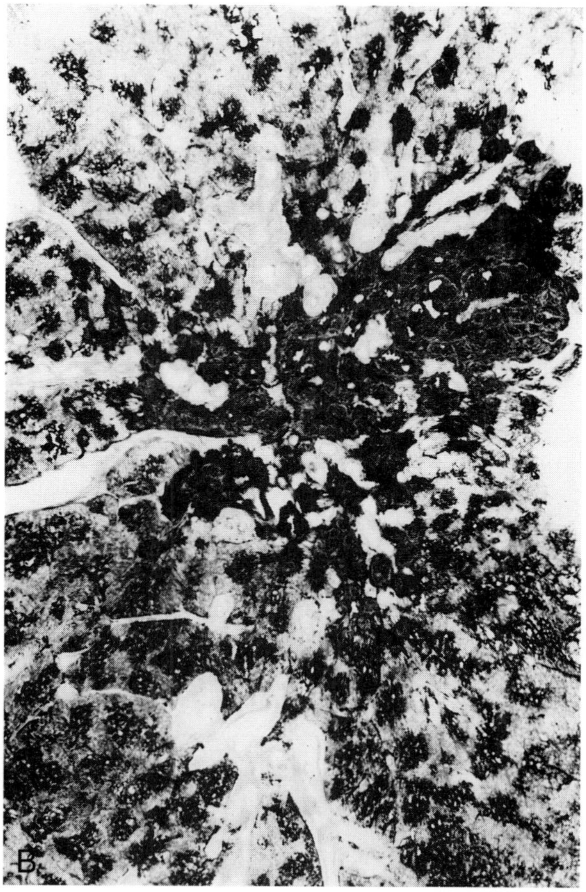

FIGURE 6.46 ***(continued)***

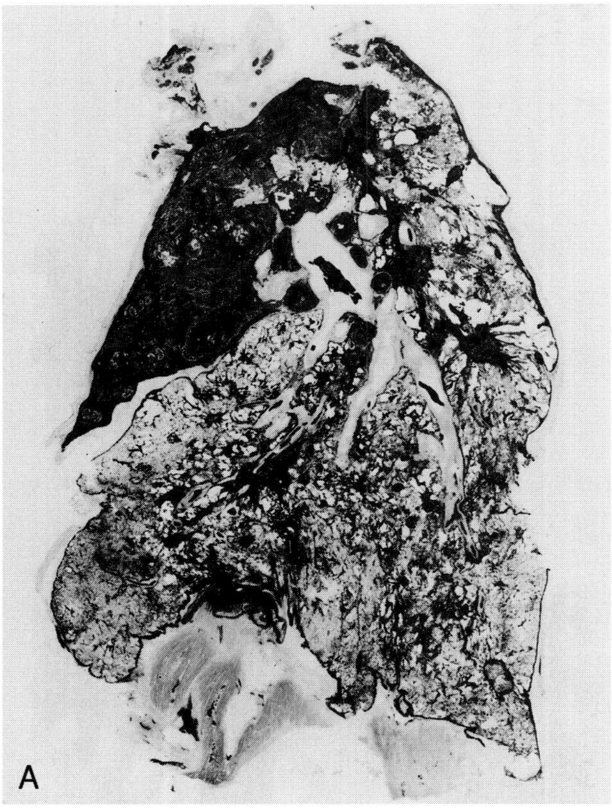

FIGURE 6.47

A. Whole lung section shows upper lobe PMF. The outlines of discrete pale nodules can be seen within the massive fibrosis. These features indicate silicosis. The lung elsewhere shows nodules and macules. **B.** Chest radiograph from same patient shows PMF in left upper lung zone set against a background of nodular opacities. ILO-80 reading for this radiograph was film quality 1; category 2/2 profusion small opacities, size/shape r/r; middle and lower zones; category B large opacities (PMF). (Reprinted with permission from Green FHY, Laqueur WA. Coal workers' pneumoconiosis. Pathol Ann 1980;15:333–409.)

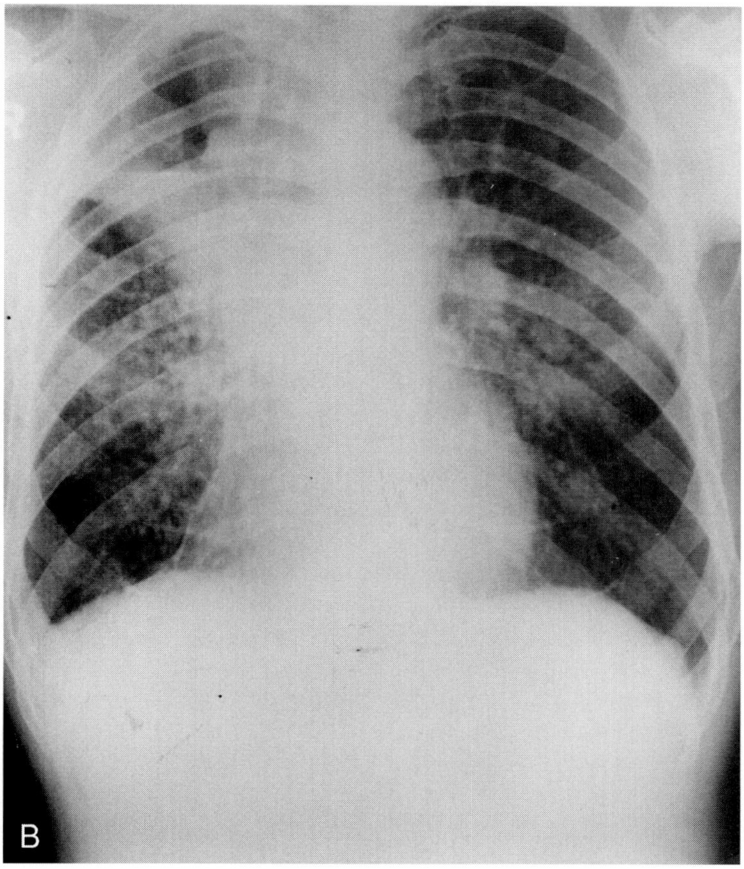

FIGURE 6.47 *(continued)*

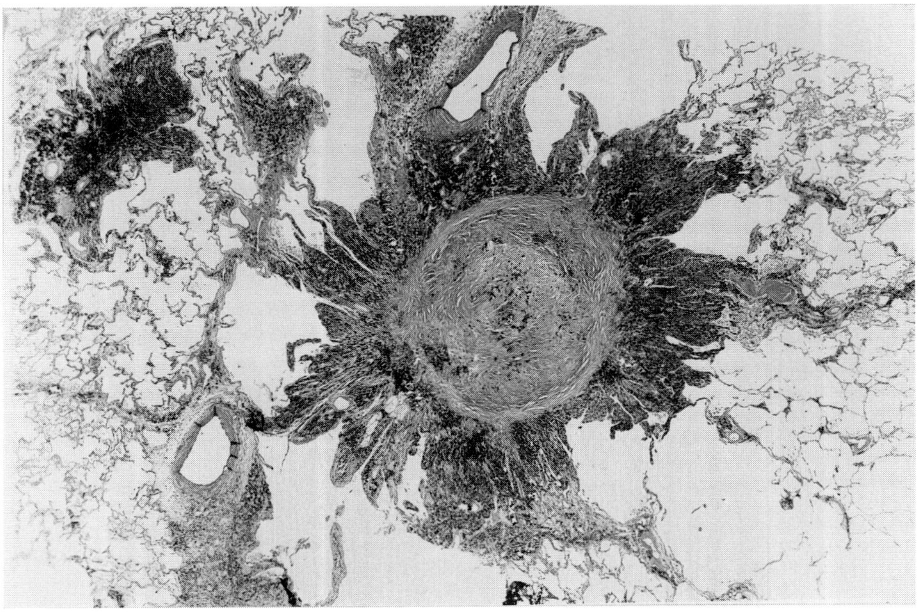

FIGURE 6.48
Silicotic nodule composed of laminated concentric collagen fibers. An irregular mantle of coal dust–containing macrophages and reticulin is characteristic of the lesion in coal workers. A coal dust macule is seen adjacent. From a 62-year-old Pennsylvania coal miner with a 25 pack-year smoking history, employed underground for 19 years, principally as coal loader.

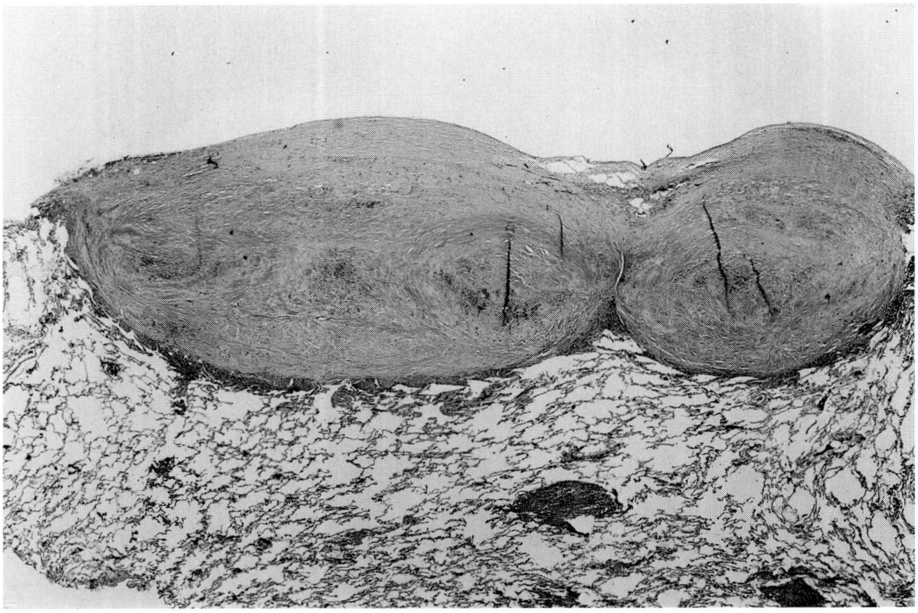

FIGURE 6.49
Subpleural silicotic nodules in a coal miner.

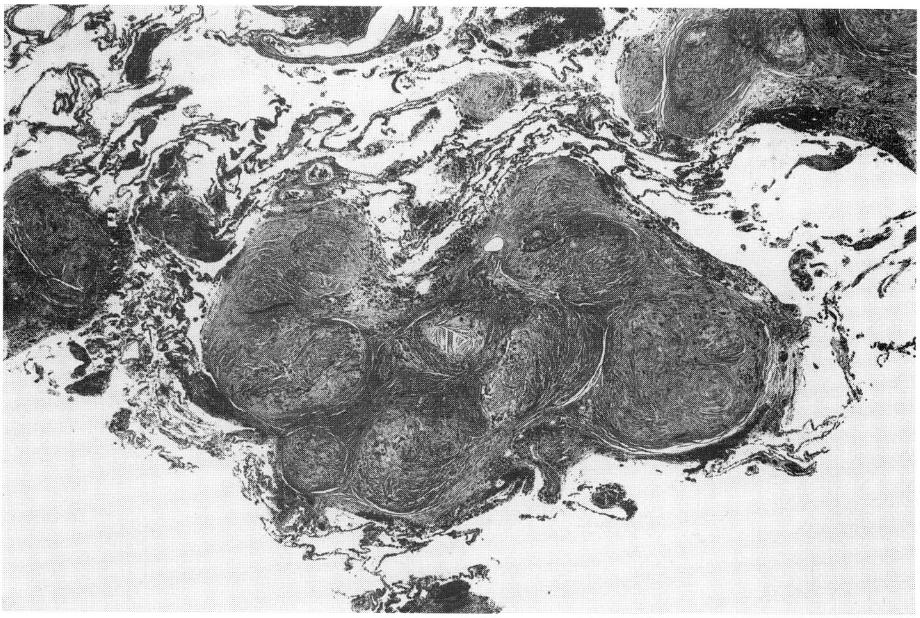

FIGURE 6.50
Conglomerate silicotic nodules. From a Pennsylvania coal miner with 29 years of underground mining and a 63 pack-year history of cigarette smoking.

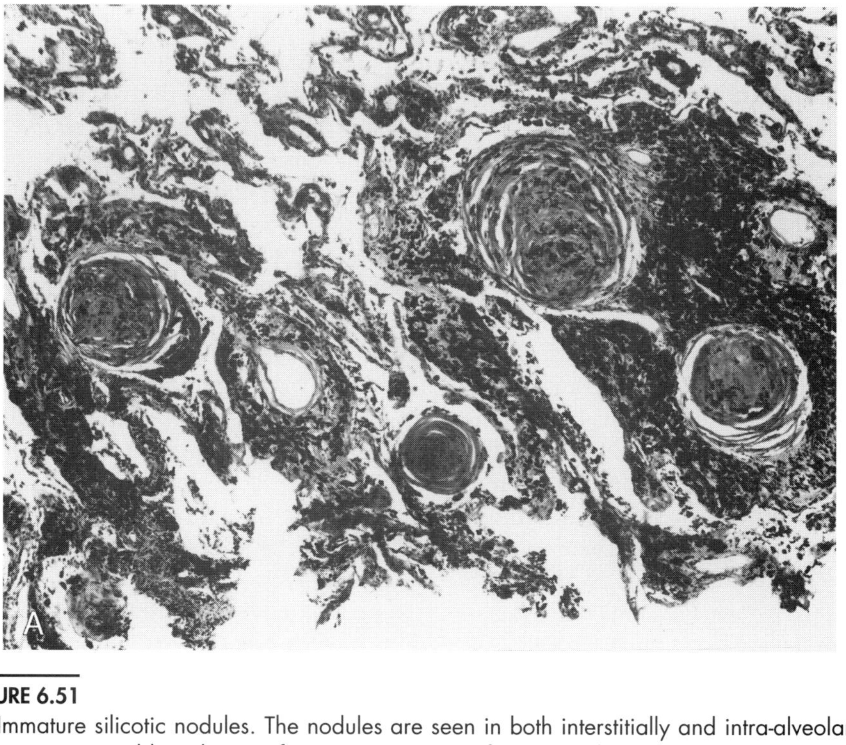

FIGURE 6.51
A. Immature silicotic nodules. The nodules are seen in both interstitially and intra-alveolarly. From a 55-year-old coal miner from West Virginia, former smoker, employed 37 years underground as cutting machine operator. **B.** High-power view of intra-alveolar nodule. The lesion shows partial incorporation into the interstitium.

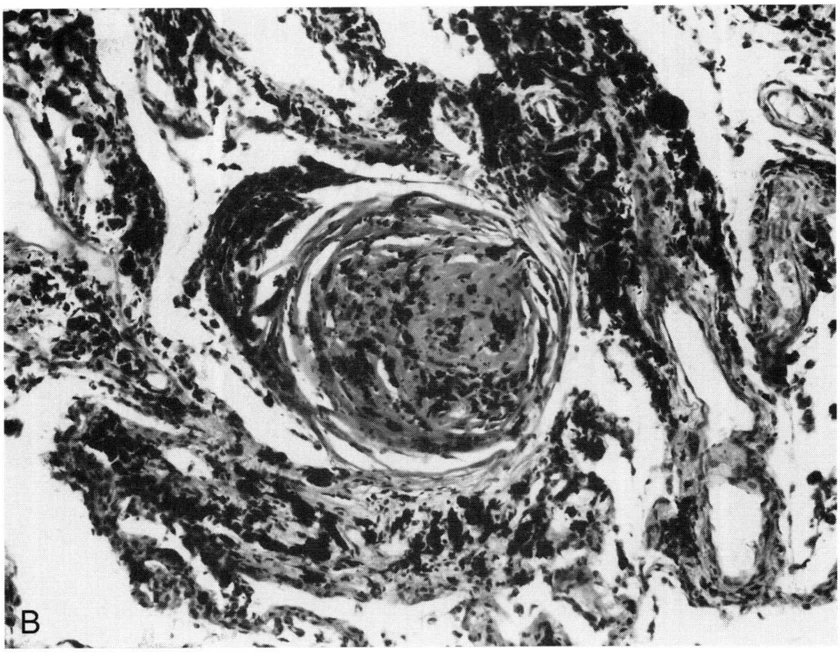

FIGURE 6.51 *(continued)*

Interstitial Lung Disease

Diffuse interstitial pulmonary fibrosis (DIPF) has been reported in the lungs of up to 18% of autopsied miners in the United States, Great Britain (127, 128), and France (129). DIPF in coal workers is associated with irregular opacities on the chest radiograph, a low gas transfer factor (128), and a relatively benign clinical course compared with that of the same condition in the general population (127). DIPF has also been reported in association with graphite pneumoconiosis (7).

Macroscopically severe cases are associated with areas of honeycombing (Fig. 6.52). Microscopically the lesions show varying degrees of fibrosis from mild interstitial fibrosis to honeycombing. The degree of pigmentation is variable (Figs. 6.53 and 6.54). In the study reported by McConnochie et al. (127), only 50% of the cases were associated with grossly visible black pigmentation. The pigmented forms of fibrosis were more likely to be associated with severe pneumoconiosis, particularly of the silicotic type, and with emphysema. The unpigmented areas of fibrosis, by contrast, were not associated with emphysema but had increased numbers of chronic inflammatory cells in the interstitium and thus resembled usual interstitial pneumonia (UIP). Pathologic changes resembling UIP were reported in a series of 38 French coal miners (129).

It seems reasonable to consider the pigmented type of interstitial fibrosis to be caused by exposure to coal mine dust. The association with silicosis implicates silica and silicates in its pathogenesis (79). The pathogenesis of the UIP type of interstitial fibrosis is less clear. Its prevalence in coal miners appears to be higher than in the general population. Coultas et al. (130) estimated the prevalence of idiopathic interstitial fibrosis in male residents of Bernalillo County, New Mexico, at 29 per 100,000 based on clinical diagnostic features and 1.8% based on the medical examiner's autopsy population. This contrasts with ap-

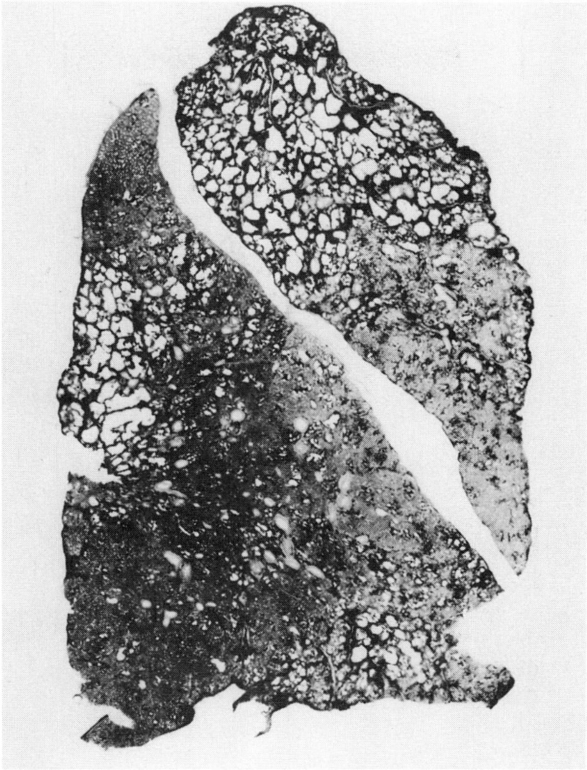

FIGURE 6.52

Interstitial fibrosis. Whole lung section shows deeply pigmented interstitial fibrosis with honeycombing and mild macular disease. From a 72-year-old miner who worked for 50 years at a variety of jobs in underground coal mines. (Reprinted with permission from Green FHY, Laqueur WA. Coal workers' pneumoconiosis. Pathol Ann 1980;v15:333–409.)

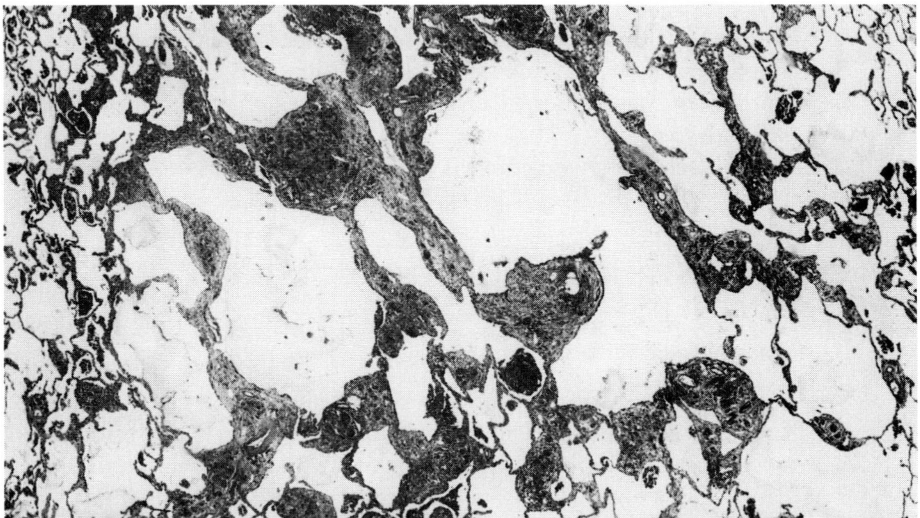

FIGURE 6.53

Pigmented interstitial fibrosis in a coal miner. The airspaces adjacent to the fibrosis are enlarged, and the dust and fibrosis are predominantly centriacinar. This type of lesion may be seen following exposure to coal mine dust and asbestos (mixed-dust exposure).

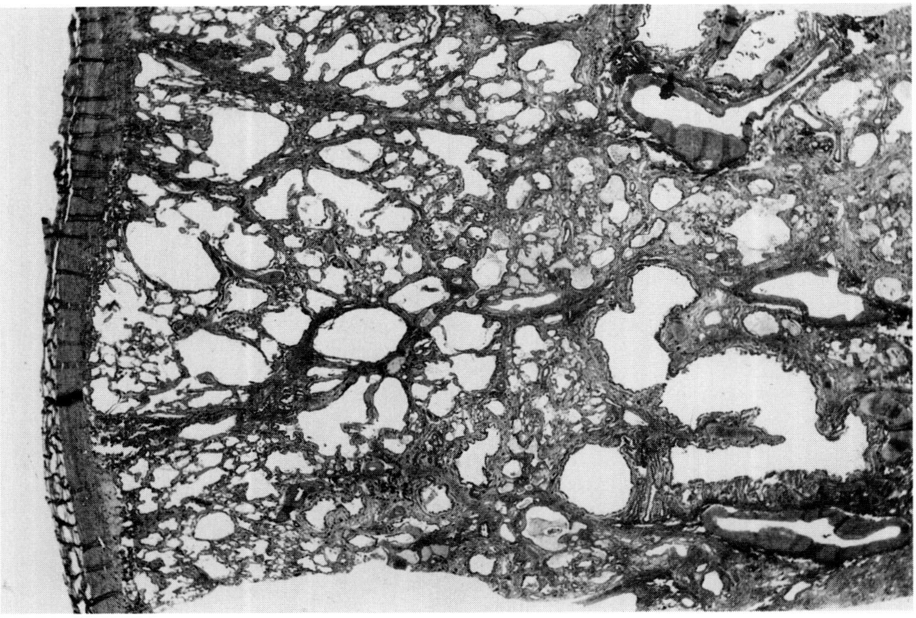

FIGURE 6.54
Diffuse interstitial fibrosis with honeycombing in lower lobe of coal miner's lung. Pigmentation is slight. No specific diagnostic features were present.

proximately 18% prevalence in U.S. and Welsh coal miners at autopsy (127, 128). It is possible that exposure to coal mine dust modifies immune and fibrogenic responses in a susceptible population, similar to the mechanisms proposed for the development of rheumatoid pneumoconiosis (see previous section). Silica in coal mine dust has also been shown to modify immune responses in exposed populations, and silica exposure is associated with autoimmune diseases such as scleroderma (131). Coal miners may also be exposed to asbestos at mine sites, particularly if they do construction work. Thus asbestosis and other defined interstitial lung diseases (e.g., sarcoidosis) should be excluded.

CHRONIC OBSTRUCTIVE LUNG DISEASE IN COAL MINERS

Epidemiologic Studies

Chronic airflow obstruction can result from several clinically and/or pathologically distinct diseases. The most important of these are asthma (reversible airway obstruction), simple chronic bronchitis (mucus hypersecretion without significant airway obstruction), chronic obstructive bronchitis (mucus hypersecretion with airway obstruction), and emphysema. Simple chronic bronchitis and chronic obstructive bronchitis associated with dust exposure are often called industrial bronchitis (74). Although one of the original terms used to describe the pneumoconiosis of coal miners was coal miners' asthma, there is no evidence that coal mine dust is capable of inducing reversible airway obstruction.

In 1985 Becklake (132) critically reviewed all the major cross-sectional and longitudinal studies since 1973 that examined the relationship between chronic airflow obstruction and exposure to dust in the workplace. She concluded that the association between exposure to mineral dust, including coal dust, and chronic airflow limitation was strong, consistent, and dose related and was independent of the effects of smoking and age. Subsequent reviews by Becklake (133) and others (134, 135) have come to essentially the same conclusion. Increasingly, chronic obstructive pulmonary disease (COPD) developing in association with dust exposure is being considered a compensable disease (136). COPD has also been associated with exposure to silica (137–140), grain dust (141), and other dusts (142–145).

Nonoccupational factors that affect lung function include age, race, gender, height, weight, physical activity, and altitude. Standard pulmonary function testing corrects for most of these variables. Smoking is a very important confounder, as approximately 75% of miners are current or former smokers and smoking is an important cause of emphysema and chronic bronchitis.

A longitudinal epidemiologic study of a large and representative group of British coal miners examined the effect of dust exposure on lung function in active and retired miners (146). The study showed a dose-related effect of dust, independent of smoking, on lung function. Furthermore, it showed that the effect of dust exposure on airflow limitation was observed in miners without radiographic evidence of pneumoconiosis. This effect was most noticeable in ex-smokers who had left the industry but was also seen in a small group of never-smoking ex-miners with chronic bronchitis. An important finding was that some miners showed greater than average decrements in lung function in response to dust exposure resulting in clinically significant pulmonary impairment. This and other studies have shown that the decline of forced expiratory volume in 1 second (FEV_1) can continue after cessation of exposure (146–149).

The rank of coal and geographic factors also influence the development of COPD. A study of U.S. miners showed that those exposed to high-rank eastern coal had greater decrements in FEV_1 than those with the same cumulative exposure to western lower-rank coal (26). Coggon et al. (150) studied mortality from CWP and COPD in 22 coal mining counties in Britain. There was no geographic correlation between the two diseases, suggesting that the characteristics of the dust that influence the development of the two diseases are different. This finding is supported by a recent study of 1286 British coal miners with no evidence of pneumoconiosis on chest radiograph (151). The investigators found that exposure to coal dust was associated with significant deficits in lung function in the absence of CWP, reinforcing the view that COPD and CWP have independent risk factors (150). These findings have implications for coal miner compensation programs (151).

The decrements in FEV_1 and forced vital capacity (FVC) associated with coal mine dust exposure have been measured in U.S. and British coal miner cross-sectional (26, 152–154) and longitudinal studies (149, 155–157). Table 6.7 lists the estimated average loss of lung function due to dust exposure over a working lifetime (45 years) at the 2 mg/m^3 exposure standard. Although these average decrements are not large in themselves and are unlikely to be associated with a compensable degree of impairment, the average hides the true picture. There is evidence that cumulative exposure may be less important than individual susceptibility to the effects of dust (146). Lewis et al. (151) have estimated that approximately 5% of miners suffer decrements of FEV_1 of 1 L or more and that

TABLE 6.7
Estimated Average Loss of Lung Function (FEV_1) Associated with Exposure to Respirable Coal Mine Dust

STUDY POPULATION	LOSS OF FEV_1 PER EXPOSURE UNIT[a] (mL)	LOSS OVER A WORKING LIFETIME[b] (mL)	REFERENCE
U.S. miners working prior to current standard (1970)	1.2	108	Henneberger and Attfield (147)
Experienced U.S. miners working during 2 mg/m^3 standard	1.4	124	Attfield and Hodous (26)
New U.S. coal miners working during 2 mg/m^3 standard	6.8	610	Seixas et al., (152)
British miners working during the 1950s, 22-year follow-up	1.5	137	Soutar and Hurley (146)
British miners working during the 1950s, 10-year follow-up	1.9	177	Marine et al., (153)

[a] Mg/m^3 per year of cumulative coal mine dust exposure.
[b] Estimated loss over a 45-year working period at the current U.S. federal dust standard (2 mg/m^3). These estimates are independent of any additional losses associated with cigarette smoking and age.

decrements of this magnitude can occur in the absence of smoking. Furthermore, the effects of dust exposure on FEV_1 appear to be much greater in younger miners (151, 152), indicating that the more susceptible miners leave the workforce (the healthy worker effect). Nonlinearity in the rates of decline associated with dust exposure have also been reported in U.S. studies (155, 158), reinforcing the view that a subset of miners are unusually susceptible to the effects of dust (147, 151). The declines in FEV_1 associated with cigarette smoking are also nonlinear, indicating that within the smoking population a subgroup of 10 to 15% will develop severe emphysema (159).

The relative roles of cigarette smoking and coal mine dust exposure in the development of COPD have been debated extensively (26,43, 46, 160). Fortunately there is now sufficient information to assess their relative contributions to rates of decline in FEV_1 (17, 156, 157, 161–163). Love and Miller (157) studied 1677 British coal miners over 11 years. They showed that an average cumulative exposure to coal mine dust of 117 gram hours per cubic meter (gh/m^3) was associated with an FEV_1 loss of 42 mL, with an additional loss of 122 mL among smokers. Attfield (156) reported dust-related losses of FEV_1 ranging from 36 to 84 mL over 11 years in 1470 U.S. coal miners, with an additional loss in FEV_1 of 100 mL for smokers. A study of coal miners from France showed rates of decline in FEV_1 of 47 mL/year for nonsmoking miners and 78 mL/year for smokers (163). The decrements associated with coal mine dust exposure thus appear to be approximately one-third to one-half those associated with cigarette smoking (78). Alcohol consumption has also been associated with declines in FEV_1 in Australian coal miners (164).

Pathologic Studies

Many anatomic studies of emphysema in coal workers have linked the postmortem severity of emphysema with antemortem functional and radiographic changes and with dust exposure (164–167, 108, 110, 128). They indicate that the severity of postmortem emphysema correlates with decrements in pulmonary function (128, 164, 167) and to some extent with smoking status (110, 165, 166). They also show that coal mining carries a risk of emphysema that is additional to the effects of age and smoking. Specifically, these and other autopsy studies have shown significant differences in emphysema scores between miners and matched controls (166–169) with positive correlations between emphysema and years worked at face (93, 164), radiographic category of pneumoconiosis (164), pathologic grade of pneumoconiosis (110, 165, 166, 170), cumulative exposure to respirable dust (110), and coal dust content of the lungs (110, 170, 171).

Although the evidence for an association between coal mining and emphysema is consistent across studies and is biologically plausible (172, 135), there are important limitations to autopsy-based research. Criticisms leveled at autopsy studies include sample selection bias, which is particularly important when the sample is selected from miners receiving compensation (167, 173) and when there is inadequate control for amount of smoking, use of inappropriate controls, and assessment of emphysema on uninflated lung (92).

Autopsy studies also indicate that centriacinar emphysema is the most common type in coal workers (93, 110, 166, 165, 168), although panacinar, scar (irregular), and paraseptal emphysema are also increased. Centriacinar emphysema was the predominant type found in 1553 South African gold miners at autopsy (139). Because focal and centriacinar emphysema involve the same anatomic locus and cannot be easily differentiated in the presence of CWP (174), most autopsy studies have not attempted to assess them as separate entities.

Although the relation between dust exposure and chronic bronchitis in coal miners is strong in epidemiologic studies, the morphologic correlates in general have been poor. A few pathologic studies used bronchial gland enlargement, including the Reid index (175), as a measure of chronic bronchitis. This index was chosen because in general it correlates with chronic bronchitis due to cigarette smoking (176, 177). Most failed to demonstrate a relation between bronchial gland size and length of employment (164, 178), severity of pneumoconiosis (164), or smoking (164) or between miner and nonminer matched controls (178). A study of 94 autopsied UK miners did, however, show the expected correlation between smoking and the Reid index (179). More important, it demonstrated a significant association between the Reid index and estimated cumulative exposure to coal mine dust. However, no significant relations were observed between gland dimensions and severity of pneumoconiosis or dust retained in the lungs. The authors considered that these apparently discrepant findings might reflect different effects for dusts containing particles of various sizes (180). Small particles (respirable) would contribute to pneumoconiosis and retained lung dust, and larger particles (inhalable) would tend to interact with the airway mucosa and be rapidly cleared by the mucociliary apparatus.

CARDIAC AND PULMONARY VASCULAR DISEASE IN COAL WORKERS

Vascular lesions related to aging, smoking, and other conditions are common in autopsy populations. It is therefore important to distinguish these changes from those associated with the macules, nodules, and PMF lesions of coal workers. Traces of atherosclerosis, replacement of elastic with collagen, and increased calcium content of the large pulmonary arteries are considered normal in aging western populations (181). This may be associated with mild dilation of the pulmonary trunk and intimal fibrosis. With increasing age the media of the muscular pulmonary arteries becomes irregular; muscle is replaced by collagen (182), and the intima shows patchy and progressive fibrosis (181). These changes are more pronounced in cigarette smokers (182). Although these changes are anatomically abnormal, they are not associated with pulmonary hypertension or cor pulmonale and thus have no obvious clinical significance.

Vascular abnormalities directly related to CWP are found in coal macules, nodules, and PMF. The small pulmonary arteries within macules may show hypertrophy of their muscular media (183, 184). The degree of pulmonary artery thickening has been shown to correlate with right ventricular hypertrophy (cor pulmonale), PMF and severity of emphysema in a postmortem study of West Virginia coal miners (184). The lesion may be responsible for the mild increases in systolic pulmonary arterial pressure observed during exercise in miners with normal ventilatory function and simple CWP (185). However, studies using the more reliable measurement of mean arterial pressure were not able to confirm this finding (186, 187). In these studies increases in mean pulmonary arterial pressure were observed only in miners with COPD.

Destructive and obliterative vascular lesions are seen in the more advanced stages of simple CWP and in PMF. They primarily involve the pulmonary arteries, but bronchial arteries, pulmonary veins, and lymphatic vessels are also affected. The affected vessels are destroyed as a result of progressive encroachment by dust and fibrous tissue. Pigmented macrophages accompany the fibrosis and frequently penetrate to the vessel lumen (Fig. 6.40). In the late stages the lumen of the vessel is obliterated. Elastic tissue stains on the larger nodules and PMF can be used to demonstrate the remains of these vessels. Secondary changes, including endarteritis, thrombosis, and chronic inflammatory cell infiltration are frequent accompaniments. Similar lesions have also been described in silicosis and other mineral dust pneumoconioses (188). Immunoglobulins and rheumatoid factor have been observed in some vessels showing inflammatory changes (103).

It is likely that the vascular lesions of PMF cause sufficient reduction in the pulmonary vascular bed to produce pulmonary hypertension (189). Lung perfusion scanning techniques in living miners with PMF have shown large deficits in perfusion in the affected areas (190). Moreover, the prevalence of cor pulmonale is much higher in miners with PMF than in miners with simple CWP (191). Cor pulmonale is a frequent cause of death for miners with categories B and C PMF (43, 46, 47). Unlike PMF, simple CWP does not lead to pulmonary hypertension and cor pulmonale (191, 192). The most likely cause of cor pulmonale in a miner with simple CWP is obstructive airway disease.

The relation between CWP and ischemic heart disease has been debated in the literature (47, 193). There is no evidence from mortality studies conducted in Great Britain and the United States that coal miners have an overall higher mortality from ischemic heart disease than the general population (49, 60). It seems reasonable to conclude that any interaction (positive or negative) between pneumoconiosis and ischemic heart disease is small.

LUNG AND STOMACH CANCER IN COAL WORKERS

When adjusted for cigarette smoking, the majority of coal miner mortality studies show that lung cancer occurs slightly less frequently in coal miners than in comparable populations (50, 58, 194). These observations in coal miners contrast with the findings of chronic inhalation studies of rats, in which overloading of the lung with relatively inert dusts, such as coal and carbon, is associated with the development of excess lung tumors (195–197). The reasons for these species differences are not known, but the differences are important in view of the fact that animal carcinogenicity studies are one of the forms of evidence used to classify substances as human carcinogens.

Only one morphologic study of lung cancer has been reported in coal workers (198). The distribution by cell type in 171 lung cancers was squamous cell, 30%; adenocarcinoma, 27%; small cell undifferentiated, 26%; large cell undifferentiated, 9%; and others, 8%. Most tumors were centered on large airways and were in the upper lobes. No effect of years of mining was observed on cell type distribution. Of the miners with lung cancer, 95% were current or former cigarette smokers. It was concluded from this study that the gross and microscopic features of lung cancer in coal workers are similar to those reported for cigarette-smoking men in the general population.

Mortality from stomach cancer appears to be elevated in coal miners in the United States (49–53) and in the United Kingdom (51). In the British study a significant relation was demonstrated between cumulative exposure to respirable coal mine dust and mortality from cancers of the digestive system. Factors such as chewing tobacco, diet, and carcinogenic compounds extractable from coal dust may all be involved (198–201).

INTERPRETATION OF THE PATHOLOGIC FINDINGS

The pathologist may be requested to estimate the degree of impairment that a miner might have suffered during life, based on the extent and severity of disease observed postmortem. It is important to stress (see Chapters 1 and 2) that an opinion based on pathologic examination alone may be misleading. Therefore, when attempting to interpret the anatomic findings, the pathologist should be familiar with the clinical details of the case as well as have a working knowledge of the many studies comparing the radiologic, physiologic, mineralogic, and pathologic features of CWP. In general there is a good correlation between the radiologic category of CWP and the severity of pneumoconiosis at autopsy (5, 81–83, 202–204). The more severe the pneumoconiosis, the better the correlation; however, in an individual case the correlation may be poor.

The radiographic category of pneumoconiosis reflects the tissue (fibrous) reaction to the dust and the dust itself. Unlike silicosis, in which radiographic category is largely determined by the fibrous tissue response, the relation between radiographic category and exposure to relatively inert dusts (e.g., barium, tin, silver, iron) depends more on the dust content of the lungs than on tissue response. For dusts with moderate fibrogenic potential, such as coal mine dust, both tissue response and dust contribute to the radiographic appearances (83). It is not surprising, therefore, that there is a positive linear relationship between lung dust burden and radiographic category of CWP (205). In a given lung the carbon and mineral fractions of the dust appear to contribute equally to the radiographic category, but weight for weight, mineral dust contributes more than carbon to the x-ray absorption characteristics of the constituent minerals (203).

Radiology and pathology differ in their abilities to detect disease in coal workers (205). Mild pathologic grades of disease do not appear on the chest radiograph. Attfield et al. (206) reported that up to 33% of chest radiographs were negative (category 0) even when the miner had moderate or severe simple macular disease on pathologic examination. The reason for this discrepancy is the variable sensitivity and specificity of the radiograph, which are affected by many factors. Individual lesions with diameters less than 3 to 6 mm may be difficult to detect on the standard chest radiograph (82, 207); thus the opacities seen in simple macular CWP largely result from the effects of summation. These images in turn are affected by background density of the lung, shape and composition of the lesions, contrast effects produced by emphysema, thickness of the chest wall, technical quality of the film, and variations among readers (47, 82). Films of poor quality tend to be read in the middle categories irrespective of their true value (205). Some of the relations among these factors are less obvious; emphysema, for example, which would be expected to reduce the reading, results in higher x-ray categories than can be justified on pathologic examination (202, 208). It appears that the loss of lung tissue is outweighed by the contrast effects produced by the enlarged airspaces.

The sensitivity of the radiograph to detect dust burden has been investigated in coal workers. In one study miners with ILO category 0/0 chest radiographs had approximately 10 times as much dust in their lungs (203) as was reported in another study of nonminer town dwellers of approximately similar age (209). The chest radiograph does not become positive for pneumoconiosis (category 1/0 or above) until dust accumulation in the lungs exceeds a threshold level, probably in the range of 5 to 10 g (203, 205). It is not surprising, therefore, that a range of severities of simple macular CWP may be observed by the pathologist in miners who have normal or equivocal chest films (81–83, 204, 210). Recent studies using computed tomography (CT) to assess coal miners have shown that CT is much more sensitive than conventional chest radiography (211, 212). In one of these studies 23% of category 0/0 radiographs using the ILO classification system were positive for pneumoconiosis on CT (211). CT is also useful for detecting emphysema (211, 212).

Despite these caveats, certain radiographic features may have specific pathologic significance. Ruckley et al. (83) compared the antemortem radiographs from 261 British coal miners with postmortem pathology and dust content of their lungs. They found that the type of lesion noted pathologically correlated closely with the radiographic classification. Radiographic category 0/0 was associated with dust macules measuring up to 0.75 mm (discussed earlier). Fine p-size rounded opacities of simple pneumoconiosis correlated with soft dust macules and with emphysema. Larger rounded opacities q- and r-size correlated with fibrotic nodular lesions. Most subjects with r-opacities demonstrated fibrotic nodules measuring 2 to 10 mm. The r-opacities in coal workers who mined low-rank coal were also highly indicative of silicosis. Vallyathan et al. (210) reported similar results from a cohort of 430 underground coal miners from Southern West Virginia: q-opacities were associated with micronodules (1 to 7 mm), and r-opacities were associated with macronodules (7–10 mm), including silicotic nodules. Other studies have shown that irregular opacities correlate with interstitial fibrosis (128, 213), with severity of postmortem emphysema (81, 166), and with reduced gas transfer factor (214).

The relation between large opacities on the chest radiograph and PMF at autopsy, though good, is far from ideal. Approximately one-third of all cases of large opacities recognized radiographically in the study by Vallyathan et al.(210) could not be substantiated as PMF on pathologic examination. Some but not all of this discrepancy can be explained on the basis of other lung pathology, such as granulomas, scars, and tumors.

Although physiologic abnormalities are almost always seen in miners with categories B and C PMF (78, 215), the correlation between the physiologic findings in simple CWP and the radiologic and pathologic features are usually poor (76, 216). Exceptions to this generalization include an apparent association between a reduced gas transfer factor and p-opacities (215) and between r-opacities and reductions in ventilatory capacity and gas transfer factor (217).

Several studies have correlated the dust content of the lungs with the pathologic grade of CWP. The ash fraction of the total dust extracted from coal miners' lungs ranges from 20 to 40% and has a mineralogic composition similar to that of the native coal mine dust (81, 85, 203, 218, 219) but may vary with rank of coal (83, 99). The proportion of ash and different minerals in the inhaled and retained coal mine dust also affect the pathologic response (87, 99).

In general there is a good correlation between the total dust and severity of disease (81, 87, 99, 100, 205). A study by Davis et al. (87) from the Institute of Occupational Medicine in Edinburgh involved the analysis of the lungs from 500 miners who worked at 25 collieries. The mean weights of total lung dust for three pathologic grades corresponding to macules, nodules, and PMF were 7.2 g, 12.5 g, and 20 g, respectively.

EXPOSURE TO OTHER CARBONACEOUS DUSTS

Carbon Black and Related Dusts

Exposure to carbonaceous dusts other than coal can cause pneumoconiosis similar in appearance to CWP. These dusts include activated carbon, graphite, lampblack, carbon black, and fumes and dusts associated with carbon electrode manufacture (220, 221, 222). Natural graphite may contain substantial quantities of quartz (3.6 to 10%), but artifical graphite, carbon black and lampblack are virtually free of silica. The population of workers who may be exposed to these substances is high. Estimates made by NIOSH in the United States indicate that as many as 2.4 million workers are exposed to natural and synthetic graphite, and 35,000 workers are exposed to carbon black (46). The prevalence of pneumoconiosis varies from country to country (9, 220). Some 25% of 3,086 European carbon black workers showed opacities of 0/1 or greater on their chest radiographs; the opacities were strongly related to indices of exposure (9). Positive associations between dust exposure, chronic bronchitis, and declines in FEV_1 were also found. Studies of North American carbon black workers by contrast have not shown these effects on pulmonary function (221). It is difficult to assess whether the differences between these studies are real or are related to different exposures or to confounding exposures with sulphur dioxide and carbon monoxide (222). The pneumoconiosis associated with exposure to these dusts is similar radiographically and pathologically (Fig. 6.18) to CWP and may progress to PMF (47). Carbonaceous dusts with low silica content usually produce a macular pattern of disease (7, 8, 223). Dusts with proportionally more silica form nodular lesions or even silicotic nodules (224).

A feature of graphite pneumoconiosis is the formation of ferruginous bodies (160, 225). These bodies have black cores, which distinguish them from asbestos bodies (see Chapter 9). Similar bodies are also seen in coal workers' lungs and occasionally in the general population.

Diesel Emissions

In the United States approximately 1.35 million people, including about 30,000 in underground mines, are exposed to diesel emissions in the workplace (226). Diesel emissions are highly complex mixtures containing gases such as nitrogen dioxide, carbon monoxide, sulphur dioxide, organic hydrocarbons, and aldehydes, as well as fine particulate matter (227). The emissions from diesel engines are richer in particulates and nitrogen dioxide than are gasoline car engines. The individual carbon particles are very small (0.01 to 0.08 µm in diameter). They tend to agglomerate into particles with a mass median aerodynamic diameter of 0.2 µm. Approximately 90% of the particulate fraction of diesel emissions is less than 1 µm in diameter; hence it is highly respirable. Vapor phase hydrocarbons and liquid condensed hydrocarbon particles (alkanes, alkenes, monocyclic and polycyclic aromatic hydrocarbons, and oxygenated organic compounds) are readily adsorbed to the particle agglomerates. Many of these compounds and their transformation products are known carcinogens. Approximately 10 to 40% of the particle mass may be adsorbed organic chemicals. Estimates of workplace exposures to the particulate fractions vary from 1 to 100 $\mu m/m^3$ in trucking and transportation to 100 to 1700 $\mu m/m^3$ in underground mines (228). In Los Angeles County diesel exhaust particles account for approximately 20% of the fine aerosol carbon particles in the atmosphere, with average ambient levels ranging from 1 to 10 $\mu m/m^3$ (229). Peak exposure levels may be considerably higher.

There have been more than 30 epidemiologic studies of the health effects of diesel emissions (230). Most focused on male workers exposed after 1950 in the trucking and transportation industries (231–244). All of these studies focused on the carcinogenic potential of diesel emissions. The studies were recently reviewed in a monograph by Cohen and Higgins (230). Epidemiologic data were consistent, finding a weak association between diesel exhaust and lung cancer, with a 1.2- to 1.5-fold increase in relative risk over that of unexposed workers. This was also found for epidemiologic studies that adequately controlled for cigarette smoking. To place this risk in perspective, the U.S. Environmental Protection Agency has estimated lung cancer risk associated with environmental tobacco smoke exposure at 1.2 to 1.6 (245). None of the studies had exposure measurements or characterized the emissions over the period of the study; hence the association between lung cancer and diesel emission exposure in humans is weak. Definitive studies with exposure details and control for confounding factors, such as cigarette smoking, asbestos, and radon gas, are required but will be very difficult to conduct. There have been no pathologic studies of diesel-exposed human populations.

Animal studies are more definitive but also reveal marked species differences in susceptibility to the carcinogenic effects of diesel emissions. Carcinogenicity in rats has been convincingly demonstrated, but no such relation has been demonstrated in hamsters or mice. Unraveling the differences in response to diesel emissions among species will be important for understanding the true hazard to humans.

The effects of diesel emissions on nonmalignant respiratory disease were recently reviewed by Cohen and Higgins (230). Most of these studies were based on death certificate data (mortality studies) or prevalence surveys of morbidity. The reviewers concluded that the studies to date do not provide strong or consistent evidence for chronic nonmalignant respiratory disease associated with exposure to diesel emissions. They caution, however, that the ability of the studies to detect an effect was weak because of methodologic difficulties.

REFERENCES

1. Gregory JC. Case of peculiar black infiltration of the whole lungs resembling melanosis. Edinburgh Med Surg J 1831;36:389–394.
2. Meiklejohn A. History of lung diseases of coal workers in Great Britain: 1. 1800–1975. Br J Ind Med 1951;8:127–137.
3. Meiklejohn A. History of lung diseases of coal workers in Great Britain: 2. 1875–1920. Br J Ind Med 1952;9:93–97.
4. Collis EL, Gilchrist JC. Effects of dust upon coal trimmers. J Ind Hyg 1928;10: 101–110.
5. Gough J, James WRL, Wentworth JE. A comparison of the radiological and pathological changes in coal workers' pneumoconiosis. J Fac Radiol (Lond) 1949;1: 28–39.
6. Levine MD, Hunter MB. Clinical study of pneumoconiosis of coal workers in the Ohio River Valley. JAMA 1957;163:1–4.
7. Gaensler EA, Cadigan JB, Sasahara AA, et al. Graphite pneumoconiosis of electrotypers. Am J Med 1966;41:864–882.
8. Watson AJ, Black J, Doig AT, Nagelschmidt G. Pneumoconiosis in carbon electrode markers. Br J Ind Med 1959;16:274–285.
9. Gardiner K, Trethowan NW, Harrington JM, et al. Respiratory health effects of carbon black: a survey of European carbon black workers. Br J Ind Med 1993;50: 1082–1096.
10. Green FHY, Althouse R, Weber KC. Prevalence of silicosis at death in underground coal miners. Am J Ind Med 1989;16:605–616.
11. Meyers RA. Coal handbook. New York: Marcel Dekker, 1981:1–17.
12. Rock RL, Svilar G, Beckman RT, Rapp DD. Evaluation of radioactive aerosols in United States underground coal mines. MSHA Informational Report. Washington: Department of the Interior.
13. Reisner MTR, Robock K. Results of epidemiological, mineralogical and cytological studies on the pathogenicity of coal mine dusts. In: Walton WM, ed. Inhaled particles IV, vol 1. New York: Pergamon Press, 1975:361.
14. Deno NC. Dihydroaromatic structure of Illinois no. 6 Monterey coal. Fuel 1980; 59:694–710.
15. MSHA. Mine injuries and worktime quarterly. Closeout edition 1992. Washington: U.S. Mine Safety and Health Administration, 1993.
16. Energy Information Administration. Coal data: a reference. Washington: U.S. Office of Coal, Nuclear, Electric and Alternate Fuels, publication DOE/EIA-0064(90), 1991.
17. National Institute for Occupational Safety and Health. Criteria for a recommended standard: occupational exposure to respirable coal mine dust. Cincinnati: National Institute for Occupational Safety and Health publication 95–106, 1995:1–336.
18. Fairman RP, O'Brien RJ, Swecker S, et al. Respiratory status of surface coal miners in the United States. Arch Environ Health 1977;32:211–215.
19. Tomb TF, Peluso RG, Parobeck PS. Quartz in United States coal mines. Ann Am Conf Gov Ind Hyg 1986;14:513–520.

20. Makimovic SD, Page SJ. Quartz dust exposures during overburden drilling at surface coal mines. Ann Am Conf Gov Ind Hyg 1986;14:361–366.
21. Green FHY, Althouse R, Frost JL, et al. Forensic investigation of coal mine fatalities. In: Wheeler RW, ed. Proceedings of the International Conference on the Health of Miners. Ann Am Conf Gov Ind Hyg 1986:117–124.
22. Stobbe T, Plummer R, Hyunwook K, Dower JM. Characterization of coal mine dust. Ann Am Conf Gov Ind Hyg 1986;14:689–696.
23. Dalal NS, Suryan MM, Vallyathan V, et al. Detection of reactive free radicals in fresh coal mine dust and their implication for pulmonary injury. Ann Occup Hyg 1989;33:79–84.
24. Mutmansky JM, Lee C. An analysis of coal and geologic variables related to coal workers' pneumoconiosis. In: Proceedings of the Lakeview Conference, October 8, 1984. Lakeview, WV: Center for Generic Respirable Disease Studies, 1984.
25. Addison J, Dodgson J. The influence of shape, size, and composition of individual dust particles on the harmfulness of coal mine dusts: development of methods of analysis. In: Proceedings of the Seventh International Pneumoconioses Conference, August 23–26, 1988, Pittsburgh. Cincinnati, OH: National Institute for Occupational Safety and Health publication 90–108, 1990.
26. Attfield MD, Hodous TK. Pulmonary function of U.S. coal miners related to dust exposure estimates. Am Rev Respir Dis 1992;145: 605–609.
27. Potts JD, McCawley MA, Jankowski RA. Thoracic dust exposures on longwall and continuous mining sections. Appl Occup Environ Hyg 1990;5:440–447.
28. Nauss KM. Diesel exhaust: a critical analysis of emissions, exposure and health effects. Cambridge, MA: Health Effects Institute, 1995:11–64.
29. Cantrell BK, Rubow KL, Watts WF Jr, et al. Pollutant levels in underground coal mines using diesel equipment. In: Bhaskar R, ed. Proceedings of the 6th U.S. Mine Ventilation Symposium. Littleton, CO: Society for Mining, Metallurgy and Exploration, 1993.
30. Ong T, Whong WZ, Xu J, Burchell B, et al. Genotoxicity studies of rodents exposed to coal dust and diesel emission particulates. Environ Res 1985;7:79–80.
31. Shirnamé-Moré L. Genotoxicity of diesel emissions: 1. Mutagenicity and other genetic effects. In: Diesel exhaust: a critical analysis of emissions, exposure and health effects. Cambridge, MA: Health Effects Institute, 221–242, 1995.
32. Green FHY, Boyd RL, Danner-Rabovsky J, et al. Inhalation studies of diesel exhaust and coal dust in rats. Scand J Work Environ Health 1983;9:181–188.
33. Lewis TR, Green FHY, Moorman WJ, et al. A chronic inhalation toxicity study of diesel engine emissions and coal dust, alone and combined. J Am Coll Toxicol 1989; 8:345–375.
34. Watson AY, Green GM. Noncancer effects of diesel emissions: animal studies. In: Diesel exhaust: a critical analysis of emissions, exposure and health effects. Cambridge, MA: Health Effects Institute, 1995:139–164.
35. Ames RG, Attfield MD, Hankinson JL, et al. Acute respiratory effects of exposure to diesel emissions in coal miners. Am Rev Respir Dis 1982;125: 39–42.
36. Reger R, Hancock J, Hankinson J, et al. Coal miners exposed to diesel exhaust emissions. Ann Occup Hyg 1982;26:799–815.
37. Fisher GL, Change DPY, Brunmer M. Fly ash collected from electrostatic precipitators: microcrystalline structure and the mystery of the spheres. Science 1976;192: 553–555.
38. Golden EB, Warnock ML, Hulett LD, Churg AM. Fly ash lung: a new pneumoconiosis? Am Rev Respir Dis 1982;125:108–112.
39. Bonnell JA, Schilling CJ, Massey PMO. Clinical and experimental studies of the effects of pulverized fuel ash. Ann Occup Hyg 1980;23:159–164.
40. Stettler LE, Groth DH, Platek FS, Donaldson HM. Fibrogenic effects and chemical characterization of coal and mineral slags used as sand substitutes. In: Wagner et al., eds. Health issues related to metal and nonmetal mining. London: Butterworth, 1983:135–160.

41. Federal Coal Mine Health and Safety Act of 1969. U.S. Public Law 91–173.
42. Jacobsen M, Rae S, Walton WH, Rogan JH. The relation between pneumoconiosis and dust exposure in British coal mines. In: Walton WH, ed. Inhaled particles 3, vol 2. Surrey, UK: Unwin Brothers, 1970:903–919.
43. Seaton A. Coal workers' pneumoconiosis. In: Morgan WKC, Seaton A, eds. Occupational lung disease, Philadelphia: WB Saunders, 1995:374–406.
44. Attfield MD, Wagner G. Respiratory disease in coal miners. In: Rom WN, ed. Environmental and occupational medicine. 2nd ed. Boston: Little, Brown, 1992: 325–344.
45. Parobek PS, Tomb TF. Respirable dust levels: surface work areas of underground coal mines and surface coal mines. Work Environ Health 1974;11:43–48.
46. Merchant JA, Taylor G, Hodous TK. Coal workers' pneumoconiosis and exposure to other carbonaceous dusts. In: Merchant JA, Boehlecke BA, Taylor G, Pickett-Harner M, eds. occupational respiratory diseases. National Institute for Occupational Safety and Health publication 86–102, 1986:329–384.
47. Parkes WR. Pneumoconiosis due to coal and carbon. In: Occupational lung disorders. London: Butterworths, 1994:340–410.
48. Enterline PE. Mortality rates among coal miners. Am J Public Health 1964;54: 758–768.
49. Rockette H. Mortality among coal miners covered by the UMWA Health and Retirement Funds. National Institute for Occupational Safety and Health publication77–155, 1977.
50. Ortmeyer CE, Costello J, Morgan WKC, et al. The mortality of Appalachian coal miners 1963–1971. Arch Env Health 1974;27:67–72.
51. Miller BG, Jacobsen M. Dust exposure, pneumoconiosis and mortality of coal miners. Br J Ind Med 1985;42:723–733.
52. Creagan ET, Hoover RN, Fraumeni JF. Mortality from stomach cancer in coal mining regions. Arch Environ Health 1974;28:28–30.
53. Matolo NM, Klauber MF, Gorishek WM, Dixon JA. High incidence of gastric carcinoma in a coal mining region. Cancer 1972;29:733–737.
54. Liddell FDK. Mortality of British coal miners in 1961–62. Br J Ind Med 1973;30: 1–14.
55. Carpenter GR, Cochrane AL, Clarke WG, et al. Death rates of miners and ex-miners with and without coal workers' pneumoconiosis in South Wales. Br J Ind Med 1956;13:102–109.
56. Cochrane AL. Relation between radiographic categories of coal workers' pneumoconiosis and expectation of life. BMJ 1973;2:532–534.
57. Ortmeyer CE, Baier EJ, Crawford GM. Life expectancy of Pennsylvania coal miners compensated for disability as affected by pneumoconiosis and ventilatory impairment. Arch Environ Health 1973;27:227–230.
58. Kuempel ED, Stayner LT, Attfield MD, Buncher CR. Exposure–response analysis of mortality among coal miners in the United States. Am J Ind Med 1995;28: 167–184.
59. Costello J, Ortmeyer CE, Morgan WKC. Mortality from lung cancer in U.S. coal miners. Am J Public Health 1974;64:222–224.
60. Costello J, Ortmeyer C, Morgan WKC. Mortality from heart disease in coal miners. Chest 1975;67:417–421.
61. Hurley JF, Copland L, Dodgson J, et al. Simple pneumoconiosis and exposure to respirable dust: relationships from twenty-five years' research at ten British coal mines. Edinburgh: Institute of Occupational Medicine report TM/79/13, 1979.
62. Reisner MTR. Results of epidemiological studies of pneumoconiosis in West German coal mines. In: Walton WH, ed. Inhaled particles 3, vol. 2. Surrey, UK: Unwin Brothers, 1971:921–931.
63. Attfield MD, Castellan RM. Epidemiological data on U.S. coal miners' pneumoconiosis, 1960 to 1988. Am J Public Health 1992;82:964–970.
64. Attfield MD, Seixas NS. Prevalence of pneumoconiosis and its relationship to dust

exposure in a cohort of U.S. bituminous coal miners and ex-miners. Am J Ind Med 1995;27:137–151.
65. McLintock JL, Rae S, Jacobsen M. The attack rate of progressive massive fibrosis in British coal miners. In: Walton WH, ed. Inhaled Particles 3, Vol 2. Surrey, UK: Unwin Brothers, 1971:933–950.
66. Bohning DE, Atkins HL, Cohn SH. Long-term particle clearance in man: normal and impaired. Ann Occup Hyg 1982;26:259–271.
67. Jacobsen M, Burns J, Attfield MD. Smoking and coal workers' simple pneumoconiosis. In: Inhaled Particles 4. London: Pergamon Press, 1975:759–771.
68. Muir DCF, Burns J, Jacobsen M, Walton WH. Pneumoconiosis and chronic bronchitis. BMJ 1977;2:424–427.
69. Shennan DH, Washington JS, Thomas DJ, et al. Factors predisposing to the development of PMF in coal miners. Br J Ind Med 1981;38:321–326.
70. Jacobsen J. Dust exposure, lung diseases and coal miners' mortality. PhD dissertation, 1976. University of Edinburgh.
71. Cochrane AL. The attack rate of PMF. Br J Ind Med 1962;19:52–62.
72. Guidelines for the use of ILO international classification of radiographs: Occupational Safety and Health Series No. 22. Geneva: International Labour Office, 1980.
73. Amandus HE, Lapp NL, Jacobson G, Reger RB. Significance of irregular small opacities in radiographs of coal miners in the USA. Br J Ind Med 1976;33:13–17.
74. Morgan WKC. Industrial bronchitis. Br J Ind Med 1978;35:285–291.
75. Jedrychowski W. A consideration of risk factors and development of chronic bronchitis in a five-year follow-up study of an industrial population. J Epidemiol Community Health 1979;33:210–214.
76. Seaton A, Lapp NL, Morgan WKC. The relationship of pulmonary impairment in simple coal workers' pneumoconiosis to type of radiographic opacity. Br J Ind Med 1972;29: 50–55.
77. Nemery B, Veriter C, Brasseur L, et al. Impairment of ventilatory function and pulmonary gas exchange in nonsmoking miners. Lancet 1987;2:1427–1430.
78. Lapp NL, Parker JE. Coal workers' pneumoconiosis. Occup Lung Dis 1992;13: 243–252.
79. Heppleston AG. Essential lesion of pneumoconiosis in Welsh coal workers. J Pathol Bacteriol 1947;59:453–460.
80. Craighead JE, Vallyathan NV. Cryptic pulmonary lesions in workers occupationally exposed to dust containing silica. JAMA 1980;244:1939–1941.
81. Davis JMG, Chapman J, Collings P, et al. Autopsy studies of coal miners lungs. Final Report on CEC Contract 6244–00/8/103. Edinburgh: Institute of Occupational Medicine, 1979.
82. Heitzman ER, Naeye RL, Markarian B. Roentgen pathological correlations in coal workers' pneumoconiosis. Ann N Y Acad Sci 1972;200:510–526.
83. Ruckley VA, Fernie J, Chapman JS, et al. Comparison of radiographic appearances with associated pathology and lung dust content in a group of coal workers. Br J Ind Med 1984;41:459–467.
84. Gross P, Hatch T. Pneumoconiosis: the requirement for lymphatic dust transport. Int Arch Gewerbepath, Gewerbehyg 1962;19:660–666.
85. Carlberg JR, Crable JV, Limitiaca LP, et al. Total dust, coal, free silica and trace metal concentrations in bituminous coal miners' lungs. Am Ind Hyg Assoc J 1971; 32:432–440.
86. LeFevre ME, Green FHY, Joel DO, Laqueur W. Frequency of black pigment in liver and spleen of coal workers. Hum Pathol 1982;13:1121–1126.
87. Davis JMG, Chapman J, Collings P, et al. Variations in the histological patterns of the lesions of coal workers' pneumoconiosis in Britain and their relationship to lung dust content. Am Rev Respir Dis 1983;128:118–124.
88. Gross P, Braun DC, deTreville RTP. The pulmonary response to coal dust. Ann N Y Acad Sci 1972;200:155–165.
89. Miller AA, Ramsden F. Carbon pneumoconiosis. Br J Ind Med 1961;18:103–113.

90. Zahorski W. Pneumoconioses dans l'industrie du graphite artificiel. Proceedings Thirteenth International Congress on Occupational Health, New York. 1961: 828–832.
91. Kleinerman J, Green FHY, Harley R, et al. Pathology standards for coal workers' pneumoconiosis: Report of the Pneumoconiosis Committee of the College of American Pathologists to the National Institute for Occupational Safety and Health. Arch Pathol Lab Med 1979;103:375–431.
92. Green FHY, Laqueur WA. Coal workers' pneumoconiosis. Pathol Ann 1980;15: 333–409.
93. Green FHY, Vallyathan V, Schleiff P, Attfield M. Emphysema in coal workers' pneumoconiosis: contribution by coal and cigarette smoking. Am Rev Resp Dis 1992;145:A321.
94. Li K, Keeling B, Churg A. Mineral dusts cause elastin and collagen breakdown in the rat lung: a potential mechanism of dust-induced emphysema. Am J Respir Crit Care Med 1996;153:644–149.
95. Heppleston AG. The pathological recognition and pathogenesis of emphysema and fibrocystic disease of the lung with special reference to coal workers. Ann N Y Acad Sci 1972;200:347–369.
96. Morgan WKC, Burgess DB, Lapp NL, et al. Hyperinflation of the lungs in coal miners. Thorax 1971;26:585–590.
97. Morgan WKC, Lapp NL. State of the art: respiratory disease in coal miners. In: Murray JF, ed. Lung disease: state of the art, 1975–1976. New York: American Lung Association, 1977:25–53.
98. Silicosis and Silicate Disease Committee. Disease associated with exposure to silica and nonfibrous silicate minerals. Arch Pathol Lab Med 1988;112:673–720.
99. Douglas AN, Robertson A, Chapman JS, Ruckley VA. Dust exposure, dust recovered from the lung and associated pathology in a group of British coal miners. Br J Ind Med 1986;43:795–801.
100. Sweet CV, Crouse W, Crabble JV, et al. The relationship of total dust, free silica and trace metal concentrations to the occupational respiratory disease of bituminous coal miners. Am Ind Hyg Assoc J 1974;35:479–488.
101. Davis JMG, Ottery J, LeRoux A. The effect of quartz and other noncoal dusts in coal workers' pneumoconiosis: 2. Lung autopsy study. In: Walton WH, ed. Inhaled Particles 4, vol 2. New York: Pergamon Press, 1975:691.
102. Jacobsen M, Maclaren WM. Unusual pulmonary observations and exposure to coal mine dust: a case control study. Ann Occup Hyg 1982;26:753–765.
103. Wagner JC, McCormick JN. Immunological investigations of coal workers' pneumoconiosis. J R Coll Physicians Lond)1967;2:49–56.
104. James WRL. The relationship of tuberculosis to the development of massive pneumoconiosis in coal workers. Br J Tuberc 1954;48:89–101.
105. Rivers D, James WRL, Davies DG, Thomson S. The prevalence of tuberculosis at necropsy in progressive massive fibrosis of coal workers. Br J Ind Med 1957;14: 39–42.
106. Hodous TK, Attfield MD. Progressive massive fibrosis developing on a background of minimal simple coal workers' pneumoconiosis. In: Proceedings of the Seventh International Pneumoconiosis Conference, August 23–26, 1988, Pittsburgh, PA. Cincinnati: National Institute for Occupational Safety and Health publication 90–108, 1990.
107. Hurley JF, Maclaren WM. Factors influencing the occurrence of progressive massive fibrosis (PMF) in miners and ex-miners. Ann Occup Hyg 1988;32(Suppl 1): 575–583.
108. Lyons JP, Campbell H. Relation between progressive massive fibrosis, emphysema and pulmonary dysfunction in coal workers' pneumoconiosis. Br J Ind Med 1981; 38:125–129.
109. Wagner JC, Wusteman FS, Edwards JH, Hill RH. The composition of massive lesions in coal miners. Thorax 1975;30:382–388.

110. Ruckley VA, Gould SJ, Chapman JS, et al. Emphysema and dust exposure in a group of coal workers. Am Rev Respir Dis 1984;129:528–532.
111. Caplan A. Certain unusual radiological appearances in the chest of coal miners suffering from rheumatoid arthritis. Thorax 1953;8:29–37.
112. Caplan A, Payne RB, Withey JL. A broader concept of Caplan's syndrome related to rheumatoid factors. Thorax 1962;17:205–212.
113. Rosenman KD, Zhu Z. Pneumoconiosis and associated medical conditions. Am J Ind Med 1995;1:107–113.
114. Benedek TG. Rheumatoid pneumoconiosis: documentation of onset and pathogenic considerations. Am J Med 1973;55:515–524.
115. Soutar CA, Turner-Warwick M, Parkes WR. Circulating antinuclear antibody and rheumatoid factor in coal pneumoconiosis. Br Med J 1974;3:145–152.
116. Benedek TG, Zawadzki ZA, Medsger TA Jr. Serum immunoglobulins, rheumatoid factor and pneumoconiosis in coal miners with rheumatoid arthritis. Arthritis Rheum 1976;19:731–736.
117. Miall WE. Rheumatoid arthritis in males: an epidemiologic study of a Welsh mining community. Ann Rheum Dis 1955;14:150–158.
118. Gough J, Rivers E, Seal RME. Pathological studies of modified pneumoconiosis in coal miners with rheumatoid arthritis (Caplan's syndrome). Thorax 1955;10:9–18.
119. Walton WH, Dodgson J, Haddon GG, Jacobsen M. The effect of quartz and other non–coal dusts in coal workers' pneumoconiosis. In: Walton WH, ed. Inhaled Particles 4, vol 2. Oxford, UK: Pergamon Press, 1977:669–690.
120. Martin JC, Daniel-Moussard H, LeBouffant L, Policard A. The role of quartz in the development of coal workers' pneumoconiosis. Ann N Y Acad Sci 1972;200: 127–141.
121. Weller W, Ulmer WT. Inhalation studies of coal–quartz dust mixtures. Ann N Y Acad Sci 1972;200:142–154.
122. Stettler LE, Platek SF, Groth DM, et al. Particle contents of human lungs. In: Basu S, ed. Electron microscopy in forensic, occupational and environmental health sciences. New York: Plenum Press, 1986:217–226.
123. Nagelschmidt G. The study of lung dust in pneumoconiosis. Am Ind Hyg Assoc J 1965;26:1–7.
124. Wallace WE, Harrison J, Keane MJ, et al. Clay occlusion of respirable quartz particles detected by low voltage scanning electron microscopy–X-ray analysis. Ann Occup Hyg 1990;34:195–204.
125. Seaton A, Dick JA, Dodgson J, Jacobsen M. Quartz and pneumoconiosis in coal miners. Lancet 1981;2:1272–1275.
126. Laqueur WA. Final report on the pathology of coal workers' pneumoconiosis and related investigations (PHS grant 65–65–9), Beckley W.V., Appalachian Regional Hospital, 1966.
127. McConnochie K, Green FHY, Vallyathan V, et al. Interstitial fibrosis in coal workers: experience in Wales and West Virginia. Ann Occup Hyg 1988;32:553–560.
128. Cockcroft AE, Wagner JC, Seal RME, et al. Irregular opacities in coal workers' pneumoconiosis: correlation with pulmonary function and pathology. Ann Occup Hyg 1982;26:767–787.
129. Brichet A, Wallaert B, Gosselin B, et al. Idiopathic-like pulmonary fibrosis in coal workers. Am J Respir Crit Care Med 1997;155:A331.B
130. Coultas DB, Zumwalt RE, Black WC, Sobonya RE. The epidemiology of interstitial lung diseases. Am J Respir Crit Care Med 1994;150:967–972.
131. Green FHY, Vallyathan V. Pathologic responses to inhaled silica. In: Castranova V, Vallyathan V, Wallace WE, eds. Silica and silica-induced lung diseases, New York: CRC Press, 1996:39–62.
132. Becklake MR. Chronic airflow limitation: Its relationship to work in dusty occupations. Chest 1985;88:608–616.
133. Becklake MR. Occupational exposures: evidence for a causal association with chronic obstructive pulmonary disease. Am Rev Respir Dis 1989;140:S85–S91.

134. Oxman AD, Muir DCF, Shannon HS, et al. Occupational dust exposure and chronic obstructive pulmonary disease: a systematic overview of the evidence. Am Rev Respir Dis 1993;148:38–48.
135. Wright JL, Cagle P, Churg A, et al. Diseases of the small airways. Am Rev Respir Dis 1992;146:240–62.
136. Industrial Injuries Advisory Council. Chronic bronchitis and emphysema. Social Security Administration Act 1992. London: Department of Social Security, 1992.
137. Cowie RL, Mabena SK. Silicosis, chronic airflow limitation and chronic bronchitis in South African gold miners. Am Rev Respir Dis 1991;143:80–84.
138. Becklake MR, Irwig L, Kielkowski D, et al. The predictors of emphysema in South African gold miners. Am Rev Respir Dis 1987;135:1235–1241.
139. Hnizdo E, Sluis-Cremer GK, Abramowitz JA. Emphysema type in relation to silica dust exposure in South African gold miners. Am Rev Respir Dis 1991;143:1241–1247.
140. Manfreda J, Johnston B, Cherniack RM. Longitudinal changes of lung function: comparison of employees of hard rock mining industry and general population. Am Rev Respir Dis 1984;129:142.
141. Kauffmann F, Drouet D, Lellouch J, Brille D. Occupational exposure and 12-year spirometric changes among Paris area workers. Br J Ind Med 1982;39:221–232.
142. Kilburn KH. Particles causing lung disease. Environ Health Perspect 1984;55:97–109.
143. Wild P, Refregier M, Auburtin G, et al. Survey of the respiratory health of the workers of a talc producing factory. Occup Environ Med 1995;52:470–477.
144. McConnochie K, Bevan C, Newcombe RG, et al. A study of Spanish sepiolite workers. Thorax 1993;48:370–374.
145. Heederik D, de Cock J, Endlich E. Dust exposure indices and lung function changes in longshoremen and dock workers. Am J Ind Med 1994;26:497–509.
146. Soutar CA, Hurley JF. Relation between dust exposure and lung function in miners and ex-miners. Br J Ind Med 1986;43:307–320.
147. Henneberger PK, Attfield MD. Coal mine dust exposure and spirometry in experienced miners. Am J Respir Crit Care Med 1996;153:1560–1566.
148. Bates DV, Pham QT, Chau N, et al. A longitudinal study of pulmonary function in coal miners in Lorraine, France. Am J Ind Med 1985;8:21–32.
149. Leigh J. 15-year longitudinal studies of FEV_1 loss and mucus hypersecretion development in coal workers in New South Wales, Australia. In: Proceedings of the Seventh International Pneumoconioses Conference, part 1, Pittsburgh. Cincinnati: National Institute for Occupational Safety and Health publication 90–108, 1990:112–121.
150. Coggon D, Inskip H, Winter P, Pannett B. Contrasting geographical distribution of mortality from pneumoconiosis and chronic bronchitis and emphysema in British coal miners. Occup Environ Med 1995;52:554–555.
151. Lewis S, Bennett J, Richards K, Britton J. A cross-sectional study of the independent effect of occupation on lung function in British coal miners. Occup Environ Med 1996;53:125–128.
152. Seixas NS, Robins TG, Attfield MD, Moulton LH. Exposure–response relationships for coal mine dust and obstructive lung disease following enactment of the Federal Coal Mine Health and Safety Act of 1969. Am J Ind Med 1992;21:715–734.
153. Marine WM, Gurr D, Jacobsen M. Clinically important respiratory effects of dust exposure and smoking in British coal miners. Am Rev Respir Dis 1988;137:106–112.
154. Soutar C, Campbell S, Gurr D, et al. Important deficits of lung function in three modern colliery populations. Am Rev Respir Dis 1993;147:797- 803.
155. Seixas NS, Robins TG, Attfield MD, Moulton LH. Longitudinal and cross-sectional analyses of exposure to coal mine dust and pulmonary function in new miners. Br J Ind Med 1993;50:929–937.

156. Attfield MD. Longitudinal decline in FEV_1 in United States coalminers. Thorax 1985;40:132–137.
157. Love RG, Miller BG. Longitudinal study of lung function in coal miners. Thorax 1982;37:193–197.
158. Hodous TK, Hankinson JL. Prospective spirometric study of newcoal miners. In: Li Y, Yao P, Schipkoter HW, et al, eds. International Symposium on Pneumoconioses, ISP '88. Dusseldorf: Stefan W. Alberg Verlag, 1990:206–211.
159. Fletcher C, Peto R. The natural history of chronic airflow obstruction. Br Med J 1977;1:1645–1648.
160. Worth G. Emphysema in coal workers. Am J Ind Med 1984;6:401–403 (editorial).
161. Rogan JM, Attfield MD, Jacobsen M, et al. Role of dust in the working environment in development of chronic bronchitis in British coal miners. Br J Ind Med 1972;30:217–226.
162. Higgins ITT. Chronic respiratory disease in coal miners. National Institute of Occupational Safety and Health publication 81–109, 1981.
163. Dimich-Ward H, Bates DV. Re-analysis of a longitudinal study of pulmonary function in coal miners in Lorraine, France. Am J Ind Med 1994;25:613–623.
164. Leigh J, Outhred KG, McKenzie HI, et al. Quantified pathology of emphysema, pneumoconiosis and chronic bronchitis in coal workers. Br J Ind Med 1983;40:258–263.
165. Lyons JP, Ryder RC, Seal RME, Wagner JC. Emphysema in smoking and nonsmoking coal workers with pneumoconiosis. Bull Eur Physiopathol Respir 1981;17:75–85.
166. Cockcroft AE, Wagner JC, Ryder R, et al. Post mortem study of emphysema in coal workers and noncoal workers. Lancet 1982;2:600–603.
167. Ryder R, Lyons JP, Campbell H, Gough J. Emphysema in coal workers' pneumoconiosis. Br Med J 1970;3:481–487.
168. Lamb D. A survey of emphysema in coal workers and the general population. Proc R Soc Med 1976;69:14 (abstract).
169. Naeye RL, Mahon JK, Dellinger WS. Effects of smoking on lung structure of Appalachian coal workers. Arch Environ Health 1971;22:190–193.
170. Vallyathan V, Green FHY, Brower P, Attfield M. The role of coal mine dust exposure in the development of pulmonary emphysema. Ann Occup Hyg 1997;41(suppl 1):352–357.
171. Leigh J, Driscoll TR, Cole BD, et al. Quantitative relation between emphysema and lung mineral content in coal workers. Occup Environ Med 1994;51:400–407.
172. Rom WN. Basic mechanisms leading to focal emphysema in coal workers' pneumoconiosis. Environ Res 1990;53:16–28.
173. Parkes W, Williamson RGB, Phillips TJG. Emphysema in coal workers. Br Med J 1970;4:430–431.
174. Heppleston AG. Emphysema and dust exposure in a group of coal workers. Am Rev Respir Dis 1984;130:949–951.
175. Reid L. Measurement of the bronchial mucous gland layer: a diagnostic yardstick in chronic bronchitis. Thorax 1960;15:132–141.
176. Thurlbeck WM, Angus GE, Pare JAP. Mucous gland hypertrophy in chronic bronchitis and its occurrence in smokers. Br J Dis Chest 1963;57:73–78.
177. Field EH, Davey EN, Reid L, Roe FJC. Bronchial mucous gland hypertrophy: its relation to symptoms and environment. Br J Dis Chest 1966;60:66–80.
178. Ryder RC, Lyons JP, Campbell J, Gough J. Bronchial mucous gland status in coal workers' pneumoconiosis. Ann N Y Acad Sci 1971;200:370.
179. Douglas AN, Lamb D, Ruckley VA. Bronchial gland dimensions in coal miners: influence of smoking and dust exposure. Thorax 1982;37:760–764.
180. Seixas NS, Hewett P, Robins TG, Haney R. Variability of particle size-specific fractions of personal coal mine dust exposures. Am Ind Hyg Assoc J 1995;56:243–250.
181. Wagenvoort CA, Wagenvoort N. Pulmonary vascular bed: Normal anatomy and

responses to disease. In: Moser KM, ed. Lung Biology in Health and Disease, Vol 14, New York, Marcel Dekker, 1979:1–109.
182. Naeye RK, Dellinger WS. Pulmonary arterial changes with age and smoking. Arch Pathol 1971;92:284–288.
183. Naeye RL, Laqueur WA. Chronic cor pulmonale: Its pathogenesis in Appalachian bituminous coal workers. Arch Pathol 1970;90:487–493.
184. Hu S-N, Vallyathan V, Green FHY, Weber KC, Laqueur W. Pulmonary arteriolar muscularization in coal workers' pneumoconiosis and its correlation with right ventricular hypertrophy. Arch Pathol Lab Med 1990;114:1063–1070.
185. Rasmussen DL. Patterns of physiological impairment in coal workers' pneumoconioses. Ann N Y Acad Sci 1972;200:455–462.
186. Lapp NL, Seaton A, Kaplan KC, et al. Pulmonary hemodynamics in symptomatic coal miners. Am Rev Respir Dis 1971;104:418–426.
187. Ulmer WT, Reichel G. Functional impairment in coal workers' pneumoconiosis. Ann N Y Acad Sci 1972;200:405–412.
188. Rüttner JR, Gassman R. Lungengefässveranderungen bei silikose und ihre Beziehungen zum cor pulmonale chronicum. In: Die Staublungenerkrankungen Band 3. (Wissenschaftliche Forschungsberichte Band 66) 1957:11.
189. Bollinelli R, LeTallec Y, Bollinelli M. Les résultats de l'exploration hémodynamique dans les silicoses pseudotumorales. J Fr Med Chir Thorac 1957;11:594–603.
190. Seaton A, Lapp NL, Chang CHJ. Lung perfusion scanning in coal workers' pneumoconiosis. Am Rev Respir Dis 1971;103:338–349.
191. Wells AC. Cor pulmonale in coal workers' pneumoconiosis. Br Heart J 1954;16:74.
192. James WRL, Thomas AJ. Cardiac hypertrophy in coal workers' pneumoconiosis. Br J Ind Med 1956;13:24.
193. Davies D. Deaths from coronary artery disease and coal workers' pneumoconiosis. Br Med J 1976;2:925–927.
194. Meijers JMM, Swaen GMH, Slangen JJM, et al. Long-term mortality in miners with coal workers' pneumoconiosis in the Netherlands: a pilot study. Am J Ind Med 1991;19:43–50.
195. Morrow PE. Dust overloading of the lungs: update and appraisal. Toxicol Appl Pharmacol 1992;113:1–12.
196. Muhle H, Creutzenberg O, Bellmann B, et al. Dust overloading of lungs: investigations of various materials, species differences and irreversibility of effects. J Aerosol Med 1990;3(Suppl 1):S111–S128.
197. Mauderly JL, Cheng Y, Snipes MB. Particle overload in toxicological studies: friend or foe? J Aerosol Med 1990;3:169–188.
198. Vallyathan V, Green FHY, Rodman NF, et al. Lung carcinoma by histologic type in coal miners. Arch Pathol Lab Med 1985;109:419–423.
199. Wu ZL, Chen JK, Ong T, et al. Induction of morphological transformation by coal-dust extract in BALB/3T3 A31–1-13 cell line. Mutat Res 1990;242:225–230.
200. Ames RG, Gamble JF. Lung cancer, stomach cancer and smoking status among coal miners. Scand J Work Environ Health 1983;9:443–448.
201. Whong WZ, Long R, Ames RG, Ong TM. Role of nitrosation in the mutagenic activity of coal dust: a postulation for gastric carcinogenesis in coal miners. Environ Res 1983;32:298–304.
202. Caplan A. Correlation of radiological category with lung pathology in coal workers' pneumoconiosis. Br J Ind Med 1962;19:171–179.
203. Rivers D, Wise ME, King EJ, Nagelschmidt G. Dust content, radiology and pathology in simple pneumoconiosis of coal workers. Br J Ind Med 1960;17:87–108.
204. Naeye RL, Dellinger WS. Coal workers' pneumoconiosis: correlation of roentgenologic and post mortem findings. JAMA 1972;220:223–227.
205. Rossiter CE. Relation between content and composition of coal workers' lungs and radiological appearances. Br J Ind Med 1972;29:31–34.
206. Attfield MD, Vallyathan V, Green FHY. Radiographic appearances of small opac-

ities and their correlation with pathology grading of macules, nodules, and dust burden in the lung. Ann Occup Hyg 1994;58(Suppl 1):783–789.
207. Spratt JS Jr, Ter-Pogossian M, Long RTL. The detection and growth of intrathoracic neoplasms: the lower limits of radiographic distinction of the antemortem size. Arch Surg 1963;86:283–288.
208. Rossiter CE, Rivers D, Bergman I, et al. Dust content radiology and pathology in simple pneumoconiosis of coal workers. In: Davies CN, ed. Inhaled particles and vapors. London: Pergamon Press, 1967:419–434.
209. Blacklock JWS, Kennaway EL, Lewis GM, Urquhart ME. Carbon content of human lungs and bronchial glands. Br J Cancer 1954;8:40–55.
210. Vallyathan V, Brower PS, Green FHY, Attfield MD. Radiographic and pathologic correlation of coal workers' pneumoconiosis. Am J Respir Crit Care Med 1996; 154:741–748.
211. Remy-Jardin M, Degreef JM, Beuscart R, et al. Coal worker's pneumoconiosis: CT assessment in exposed workers and correlation with radiographic findings. Radiology 1990;177:363–371.
212. Gevenois PA, Dargent F, Dedeire S, et al. Low grade coal worker's pneumoconiosis. Acta Radiol 1994;35:351–356.
213. Lyons JP, Ryder RC, Campbell H, et al. Significance of irregular opacities in the radiology of coal workers' pneumoconiosis. Br J Ind Med 1974;31:36–44.
214. Cockcroft A, Andersson N. Radiological irregular opacities and coalwork exposure: a case-reference study. Br J Ind Med 1987;44:484–487.
215. Musk AW, Cotes JE, Bevan C, Campbell MJ. Relationship between type of simple coal workers' pneumoconiosis and lung function: a nine-year follow-up study of subjects with small rounded opacities. Br J Ind Med 1981;38:313–320.
216. Lamb D. Physiological/pathological correlations in coal workers' pneumoconiosis. Bull Physiopathol Respir 1975;11:471–478.
217. Cockcroft A, Berry G, Cotes JE, Lyons JP. Shape of small opacities and lung function in coal workers. Thorax 1982;37:765–769.
218. Faulds JS, King EJ, Nagelschmidt G. The dust content of the lungs of coal workers from Cumberland. Br J Ind Med 1959;16:43–50.
219. Einbrodt HJ. Untersushungen über die Straubreteneion in der menschlichen Lunge. Beitr Silikose-Forschung H, 1965;87:S1–105.
220. Gardiner K. Effects of respiratory morbidity of occupational exposure to carbon black: a review. Arch Environ Health 1995;50:44–60.
221. Robertson JM. Epidemiologic studies in North American carbon black workers. In: Mauderly JL, McCunney RJ, eds. Particle overload in the rat lung and lung cancer: implications for human risk assessment. Washington, DC: Proceedings of a conference held at the Massachusetts Institute of Technology, Taylor & Francis, 1995.
222. Gardiner K, Trethowan NW, Harrington JM, et al. Occupational exposure to carbon monoxide and sulphur dioxide during the manufacture of carbon black. Ann Occup Hyg 1992;36:363–372.
223. Gross P, Nau CA. Lignite and steam derived activated carbon: the pulmonary response to their dusts. Arch Environ Health 1967;14:450–460.
224. Gloyne SR, Marchall G, Hoyle C. Pneumoconiosis due to graphite dust. Thorax 1949;4:32–38.
225. Town JE. Pseudoasbestos bodies and asteroid giant cells in a patient with graphite pneumoconiosis. Can Med Assoc J 1968;98:100–104.
226. National Institute for Occupational Safety and Health. Carcinogenic effects of exposure to diesel exhaust. NIOSH Current Intelligence Bulletin 50. Atlanta: Centers for Disease Control publication 88–116, 1988.
227. Winer AM, Busby Jr WF. Atmospheric transport and transformation of diesel emissions. In: diesel exhaust: a critical analysis of emissions, exposure and health effects. Cambridge, MA: Health Effects Institute, 1995:83–106.
228. Watts Jr WF. Assessment of occupational exposure to diesel emissions. In: Diesel

exhaust: a critical analysis of emissions, exposure and health effects. Cambridge, MA: Health Effects Institute, 1995:107–124.
229. Cass GR, Gray HA. Regional emissions and atmospheric concentrations of diesel engine particulate matter: Los Angeles as a case study. In: Diesel exhaust: a critical analysis of emissions, exposure and health effects. Cambridge, MA: Health Effects Institute, 1995:125–138.
230. Cohen AJ, Higgins MWP. Health effects of diesel exhaust: epidemiology. In: Diesel exhaust: a critical analysis of emissions, exposure and health effects. Cambridge, MA: Health Effects Institute, 1995:251–292.
231. Ahlberg J, Ahlbom A, Lipping H, et al. Cancer among professional drivers: a problem-oriented register-based study. Lakartidningen 1981;78:1545–1546.
232. Boffetta P, Harris RE, Wynder EL. Case-control study of occupational exposure to diesel exhaust and lung cancer risk. Am J Ind Med 1990;17:577–591.
233. Boffetta P, Stellman SD, Garfinkel L. Diesel exhaust exposure and mortality among males in the American Cancer Society prospective study. Am J Ind Med 1988;14: 403–415.
234. Burns PB, Swanson GM. The occupational cancer incidence surveillance study (OCISS): Risk of lung cancer by usual occupation and industry in the Detroit metropolitan area. Am J Ind Med 1991;19:655–671.
235. Hall NEL, Wynder EL. Diesel exhaust exposure and lung cancer: a case-control study. Environ Res 1984;34:77–86.
236. Hayes RB, Thomas T, Silverman DT, occupational cancer incidence surveillance study. Lung cancer in motor exhaust-related occupations. Am J Ind Med 1989;16: 685–695.
237. Howe GR, Fraser D, Lindsay J, et al. Cancer mortality (1965–1977) in relation to diesel fume and coal exposure in a cohort of retired railway workers. J Natl Cancer Inst 1983;70:1015–1019.
238. Menck HR, Henderson BE. Occupational differences in rates of lung cancer. J Occup Med 1976;18:797–801.
239. Schenker MB, Smith T, Muñoz A, et al. Diesel exposure and mortality among railway workers: result of a pilot study. Br J Ind Med 1984;41:320–327.
240. Siemiatycki J, Gérin M, Stewart P, et al. Associations between several sites of cancer and ten types of exhaust and combustion products. Scand J Work Environ Health 1988;14:79–90.
241. Steenland NK, Silverman DT, Hornung RW. Case-control study of lung cancer and truck driving in the Teamsters Union. Am J Public Health 1990;80:670–674.
242. Williams RR, Stegens NL, Goldsmith JR. Associations of cancer site and type with occupation and industry from the Third National Cancer Survey Interview. J Natl Cancer Inst 1977;59:1147–1185.
243. Garshick E, Schenker MB, Muñoz A, et al. A retrospective cohort study of lung cancer and diesel exhaust exposure in railroad workers. Am Rev Respir Dis 1988;137: 820–825.
244. Garshick E, Schenker MB, Muñoz A, et al. A case-control study of lung cancer and diesel exhaust exposure in railroad workers. Am Rev Respir Dis 1987;135: 1242–1248.
245. U.S. Environmental Protection Agency. Respiratory health effects of passive smoking: lung cancer and other disorders, Washington: Office of Air and Radiation publication EPA/700/6–90/006F, 1992.

CHAPTER 7

Diseases Due to Silica

❖ Allen R. Gibbs
❖ J. C. Wagner

Silicosis, the lung disease caused by the inhalation of free silica, is one of civilization's oldest recognized occupational diseases (1); it was described in Egyptian mummies. In recent times the first recognition was among the Sheffield knife grinders in the 1820s. However, despite recognition, silicosis continues to occur when the quartz content of the dust is not appreciated and because the amount of dust generated is greatly increased by mechanization, as in mining with the introduction of pneumatic drills. Examples of unexpected causes of silicosis include the preparation of scouring powders and sandblasting. It also still occurs in developing countries where there is a general lack of industrial hygiene. It is not confined to developing countries: a recent paper described accelerated silicosis occurring in a small group of Scottish stonemasons who were exposed to levels of respirable quartz up to 130 times the workplace standard (2).

It is not possible to give accurate figures for the prevalence of silicosis, since there are few national case registries. However, in 1970 it was estimated that more than 1 million workers in the United States possibly were exposed to free silica (3). A radiographic survey of British foundrymen published in 1971 disclosed a 34% and 14% prevalence of simple pneumoconiosis in fettles and foundry floor men, respectively (4). The Surveillance of Work- Related and Occupational Respiratory Disease (SWORD) scheme of occupational respiratory disease reported by clinicians in the United Kingdom reported that out of 3300 work-related respiratory diseases in 1994, 341 were pneumoconiosis, of which 11% were attributed to silica (5). From 1984 to 1994 cases of pneumoconiosis that were diagnosed by the Special Medical Boards of Great Britain and that were likely to be due to silica exposure ranged from 17 to 48 per year (6). Therefore it is important for the pathologist to recognize the situations in which significant exposure to free silica is likely to arise and to be conversant with the macroscopic and microscopic appearances it engenders.

Although exposure to free silica can result in severe pulmonary fibrosis, it rarely causes death by itself. Before the advent of antituberculous drugs in the 1950s the most common cause of death among workers with silicosis was tuberculosis. There is an unexplained synergism between exposure to free silica and the development of tuberculosis.

In the first part of this chapter we outline the mineralogy and sources of exposure to silica. We next describe the range of pathologic appearances encountered when subjects have been chronically and acutely exposed to significant quantities of dust containing a high percentage of free silica—so-called nodular or classic silicosis and acute silicoproteinosis—and to dusts containing free silica combined with less fibrogenic agents such as iron oxide, called mixed-dust fibrosis. Finally we discuss the pathogenesis of silica-induced lesions and briefly comment on clinical and radiographic features.

MINERALOGY

Free or uncombined silica, as distinguished from silicates (see Chapter 8), occurs naturally in noncrystalline (amorphous) and several crystalline forms. The latter include quartz, tridymite, cristobalite, coesite, and stishovite (7). Quartz is the most abundant natural silica mineral, present in almost all types of igneous, sedimentary, and metamorphic rocks. It occurs in sand, quartzite, sandstone, and granite. Quartz possesses several useful industrial properties, including hardness, chemical stability, high electrical resistance, and heat resistance.

All the crystalline forms except stishovite, which is octahedral, have a tetrahedral structure. This has an important bearing on fibrogenic potential, since stishovite is the only form that is nonfibrogenic (8). Tridymite and cristobalite are less common than quartz; they may be formed during industrial processes when quartz or amorphous silica is heated or naturally in volcanic rocks. Stishovite and Coesite are high-temperature and high-pressure products found naturally in meteorite craters (8, 9).

Amorphous silica occurs as diatomite (kieselguhr) and vitreous silica. It is nonfibrogenic but may become fibrogenic if heated, since tridymite and cristobalite may be formed. The amount formed depends on the temperature and length of time heated (10).

In practice most cases of silicosis and mixed-dust fibrosis are associated with exposures to quartz. Although studies of the effect of particle size and surface area on the development of fibrosis have not been consistent because they are intimately linked with particle retention, some investigators have found that quartz particles less than 1μm in size are most pathogenic (11).

SOURCES OF EXPOSURE

Exposure to silica can occur in (*a*) industrial processes directly involved with siliceous materials or (*b*) during mineral extraction processes in which the residual rock contains uncombined silica. Therefore significant exposure to free silica can occur in a wide range of occupations (10, 12) (Table 7. 1). Environmen-

TABLE 7.1
Occupations with Exposure to Crystalline Silica

Mining, quarrying, and tunneling through siliceous rock
Stonecutting, engraving, and polishing
Manufacture and use of silica-containing abrasives and fillers
Foundry work
Manufacture of ceramics and refractories
Sandblasting and grinding

tal exposure to silica is widespread, since quartz is the most abundant mineral on the earth's surface and is airborne in both the country and the city. It is an important constituent of PM_{10} (airborne particulate matter less than 10 μm in aerodynamic diameter), which is considered to be important in the genesis of respiratory diseases caused by air pollution. In some windy, dusty areas early changes of silicosis and mixed-dust fibrosis may be observed in the lung tissues of the inhabitants.

Mining, Quarrying, and Tunneling of Siliceous Rocks

Various processes may produce dusts with a high quartz content during the mining of gold, tin, copper, platinum, mica, talc, bentonite, barium, coal, fire clays, and fluorspar. The quarrying of granite, slate, or sandstone may produce significant quartz exposure. Tunneling or excavating through rocks with a high quartz content can result in silicosis.

Stonecutting, Engraving, and Polishing

Sandstone and granite, which have a high content of quartz, are the main materials used. The cutting, smoothing, engraving, and cleaning of these stones, which is very dusty, is often carried out in poorly ventilated premises, resulting in considerable exposure to quartz. Sandblasting is particularly hazardous (13).

Use of Abrasives and Fillers

Polishes, scouring powders, and sandpapers may contain quartz, and their manufacture may be associated with a significant dust hazard. Silica flour (finely powdered quartz) used in abrasives, paints, rubbers, and plastics has caused rapidly progressive silicosis (14).

Foundry Work

Since foundry work is carried out at high temperatures, exposure to quartz and cristobalite may occur. Molten metals are poured into molds composed of sand and clay. These molds may be coated with a powder high in free silica. The casting is knocked out of the mold, and the material adhering, which contains cristobalite and quartz, is removed (fettling) by blasting, hammering, and chiseling. Other materials to which foundry workers are exposed include iron oxide, clays, carbon, metal fumes, and isocyanates. The pneumoconiosis encountered in these workers is usually mixed-dust fibrosis rather than classic silicosis (15).

Ceramic Industry

The manufacture of china and earthenware uses raw materials such as china clay, china stone, ball clays, and powdered flint. Refined china clay contains very little silica, but china stone and ball clays have a significant content. The main risk of exposure to silica is in the crushing and milling of these clays and calcined flint before shaping, fettling, firing, and glazing. Also, high concentrations of quartz, tridymite, and cristobalite may result during the production of refractory bricks and cements, since this requires crushing, milling, shaping, and firing of sandstone.

Other Industries

The use of sand to grind and polish glass continues in a few small plants only. Boiler scaling may result in exposure to a variety of dusts including quartz, iron, and carbon. Vitreous enameling is also associated with exposure to free silica. Exposure to calcined diatomaceous earth, used in filters, fillers, abrasives, adsorbents, and insulation products, may lead to silicosis.

PATHOLOGIC REACTIONS

Nodular (Classical) Silicosis

Nodular silicosis is characterized by the presence within the lung of discrete, rounded, whorled, hyalinized, fibrous nodules that are sharply separated from the surrounding lung tissue. It is consequent to exposure to dust with a high free-silica content, an often-quoted figure being more than 18% (16). At least 20 years of exposure to the dust is required before this form of silicosis becomes clinically apparent as *chronic silicosis.* Rarely clinical disease becomes manifest within 3 to 10 years of exposure; the term *accelerated silicosis* is often used for this phenomenon. The pathology is similar in both circumstances except the nodules are less well developed and there is more pronounced interstitial fibrosis in the accelerated form (2). When the nodules are all 10 mm or less, the disease is termed *simple silicosis* or *simple pneumoconiosis. Complicated pneumoconiosis* (progressive massive fibrosis, or PMF), defined as the presence of nodules measuring 1 cm or greater, is not uncommon and may occur in any part of the lung but is more common in the upper zones.

Macroscopic Appearances. When lungs of silicotics are examined, the pleura is usually found to be thickened by fibrous tissue, and there are frequent dense adhesions, particularly over the upper lobes. This may give rise to considerable difficulty in removal of the lungs from the thoracic cavity at autopsy. The visceral pleura frequently contains so-called candle wax lesions up to 10 mm in diameter. They are gray waxy nodules often surrounded by a peripheral rim of black carbonaceous material. They are similar to intrapulmonary silicotic nodules by light microscopy (17).

The hilar lymph nodes are usually enlarged, fixed, pigmented, hard, and frequently calcified (Figs. 7.1 and 7.2). Calcification is responsible for the radiographic eggshell appearance. This feature is rarely seen in other conditions except tuberculosis and sarcoidosis (12). Cut sections of the nodes frequently exhibit a whorled gray pattern. The lymph nodes commonly show these changes when there are few or no whorled nodules within the lung parenchyma. Lesions limited to the lymph nodes without involvement of the lung should not be called silicosis. The lungs on cut section reveal rounded, whorled, well-demarcated gray nodules (Fig. 7.3). They are hard, often calcified, and most prevalent in the upper and posterior areas of the lung. Nodules are often numerous under the pleura, even when few or none are present within the remainder of the pulmonary parenchyma. They usually measure 3 to 6 mm in diameter, but they may

FIGURE 7.2
Chest radiograph of a North Wales slate worker showing rounded and irregular opacities and massive fibrosis. The nodes show eggshell calcification (ILO classification r 2/3 and C).

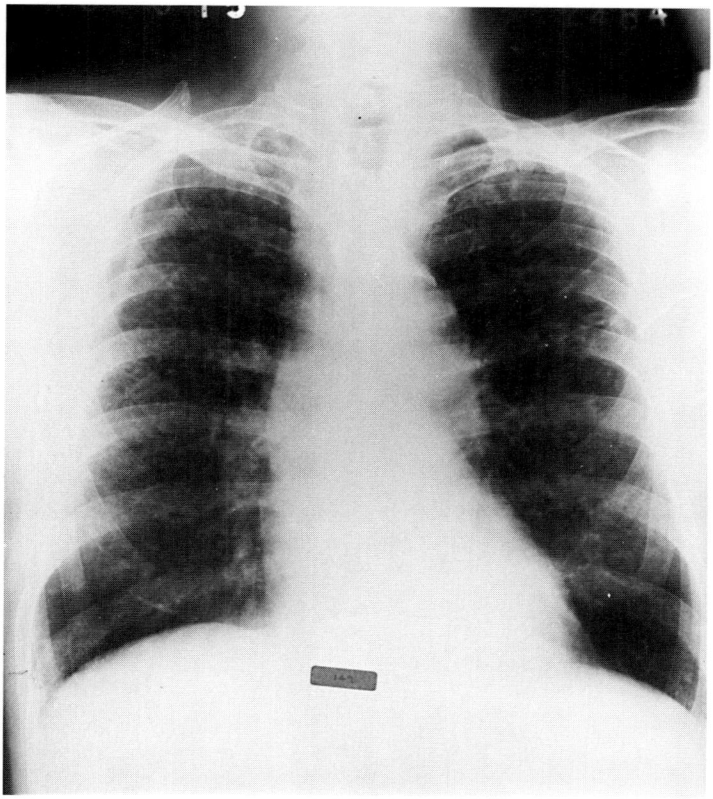

FIGURE 7.1
Chest radiograph of a North Wales slate worker showing numerous rounded opacities (ILO classification r, 1/2).

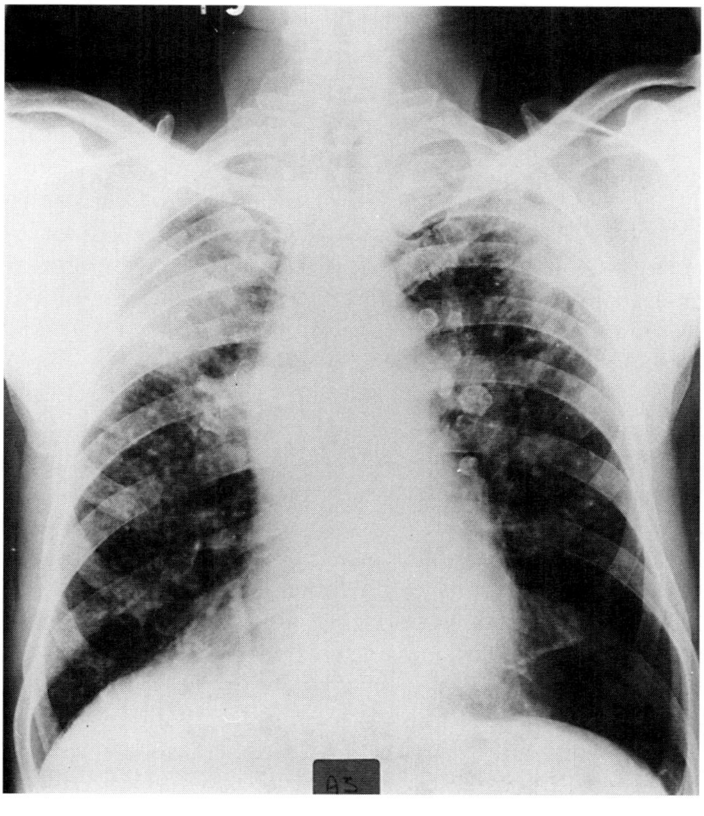

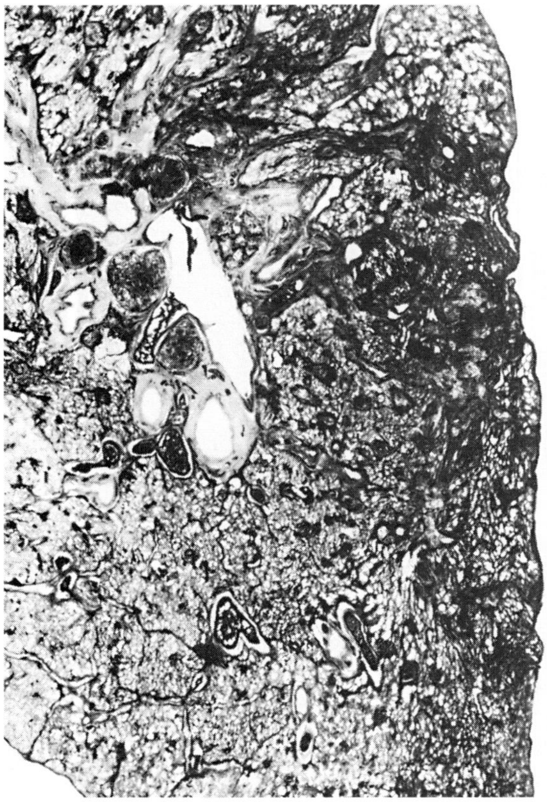

FIGURE 7.3
Part of a Gough-Wentworth whole lung section of a tin miner showing whorled, fibrotic enlarged lymph nodes and numerous silicotic nodules with conglomeration in the lung parenchyma.

be smaller or larger. Nodules frequently conglomerate to form large masses of PMF, and these may occupy most of a lobe and even cross the fissure into the adjacent lobe (Figs. 7.2, 7.4, and 7.5). Cavitation sometimes takes place within these large lesions as a result of either ischemia or mycobacterial infection. PMF lesions usually but not necessarily parallel the profusion of nodules or amount of dust in the background lung, and sometimes they occur when there are few nodules in the background pulmonary parenchyma.

Microscopic Appearance. Initially dust is observed free or within macrophages around respiratory bronchioles, pulmonary arterioles, and paraseptal and subpleural tissues. At first reticulin and collagen are formed irregularly, but this gradually becomes rounded at the center of the dust collections. With further development the central zone becomes more fibrotic, and the dust-containing macrophages are found at the periphery of the nodule. As expansion of the nodule proceeds, the central fibrous zone develops with hyalinization and a concentric laminar arrangement, and the dust- containing elements are pushed farther from the central zone. The fully developed nodule therefore consists of a concentric fibrous laminar core with variable calcification and hyalinization and a dust-laden cellular peripheral zone of variable width (17, 18) (Figs. 7.6–7.10). The dust is best observed under polarized light when the min-

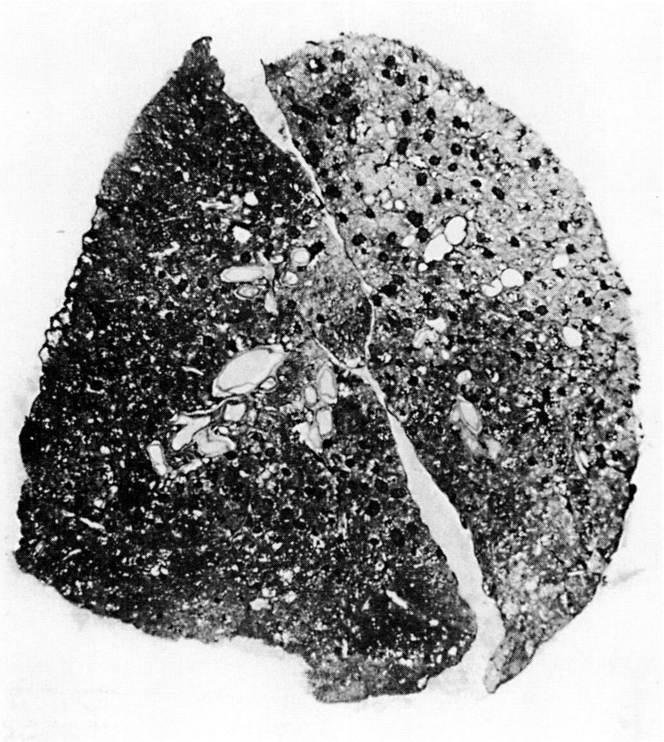

FIGURE 7.4
A Gough-Wentworth whole lung section of a tin miner showing well-demarcated rounded nodules most marked in the upper zones.

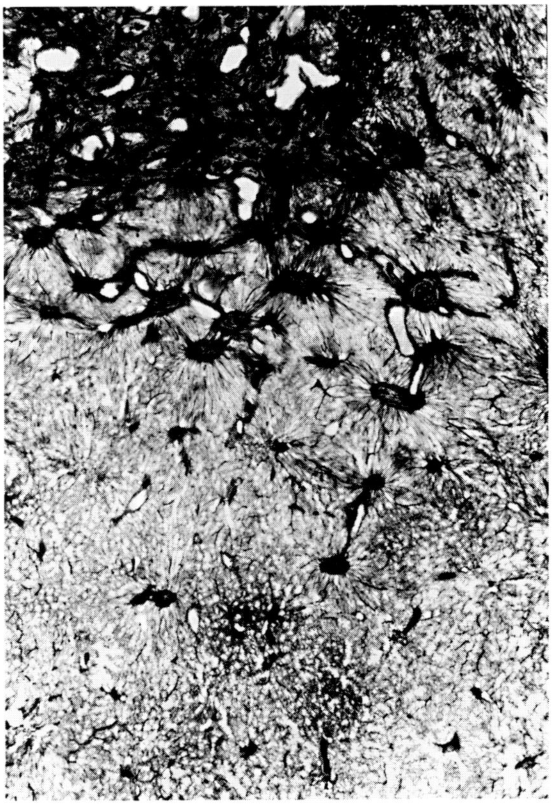

FIGURE 7.5
Part of a Gough-Wentworth whole lung section of a granite mason showing part of a PMF lesion that appears to have formed by conglomeration of nodules. The lung also shows scattered, well-demarcated whorled nodules.

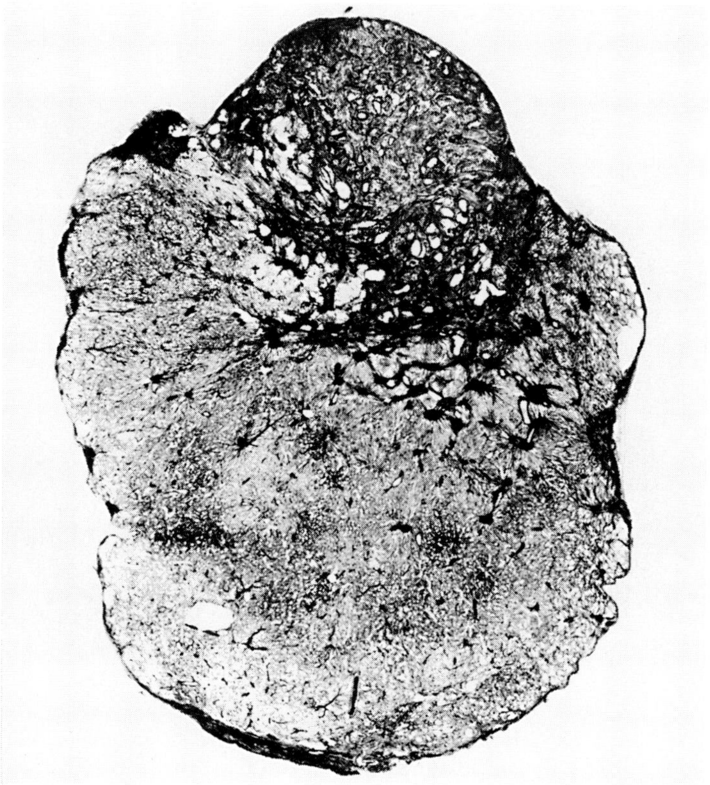

FIGURE 7.6

The entire Gough-Wentworth whole lung section in FIGURE 7.5. The PMF lesion occupies almost the whole of the upper lobe.

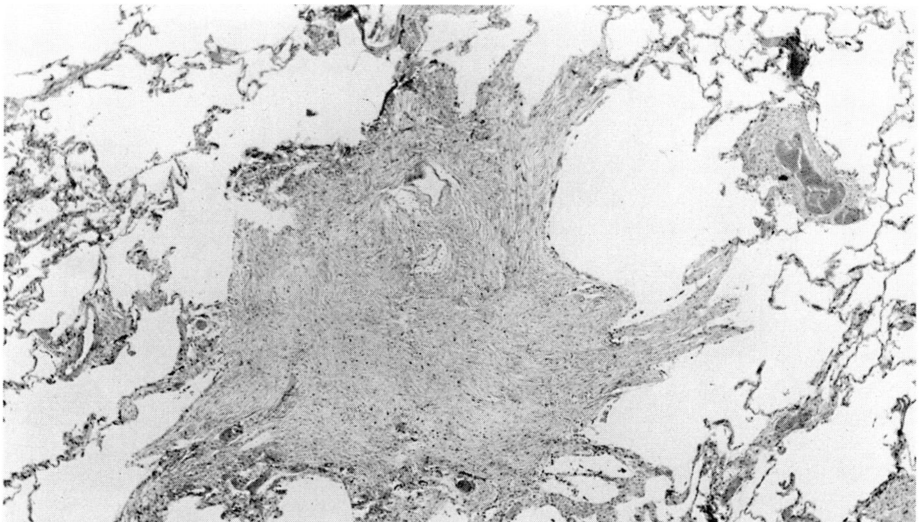

FIGURE 7.7

Lung of a slate worker with interstitial dust accumulation and connective tissue reaction, Collagen fibers are randomly oriented. (hematoxylin and eosin, (10.)

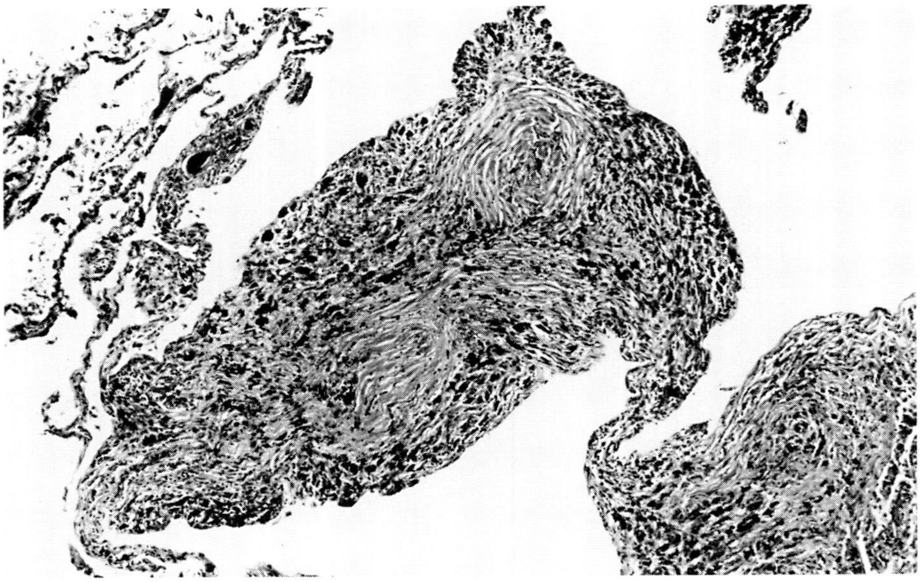

FIGURE 7.8
Lung of a slate worker with interstitial dust accumulation showing beginnings of circumferential orientation of collagen. (Hematoxylin and eosin, (36.)

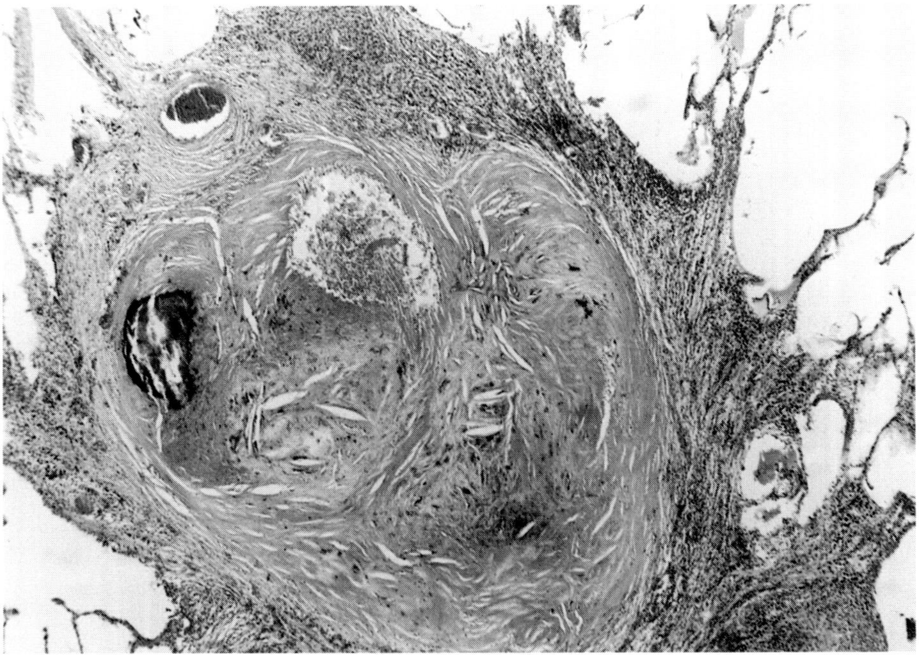

FIGURE 7.9
Lung of a slate worker with well-developed silicotic nodule that shows central hyalinized, calcified, circumferential collagen surrounded by a peripheral rim of dust containing macrophages (Hematoxylin and eosin, (20.)

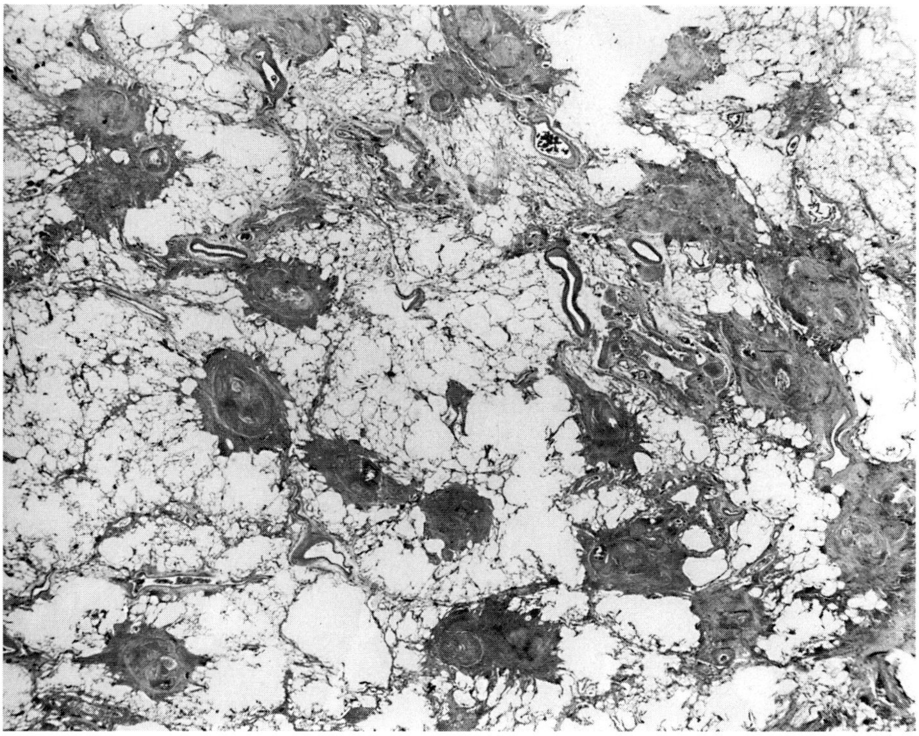

FIGURE 7.10
Lung of a slate worker with well-developed silicotic nodules. There are also foci of centrilobular emphysema present. (Hematoxylin and eosin, (2.)

eral particles exhibit strong birefringence. However, the strong birefringence is not due to quartz, as is commonly believed, but rather to associated minerals such as mica; quartz is only weakly birefringent. As the lesions progress, the respiratory bronchioles, pulmonary arterioles, and perivascular lymphatics become further enmeshed by the fibrotic process. The result is destruction of their architecture, often leaving some fragmented elastic fibers as the only evidence of their previous existence. If the process is rapid, obstruction of the pulmonary arteriolar lumen may lead to ischemic necrosis of the center of the nodule. This is most likely to happen in the larger nodules.

PMF lesions, unlike coal workers' pneumoconiosis, consist of fused whorled silicotic nodules (Figs. 7.5 and 7.11). Cavitation as a result of either ischemia or mycobacterial infection is fairly frequent. In the latter instance the typical granulomas composed of compact clusters of epithelioid cells and giant cells may not accompany silicosis. Whenever necrosis and cavitation are conspicuous in silicosis, the tissues and microbiologic cultures should be carefully screened for acid-fast bacilli.

If pulmonary hypertension has resulted from the silica exposure, the pulmonary arterioles and small muscular pulmonary arteries show medial hypertrophy and longitudinal smooth muscle fibers in the intima (not normally observed in muscular pulmonary arteries). The pulmonary veins and venules may manifest medial hypertrophy, intimal fibrosis, and intimal longitudinal smooth muscle bundles. Bronchopulmonary arterial and venous anastomoses may also be present (19).

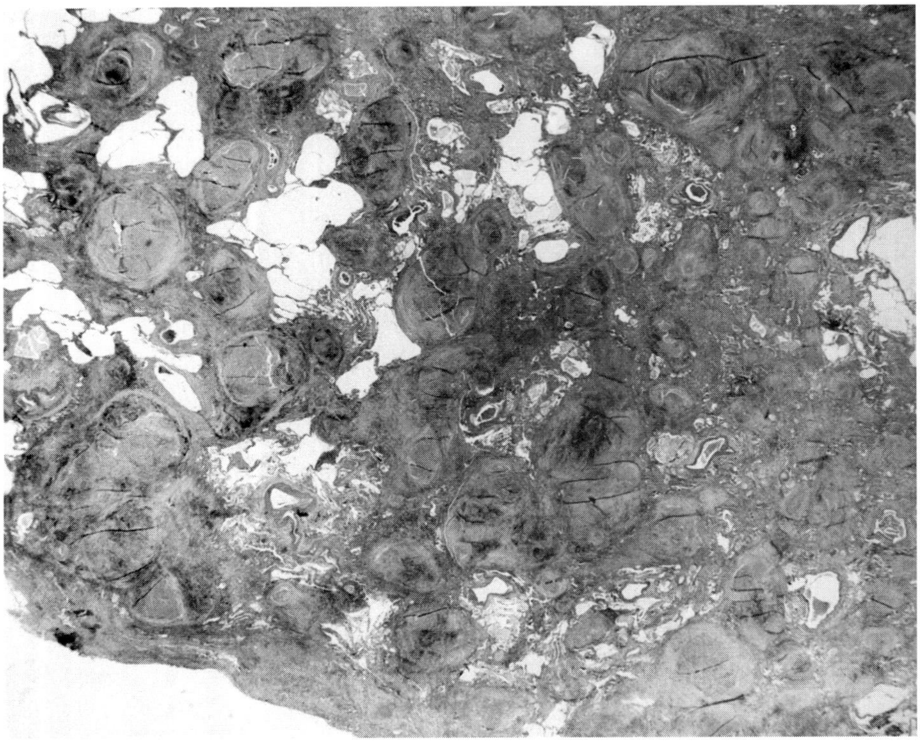

FIGURE 7.11
Lung of a slate worker with PMF that appears to have developed by conglomeration of individual nodules. (Hematoxylin and eosin, (2.)

In contrast to coal workers' pneumoconiosis, neither focal (20) nor centrilobular emphysema (21) appears to be a consequence of classic silicosis. By the term *focal emphysema* we mean dilated respiratory bronchioles and their adjacent alveoli at the center of the lobule around the dust focus. Irregular (scar) emphysema may be observed, but not consistently, around the larger nodules and PMF lesions.

Recently two cases of *rounded atelectasis* in Japanese men, confirmed at autopsy, were described in association with silicosis (22).

Silicosis and Tuberculosis

It has been known since the beginning of this century that patients with silicosis have a greatly increased risk of tuberculosis (23, 24). This also applies to other mycobacteria. Bruce (25) found that the frequency of tuberculosis increased with the stage of silicosis and that there was a greater prevalence and poorer prognosis in classic silicosis than in mixed-dust fibrosis. Despite the reduction in prevalence of tuberculosis in the general community, there still remains a high risk of tuberculosis developing in the person with silicosis (26). It is probable that silicosis leads to a reduction in cell-mediated immunity, since there are reduced numbers of T cells and increased numbers of B cells circulating with increased serum immunoglobulins in workers with silicosis (27).

When silicosis is complicated by tuberculosis, the nodules evince marked central necrosis, and if the lesions contain black dust, laminations, that indicate the site of a dust-laden histiocytic capsule may be observed. The edge of the lesion may contain recognizable epithelioid granulomas. However, if the lesion has been quiescent, the edge may show collagenization only, making the diagnosis difficult.

Rheumatoid Pneumoconiosis

Caplan first drew attention to an unusual pattern of pneumoconiosis in coal workers with rheumatoid arthritis (28). In these subjects well-developed scattered large radiologic opacities developed quickly, particularly in the peripheral areas of the lung. Gough et al. (29) described the histopathologic appearances of these lesions. Grossly the nodules consist of laminated alternating light and dark areas with central necrosis usually situated subpleurally. They usually measure between 0.5 and 5 cm and are often set in a background of only slight pneumoconiosis.

Microscopically there is central necrosis, with dust arranged free and in lines and circles (Figs. 7.12 and 7.13). Surrounding the necrotic area is a layer of palisaded histiocytes, polymorphs, neutrophils, fibroblasts, and collagen. Often the inflammatory cells within this zone show signs of disintegration, which helps to differentiate the lesion from tuberculosis. The most peripheral part of the nodule contains lymphocytes and plasma cells that also cluster around small vessels. The central necrotic area frequently undergoes calcification. These lesions have been described in silicosis very infrequently (30–32) (Fig. 7.13). In old lesions where inflammatory activity has disappeared, no distinction from healed tuberculosilicotic lesions can be made.

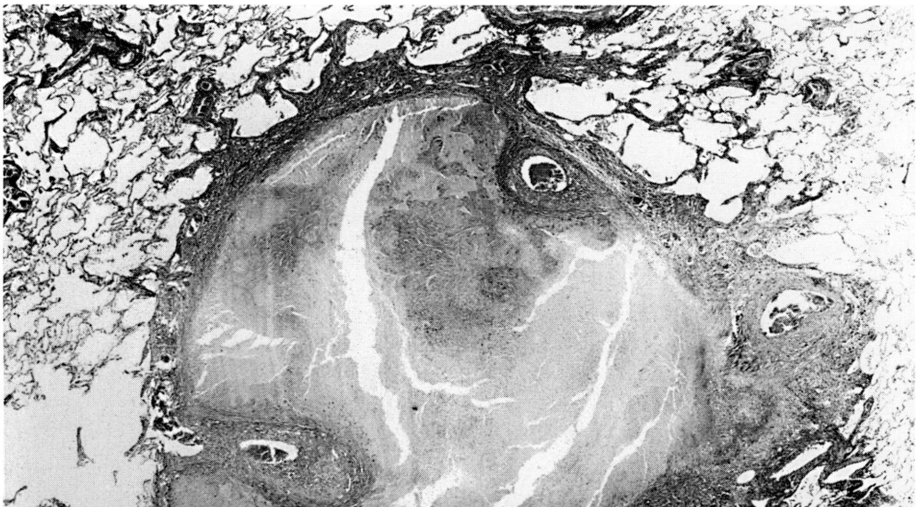

FIGURE 7.12

Lung of a slate worker with rheumatoid arthritis that shows well-demarcated Caplan-type nodule with central necrosis and a peripheral rim of histiocytes, fibrosis, and dust-laden macrophages. (Hematoxylin and eosin, (20.)

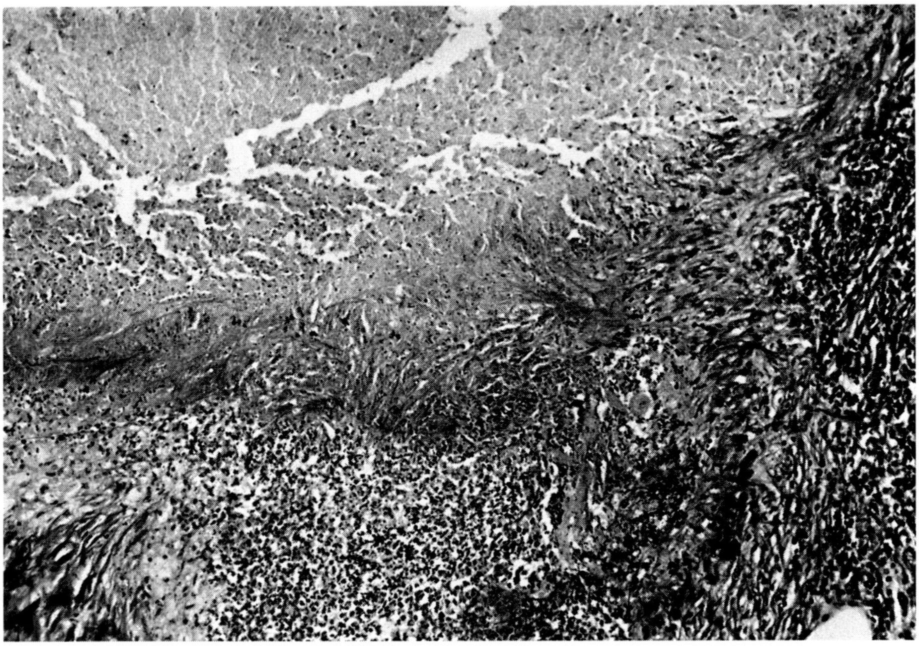

FIGURE 7.13
Lesion shown in FIGURE 7.12 showing the palisading of histiocytes at the periphery of the lesion. (Hematoxylin and eosin, (60.)

Silica and Collagen Vascular Diseases

A number of case reports over the years have linked exposure to silica and/or silicosis to systemic sclerosis, rheumatoid arthritis, and systemic lupus erythematosus. However, studies conflict. A cohort study of Finnish granite workers demonstrated higher prevalence of rheumatoid arthritis, which was clinically severe, in the granite workers than in the general population (33). However, a case control study reported by Sluis-Kremer et al. (34) found that silica dust exposure did not predispose to rheumatoid arthritis. Similarly there have been conflicting findings for scleroderma (17), but a case control study of scleroderma carried out in white South African gold miners reported a consistent heavy pattern of exposure to silica exposure but not an increase in radiologically detectable silicosis (35).

Silicosis and Lung Cancer

There has been controversy over the relationship between crystalline silica exposure and the risk of development of lung cancer. The International Agency for Research on Cancer (IARC) reviewed the human and experimental literature up to 1986 and concluded that there was sufficient evidence for the carcinogenicity of crystalline silica in experimental animals but limited evidence for the carcinogenicity of crystalline silica in man (36). The agency classified silica under 2A i.e., probably carcinogenic in humans (37). In fact neither the animal nor the human evidence for carcinogenicity is very convincing.

Evidence in experimental animals that silica may be a carcinogen was described by Wagner et al, (38) after intrapleural inoculation, using silica as a control for asbestos. These tumors were not malignant mesotheliomas but were found to be some form of hemopoietic tumor. Subsequent work has shown that these were malignant histiocytic tumors (39). It must be stressed that this type of tumor is especially associated with the Wistar rat and is statistically reduced by neonatal thymectomy (40). This suggests an association with a virus, such as the Kilham virus. This work has never supported the thesis that silica may be carcinogenic to cells of the lung or pleura.

Some other animal studies have found that silica can behave as a direct-acting carcinogen or cocarcinogen, but again this has been very species dependent, happening in rats but not mice, hamsters, or guinea pigs, and there is no evidence of a dose–response relation (41). There is a large amount of evidence to indicate that particle overload experiments, in which the alveolar macrophages become overloaded to the point that they cease removing particles from the lung, result in the rat producing an additional biological response in the form of tumors, but this does not occur in other animal species (42). Therefore these tumors appear to be specific for rats and not a good model for human risk evaluation.

The epidemiologic evidence is also weak, mainly because of the lack of good cohort studies that adequately allowed for smoking and other exposures to radon, asbestos, and polycyclic aromatic hydrocarbons. Since the IARC review more than thirty papers examining the relation between silica, silicosis, and lung cancer have been published. However, in the opinion of Weill and McDonald (43) only "eleven studies were identified as being of reasonably satisfactory design and presentation, and primarily concerned with the effects of exposure to crystalline silica on the risk of lung cancer." Nine of the studies showed some excess of lung cancer, and these included refractory brick workers, diatomaceous earth workers, pottery workers, foundry workers, and various mine workers and granite workers. However, only one of these studies showed a significant excess, correlation with severity of exposure, and absence of confounders, and even in this study there was possible early exposure to asbestos in some parts of the plant (44). Two of these eleven studies failed to demonstrate any excess risk; these were in ceramic and slate quarry workers. Overall the studies suggest that in the absence of silicosis there is little or no excess risk of developing cancer, but this should be further investigated. However, a postmortem case control study of South African miners exposed to silica found no differences for any of the exposure indicators (which included cumulative dust exposure, total dusty shifts, weighted average intensity of exposure, total underground shifts, shifts in high dust, and the presence or severity of silicosis) between cases of lung cancer and controls without lung cancer (45). Gibbs has examined the lungs obtained from postmortems of 221 North Wales slate workers in whom there was a high prevalence of silicosis and a high prevalence of lung cancer (14.5%) and found no correlation between the risk of lung cancer and the severity of nodular or interstitial fibrosis (46). Further studies are necessary to determine whether exposure to silica or one of its polymorphs raises the risk of lung cancer and whether there is a relation with silicosis. These should be cohort studies that account for the type and amount of exposure to crystalline quartz, adequate exclusion or allowance for confounders, and good smoking data; ideally that estimate fibrosis radiologically and/or pathologically; and that incorporate lung burden data. As Hardy and Weill (47) state, "Legitimate scientific debate exists as to whether crystalline silica causes cancer in humans. IARC may have concluded 'probably,' but other scientists equally familiar with the data say 'maybe not.'"

Acute Silicoproteinosis

Acute silicoproteinosis is a rapidly fatal form of silicosis that shows features quite dissimilar from those of the more common nodular type. The pathology in the acute form is similar to that in alveolar lipoproteinosis. Acute silicoproteinosis usually follows exposure to large quantities of finely particulate silica, for example in sandblasting, silica flour workers, and the ceramic industry (13, 14, 48–50). The disease becomes apparent within about 3 years of exposure, and death from hypoxia frequently supervenes. Radiologically the lungs show a ground glass appearance (12).

Pathology. Macroscopically the lungs are heavy and firm, and on cutting, fluid exudes from the surface. Microscopically there is a striking relatively uniform filling of alveoli by an eosinophilic, amorphous, and granular periodic acid-Schiff (PAS) positive and lipid-rich exudate (48) (Fig. 7.14). The exudate contains acicular clefts due to dissolved lipid crystals. Alveolar lining cells are plump and granular. There is a variable amount of interstitial pneumonitis and collagenization. Sparse, poorly demarcated silicotic nodules may be present (50), but well-circumscribed concentric nodules are usually absent (51). Polarization of the section may reveal small doubly refractile crystalline material, but this is not always true, since the particles may be below the resolution of the light microscope. In that circumstance the tissue should be submitted for electron microscopic and energy-dispersive x- ray analysis. In some cases poorly formed loose granulomas that superficially resemble those of sarcoidosis have been described (13). Ultrastructural examination of these cases has shown that the alveolar spaces contain desquamated type 2 cells, macrophages containing osmiophilic lamellated bodies derived from the type 2 pneumocytes, silica particles, and lipid

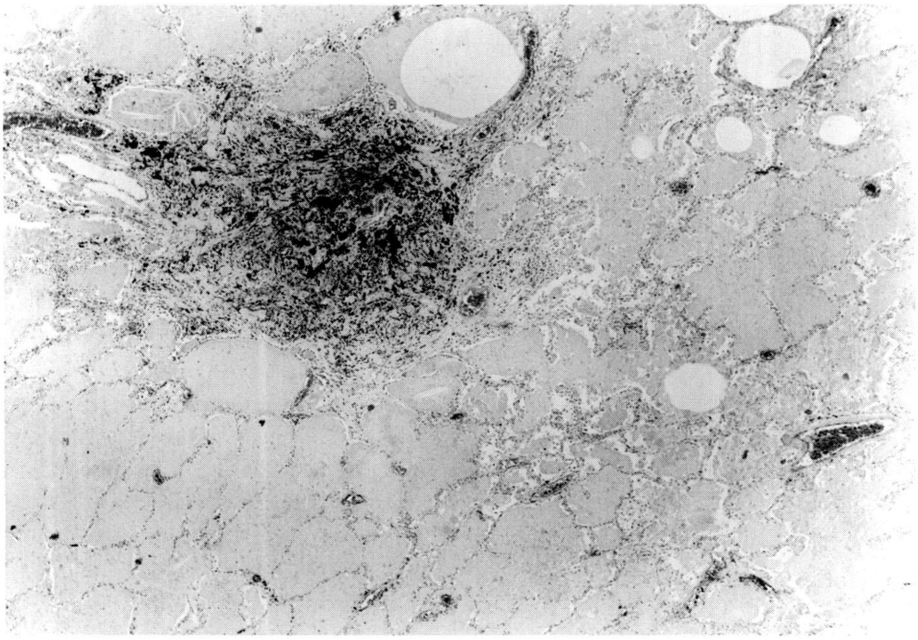

FIGURE 7.14
Alveolar lipoproteinosis in a worker exposed to high levels of quartz. (Hematoxylin and eosin, (10.)

membranous aggregates with hyperplastic type 2 pneumocytes lining the alveolar walls (52). This pathologic picture has been produced experimentally by exposing animals to high concentrations of finely particulate quartz, tridymite, and cristobalite (53–55).

Mixed-Dust Fibrosis

Mixed-dust fibrosis is the pulmonary response to the simultaneous inhalation of dusts containing free silica and less fibrogenic dusts in some industrial process (56). This can occur in a number of settings:

- Iron and steel foundries (15). The main exposure is to free silica (quartz, tridymite, or cristobalite) and iron oxide.
- Hematite mining (57). The main exposure is to free silica and iron oxide.
- Slate industry (58). The main components of the dust are quartz and mica.
- China clay industry (59). Some workers in the clay industry have been exposed to china stone, which is composed of quartz and kaolinite.
- Shale mining (60, 61). Exposure is to quartz, mica, and kaolin.
- Ceramic industry. Exposure to ball clays, either in the production of ceramics, pottery, or refractory wares or in the production of the mineral, may cause a mixed-dust fibrosis (62). The exposure is to quartz, kaolinite, and mica.
- Coal mining. Coal workers exposed to significant concentrations of quartz within the coal dust develop lesions that are intermediate between the typical coal nodule and silicotic nodule, and this can be considered a mixed-dust fibrosis. It is sometimes called anthracosilicosis.

The clinical manifestations of mixed-dust fibrosis are similar to classic silicosis but take longer to develop. Irregular opacities are seen on radiography. Even though the proportion of free silica is greater than 20% in many of these exposures, it is thought that other minerals, such as mica, may dampen the effect of the quartz so that classic silicosis does not develop.

Pathology. Macroscopically the pleura shows diffuse thickening, and nodules may be palpable. On cutting the lungs reveal a variable number of stellate nodules that lack the concentric whorled pattern of the classic silicotic nodule. They are more prevalent in the upper zones of the lungs and are often seen earliest below the pleura. The color of the lesions depends on the nature of the nonquartz dust, since this is in the majority–red in the case of iron oxide, white with kaolin, and black with coal. Hilar lymph nodes are enlarged and may show some whorled fibrosis, but it is not as conspicuous as in classic silicosis. The classic eggshell calcification as observed in classic silicosis is not always present.

Microscopically the mixed-dust lesion is characterized by a stellate linear arrangement of reticulin and collagen fibers admixed with dust-laden macrophages (Fig. 7.15) (see Chapter 6). There is little pigmentation in the central zone of the lesion, and the pigment is concentrated mostly around the periphery. If exposure is to relatively little free silica, little fibrosis develops. Conversely, if exposure is to relatively high quartz concentrations, typical silicotic nodules can accompany the mixed-dust lesions. Frequently several types of nodules are seen: silicotic nodules, mixed-dust lesions, and nodules intermediate between the two.

It is sometimes possible to identify more than one type of dust particle on light

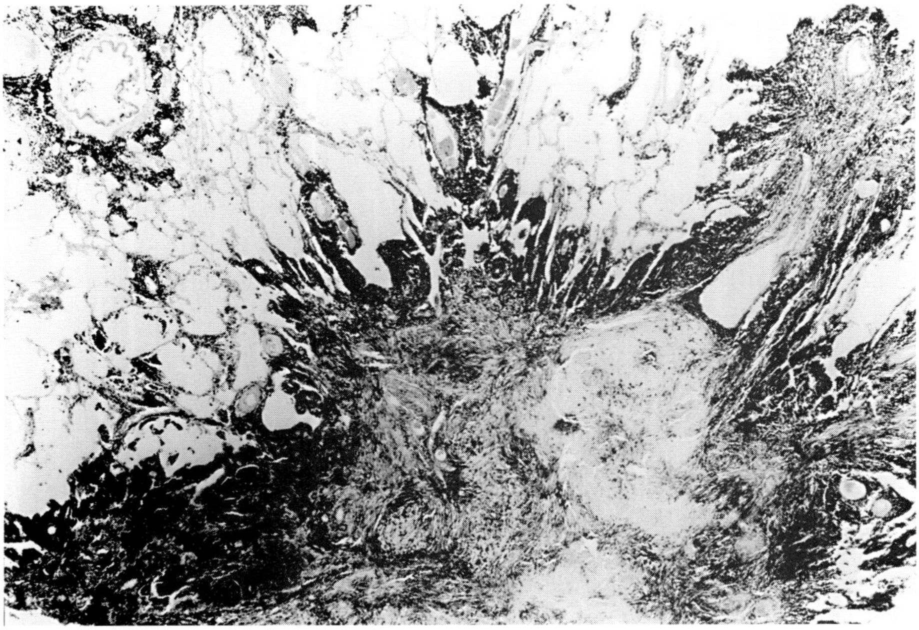

FIGURE 7.15
Part of a mixed-dust lesion in a hematite worker. (Hematoxylin and eosin, (16.).

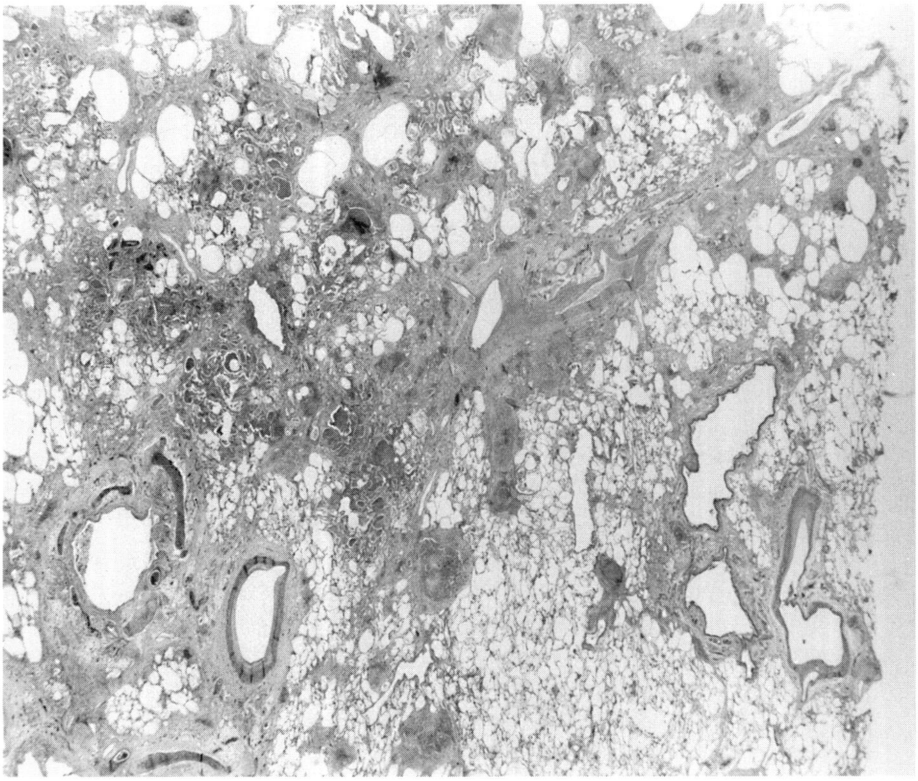

FIGURE 7.16
Lung of a slate worker showing silicotic nodules and interstitial fibrosis. (Hematoxylin and eosin, (2.)

microscopy, particularly under polarized light. Quartz is weakly doubly refractile; carbon, nonrefractile; kaolin and mica, strongly birefringent. However, mineralogic analysis is required to give accurate identification of the materials present within the lung.

Massive fibrotic lesions can occur in mixed-dust fibrosis. They tend to show an irregular arrangement of connective tissue fibers intermingled with dust and dust-laden macrophages rather than the conglomerated concentric nodules that are observed in classic silicosis. Cavitation can be a result of either ischemia or mycobacterial infection. The risk of the latter is less than in cases of classic silicosis.

Interstitial Fibrosis

Significant interstitial fibrosis is found in a surprisingly high proportion of lungs obtained from subjects exposed to free silica in combination with less fibrogenic materials. More than a fifth of the lungs from North Wales slate workers have severe interstitial fibrosis (58). A number show honeycombing (Fig. 7.16). The reason for this is unknown.

PATHOGENESIS

The fibrogenic property of free silica depends on a tetrahedral arrangement of silicon tetroxide (SiO_4) groups (8, 9, 63). Both animal and human studies have shown a dose–response relation between exposure to crystalline silica and the development of fibrosis. The changes of silicosis are seen when the percentage of silica within the dust exceeds 18 (64). Particles reach the lung parenchyma when they are less than 5 µm in diameter, but particles less then 1µm in diameter are the most pathogenic (11, 65). Particles deposited in the small airways and alveoli are rapidly ingested by macrophages that are attracted to the site by complement activation (66). Accumulations of macrophages in response to deposition and retention of mineral particles can be observed in lung biopsies and in bronchoalveolar lavages (BAL). The particles are incorporated in the lysosomes of the cells, and these may rupture, perhaps killing the cell and releasing the silica particles. Damage to the lung may occur directly as a consequence of the cytotoxicity of the silica particles or indirectly via the production of oxidants.

Three main theories have been proposed to explain the cytotoxicity of crystalline silica (67):

1. Silanol(SiOH) groups on the surface of the particles may form hydrogen bonds with the oxygen or nitrogen groups in biologic membranes, causing disruption and cell death.
2. The negative surface charge associated with SiO^- groups is important. Pretreatment of crystalline silica with aluminium lactate, which neutralizes the negative surface charge, can reduce in vitro and in vivo cytotoxicity (67, 68, 69). Other minerals in coal, such as illite and kaolin, may also reduce the cytotoxicity of crystalline silica.
3. Radical sites that are injurious to lung tissue may be present on the surface of the silica particles. Freshly fractured silica from crushing, drilling, or grinding contains more surface radicals and causes more lipid peroxidation and membrane damage than aged silica (67). Freshly fractured silica is also more potent in stimulating alveolar macrophages to produce oxidant species.

In vitro and in vivo studies have shown that in addition to the direct cytotoxicity and the generation of oxygen radicals by the damaged macrophages, other inflammatory and fibrogenic factors may be produced by the macrophages. These include leukotriene B_4 (a chemotactic factor for neutrophils), fibronectin and alveolar macrophage–derived growth factor (respectively competence and progression factors for fibroblast growth), and cytokines such as interleukin (IL) 1, IL-2, interferon, and tumor necrosis factor (70, 71). The human corollary to these findings is that examinations of the BAL fluid from asymptomatic granite workers have shown increased percentages of macrophages, lymphocytes, and neutrophils (72) and alveolar macrophages from the BAL fluid of persons with silicosis spontaneously release oxidants and increased quantities of fibronectin and alveolar macrophage–derived growth factor (73).

Experimental animal studies have shown that deposition of crystalline silica particles is associated with accumulation of neutrophils as well as macrophages, which is not surprising, considering the events outlined earlier in this chapter. Activated neutrophils can secrete collagenase, elastase, other proteolytic enzymes, and oxidants, which can degrade connective tissue components of the lung (66, 74).

Changes also occur in the lymphocyte population. In the rat model of silicosis a significant influx of T-helper cells into the lung is stimulated by the release of inflammation mediators such as IL-1macrophages, and neutrophils (75). This is associated with decreased numbers of circulating T cells and increases in circulating B cells, which may be one of the reasons for the predisposition of humans to develop mycobacterial infection (27). In subjects exposed to crystalline silica there are significant increases of hypergammaglobulinemia, rheumatoid factor, and immune complexes, but these do not correlate well with severity of disease (75).

The epithelial cells are also involved in the events following crystalline silica deposition. Damage to type 1 pneumocytes occurs within a few days of exposure, which allows silica to reach the interstitium (76). There is evidence to suggest that fibrosis is a consequence of prolonged retention of particulates within the interstitium, and therefore it is probable that the interstitial macrophage plays a larger role than the alveolar macrophage in the development of fibrosis (77). Hyperplasia and activation of type 2 pneumocytes occurs with increased production and release of surfactant (78). When the exposures to silica are very intense, these changes may manifest in the form of silicoproteinosis.

Particulate-induced fibrosis results from complex interactions between the particles, interstitial and alveolar macrophages, neutrophils, lymphocytes, epithelial cells, fibroblasts, and complex cytokine networks.

MINERAL CONTENT

There is little published information comparing the pathology with mineral content of the lungs. We have found in a group of workers exposed to both china clay (kaolin) and china stone that both nodular and interstitial fibrosis developed. In these workers nodular fibrosis correlated with quartz content, and interstitial fibrosis correlated with kaolinite content (59). The quartz content of the lung in this group of workers ranged from 1 to 20%, and the kaolinite content ranged from 15 to 89%. Up to 44.8 mg of dust per gram of dried lung tissue was found in the lung. No correlation between lung dust content and the development of PMF was found in this group.

In a group of North Wales slate workers with silicosis, lung dust concentration ranged from 2.4 to 75.2 mg/g of dried lung tissue, and the composition of the lung dust varied from 4 to 30% quartz and up to 92% micas (26, 58).

CLINICAL AND RADIOGRAPHIC FEATURES

Exposure to dust that contains free silica can cause a persistent productive cough, but this does not correlate with either the presence or severity of radiologic opacities (79, 80). However, dyspnea does (20, 79). Airflow obstruction is uncommon in simple silicosis (79) but is associated with complicated silicosis (80). Complicated silicosis may also lead to pulmonary hypertension and cor pulmonale.

Radiographic signs take at least 20 years to develop unless exposure to free silica has been very heavy, for example in silica flour workers (81, 82). Rarely manifestations of silicosis may appear after a post-exposure interval of many years (12, 83).

Simple silicosis is characterized radiographically by rounded, moderately dense, sometimes calcified nodular opacities that predominate in the upper zones of the lung (Fig. 7.1). This is frequently accompanied by eggshell calcification of the hilar lymph nodes, a finding strongly suggesting silicosis (84). When the exposure is to mixed dust, the opacities are frequently irregular; this is also true when emphysema is present.

Radiographs appear to produce a faithful image of nodules and conglomerate masses, both in coal workers' pneumoconiosis and in silicosis (85). In general solitary lesions can be discerned on chest radiograph only when they are greater than 3 mm in diameter (86), but when multiple lesions are present, there is a summation effect, and they can be detected at smaller sizes (87). There appears to be a direct correlation between the severity of silicosis as assessed radiographically and total dust exposure, but individual susceptibility also appears to affect the radiographic appearance (88).

Conglomeration of isolated nodules may lead to lesions measuring more than 1 cm in diameter (PMF). These generally appear as sharply demarcated large masses and are often bilateral (Fig. 7.2). In the usual case of PMF there is a background of severe simple pneumoconiosis (Fig. 7.2). Rheumatoid pneumoconiosis, which presents as rapidly enlarging large opacities, usually occurs against a background of mild simple pneumoconiosis. Progression from simple to complicated silicosis can occur after cessation of exposure (12).

REFERENCES

1. Corn JK. Historical aspects of industrial hygiene: silicosis. Am Ind Hyg Assoc J 1980; 41:125–133.
2. Seaton A, Legge JS, Henderson J, Kerr KM. Accelerated silicosis in Scottish stonemasons. Lancet 1991; 337:341–344
3. Criteria for a recommended standard occupational exposure to crystalline silica. Washington: U.S. Department of Health Education and Welfare, 1974.
4. Lloyd Davies TA. Respiratory disease in foundrymen: report of a survey. London: HM Stationery Office, 1971.
5. Ross DJ, Sallie BA, McDonald JC. SWORD '94: surveillance of work related and occupational respiratory disease in the UK. Occup Med 1995;45:175–178.
6. Health and Safety Statistics 1994–1995. Suffolk: Health and Safety Commission HSE Books, 1994.

7. Silica minerals. Encyclopedia Britannica Macropaedia, vol 9. 1979:751–765.
8. Brieger H, Gross P. On the theory of silicosis: 3. Stishovite. Arch Environ Health 1967;15:751–757.
9. Brieger H, Gross P. On the theory of silicosis: 1. Coesite. Arch Environ Health 1966; 13:38–43.
10. Parkes WR. Occupational lung disorders. Oxford: Butterworth Heinemann, 1994: 841–867.
11. Reiser KM, Last JA. Silicosis and fibrogenesis: fact and artifact. Toxicol 1979;13: 51–72.
12. Seaton A. Silicosis. In: Morgan WKC, Seaton A, eds. Occupational lung diseases. Philadelphia: Saunders, 1995:222–267.
13. Suratt PM, Winn WC, Brody AR, et al. Acute silicosis in tombstone sandblasters. Am Rev Respir Dis 1977;115:521–529.
14. Banks DE, Morring KD, Boehlecke BA, et al. Silicosis in silica flour workers. Am Rev Respir Dis 1981;124:445–450.
15. McLaughlin AIG. Pneumoconiosis in foundry workers. Br J Tuberc Dis Chest 1957; 51:297–309.
16. Nagleschmidt G. The relation between lung dust and lung pathology in pneumoconiosis. Br J Ind Med 1960;17:247–259.
17. Craighead JE, Kleinerman J, Abraham JL, et al. Diseases associated with exposure to silica and nonfibrous silicate minerals. Arch Pathol Lab Med 1988;112:673–720.
18. Simpson FW. The histopathology of silicosis. In: Silicosis in South Africa. Meetings of the Transvaal Mine Medical Officers Association, 1930:1–8.
19. Wagenvoort CA, Wagenvoort N. Hypoxic pulmonary vascular lesions in man at high altitudes and in patients with chronic respiratory disease. Pathol Microbiol 1973;39:276–282.
20. Heppelston AG. The pathological anatomy of simple pneumoconiosis in coal workers. J Pathol Bacteriol 1953;66:235–246.
21. Leopold JG, Gough J. The centrilobular form of hypertrophic emphysema and its relation to chronic bronchitis. Thorax 1957;12:219–235
22. Honma K, Shida H, Chiyotani K. Rounded atelectasis associated with silicosis. Wien Klin Wochenschr 1995;107:585–589.
23. Watkins-Pritchard W, Moir J. Report No. 8 to South African Institute for Medical Research, 1916.
24. Riddell AR. The clinical aspects of simple silicosis and silicosis with tuberculosis. Am Rev Tuberc 1934;29:36–42.
25. Bruce T. Silicotuberculosis. Scand J Respir Dis 1968;65(Suppl):139.
26. Glover JR, Bevan C, Cotes JE, et al. Effects of exposure to slate dust in North Wales. Br J Ind Med 1980;37:152–162.
27. Watanabe S, Shirakami A, Takeichi T, et al. Alterations in lymphocyte subsets and serum immunoglobulins levels in patients with silicosis. J Clin Lab Immunol 1987; 23:45–51.
28. Caplan A. Certain unusual radiological appearances in the chest of coal miners suffering from rheumatoid arthritis. Thorax 1953;8:29–37.
29. Gough J, Rivers D, Seal RME. Pathological studies of modified pneumoconiosis in coal miners with rheumatoid arthritis (Caplan's syndrome). Thorax 1955;10:9–18.
30. Chatgidakis CB, Theron CP. Rheumatoid pneumoconiosis (Caplan's syndrome). Arch Environ Health 1961;2:397–408.
31. Lamvik J. Rheumatoid pneumoconiosis: a case of Caplan's syndrome in a chalk mine worker. Acta Pathol Microbiol Scand 1963;57:169–174.
32. Ezenwa AO. Prevalence of rheumatoid pneumoconiosis (Caplan's syndrome) in metal miners. Can Med Assoc J 1979;120:1492–1494.
33. Klockars M, Koskela RS, Jarvinen E, et al. Silica exposure and rheumatoid arthritis: a follow up study of granite workers 1940–81. BMJ 1987;294:997–1000.
34. Sluis-Kremer GK, Hessel PA, Hnizdo E, Churchill AR. Relationship between silicosis and rheumatoid arthritis. Thorax 1986;41:596–601.

35. Sluis-Kremer GK, Hessel PA, Hnizdo E, et al. Silica, silicosis, and progressive systemic sclerosis. Br J Ind Med 1985;42:838–843.
36. International Agency for Research on Cancer. Monographs on the evaluation of the carcinogenic risks to humans: silica and some silicates. vol 42. Lyon: IARC, 1987.
37. International Agency for Research on Cancer. Overall evaluations of carcinogenicity: an updating of IARC volumes 1–42, Suppl 7. Lyon: IARC, 1988.
38. Wagner JC. The pathogenesis of tumours following the intrapleural injection of asbestos and silica. In: Nettesheim P, Hanna MG Jr, Deatherage JW Jr, eds. Morphology of experimental respiratory carcinogenesis, Oak Ridge, TN: US Atomic Energy Commission, 1970:347–358.
39. Harvey JJ. Tumours induced experimentally by silica; establishment and characterisation of malignant cell lines in vitro. In: Goldsmith DF, Winn DM, Shy CM, eds. Silica, silicosis and cancer: controversy in occupational medicine. New York: Praeger, 1986:229–242.
40. Wagner MMF, Wagner JC, Davies R, Griffiths DM. Silica induced malignant histiocytic lymphoma incidence linked with strain of rat and type of silica. Br J Cancer 1980;41:908–917.
41. Holland LM. Crystalline silica and lung cancer: a review of recent experimental evidence. Regul Toxicol Pharmacol 1990;12:234–235.
42. Levy LS. The "particle overload" phenomenon and human risk assessment. Indoor Environ 1995;4:254–262.
43. Weill H, McDonald H. Exposure to crystalline silica and risk of lung cancer: the epidemiological evidence. Thorax 1996;51:97–102.
44. Checkoway H, Heyer NJ, Demers PA, Breslow NE. Mortality among workers in the diatomaceous earth industry. Br J Ind Med 1993;50:586–597.
45. Hessel PA, Sluis-Kremer GK, Hnizdo E. Silica exposure, silicosis, and lung cancer: a necropsy study. Br J Ind Med 1990;47:4–9.
46. Gibbs AR. Lung cancer in North Wales slate workers. Eur Respir J 1995;8:30s.
47. Hardy TS, Weill H. Crystalline silica: risks and policy. Environ Health Perspect 1995;103:152–155.
48. Bueschner HA, Ansari A. Acute silicoproteinosis. Dis Chest 1964;55:274–284.
49. Xipell J M, Harn KN, Price CG, Thomas DP. Acute silicoproteinosis. Thorax 1977; 32:104–111.
50. Roeslin N, Lassabe-Roth C, Morand G, Batzenschlager A. La silico-proteinose aique. Arch Mal Prof 1980;41:15–18.
51. Gardner LU. Pathology of the so-called "acute" silicosis. Am J Publ Health 1933;23: 1240–1249.
52. Hoffman EO, Lamberty J, Pizzolato P, Coover J. The ultrastructure of acute silicosis. Arch Pathol 1973;96:104–107.
53. Gross P, de Treville RTP. Alveolar proteinosis: its experimental production in rodents. Arch Pathol 1968;86:255–261.
54. Heppleston AG, Wright NA, Stewart JA. Experimental alveolar lipoproteinosis following the inhalation of silica. J Pathol 1970;101:293–307.
55. Corrin B, King E. Experimental endogenous lipid pneumonia and silicosis. J Pathol 1967;97:325–330.
56. Harding HE, Gloyne SE, McLaughlin AIG. Industrial lung diseases in iron and steel foundry workers. London: HM Stationery Office, 1950.
57. Stewart MJ, Faulds JS. Pulmonary fibrosis in haematite miners. J Pathol Bacteriol 1934;39:233–253.
58. Gibbs AR, Craighead JE, Pooley FD, Wagner JC. The pathology of slate workers' pneumonoconiosis in North Wales and Vermont. In: Dodgson J, McCallum RI, Bailey MR, Fisher DR, eds. Inhaled particles VI. Annals of Occupational Hygiene 1988; 32:273–278.
59. Wagner JC, Pooley FD, Gibbs AR, et al. Inhalation of china clay and china stone dusts: the relationship between the mineralogy of dust retained in the lung and associated pathology. Thorax 1986;41:190–196.

60. Kung VA. Morphological investigations of fibrogenic action of Estonian oil shale dust. Environ Health Perspect 1979;30:153–156.
61. Seaton A, Lamb D, Rhind Brown W. Pneumoconiosis of shale miners. Thorax 198 1;36:412–418.
62. Thomas RW. Silicosis in the ball clay and china clay industries. Lancet 1952;1: 133–135.
63. Stober W, Brieger H. On the theory of silicosis: 4. The topochemical interaction. Arch Environ Health 1968;16:706–708.
64. Heppleston AG. Minerals, fibrosis and the lung. Environ Health Perspect 1991;94: 149–168.
65. Kysela R, Jirakara D, Holusa R, Skoda V. The influence of the size of quartz dust particles on the reaction of lung tissue. Ann Occup Hyg 1973;16:103–109.
66. Bégin R, Cantin A, Masse S. Recent advances in the pathogenesis and clinical assessment of mineral dust pneumoconioses: asbestosis, silicosis and coal pneumoconiosis. Eur Respir J 1989;2:988–1001.
67. Castranova V. Generation of oxygen radicals and mechanisms of injury prevention Environ Health Perspect 1994;102 (Suppl 10):65–68.
68. Nolan RP, Langer AM, Harington JS, et al. Quartz hemolysis as related to its surface functionalities. Environ Res 1981;26:503–520.
69. Brown GM, Donaldson K, Brown DM. Bronchoalveolar leukocyte responses in experimental silicosis: modulation by a soluble aluminium compound. Toxicol Appl Pharmacol 1989;101:95–105.
70. Martin TR, Raugi G, Merritt TL, Henderson WA. Relative contribution of leukotriene B_4 to the neutrophil chemotactic activity produced by the resident human alveolar macrophage. J Clin Invest 1987;80:1114–1124.
71. Lapp NL, Castranova V. How silicosis and coal workers' pneumoconiosis develop: a cellular assessment. Occup Med 1993;8:35–56.
72. Christman JW, Emerson RJ, Graham WGB, Davis GS. Mineral dust and cell recovery from the bronchoalveolar lavage of healthy Vermont granite workers. Am Rev Respir Dis 1985;135:393–399.
73. Rom WM, Bitterman PB, Rennard SI, et al. Characterization of the lower respiratory tract inflammation of nonsmoking individuals with interstitial lung disease associated with chronic inhalation of inorganic dusts. Am Rev Respir Dis 1987;136: 1429–1434.
74. Brown GM, Donaldson K. Degradation of connective tissue components by lung derived leukocytes in vitro: role of proteases and oxidants. Thorax 1988;43:132–139.
75. Scheule RK, Holian A. Immunologic aspects of pneumoconiosis. Exp Lung Res 1991;17:661–685.
76. Driscoll KE, Lindenschmidt RC, Maurer JK, et al. Pulmonary response to silica or titanium dioxide: inflammatory cells, alveolar macrophage derived cytokines and histology. Am J Respir Cell Mol Biol 1990;2:381–390.
77. Bowden DH, Hedgecock C, Adamson IYR. Silica induced pulmonary fibrosis involves the reaction of particles with interstitial rather than alveolar macrophages. J Pathol 1989;158:73–80.
78. Miller BE, Dethloff DA, Hook GER. Silica induced hypertrophy of type II cells in the lungs of rats. Lab Invest 1986;55:153–163.
79. Koskinen H. Symptoms and clinical findings in patients with silicosis. Scand J Environ Health 1985;11:101–106.
80. Irwig LM, Rocks P. Lung function and respiratory symptoms in silicotic and nonsilicotic gold miners. Am Rev Respir Dis 1978;117:429–435.
81. Jones RN. Silicosis: In: Rom WN et al., eds. Environmental and occupational medicine. Boston: Little, Brown, 1983:197–206.
82. Bank DE, Morring KL, Boehlecke BE, et al. Silicosis in silica flourworkers. Am Rev Respir Dis 1981;124:445.
83. Symanski H. Delayed onset of sandstone pneumoconiosis. Am J Ind Med 1981;2: 101–102.

84. Davies TW. Silicosis in slate quarry miners. Tubercle 1939;20:543–555.
85. Heitzman ER. The lung: radiologic–pathologic correlations. 2nd ed. St. Louis: Mosby, 1984:319–322.
86. Spratt JS, Teo-Pogassian M, Long RTL. The detection and growth of intrathoracic neoplasms. Arch Surg 1963;86:283–288.
87. Newell RR, Garneau R. The threshold visibility of pulmonary shadows. Radiology 1951;56:409–415.
88. Beadle DG. The relationship between the amount of dust breathed and the development of radiological signs of silicosis: an epidemiologic study in South African gold miners. In: Walton WH, ed. Inhaled particles 3. Surrey, UK: Unwin Brothers, 1971: 953–964.

CHAPTER 8

Diseases Due to Nonasbestos Silicates

❖ Francis H. Y. Green
❖ Andrew Churg

MINERALOGY

Silicates consist of silicon dioxide (SiO_2) combined in varying proportions with one or more cations such as magnesium, calcium, and aluminum (Fig. 8.1). They are distinguished from the various forms of pure crystalline silicon dioxide (e.g., quartz, cristobalite, tridymite), which are often called *silica*. The old terms *combined silica* for the silicates and *free silica* for the different types of silica make this point (1). Since there are significant differences between the frequency and severity of reactions to silicates and silica, the distinction is important. Asbestos, a fibrous silicate, also produces a fairly distinctive set of reactions (see Chapters 9 and 10). It is not discussed further here; the term *silicate* in the remainder of this chapter specifically excludes asbestos. Table 8.1 shows the chemical composition of some silicates that have been reported to produce disease in humans.

About one-third of all mineral species are silicates (2), and silicates make up a substantial portion of the earth's rocks and soil. Indeed, considering their ubiquity, it is remarkable how little disease is actually attributable to pure silicate exposure. A variety of mineralogic subclasses of silicates (Table 8.1, Fig. 8.1) are based largely on crystal structure (3), but it is unclear what effect, if any, crystal structure plays in producing pathologic reactions.

Silicate minerals are the predominant mineral species in human lung tissue. The mean concentration of silicates in the lung at death of 87 city dwellers from Cincinnati, Ohio, was 199×10^6 particles per gram of dry lung tissue (4) (Table 8.2). This dust burden was not associated with lung disease of any kind, reinforcing the impression that silicates are relatively innocuous.

Most of the commercially important nonasbestos silicates are nonfibrous; examples include talc, mica, kaolin, and clays (Fig. 8.1). A few exist in fibrous form (defined as a length-to-width [aspect] ratio greater than 3:1); examples of these include wollastonite, attapulgite, zeolites, and sepiolite (Fig. 8.1C). Some of the platy silicates, such as talc and mica, may appear as fibers when viewed on edge; however, this appearance is best described as acicular rather than fibrous (Fig. 8.1*D*).

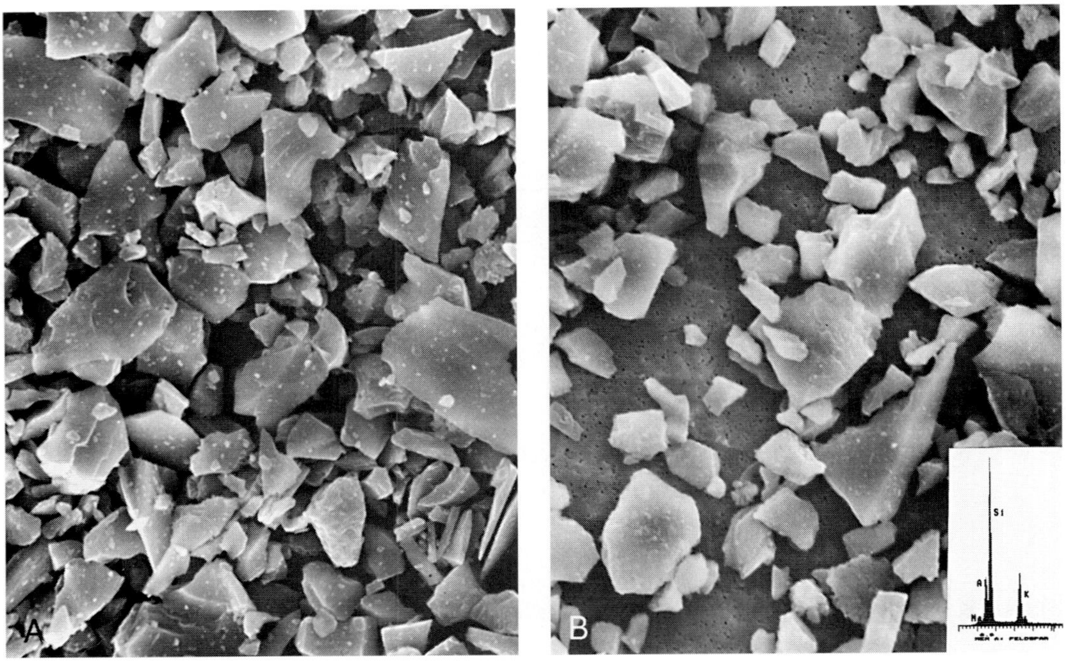

FIGURE 8.1
Scanning electron micrographs of size-fractionated respirable particles of silicate minerals and quartz; 90% of the particles are less than 5 mm in diameter. **Insets.** X-ray spectra. (×2000.) **A.** Quartz (SiO_2). Most common of the silica polymorphs, it is composed of stable quartz tetrahedra. Silica is not a silicate mineral. **B.** Feldspar, a major constituent of igneous rocks also common in sedimentary deposits. Many types exist; this one is an alkali feldspar containing sodium and potassium. **C.** Wollastonite ($CaSiO_3$). Associated with metamorphosed limestones, it has been exploited as an asbestos substitute because it is semifibrous. **D.** Talc ($Mg_3(OH)_2Si_4O_{10}$). Talc forms thin plates that appear acicular when viewed on edge. Asbestos (tremolite) contamination (not shown) is common. **E.** Kaolinite [$A1_4(Si_4O_{10})OH_8$]. A sheet silicate and the most common of the clay minerals, kaolinite is formed in weathering of feldspars and other silicates. **F.** Bentonite, a clay silicate containing varying amounts of cations calcium, sodium, magnesium, iron, and aluminum that exchange readily.

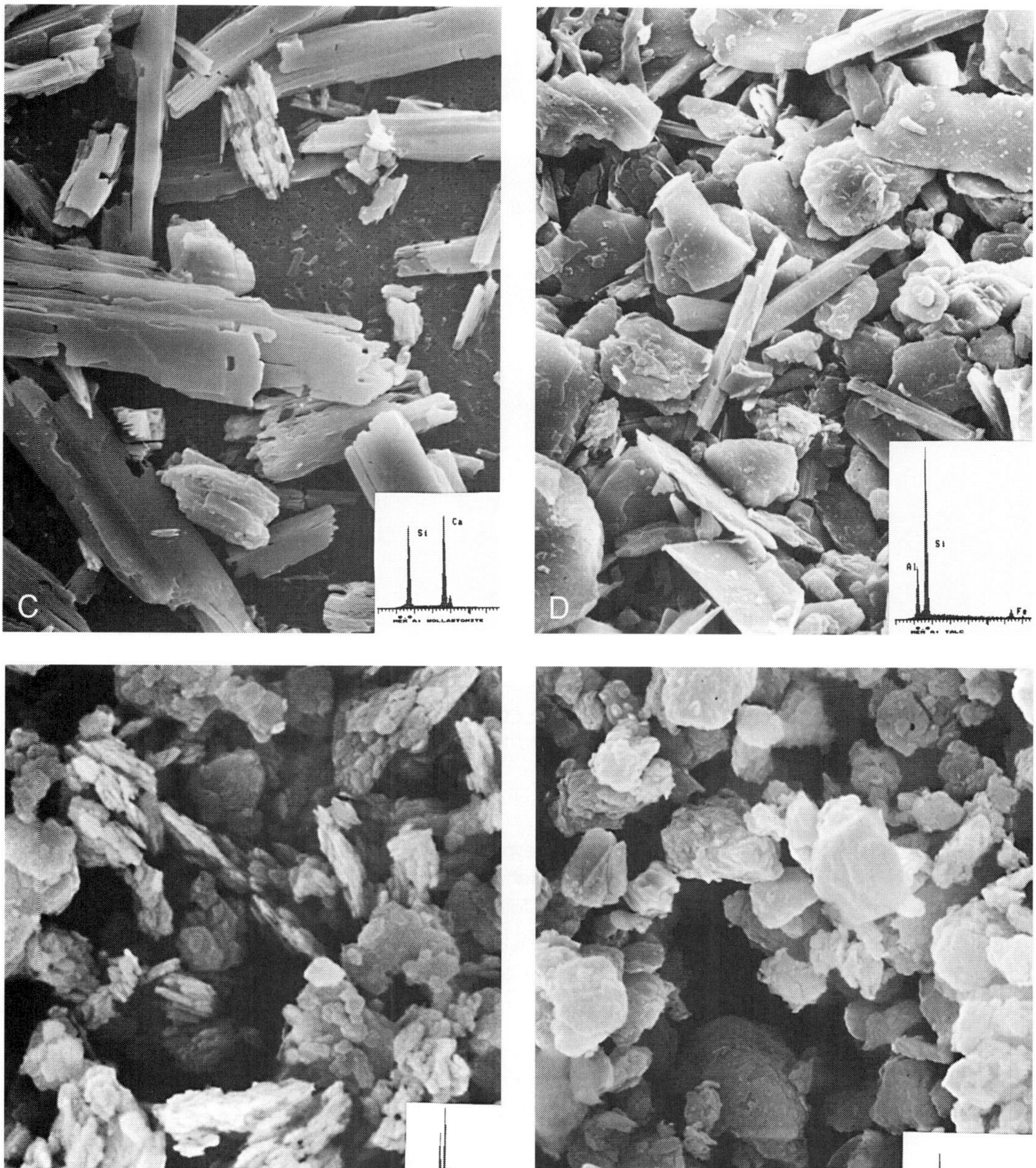

FIGURE 8.1 *(continued)*

TABLE 8.1
Classification and Composition of Silicate Minerals of Pathologic Importance

MINERAL	MAJOR CATIONS
Sheet silicates	
Talc	Mg
Mica (usually muscovite)	K, Na, Al
Vermiculite	Al, Mg, Ca, Fe
Kaolin	Al
Fuller's earth	
Montmorillonite	Ca, Na, Mg, Fe
Sepiolite	Mg
Attapulgite	Mg, Al
Framework silicates	
Feldspars	
Albite	Al, Na
Orthoclase	Al, K
Zeolites (e.g., erionite)	Na, Ca, Mg, Al
Chain silicates	
Wollastonite	Ca
Orthosilicates	
Mullite	Al

TABLE 8.2
Silicate Minerals in Lung Tissue

MINERAL SPECIES	TOTAL COUNT[a]	PERCENT	SIZE (μm)[b]
All exogenous	476 ± 380	100.0	0.60 ± 2.35
All silicates	179 ± 144	38.0	0.74 ± 2.28
Mg silicates	9 ± 8	2.5	1.05 ± 2.89
Silica	94 ± 70	21.0	0.66 ± 2.25
Rutile (TiO_2)	15 ± 12	3.0	0.34 ± 1.77

[a] $\times 10^6$ per gram of dry lung.
[b] Geometric median plus or minus geometric standard deviation.
Adapted from Stettler LE, Platek SF, Riley RD, et al. Lung particulate burdens of subjects from the Cincinnati, Ohio, Urban area. Scanning Micros 1991;5:85–94.

The nonasbestos silicates most frequently implicated in pulmonary disease are the sheet silicates, which cleave into broad plates, reflecting a crystal structure with a high ratio of diameter to height. These include talc, mica, and kaolinite (3) (Fig. 8.1). It is unknown whether this implies that sheet silicates are more dangerous than other mineralogic types or is merely a reflection of the fact that sheet silicates happen to be the form most widely used commercially. In vitro assays indicate that silicate minerals are generally cytotoxic (5–10), but the degree of cytotoxicity varies from almost naught to levels that equal or exceed that of free crystalline silica (10). There appears to be a relatively poor correlation between in vitro cytotoxicity and in vivo fibrogenicity (10); thus the value of cytotoxicity assays as predictors of fibrogenesis is limited.

Identification of silicate minerals in lung tissue can be achieved by many of the techniques discussed in Chapter 3. For specific identification, energy-dispersive x-ray spectroscopy applied to tissue sections or to tissue digestates has been widely used, as has x-ray diffraction. However, simple light microscopic examination often suggests the nature of the exposure. Pathologically important silicate minerals usually appear in tissue sections as polygonal particles, plates, and needles that may be colorless or pale yellow to brown and are strongly birefringent. The presence of large numbers of birefringent particles should suggest silicate exposure (Figs. 8.2–8.5). The needlelike shape, which is often incorrectly cited as a marker of silica, is not specific, since plates cut on edge also appear as needles (11) (Fig. 8.1*D*). Crystalline silica is only weakly birefringent in tissue sections, and the bright particles seen by polarization in the usual case of silicosis are actually accompanying silicate minerals. Particle size can also be useful in evaluating silicate exposures, since most particles much larger than about 5 μm

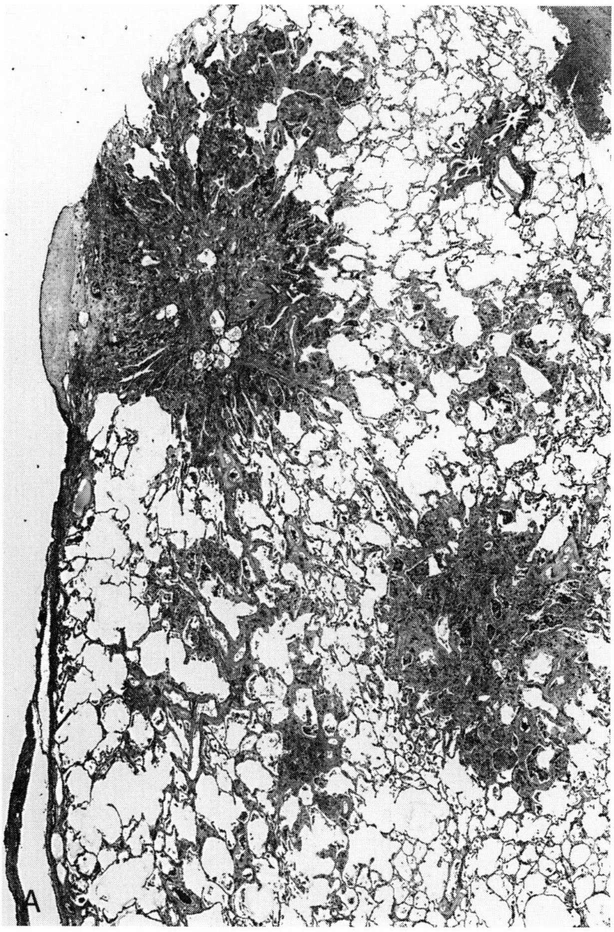

FIGURE 8.2
Lung of a 57-year-old white male pipe and cigarette smoker who worked for approximately 30 years manufacturing rubber parts for automobiles. Patient had carcinoma of the right upper lobe; chest radiograph at this time was negative for pneumoconiosis. Analysis of ashed lung sample revealed a total particle concentration of 15,900 × 10⁶ per gram of dry lung, of which 88% were aluminum silicates consistent with mica. **A.** Low-power view shows macules, nodules and patchy interstitial fibrosis. The pleura is thickened over the larger nodule.

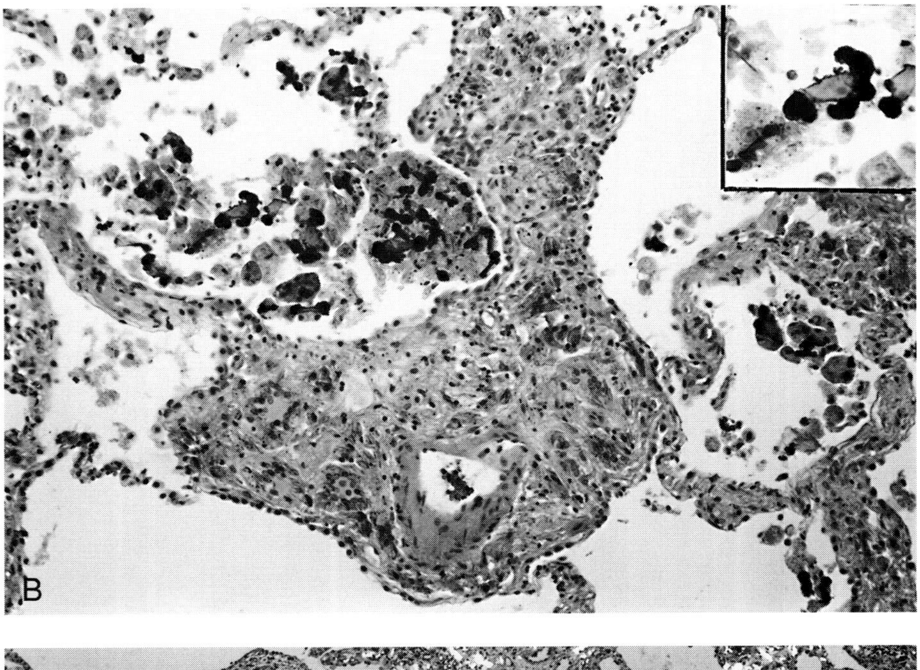

FIGURE 8.2 *(continued)*

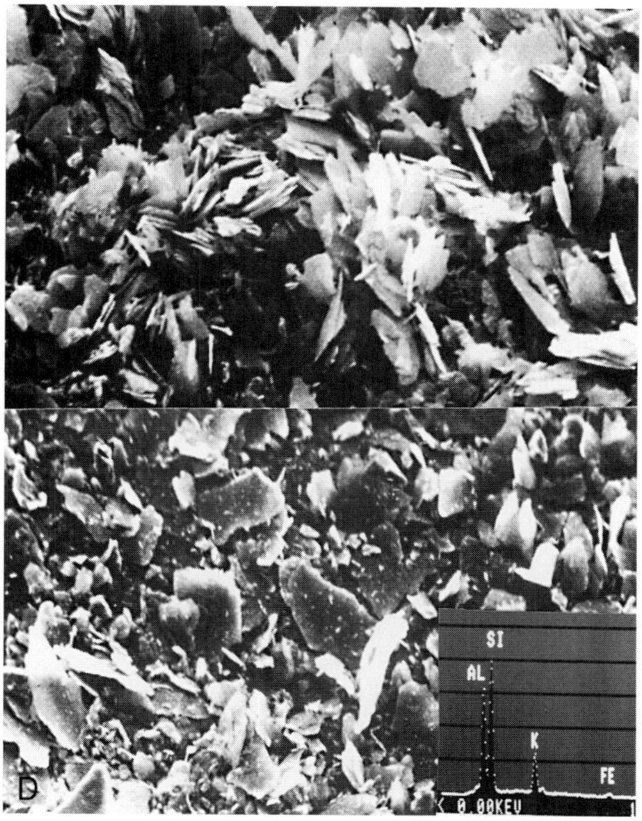

FIGURE 8.2 ***(continued)***

B. Close-up of macule shows giant-cell granulomatous reaction in the interstitium. Numerous ferruginous bodies formed on mica (**inset**) are also present. **C.** Area of interstitial fibrosis viewed with partially crossed polarizers shows numerous platy, highly birefringent particles consistent with mica. The presence of numerous large refractile particles and ferruginous bodies of this type suggests silicate minerals. **D.** Scanning electron micrograph of dust extracted from lung (top) compared with sample of mica from workplace (bottom). This particular material reportedly had been used for the past 30 years. **Inset**. x-ray spectrum of lung dust. (Analyses performed by J. Tucker and L. Stettler. Courtesy relatives of the patient.)

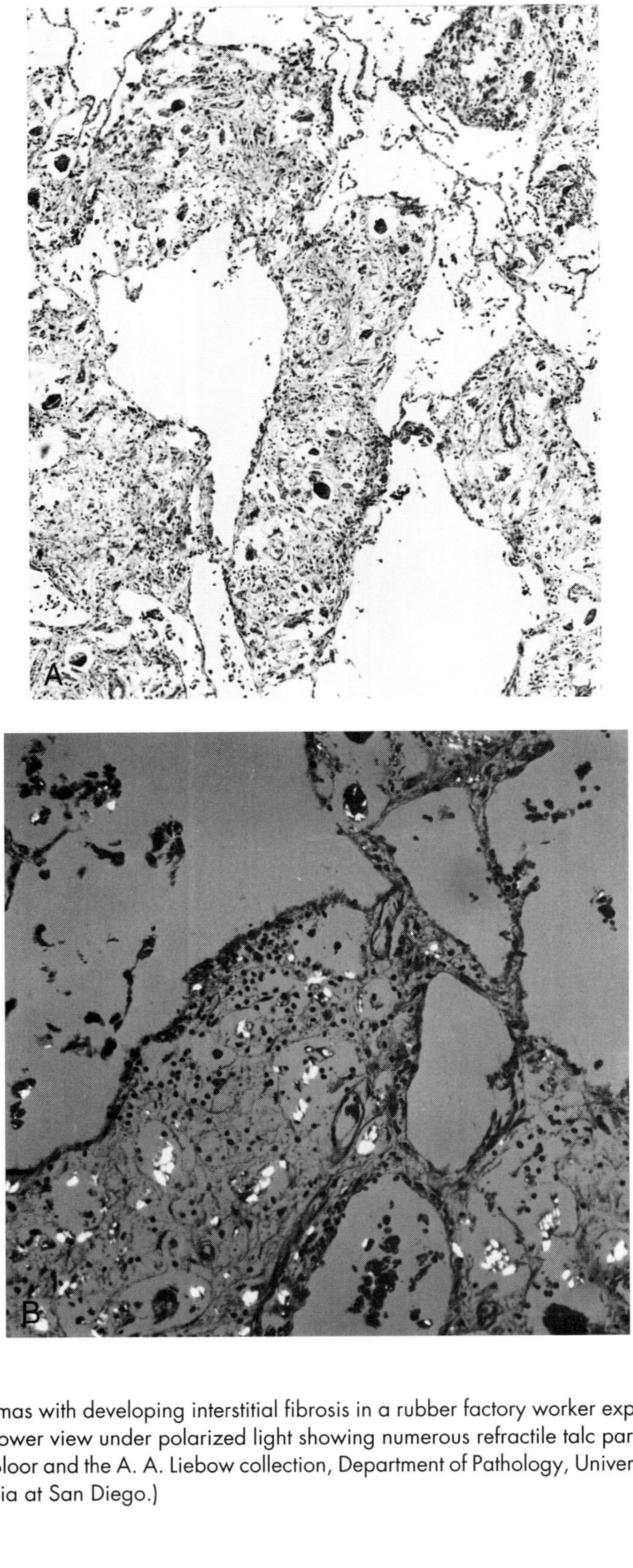

FIGURE 8.3

A. Granulomas with developing interstitial fibrosis in a rubber factory worker exposed to talc. **B.** Higher-power view under polarized light showing numerous refractile talc particles. (Courtesy Dr. C. Bloor and the A. A. Liebow collection, Department of Pathology, University of Southern California at San Diego.)

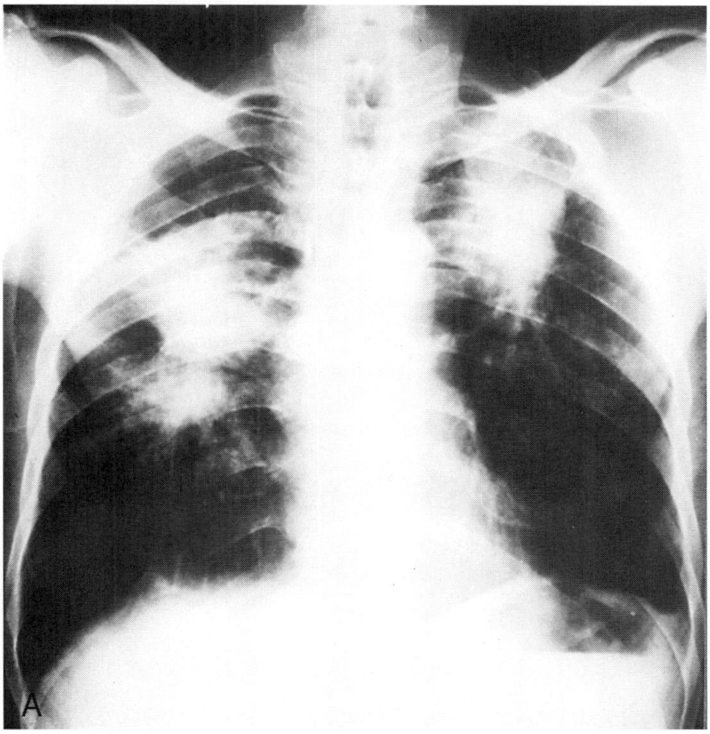

FIGURE 8.4

A. Chest radiograph of a 62-year-old man who worked 34 years in a Georgia kaolin-processing plant. Bilateral massive opacities are seen. Patient was a cigarette smoker (22 pack-years). Pulmonary function tests showed both obstructive and restrictive lung disease. **B.** Biopsy of mass lesion shows irregularly arranged collagen fibers and fine dust, macrophages, and occasional lymphocytes and plasma cells. **C.** Blood vessel within area of massive fibrosis shows narrowing and infiltration by dust-containing macrophages. **D.** Section from area adjacent to mass lesion shows diffuse interstitial fibrosis. **E.** Higher-power view shows numerous particles of highly birefringent dust. **F.** Electron microscopy and electron diffraction (**inset**) confirmed that the particles were kaolin. (Reprinted with permission from Sepulveda MJ, Vallyathan V, Stettler LE, et al. Kaolin pneumoconiosis in a Georgia mill. In: Wagner WL, Rom WN, Merchant JA, eds. Health issues related to metal and nonmetallic mining. Ann Arbor, MI: Ann Arbor Science, 1983:331–348.)

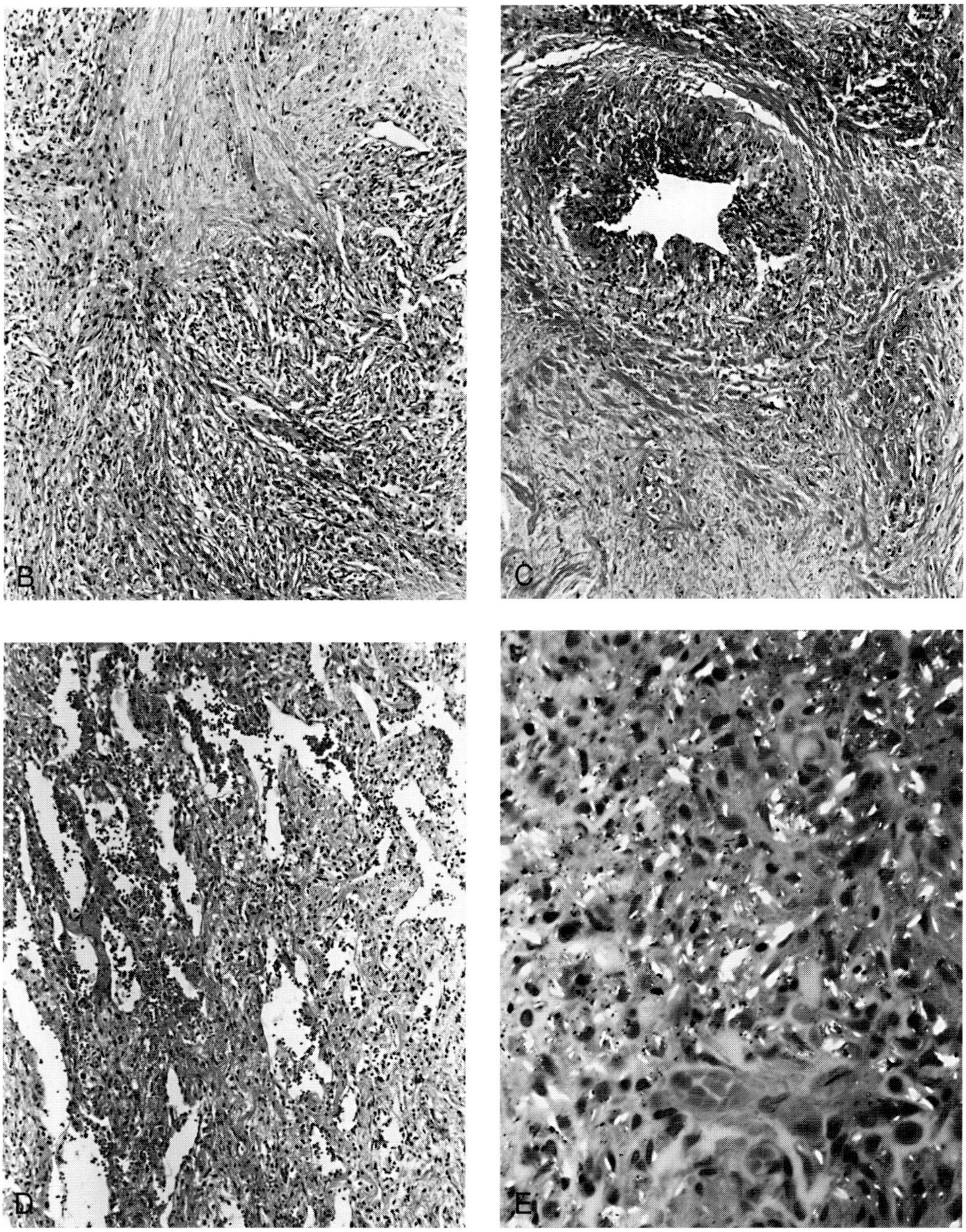

FIGURE 8.4 *(continued)*

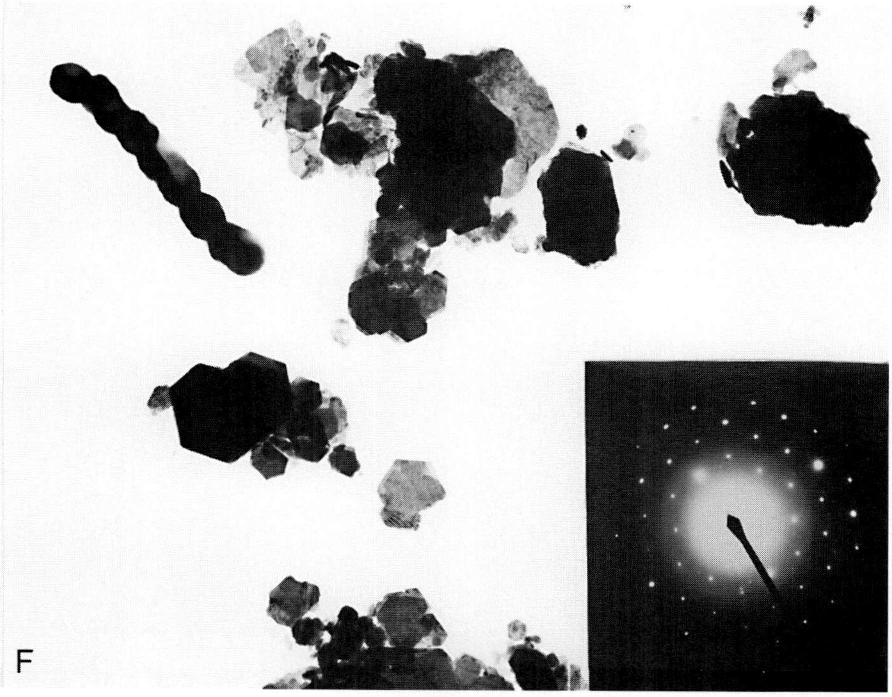

FIGURE 8.4 (*continued*)

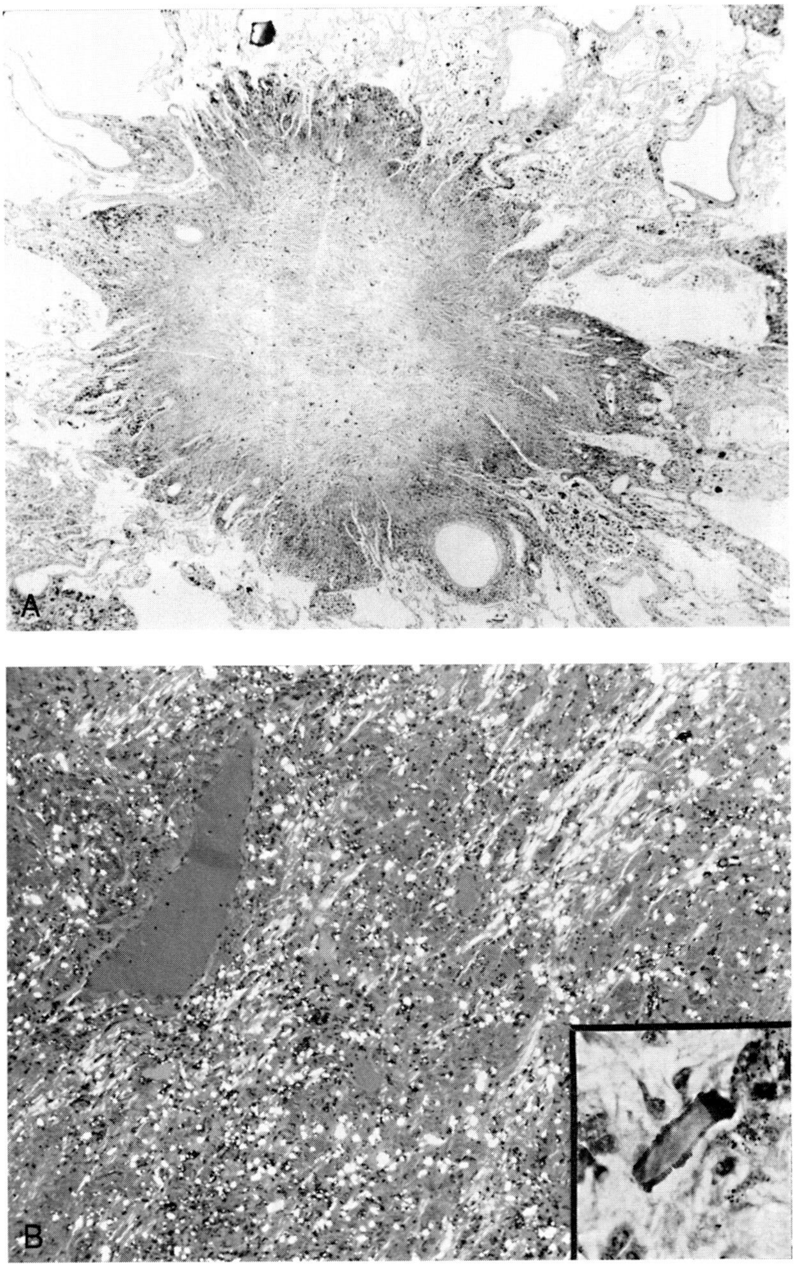

FIGURE 8.5
Pathologic changes in the lungs of a worker employed in the manufacture of roofing materials. He used mica, kaolin, and silica in making the roofing materials, and analysis of this lung revealed these same minerals. **A.** Nodular lesions with medusa head configuration typical of mixed-dust fibrosis. **B.** Higher-power view taken under polarized light shows numerous birefringent plates, a finding typical of silicate exposure. **Inset.** Ferruginous body formed on a sheet silicate. Another ferruginous body from this case is shown in colorplate 2. **C.** Another area from the same slide shows granulomas progressing to interstitial fibrosis. **D.** The same field under polarized light.

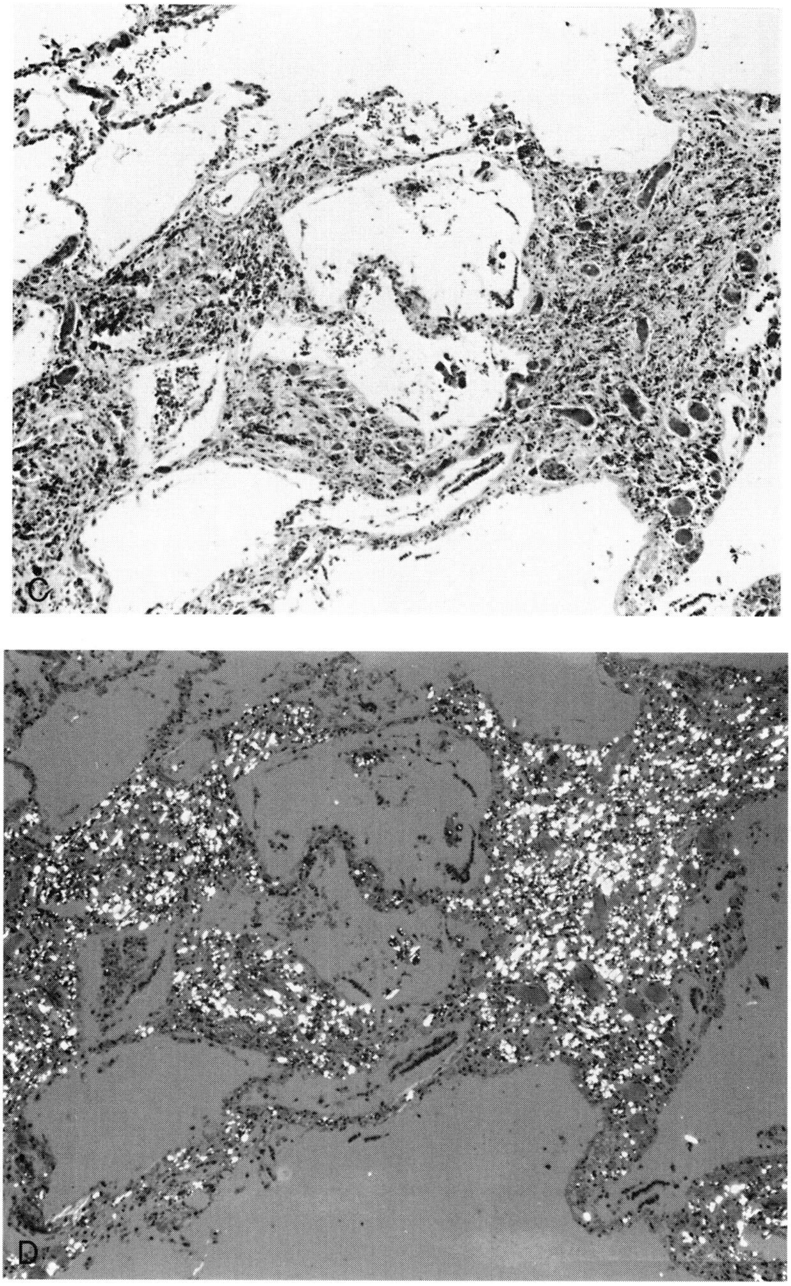

FIGURE 8.5 *(continued)*

do not reach the alveoli, and the presence of numerous very large mineral plates in the interstitia without particles in the alveolar spaces raises the possibility of intravenous drug abuse (12) (so-called intravenous talcosis, discussed later in this chapter and in Chapter 13).

Sheet silicates also tend to form ferruginous bodies with broad yellow plate-like or broadly fibrous cores (13). These structures are discussed in detail in Chapter 9 and are illustrated in colorplate 2 and Figures 8.2 and 8.5. Because relatively few minerals become ferruginated and because of the distinctive appearance of ferruginous bodies formed on sheet silicates, their identification in tissue sections may permit an accurate estimate of the nature of the dust exposure.

PATHOLOGIC REACTIONS TO SILICATE MINERALS

The very existence of pathologic reactions to silicates is controversial, and there are considerable differences in the lesions that various authors believe may be attributed to specific silicates (1, 14). In large part this dispute has arisen because the ores from which commercially important silicate minerals are derived often contain other minerals of marked pathogenicity. Much of the older literature reporting supposed silicate pneumoconioses cannot be interpreted, either because the problem of coexposures has been ignored (indeed, sometimes it is unclear whether the term *silica* actually means silica or silicates) or because analytic data are insufficient to ensure that exposure was actually to a pure silicate.

The important contaminating minerals in this regard are silica, usually quartz, and asbestos. Talc in particular is likely to contain one or both, and this problem is so well recognized that some authors use the names *talcosilicosis* and *talcoasbestosis* to describe the resulting pneumoconioses. Cosmetic-grade talc is usually free of asbestos, although this may not always have been true (15–17). The mineral sold as industrial-grade talc on occasion is more tremolite asbestos than talc (1, 18). Talc used in the rubber, plastic, and paper industries contains varying amounts of dolomite, calcite, chert, clays, serpentines, chlorite, actinolite, iron, manganese, and carbonaceous material (19). Silica is a contaminant of many ores, and the manifestations of exposure to quartz-containing mica, kaolin (20), or feldspars (21), as well as talc, may be those of silicosis or mixed-dust (i.e., silica plus another dust) pneumoconiosis (see Chapter 7). The magnitude of the problem may be judged from a review of mica pneumoconiosis by Skulberg et al. (22): of 202 cases of pneumoconiosis in workers known to be exposed to mica, 167 were considered to be silicosis or mixed dust pneumoconiosis.

A second reason for the controversy surrounding silicate pneumoconiosis is that even if the ability of these minerals to cause disease is accepted, it is clear that they do so only infrequently and then only in response to high exposure levels, particularly in comparison with the much more potent agents silica and asbestos. Only talc, mica, and kaolin have been reported as pathologic agents in more than a handful of cases, and even here the numbers are small. The study of Skulberg et al. (22) illustrates this point, since their fairly comprehensive review of the literature revealed only 66 cases that could be definitely or probably ascribed to mica alone, and in only 6 cases were detailed clinical, pathologic, and mineralogic descriptions provided. Many commercially used silicate minerals are associated with no reports of pneumoconiosis at all (1).

Nonetheless, examination of the relatively recent literature reveals cases in which analysis of the nature of the mineral exposure has ruled out a significant contribution by contaminating dusts (23–25). Moreover, some of the pathologic reactions caused by these dusts are distinctive (discussed later), and they are not seen in workers who are exposed to quartz or asbestos. Hence we believe that silicate pneumoconiosis, albeit uncommon, does occur and can be diagnosed by pathologic techniques.

We rely on what appear to be properly documented reports and on our own experience in describing pathologic reactions produced by silicates. It appears that silicate minerals produce a limited range of reactions in the lung. Hence we have grouped the discussion by pathologic processes. However, the frequency of these reactions differs from mineral to mineral, and because of the limited numbers of cases reported, it is not clear whether all minerals produce all lesions. The pathologic response to intravenous talc is discussed primarily in Chapter 13.

CLINICAL AND EPIDEMIOLOGIC FEATURES OF SILICATE PNEUMOCONIOSIS

Although many nonfibrous silicate minerals are used in industry, very few have been studied epidemiologically. This is due in part to small sample sizes, but the primary difficulty lies in finding populations of workers with relatively pure exposure, that is, free of silica and asbestos. Many studies have been flawed by inadequate mineralogic analysis of the raw mineral. A summary of the major findings from epidemiologic studies of silicate exposed workers is given in Table 8.3.

There appear to be no unique clinical features of silicate pneumoconiosis; when inhaled in high enough concentrations over long periods, all silicates probably can produce a relatively benign form of pneumoconiosis. Less commonly silicate exposure produces severe diffuse interstitial fibrosis or massive fibrosis (Fig. 8.4), and a case of rheumatoid pneumoconiosis has been described in a worker exposed to talc (1). In general the latency period is longer and rate of progression slower than is seen with asbestosis or silicosis. When the disease arises after a relatively short latency period or progresses rapidly, concomitant exposure to asbestos, free silica, or some other disease should be suspected.

The clinical features of silicate pneumoconioses vary; simple forms of pneumoconiosis, particularly those showing nodular opacities, are usually symptom free and produce few if any changes in pulmonary function. When the radiologic pattern is reticular or reticulonodular, indicating interstitial fibrosis, symptoms and signs of restrictive lung disease may be seen (see Chapter 1). Chronic obstructive pulmonary disease (COPD), including industrial bronchitis (26), may occur in response to many mineral dusts (see Chapter 6), and silicates are no exception. Dust-related declines in forced expiratory volume in 1 second (FEV_1) and forced vital capacity (FVC) have been documented in workers exposed to sepiolite (27), talc (28), and mixed dust (29). Progressive massive fibrosis usually produces clinically apparent disturbances in pulmonary function. These may be primarily obstructive, primarily restrictive, or both. In severe cases cor pulmonale may supervene. There is no evidence that in the absence of asbestos or other confounding exposures, any of the nonfibrous silicates increase the risk for respiratory cancers, although research on this question is continuing.

TABLE 8.3
Epidemiologic Studies of Workers Exposed to Silicate Minerals

PRINCIPAL EXPOSURE	OTHER EXPOSURES	STUDY	POPULATION	STUDY DESIGN	MAJOR FINDINGS AND COMMENTS
Attapulgite (Fuller's earth)	4–8% quartz, 1–5% dolomite	Waxweiler et al. (135)	2,302 Attapulgite clay miners	Mortality	Overall deficit in deaths from all causes and from nonmalignant respiratory disease. Excess lung cancer deaths in whites, decreased in blacks. Cancer results inconclusive.
Bentonite (Fuller's earth)	5–10% free silica (cristobalite)	Phibbs et al. (136)	Nonrandom sample of 32 bentonite workers	Survey	Simple pneumoconiosis in 14 and PMF in 2 workers. Changes probably due to free silica.
Kaolin	Minimal	Edenfield (30)	1,130 Georgia kaolin workers	Cross-sectional	Overall, 2.5% showed x-ray evidence of simple pneumoconiosis, 1.1% had complicated pneumoconiosis. No symptoms with simple disease.
Kaolin	1–2% free silica	Warraki and Herant (31)	914 Egyptian men, kaolin processing plant	Cross-sectional	1% had radiographic evidence of pneumoconiosis with >15 years exposure. No pneumoconiosis seen with <15 years exposure.
Kaolin	Minimal	Sheers (32)	1,394 Cornish china clay workers	Cross-sectional	X-ray prevalence of pneumoconiosis depended on duration and intensity of exposure, ranging from 2–23%; 12 cases of complicated pneumoconiosis.
Kaolin	Quartz (<4.5%) cristobolite	Lesser et al. (20)	9 selected workers at firebrick factory	Hospital series	7 simple pneumoconiosis, 2 complicated. Moderate obstructive and restrictive airway disease. Calcined kaolin more hazardous.
Kaolin	4% TiO_2	Sepulveda et al. (33)	65 current and former Georgia, U.S. kaolin mine and mill workers	Cross-sectional	X-ray prevalence of pneumoconiosis 13% in current and 19% in former workers. Minimum latency 15 years. PMF in half of cases with pneumoconiosis.
Kaolin	<1% silica	Kennedy et al. (34)	459 Georgia, U.S., kaolin mining and processing workers	Morbidity	Overall prevalence of pneumoconiosis 9.2%. Small irregular opacities predominated; PMF seen in 8 cases. Simple pneumoconiosis not associated with functional abnormalities. PMF associated with mild restrictive disease.
Mica	Various, quartz, feldspar, pegmatite	Dreessen et al. (137)	57 men exposed to relatively pure mica; 31 men and 78 women fabricating sheet mica; 741 men mining and sorting pegmatite contaminated with quartz and feldspar	Cross-sectional morbidity	No pneumoconiosis in sheet mica fabrication. Pneumoconiosis seen in other groups at exposure levels >10 mppcf. Latencies of 5–10 years observed in workers exposed to >50 mppcf.

TABLE 8.3
(continued)

PRINCIPAL EXPOSURE	OTHER EXPOSURES	STUDY	POPULATION	STUDY DESIGN	MAJOR FINDINGS AND COMMENTS
Mica	Negligible	Vestal et al. (120)	79 men employed in North Carolina, mica-grinding plants	Cross-sectional morbidity	Prevalence of pneumoconiosis 11%. Exposures very high.
Mica	<1% quartz	Heinmann et al. (138)	61 Indian muscovite workers; most exposures were less than 5 years	Cross-sectional morbidity	44% had minor radiographic changes interpreted as being due to mica exposure.
Mica	Negligible	Smith (52)	302 male mica insulators	Cross-sectional morbidity	No pneumoconiosis. 1.6% had pleural calcification.
Montmorillonite (Fuller's earth)	Quartz, muscovite, glauconite, (1–2%)	McNally and Trostler (139)	49 men employed at Fuller's earth plant in Illinois	Survey	Pneumoconiosis similar to silicosis seen on chest radiograph. Inadequate study design. Positive findings could have been due to free silica exposure.
Meerschaum Sepiolite	Tremolite and zeolite	Baris et al. (54)	63 Turkish sepiolite workers	Survey	No pleural changes. 10 workers showed pulmonary fibrosis that may have been due to other exposures.
Sepiolite	None recorded	McConnochie et al. (27)	Total worker population (n = 218) of Spanish sepiolite plant	Cross-sectional morbidity	Dust-related declines in FEV_1 and FVC. No changes on chest radiograph.
Slate (Muscovite and quartz)	Feldspar, kaolin, chlorite, hematite	Craighead et al. (140)	Autopsy study of 12 slate quarriers in Vermont	Autopsy series from Vermont field survey	A pneumoconiosis distinct from silicosis was identified.
Talc	Minimal	Hogue and Mallette (141)	20 rubber workers with 10–36 years' exposure	Cross-sectional morbidity	No clinical, radiologic, or pulmonary functional abnormalities.
Talc	Free silica	Scansetti et al. (142)	236 Italian talc miners	Cross-sectional morbidity	High incidence of mild pneumoconiosis. Inadequate control for age, smoking, and attrition. Some miners (drillers) may have received high silica exposure.
Talc	Not known	Wild et al. (28)	166 French talc millers	Cross-sectional morbidity	Exposure-related declines in FEV_1 and FVC. Significant relation between small radiologic opacities and dust exposure.

TABLE 8.3
(continued)

PRINCIPAL EXPOSURE	OTHER EXPOSURES	STUDY	POPULATION	STUDY DESIGN	MAJOR FINDINGS AND COMMENTS
Talc	Free silica, no asbestos	Rubino et al. (43)	Male talc miners and millers	Prospective mortality	No association between cause of death and cumulative exposure for millers. Excess deaths from nonmalignant respiratory disease in miners attributable to silica exposure.
Talc	Chlorite, calcite, pyrite, quartz <3.5%	Delaude (143)	94 French talc workers with tenures of 11–36 years	Cross-sectional morbidity	15 workers with pneumoconiosis (8 minimal), 1 worker with reduced pulmonary function. Smoking enhanced rate of chronic bronchitis.
Talc	Free silica (0.2–4%)	Messite et al. (144)	15 New York talc miners and 46 talc millers	Cross-sectional morbidity	Low prevalence of radiographic changes (0/15 miners, 2/46 millers) with historic high exposures (47–1090 mppcL) in the mill.
Talc	<1% free silica	Selevan et al. (44)	Vermont talc miners	Mortality	Increased mortality from pneumoconiosis.
Talc	<1% free silica	Gamble et al. (38)	121 New York state talc miners and millers compared with potash miners	Cross-sectional morbidity	31% pleural thickening in talc workers with >15 years exposure compared with 4.4% in potash miners. More symptoms, less function than in potash miners.
Talc	Not known	Fine et al. (41)	80 talc-exposed rubber workers, 189 rubber workers not exposed to talc	Cross-sectional morbidity	Increased prevalence of respiratory symptoms, cough, phlegm, and wheezing in talc-exposed workers. No radiographic abnormalities. Mild obstructive disease in workers with 10 years or more of exposure to talc.
Talc	Tremolite, anthophyllite in New York talc	Gamble and Greife (39)	Talc miners and millers from 4 U.S. talc-producing plants	Cross-sectional morbidity	Low prevalence of pneumoconiosis. Dose-related pleural thickening, overall prevalence 9% with talc either with or without asbestos. No consistent association of exposure with respiratory symptoms or function.
Talc	Tremolite, anthophyllite	Kleinfeld et al. (42)	260 New York state talc miners	Mortality	Fourfold excess of deaths from lung cancer. No excess of gastrointestinal malignancies. 27% of deaths related to pneumoconiosis.
Vermiculite	Fibrous tremolite	McDonald et al. (58)	406 vermiculite miners from Montana	Retrospective cohort study	Excess mortality from respiratory cancer, nonmalignant respiratory disease, and mesothelioma.
Wollastonite	2% free silica	Shasby et al. (57)	87 current and 5 former wollastonite miners and millers	Cross-sectional morbidity	No excess of respiratory symptoms, radiographic or pulmonary function abnormalities.

Mppcf, million particles per cubic foot.
MppcL, million particles per cubic liter.

KAOLIN

Kaolin comprises a group of commercial clays in which the aluminum silicate kaolinite predominates. Kaolin, which is derived from the breakdown of igneous feldspar minerals, contains varying amounts of silica, mica, and residual feldspar. Calcined kaolin also contains mullite and cristobalite. Major kaolin deposits occur in Cornwall, Georgia and the Carolinas in the United States, Japan, Egypt, Czechoslovakia, and Germany (14). China clay, ball clay, halloysite clay, and fire clay are all forms of kaolin.

In the United States approximately 4000 workers are involved in mining kaolin, primarily open cast, and 9000 others work in kaolin processing plants (19). Kaolin is used in many industries, mostly in the manufacture of paper, rubber, plastic, ceramics, and pharmaceuticals. In the paper industry it is used as a filler to provide body and a smooth surface coating. It is used extensively in plastics and rubber as a filler, as an extender in paints, and in the manufacture of china, stoneware, insulation, and refractories. Lesser amounts are used in the manufacture of textiles, drugs, toothpaste, floor tiles, detergents, and insecticides.

The major findings from epidemiologic studies in which kaolin was the primary exposure are presented in Table 8.3 (20, 30–34). Kaolin pneumoconiosis appears to have a low to moderate prevalence among exposed workers. Small nodular opacities similar to those seen in coal workers are reported as being characteristic of kaolin exposure in Cornish china clay workers (32). On the other hand, kaolin workers in middle Georgia appear to develop primarily small irregular opacities in the mid zones of the lungs (34). The very few pulmonary function studies in kaolin workers indicate that simple pneumoconiosis is not associated with abnormalities of pulmonary function (34). However, workers with progressive massive fibrosis (PMF) are usually symptomatic, with chest tightness, productive cough, and exertional dyspnea (20, 35). One study of Georgia kaolin workers with PMF showed mild decrements in FVC interpreted as evidence of mild restriction (34). Another reported both obstructive and restrictive abnormalities (33). Tuberculosis may complicate kaolinosis (35) but probably occurs primarily in kaolin workers who receive substantial silica exposure.

TALC

The properties of softness, large surface area, slipperiness, chemical inertness, oil absorptiveness, and high refractoriness have made talc a valuable resource with more than 100 applications. World production of talc is approximately 5 million to 6 million tons per year (36). In 1978 there were approximately 400 workers in underground and open cast mines and approximately 700 workers in preparation plants in the United States (19). Approximately 200 of these workers were exposed to fibrous talc. The number of exposed workers in secondary industries is unknown, as is the number of persons at risk from use or misuse of cosmetic products. The majority of talc is used in the manufacture of ceramics, paints, paper, refractories, building materials, insecticides, rubber, plastics, cosmetics, pharmaceuticals (19), and confectionery (37).

The major findings from epidemiologic studies in which talc was the primary exposure are presented in Table 8.3. These data indicate that prolonged high exposures produce radiographic evidence of pneumoconiosis with few functional abnormalities in the early stages. The latency for talc pneumoconiosis is usually greater than 15 years, and the disease progresses slowly. Rapidly progressive forms of pneumoconiosis have been described, but they are rare and probably due to combined exposure to silica.

The radiographic features of talc pneumoconiosis vary. Nodular or reticular opacities predominating in the mid zones are most often seen when the exposure is relatively pure or contaminated with silica. An interstitial disease pattern with linear and reticular opacities in the lower zones is sometimes called *talcosis*. Mild forms of talc pneumoconiosis having a granulomatous pathologic pattern are reported to show a miliary pattern of small opacities on chest radiograph (38). Visceral and parietal pleural changes, including diffuse thickening of the visceral pleura, obliteration of the costophrenic angles, and thoracic and diaphragmatic pleural plaques, are common in talc-exposed workers. The plaques may calcify. Pleural changes are seen in workers exposed to talcs contaminated with asbestos and those free of asbestos (39).

Clinically talc pneumoconiosis is initially symptom free, but as it progresses, it may resemble a mild form of asbestosis (14), and it is accompanied by a reduction in lung volume and diffusing capacity (40). Chronic cough with productive clear sputum and wheezing (industrial bronchitis) has been described in talc workers (41).

Mortality studies of talc-exposed workers show an excess of deaths from nonmalignant respiratory disease in those exposed to talcs with (42) and without contaminating asbestos (43, 44) and silica (45). The carcinogenic potential of talc has received considerable attention. A fourfold increased rate of lung cancer has been reported in New York talc miners and millers (42). This excess was attributed to the high levels of tremolite or anthophyllite asbestos in the ore. However, no dose–response relationship was demonstrated, and it has been suggested that exposure to radon daughters in other mines may have been a confounding factor (46). Lung cancer mortality was also significantly higher (standardized mortality rate [SMR] 2.54) in pottery workers exposed to both silica and talc (46). Mortality studies conducted on workers exposed to asbestos-free talc fail to show consistent effects of talc on lung cancer mortality (43, 44, 46, 47). Mesothelioma has not been described in workers exposed to talc although tremolite is a potent inducer of this tumor in animals (48) and mesothelioma occurs in vermiculite workers exposed to tremolite (49, 50). No mesotheliomas were observed in a series of 136 patients, followed for 14 to 40 years, who received talc pleurodesis (51).

MICA

Mica is used primarily for electrical and thermal insulation. Lesser uses include manufacture of building products and filler in asphalts, enamels, mastics, textured paints, cements, adhesives, and oil well drilling mud. Ground mica is used for lubrication of molds in the rubber and plastics industry. The number of workers employed in the mining and processing of mica is small, estimated at 382 in the United States in 1978 (19). Most epidemiologic studies of mica workers were conducted before widespread use of standardized radiographic classification systems; hence they are difficult to interpret. Data presented in Table 8.3 indicate that mica dust exposure is associated with radiographic evidence of pneumoconiosis and pleural calcification (52, 53).

The clinical and radiologic features have not been well described. Case reports indicate that the mid and lower zones of the lung may be primarily involved with reticular and reticulonodular opacities (52,53). In neither report was the possibility of confounding exposures eliminated.

FULLER'S EARTH

Fuller's earth comprises several clays with absorbing properties. It is a loose term that may be applied to clays with different chemical compositions. The four major clays with the physical properties of fuller's earth are calcium montmorillonite, sodium montmorillonite (bentonite), sepiolite, and attapulgite (palygorskite). Large deposits are found in the United States, Europe, and elsewhere. There are approximately 800 to 1000 miners and millers of fuller's earth in the United States (19). Fuller's earth is primarily mined by open cast methods, desiccated in rotary dryers, and size-sorted by air flotation or elutriation. These operations may be very dusty (1). The exact composition and the amount of free silica in the clay deposits varies from 0 to 20%; hence epidemiologic or pathologic findings based on a population exposed to a specific clay deposit may not be applicable to other situations.

Calcium and sodium montmorillonites are used in the oil industry for refining, in drilling muds, and as a foundry sand bond. They are also used as a filtering agent and to prevent seepage in waste disposal and containment systems. Lesser uses include colloid fillers for paints, fire retardant materials, cosmetics, and pharmaceuticals.

Attapulgite clay is mined in Florida and Georgia in the United States. It differs from the other clays in that it is fibrous. It has numerous industrial uses: its great absorptive and binding properties are used to purify a variety of products, from oils, fats, and vitamins to industrial wastes (including nuclear waste) and sewage. Approximately 65% of attapulgite is used as an absorbent; pesticides and related products consume 15%, and 5% is used in oil treatment. Miscellaneous uses (15%) include catalytic applications, petroleum refining oil well drilling mud, and stabilization and thickening of putties, glazes, and adhesives (19).

Sepiolite is an absorbent clay primarily used as pet litter. It is mined commercially in Spain (27) and Turkey (54), and exploitable deposits exist in Nevada. It consists of fine crystals that are a transition between chain and layered silicates. The compact form, meerschaum, is carved into pipes and cigarette holders.

The few epidemiologic and clinical studies of workers exposed to fuller's earth are summarized in Table 8.3. It appears from these reports that pneumoconiosis, including PMF, occurs in workers exposed to high dust concentrations. It is not possible to determine from the literature whether the pneumoconiosis is due to the clay minerals or contaminating free silica. Sepiolite has been linked to endemic pleural plaques in Bulgaria (55), although asbestos and zeolites were not excluded as causative agents.

OIL SHALE

Oil shales consist largely of the silicates kaolin and mica with lesser amounts of illite, limestone, and free silica, depending on the source of origin (14, 56). Four cases of shale miner's pneumoconiosis, two with PMF, were reported from the now defunct Scottish oil shale industry (56). The disease radiographically and pathologically resembled coal workers' pneumoconiosis, and mineral dust extracted from the lungs of three miners had a similar composition to that obtained from soft coal miners.

WOLLASTONITE

Wollastonite is an acicular chain silicate (Fig. 8.1*C*) that can substitute for asbestos in several applications. A single epidemiologic study encompassed the majority of wollastonite workers in the United States (57) (Table 8.3). The study did not find any adverse health effects, though the population was small and the latency periods for most workers too short to detect pneumoconiosis or malignancy.

VERMICULITE

Vermiculite exfoliates when heated to produce a low-density material for use in construction materials, agricultural products, and other purposes. Commercial deposits are mined in Montana and South Carolina in the United States, and these deposits are contaminated with the asbestos mineral fibrous tremolite–actinolite, which in this setting may be a long fiber with a high aspect ratio. It is also mined in South Africa. Epidemiologic studies of workers in the Montana mine and mill (58–60) and workers at an Ohio fertilizer plant that used vermiculite from Montana and South Africa (61) show a high prevalence of pleural and pulmonary interstitial abnormalities and increased mortality from nonmalignant respiratory disease and lung cancer (49, 58). Four cases of mesothelioma have been reported. Mortality from lung cancer in the workers from Montana showed a linear relationship with individual cumulative fiber exposure (49, 58). The authors concluded that the findings were more likely to be due to the effects of asbestos than vermiculite. The histologic appearances of the lungs at autopsy from a vermiculite worker in the latter cohort are shown in Figure 8.6.

OTHER SILICATES

Case reports and case series describing pneumoconiosis in association with exposures to feldspars (Fig. 8.7), nepheline (14, 62), mullite (63), cement (64), sillimanite (14), and pumice (65) have appeared in the literature; however, detailed studies have not been conducted. There is no reason to believe that these silicates are materially different in their pathogenicity from the ones already described.

MINERAL DUSTS IN AGRICULTURE

Farming is a dusty occupation. Concentrations of respirable particulates within farm tractor cabs may exceed 10 mg/m^3 (66). Soil consists of a mixture of organic and inorganic materials that in theory should contain representative portions of all major mineral classes in the earth's crust. In practice most agricultural soils consist largely of silicate minerals, with lesser amounts of other mineral classes depending on the local geologic history. The amount of crystalline silica (quartz) varies from 1 to 20% (67). X-ray diffraction analysis of respirable farm dust from Alberta, Canada, showed that the most common minerals were feldspar, quartz, illite, kaolinite, chlorite, montmorillonite, anhydrite, and calcite (67). In addition, variable amounts of dolomite, pyrite, goethite, halite, marcasite, smectite, hornblende, and gypsum were identified. Fibrous mineral species are uncommon in soil but may be important locally, as with richterite and anthophyllite asbestos in Finland (68, 69), tremolite in Cyprus (70), and erionite in Turkey (71) and Nevada (72).

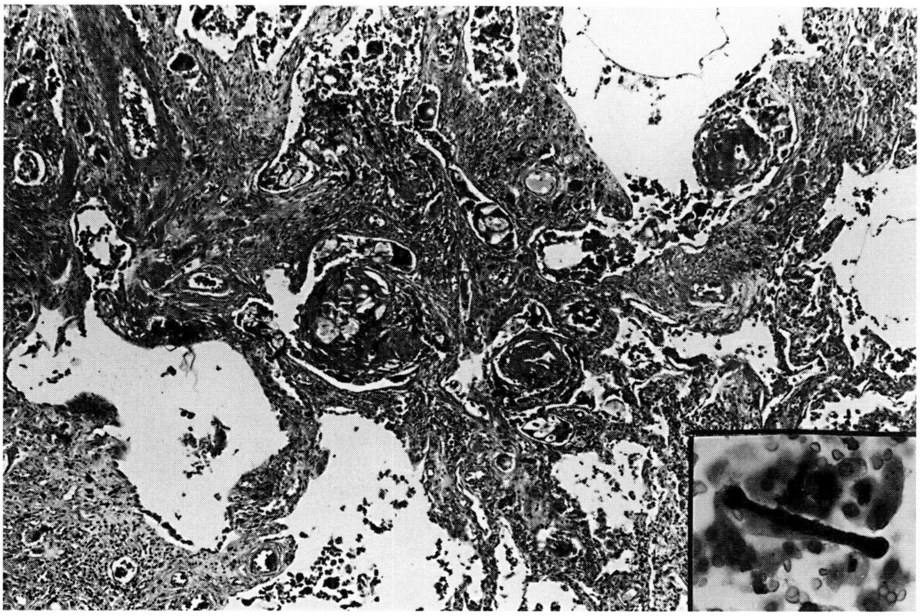

FIGURE 8.6
Section of lung obtained at autopsy from a man employed at a vermiculite mine and mill in Montana. The vermiculite ore was heavily contaminated with tremolite asbestos. The lung shows numerous asbestos bodies and severe diffuse interstitial fibrosis representing tremolite-induced asbestosis, along with a giant-cell intra-alveolar granulomatous reaction in which birefringent vermiculite particles can be seen. **Inset.** Asbestos body.

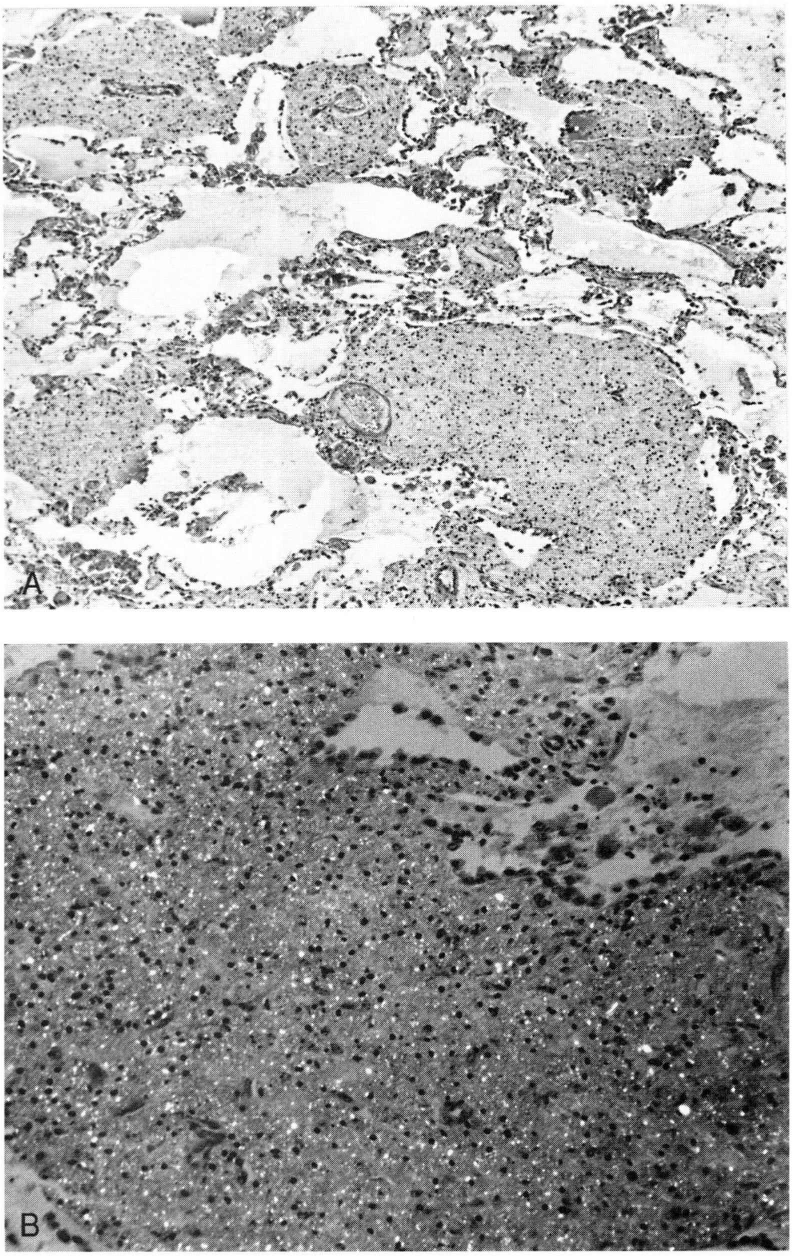

FIGURE 8.7
Ordinary and polarized light micrographs of interstitial granulomatous-to-nodular lesions from the lungs of a worker exposed to dust in tunnel drilling. Analysis revealed that almost all the dust was the feldspar orthoclase. Chest radiograph revealed finely nodular lesions. **A.** Low-power view. **B.** High-power view shows numerous macrophages that contain fine granular dust;.

In addition to naturally occurring minerals, soil contains mineral dusts derived from commercial agricultural products. Minerals such as talc, zeolite, kaolin, attapulgite clay, and vermiculite are used as fillers and carriers for pesticides, as additives to livestock feeds, and in the treatment of animal wastes (73). Industrial grades of these minerals are commonly contaminated with fibrous particles, notably tremolite asbestos (16, 74). Synthetic silicates, which may be very small (about 18 nm), are used in the animal feed industry as liquid carriers and anticaking agents (75).

In dry and windy regions dusts derived from farming may be a source of regional air pollution (67, 76). Loss of ground cover, exposed rocky outcrops, and unpaved roads also increase the likelihood of mineral particles becoming airborne. The composition of the airborne dust primarily depends on the geochemistry of the soils but is also influenced by factors such as the predominant farming pattern (e.g., crops, forage, pasture) and use of irrigation.

The few case reports and case series describing pneumoconiosis in farmers provide evidence that the primary hazard is from silica (quartz) and silicate minerals (77–80) and that exposures are to a mixture of minerals. To this extent the disease can be classified as a mixed-dust pneumoconiosis (see Chapter 7). Diffuse interstitial fibrosis, foreign-body granulomas, alveolar lipoproteinosis, and constrictive bronchiolitis have all been described in workers in the agricultural industry exposed to predominantly silicate mineral dusts (75, 77, 81).

In general the silicate minerals are weakly fibrogenic, and prolonged and intense exposures are required for clinical disease. There is evidence that quartz is less fibrogenic when it is weathered, mixed with other minerals, or coated with organic compounds and surfactant (82–84).

Soil samples from the Mexican city Mexicali have been shown to be potent activators of complement and capable of inducing interstitial fibrosis in exposed rats (85). The soil from this region consists predominantly of potassium aluminium silicates (illite) (75%) and silica (approximately 20%) and is geographically related to soils in southern California that are linked to pneumoconiosis in the farm population (77).

Biogenic silica fibers are common to many plants important to agriculture, including, for example, sugar cane, flax, and grasses. The fibers have structural similarities to asbestos (86) and can promote mesothelial tumors in rats (87). Their role in fibrogenesis has not been studied; however, it is likely, based on their physical characteristics, that they can cause pulmonary fibrosis. Exposure to biogenic silica fibers has been linked to excess deaths from lung cancer (88), mesothelioma (89), and esophageal cancer (90, 91).

Studies of Farm and Wild Animals

Studies of animals exposed on the farm, in the zoo, or in the wild provide evidence that airborne mineral dusts cause pneumoconiosis. As such, they provide an important source of information for assessing risks to human populations. Increased pulmonary dust burdens of silicate minerals and/or silicate pneumoconiosis have been described in dogs (92, 93), pigs (94), pheasants (95), kiwis (96), camels (97), horses (98), and water buffaloes (99).

Schwartz et al. (98) reported findings on nine horses from the Monterey–Carmel peninsula of California that had exercise intolerance and varying degrees of respiratory distress. Morphologic examination of pulmonary tissue obtained at biopsy or autopsy showed a granulomatous interstitial pneumonitis associated with birefringent particles on polarizing microscopy. X-ray microanalysis of lung tissue from five horses, as well as a sample of soil from one stable, showed in the granulomas large numbers of particles of aluminum silicates and silica smaller than a micrometer.

A simple silicate pneumoconiosis has been reported in animals dying in the San Diego Zoo (100). Some 100 autopsies from 11 mammalian and 8 avian species were studied by light and electron microscopy and x-ray microanalysis. Interstitial fibrosis associated with mineral dust deposits were found in 20% of lungs. The particles were 90% silicates, which x-ray diffraction showed to be predominantly muscovite mica and its hydrothermal degradation product, illite clay. A similar mineralogic profile was found on analysis of atmospheric air samples taken at the zoo.

Silicate pneumoconiosis has also been described in 94 of 134 autopsied camels from the Somali desert (97). In addition to diffuse interstitial fibrosis, classic hyalinized nodules of silicosis were seen in six cases. X-ray microanalysis showed a mixed dust exposure containing silica and silicates of aluminum, potassium, and iron.

Four cases of silicate pneumoconiosis were described in pigs raised near chalk quarries and cement works in Italy (94). Interstitial and peribronchial fibrosis associated with deposition of dust was the characteristic lesion. X-ray microanalysis of the dust revealed particles composed mainly of silicon, calcium, potassium, sulphur, aluminum, and iron. Air samples from the region showed similar particles.

Human Studies

Sherwin et al. (77) reported a silicate pneumoconiosis in seven patients (five vineyard workers, one produce farmer, and one rural resident) living in the central valley of California. Six of the seven were nonsmokers at the time of death. All five vineyard workers died of respiratory failure. Interstitial fibrosis, chronic inflammation, and foreign-body granulomas to varying degrees were the primary pathologic abnormalities. The lesions were associated with deposition of birefringent particles. Scanning electron microscopy combined with x-ray microanalysis of respirable-sized (less than 5 μm) particles from the lungs of four of the patients and corresponding soil samples showed that silicates of the mica group predominated.

A mild silicate pneumoconiosis has been reported in a 53-year-old farmer in Norway undergoing lung resection for a carcinoid tumor (78). The lung adjacent to the tumor showed patchy pleural fibrosis with peribronchial and interstitial fibrosis. These lesions were associated with mineral dust particles, observed by polarizing microscopy, that showed fibrous, needle-shaped and platy morphology. Nonasbestos ferruginous bodies were also observed. Examination of ashed lung samples by x-ray elemental and x-ray diffraction analysis showed that muscovite mica, talc, silica, and feldspar were the most abundant minerals. Fibrous mullite and anthophyllite asbestos were present in concentrations of 4.5×10^6 and 2.7×10^6 fibers per gram of dried lung tissue, respectively. Analysis of soil from the farmer's potato storehouse revealed mica along with quartz and plagioclase feldspar but no talc. Rutile fibers were also detected in the dust. The authors concluded that the mica, silica, and feldsparlike particles came from soil derived from schists, which are the most abundant rocks in the region.

Spain et al. (75) described a case of constrictive bronchiolitis without organizing pneumonia in a 38-year-old nonsmoking, previously healthy woman who worked for 2 years in the production of animal feeds. The composition of the feed was complex, including grains, enzymes, and bacterial products in addition to large quantities of amorphous silica, silicates, and synthetic silicates. The synthetic compound was composed of very fine and highly respirable ultrafine particles (about 18 nm). Open lung biopsy revealed a constrictive bronchiolitis without organizing pneumonia. Birefringent silicate particles were identified in the walls of the respiratory bronchioles. The patient did not respond to corticosteroid therapy, and the investigators concluded that exposure to silicate minerals was the primary causative factor in the disease. Other case reports of silicate pneumoconiosis in farmers have been reported (79–81).

An ongoing study of Hispanic farm workers of the central valley of California shows that the primary site of deposition of the mineral dust is in the proximal respiratory bronchioles (101). Mineral dust small airway disease, macules, and lymph node fibrosis were all significantly associated with a history of farming. Total mineral and total silica dust were also positively associated with farming and with small airway disease.

SPECIFIC PATHOLOGIC REACTIONS TO SILICATES

Macules

Macules are collections of dust and dust-laden macrophages associated with little fibrosis. The macules are found around respiratory bronchioles and accompanying vessels (Figs. 8.2, 8.8, and 8.9). By definition macules are nonpalpable because they do not contain much fibrous tissue. Analogous (unnamed) collections of dust may be seen in interlobular septa and under the pleura, all of which are sites of lymphatic drainage. Macules have been specifically described in workers exposed to kaolin (102), mica (100), feldspars (65, 103), talc (104), and fuller's earth (105, 106) (Table 8.4), but they probably occur with all silicate exposures. The scanty literature suggests that macules in those exposed to talc (104) tend to develop more fibrosis than occurs in the macules of coal miners, and this is our impression also. If the dust has a distinctive color, macules may be visible grossly as collections of pigment in the centers of the acini. Macules caused by kaolin, for example, may have a gray to gray–brown color (63). Macules sometimes give rise to radiographic appearance of fine nodular opacities. Because macules are small, these appearances probably reflect summation effects.

Mineral Dust–Induced Small Airway Disease

Mineral dust–induced small airway disease is a common finding in workers exposed to silica and silicate minerals (107). The lesion consists of fibrous thickening of the walls of membranous and respiratory bronchioles and alveolar ducts, usually with large amounts of accompanying dust and often with considerable distortion of the airway lumen. Workers with this lesion have significantly lower values of FEV_1 and FEF_{25-75} and higher residual volume (RV) and total lung capacity (TLC) than controls matched for age, sex, and smoking. Mineral dust small airway disease is seen following exposures to feldspars, kaolin, mica, mixed dusts, and talc (Table 8.4) and is the primary abnormality in agricultural workers exposed to crustal silicates (101).

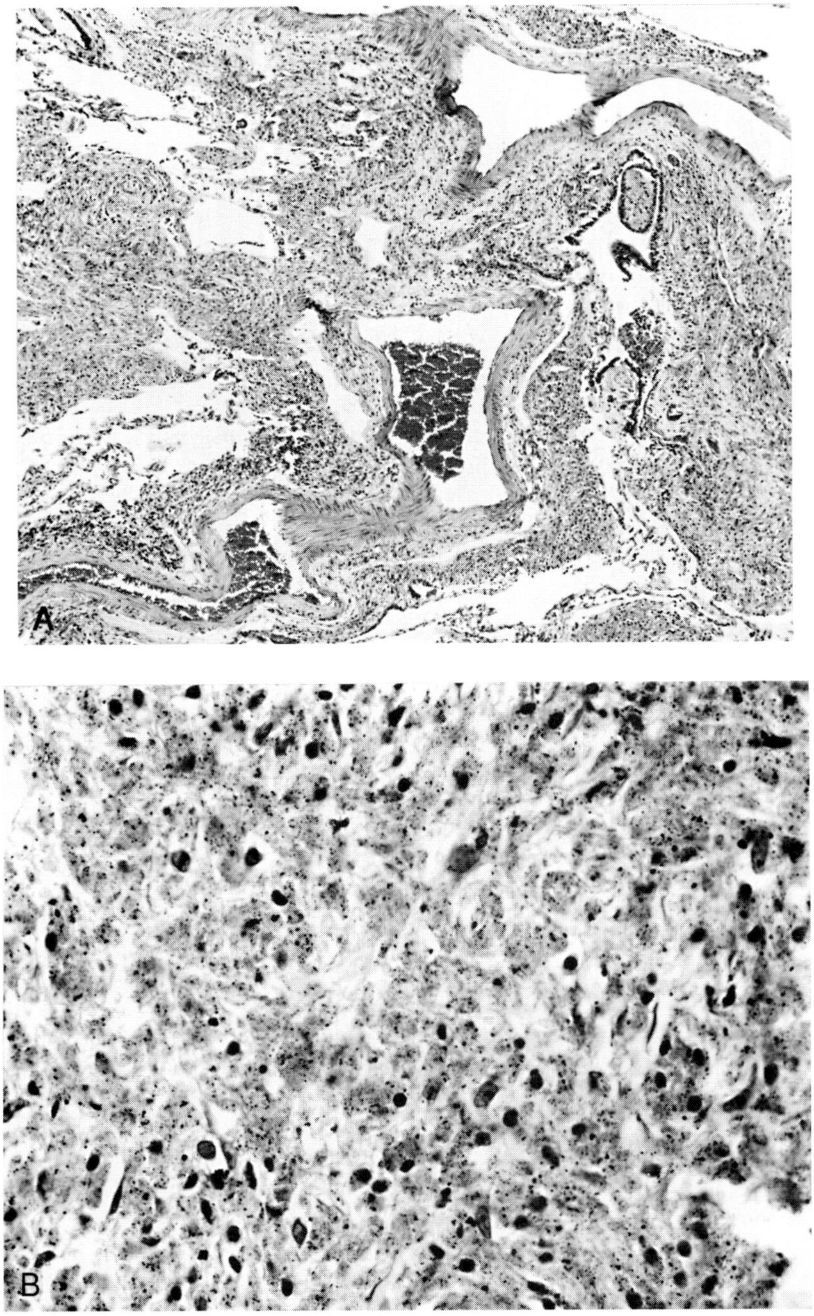

FIGURE 8.8

A. Macular lesion in a worker exposed to china clay. The macule was gray–brown by light microscopy. **B.** Higher-power view shows numerous pigment-laden macrophages. There was essentially no fibrosis in the lesion. (Courtesy Dr. A. Gibbs, Department of Pathology, Llandough Hospital, Penarth, Wales.)

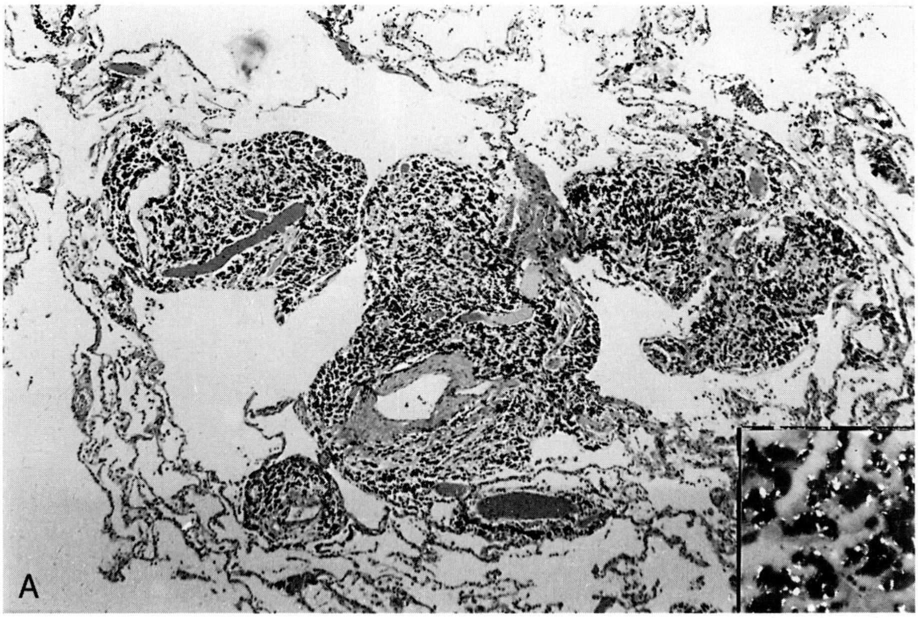

FIGURE 8.9

A. Section of lung from a 76-year-old man employed for 38 years in a foundry. Analysis of the mineral content of the lung revealed a total of 13×10^9 particles per gram of dry lung, of which 23% were kaolin, 19% mica, 26% silica, and 25% iron. In this macular lesion the dust is primarily in the perivascular and peribronchiolar interstitial tissues but also extends into the alveolar walls. **Inset.** Area viewed by polarized light. Numerous birefringent particles are visible together with carbonaceous dust. There was mild centriacinar (focal) emphysema associated with the macules. **B.** Scanning electron micrograph of deparaffinized section viewed by backscattered imaging to show mineral particles in perivascular connective tissue. **Inset.** X-ray spectrum of particle showing silicate chemistry. **C.** X-ray map of same area as **B** shows distribution of silicon.

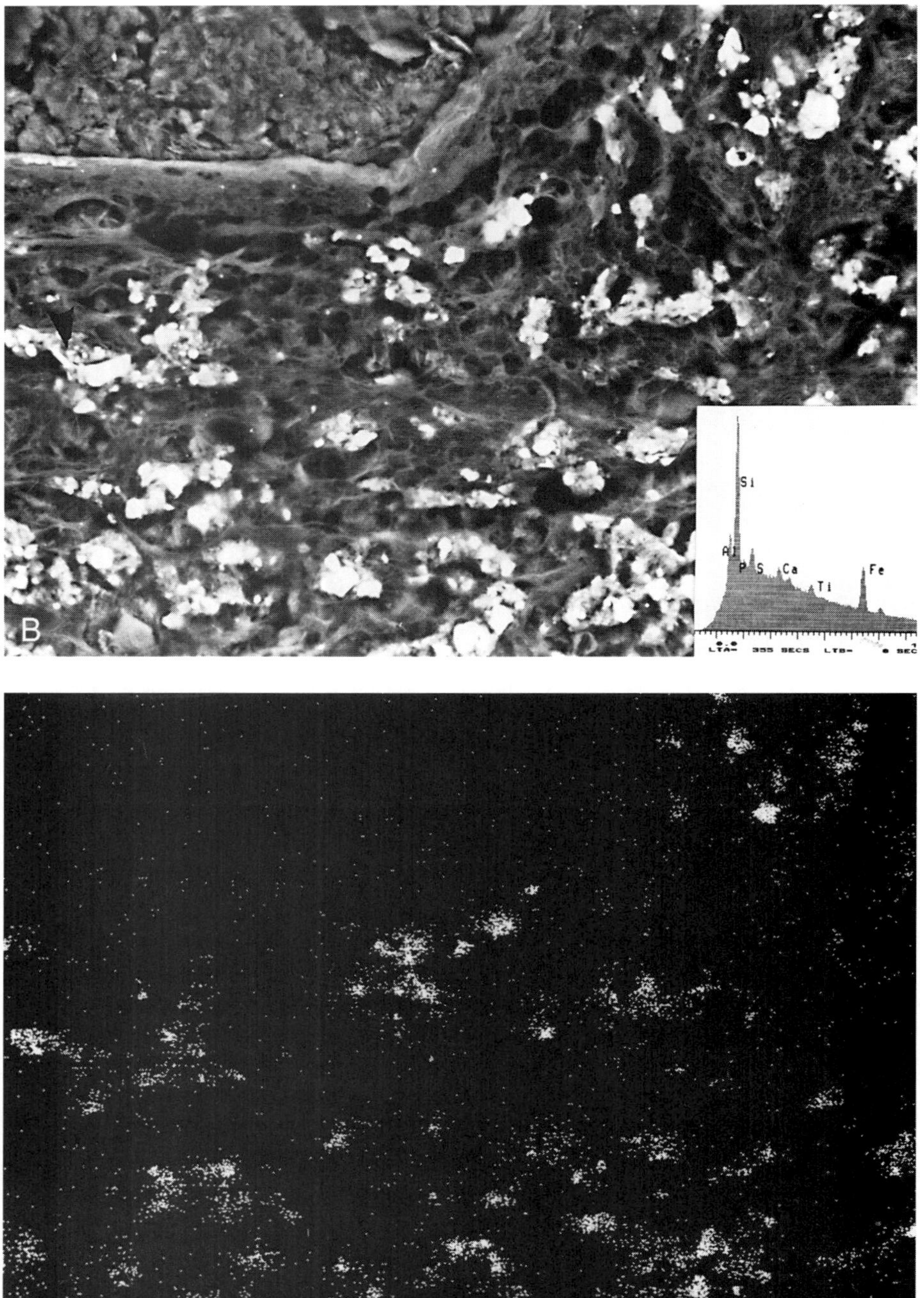

FIGURE 8.9 *(continued)*

TABLE 8.4
Pathologic Reactions to Nonfibrous Silicate Minerals Contrasted with Asbestos and Silica (Quartz)

MINERAL	MACULES	GRANULOMAS	NODULES	MASSIVE FIBROSIS	DIFFUSE INTERSTITIAL FIBROSIS	MINERAL DUST SAD	PLEURAL FIBROSIS
Asbestos	–	–	–	±	+	+	+
Silica	–	–	+	+	+	+	+
Attapulgite	N/A	N/A	N/A	N/A	+[a]	N/A	N/A
Feldspars	+	+[b]	+	+	+	+	N/A
Fuller's earth	+	N/A	+	+	N/A	N/A	N/A
Kaolin	+	+[b]	+	+	+	+	+
Mica[c]	+	+	+	+	+	+	+
Mullite	N/A	N/A	N/A	N/A	+	N/A	N/A
Mixed dust	+		+	+	+	+	+
Sepiolite	N/A	N/A	N/A	N/A	+[a]	+[a]	N/A
Shale	+	N/A	+	+	N/A	N/A	+
Talc	+	+	+	+	+	+	+[d]
Wollastonite	N/A	N/A	N/A	N/A	+[a]	N/A	N/A
Zeolite	N/A	N/A	N/A	N/A	N/A	N/A	+

[a] Implied from radiographic or pulmonary function data.

[b] These granulomas appear as collections of dust-containing macrophages, but giant cells are apparently not formed.

[c] Largely muscovite mica.

[d] Pleural fibrosis in those with talc exposure may be caused by contaminating asbestos.

N/A, not known or not reported.

SAD, small airway disease.

Granulomas

Foreign-body granulomas (Fig. 8.3) may be seen in the lungs of those exposed to mica (77, 108, 109) and talc, both of industrial type and cosmetic grade in the form of talcum powder (23, 104, 109, 110), and animals exposed to volcanic silicates (111) (Table 8.4). They are also common in individuals exposed to talc through intravenous drug abuse (see Chapter 13). Musk et al. (63) describe granulomas in the lungs of a worker exposed to nonfibrous mullite used as cat litter. These granulomas have foreign-body type of giant cells containing crystalline material. Lapenas et al. (102) illustrate what appear to be corresponding collections of particles in kaolin workers; however, the cellular infiltrate is composed of macrophages of the usual size rather than giant cells. We have also seen a similar reaction to feldspars (Fig. 8.7). In some instances the granulomas appear to be related to macules, but in others they are found in the interstitium without any obvious relation to structures of the bronchovascular bundle.

Foreign body granulomas of this type are a distinctive lesion. To us they provide strong evidence for the specificity of silicate pneumoconioses, since they are not seen in those exposed purely to silica or asbestos, although a giant cell reaction is sometimes seen in response to long asbestos fibers and bodies (see Chapter 9). Granulomas appear to be an important stage in the genesis of some silicate pneumoconioses, as they appear to progress to become nodules or diffuse interstitial fibrosis (Figs. 8.3 and 8.5). This impression is supported by studies in experimental animals exposed to talc, mica, and kaolin (112).

Nodules

The lesion most commonly described in those exposed to silicates is the nodule (Table 8.4). Nodules have been reported after exposure to both industrial and cosmetic talc (11, 18, 23, 104, 109, 110, 113, 114), mica (22), kaolin (115, 116), feldspars (62), and montmorillonite clays (1). Pathologic nodules appear to correspond to the radiographic nodules seen in many of these workers, and both pathologic and radiographic nodules show a predilection for the upper and middle zones.

Grossly nodules range in size from 2 or 3 mm to 1 cm and vary from gray to gray–brown, blue, or black (35, 102). The kaolin-associated lesions appear to be brown to gray, but different ore bodies of the same mineral apparently have somewhat different colors; and color in this instance is probably not a reliable guide to diagnosis. In contrast to the macules, the nodules are palpable and often very hard; sometimes the small lesions are more readily found by palpation than inspection. Nodular lesions of similar appearance are seen in hilar nodes (35, 102, 103). In and of themselves the nodal lesions do not constitute a pneumoconiosis, and the term *pneumoconiosis* should be used only when parenchymal disease is also present.

Microscopically the nodule has several morphologically different forms. Some consist of lesions with irregularly collagenized, sometimes noncollagenized, centers and irregular (medusa head) pigmented peripheries (Fig. 8.5). These resemble mixed-dust nodules, but some apparently occur in workers exposed to quartz-free dust, for example the kaolin-exposed patients described by Hale (117), the talc-induced lesions reported by Roub et al. (118), and the mica-associated reactions published by Davies and Cotton (108). Wagner et al. (116) note that nodular lesions in workers exposed to china clay containing both kaolin and silica tended to reflect increased amounts of silica in the lungs, whereas interstitial fibrosis was more typical for those with relatively pure kaolin exposure. In our experience nodules with distinct hyalinized centers contain more silica than those without such centers, and it is unclear at what point they should be called nodules of mixed-dust fibrosis.

The other form of nodule consists of masses of dust particles with greater or lesser amounts of intermingled collagen and foreign-body giant cells (Figs. 8.2 and 8.10). These types of lesions, which have been seen after exposure to talc, mica, kaolin, montmorillonite, and feldspars, may represent a fibrotic stage of the granulomas previously described. These nodules are much more clearly manifestations of silicate disease as opposed to the type with hyalinized centers. Furthermore, the morphologic separation between macule, interstitial fibrosis, and nodules may be arbitrary and can be influenced considerably by the plane of section. However, the important point is to recognize these structures as features of silicate pneumoconioses.

Massive Fibrosis

Massive fibrosis (complicated pneumoconiosis) has been reported after exposure to industrial and cosmetic talc (23, 109, 113, 119) (Fig. 8.10), kaolin (102, 115–117, 120) (Fig. 8.4), mica (22, 108, 118), feldspars (62), and other silicates (121, 122) (Table 8.4). Massive fibrosis has also been seen in intravenous drug abusers (121, 122) (see Fig. 13.11). In most instances massive fibrosis appears to arise in a setting of multiple large and small nodules, and some mass lesions form by coalescence of multiple smaller nodules, as in silicosis; however, it is not clear whether this is always true. Grossly the mass lesions are usually sharply defined and generally bilateral. They may replace most of a lobe (Fig. 8.4). Although in many cases the lesions are upper or mid zonal (the usual distribution for mass lesions secondary to coal or silica exposure), lower-zone mass lesions also occur. As a rule they are extremely hard and difficult to cut. As with the smaller nodules, their color varies with the specific mineral and ore involved.

Microscopically the mass lesions consist of myriad refractile particles, some free and some within macrophages, intermixed with collagen (Fig. 8.4). The particulate load is usually obvious, although Miller et al. (110) report a case of massive fibrosis caused by talc in which they claim most of the particles were submicroscopic and none could be seen by light microscopy. It is unclear whether polarization was employed in this instance, since our experience is that polar-

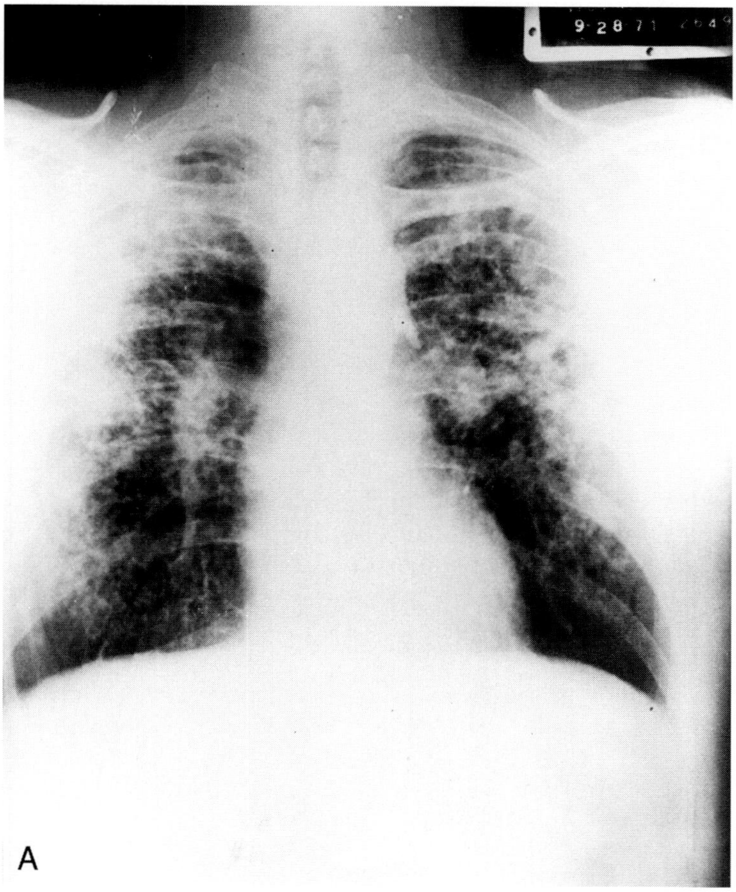

FIGURE 8.10

A. Chest radiograph from worker exposed to cosmetic-grade talc for 27 years. The film, taken 5 years before death from respiratory insufficiency, shows pleural thickening and interstitial and nodular opacities with bilateral large opacities (PMF). **B.** Whole lung section shows pleural thickening, nodular and interstitial fibrosis, and PMF. **C.** Section from nodule shows irregularly arranged collagen and dust. (Reprinted with permission from Vallyathan NV. Talc pneumoconiosis. Respir Ther 1980;6:34–39.)

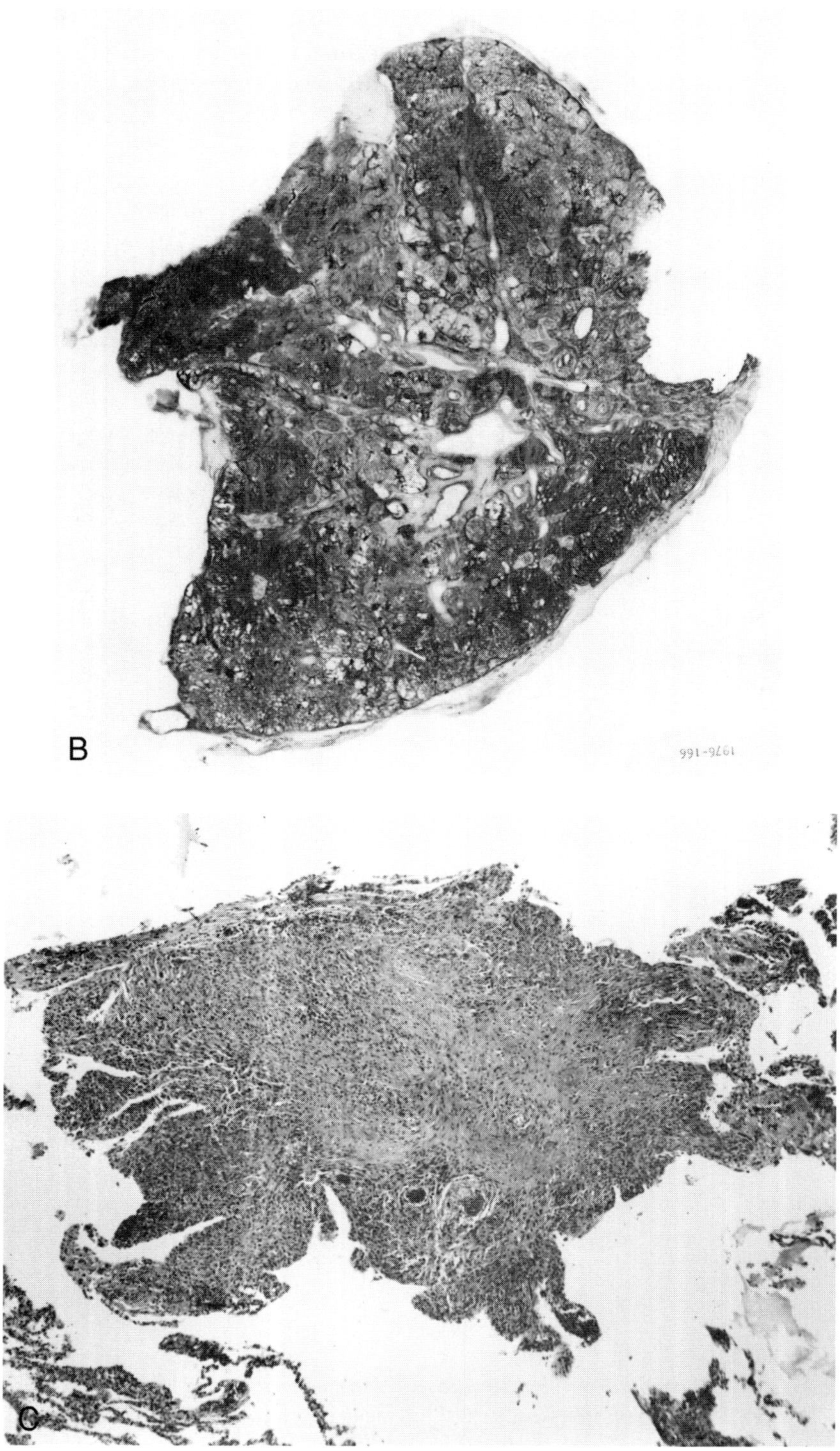

FIGURE 8.10 *(continued)*

ization of silicate-induced mass lesions almost invariably reveals large numbers of particles.

Vasculitis and vascular obliteration similar to that seen in coal workers (see Chapter 6) are also seen in PMF due to silicates (123) (Fig. 8.4). In the few instances when the pulmonary dust burden was measured, the total load was in the range of 20 to 40 g (62, 117), a very large amount in keeping with the idea that massive fibrosis may be a reaction to extremely high dust burdens.

Diffuse Interstitial Fibrosis

Diffuse interstitial fibrosis is mentioned or described in reports of those exposed to talc (23, 104 ,113, 124, 125), including cosmetic talc (114, 119, 126), intravenously delivered talc (121, 122) (see Chapter 13), mica (22, 24, 100, 108, 127), nonfibrous mullite (63), kaolin (116, 128), zeolite (72), montmorillonite (Fuller's earth) (25), and attapulgite (129) (Table 8.4). One of the problems with the term *diffuse interstitial fibrosis* is that it has been used to describe two different processes in conjunction with silicate exposure. In one the fibrosis links clearly defined nodules; in the other the fibrosis is more like that of usual interstitial pneumonia and nodules are scanty or absent, at least in the areas of diffuse fibrosis. When the process is similar to usual interstitial pneumonia, the gross appearance is lower-zone severe fibrosis and honeycombing.

Microscopically, diffuse fibrosis appears as interstitial inflammation and fibrosis, again accompanied by numerous refractile particles and sometimes giant cells (Figs. 8.2, 8.4–8.6, and 8.11). As with nodules, at least some examples of diffuse fibrosis appear to reflect progression of lesions that start as interstitial granulomas, but in this instance fibrose in a linear rather than a nodular fashion. Ferruginous bodies formed on talc or mica, which may be prominent when these are the dusts involved, should not be mistaken for asbestos bodies (Figs. 8.2 and 8.5; see Chapter 9 and colorplate 2).

Diffuse fibrosis secondary to talc exposure is the best defined of this group and the most controversial. This condition, to which the term *talcosis* is often applied, is typically but not always lower zonal (113, 124, 125). It very much resembles usual interstitial pneumonia or asbestosis clinically, radiographically, and pathologically. Indeed, one of the major problems in this regard is whether talcosis of this type is really asbestosis caused by tremolite in the talc (1, 14, 18, 125). Some of the older cases, particularly in workers mining the New York state talc, which is known to be heavily contaminated with tremolite, probably are forms of asbestosis (18, 123), and the patients may even show typical asbestos bodies in their lungs (18). However, recent reports of individuals who inhaled industrial or cosmetic talc containing little or no asbestos (104, 110, 113, 114, 124) and the appearance of the same condition in drug abusers exposed to the pure talc used for filler in oral pharmaceuticals (see Chapter 13) seem to leave little room for such arguments. Vallyathan and Craighead (104) analyzed the lung content of several such cases and showed that there appears to be crude correlation between mineral content measured by silicon content and extent of disease. Figure 8.11 illustrates a case of inhalational talcosis in which analysis of the mineral content ruled out an asbestos causation.

Diffuse interstitial fibrosis in mica-exposed workers may be either lower zonal and resemble usual interstitial pneumonia or predominantly upper zonal, in which case the process is more in the form of a fibrous bridging of nodules (104). The degree of interstitial fibrosis in workers exposed to nearly pure kaolin (china clay) appears to correlate well with total dust content of the lungs (116).

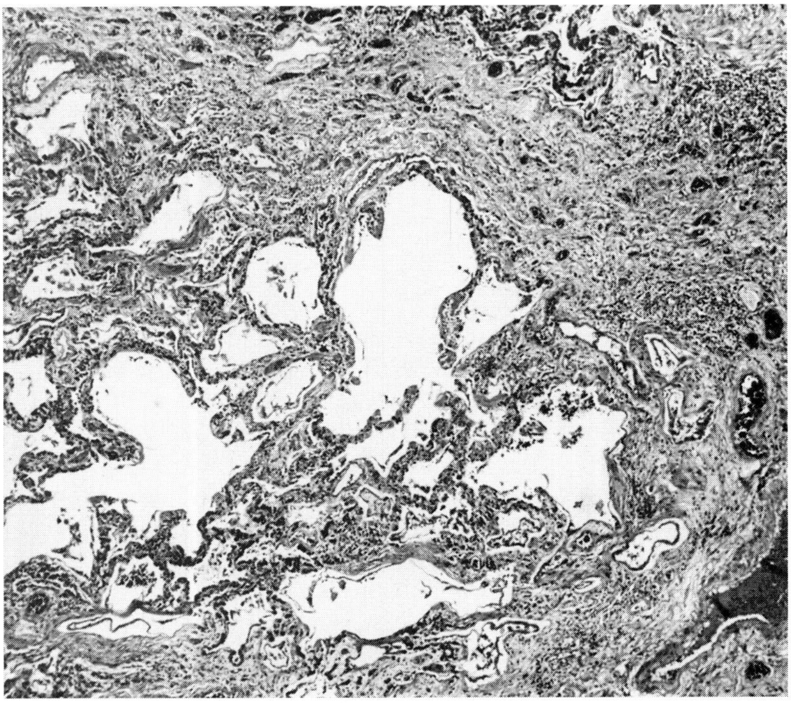

FIGURE 8.11
Severe diffuse interstitial fibrosis secondary to talc inhalation in a worker employed many years in a rubber factory. The patient had lower-zone disease that was grossly identical to asbestosis or usual interstitial pneumonia. Analysis of his lung tissue revealed talc but no asbestos. (Courtesy Dr. F. Askin, Department of Pathology, Johns Hopkins School of Medicine, Baltimore.)

Interstitial fibrosis in workers exposed to sepiolite (54) has also been reported, but this group was also exposed to zeolites and asbestos. There are virtually no pathologic descriptions of sepiolite and the remainder of the dusts mentioned earlier. However, the fact that pure silicate exposure can produce diffuse interstitial fibrosis seems inescapable, and some animal studies lend support to this idea (6, 130). Interstitial fibrosis may be accompanied by other silicate-induced lesions.

A mineralogic study of lung tissues from 25 patients diagnosed as having idiopathic pulmonary fibrosis (IPF) showed that the IPF group had significantly higher silicon-to-sulfur (Si–S) ratios than 25 samples from normal lungs (131). Moreover, 12 of the patients had Si–S ratios in the range associated with pneumoconiosis. Six of these 12 patients on subsequent investigation revealed histories consistent with exposure to silica or silicates. Cryptogenic exposures to silica and/or silicates may be a cause of so-called idiopathic pulmonary fibrosis and should be considered in the clinical setting.

Pleural Thickening

Pleural thickening is also seen with silicate exposure (Table 8.4). In talc workers the process is usually ascribed to contaminating asbestos, not necessarily correctly (1). It is seen with approximately equal frequency in workers exposed to asbestiform and nonasbestiform talcs (39). Similar changes have been described in individuals exposed to zeolites (72), kaolin (117, 102), sepiolite (55), and wollastonite (132), the latter two by radiograph only. We have seen pleural fibrosis after mica exposure (Fig. 8.2).

Other Pathologic Reactions to Silicate Exposure

A case of hypersensitivity pneumonitis has been described in a 25-year-old nonsmoking ceramic tile worker exposed to dusts of clay, quartz, wollastonite, and zirconium silicate (133). Gibbs et al. (23) describe a sarcoidlike reaction in a rubber plant worker exposed to talc. Mineralogic analysis of lung revealed 13.3 mg of dust per gram of dry lung; 73% of the particles were consistent with talc. It is problematic whether this case is an unusual variant of talcosis or a case of sarcoid in a talc-exposed worker.

Endemic elephantiasis of the lower legs in Ethiopia has been linked to adsorption of basaltic soils through the skin of the feet (134). These soils are highly adherent to skin, and it is thought that the silicate minerals are toxic to the lymphatic vessels.

REFERENCES

1. Parkes WR. Occupational lung disorders. 2nd ed. London: Butterworths, 1982.
2. Sinkankas J. Mineralogy. New York: Van Nostrand Reinhold, 1964.
3. Deer WA, Howie RA, Zussman J. An introduction to the rock-forming minerals. London: Longmans, 1962.
4. Stettler LE, Platek SF, Riley RD, et al. Lung particulate burdens of subjects from the Cincinnati, Ohio urban area. Scanning Micros 1991;5:85–94.
5. Huuskonen MS, Toasavainen A, Koskninen, et al. Wollastonite exposure and lung fibrosis. Environ Res 1983;30:291–304.
6. Lord GH. The biological effects of talc in the experimental animal: a literature review. Food Cosmet Toxicol 1978;16:51–57.
7. Vallyathan V, Green FHY, Mentnech MS, et al. Mt. St. Helens volcanic ash: hemolytic activity. Environ Res 1983;30:349–360.
8. Beck BD, Brain JD. Predicting the pulmonary toxicity of particulates using damage indicators in lung lavage fluid. In: Wagner WL, Rom WN, Merchant JA, eds. Health issues related to metal and nonmetallic mining. Ann Arbor, MI: Ann Arbor Science,1983:83–104.
9. Brain JD, Beck BD. Assessment of particulate toxicity. In: Wagner WL, Rom WN, Merchant JA, eds. Health issues related to metal and nonmetallic mining. Ann Arbor, MI: Ann Arbor Science, 1983:51–62.
10. Vallyathan V, Reasor M, Schwegler D, et al. Comparative in vitro cytotoxicity and relative pathogenicity of mineral dust. Ann Occup Hyg 1988;32:279–89.
11. Berner A, Gylseth B, Levy F. Talc dust pneumoconiosis. Acta Pathol Microbiol Scand A 1981;89:17–21.
12. Abraham J, Brambilla C. Particle size for differentiation between inhalation and injection pulmonary talcosis. Environ Res 1980;21:94–96.
13. Crouch E, Churg A. Ferruginous bodies and the histologic evaluation of mineral dust exposure. Am J Surg Pathol 1984;8:109–116.
14. Seaton A. Silicates and disease. In: Morgan WKC, Seaton A, eds. Occupational lung diseases. 2nd ed. Philadelphia: WB Saunders,1984:295–322.
15. Cralley LJ, Key MM, Groth DH, et al. Fibrous and mineral content of cosmetic talcum products. Am Ind Hyg Assoc J 1968;28:350–354.
16. Rohl AN. Asbestos in talc. Environ Health Perspect 1974;9:129–132.
17. Pooley FD, Rowlands N. Chemical and physical properties of British talc powders. In: Walton WH, ed. Inhaled particles 4. London: Pergamon Press, 1977:639–646.

18. Scancarello G, Romeo R, Sartorelli E. Respiratory disease as a result of talc inhalation. J Occup Environ Med 1996;38:610–614.
19. Gamble JF. Silicate pneumoconiosis. In: Merchant JA, Bochlecke BA, Taylor G, Pickett Harner M, eds. Occupational respiratory diseases. U.S. Dept. of Health and Human Services Publication 86–102, 986:243–286.
20. Lesser M, Zia M, Kilburn KH. Silicosis in kaolin workers and fire-brick makers. South Med J 1978;71:1242–1246.
21. Ng TP, Allan WGL, Tsin TW, O'Kelley FJ. Silicosis in jade workers. Br J Ind Med 1985;42:761–764.
22. Skulberg KR, Gylseth B, Skaug V, Hanoa R. Mica pneumoconiosis: a literature review. Scand J Work Environ Health 1985;11:65–74.
23. Gibbs AE, Pooley FD, Griffiths DM, et al. Talc pneumoconiosis: a pathologic and mineralogic study. Hum Pathol 1992;23:1344–1354.
24. Landas SK, Schwartz DA. Mica-associated pulmonary interstitial fibrosis. Am Rev Respir Dis 1991;144:718–721.
25. Gibbs AR, Pooley FD. Fuller's earth (montmorillonite) pneumoconiosis. Occup Environ Med 1994;51:644–646.
26. Morgan WKC. Industrial bronchitis and other nonspecific conditions affecting the airways. In: Morgan WKC, Seaton A, eds. Occupational lung diseases. 2nd ed. New York: WB Saunders, pp. 521–540, 1984;.
27. McConnochie K, Bevan C, Newcombe RG, et al. A study of Spanish sepiolite workers. Thorax 1993;48:370–374.
28. Wild P, Refregier M, Auburtin G, et al. Survey of the respiratory health of the workers of a talc producing factory. Occup Environ Med 1995;52:470–477.
29. Heederik D, de Cock J, Endlich E. Dust exposure indices and lung function changes in longshoremen and dock workers. Am J Ind Med 1994;26:497–509.
30. Edenfield RW. A clinical and roentgenological study of kaolin workers. Arch Environ Health 1960;1:392–403.
31. Warraki S, Herant Y. Pneumoconiosis in china-clay workers. Br J Ind Med 1963; 20:226–230.
32. Sheers G. Prevalence of pneumoconiosis in Cornish kaolin workers. Br J Ind Med 1964;21:218–225.
33. Sepulveda MJ, Vallyathan V, Stettler LE, et al. Kaolin pneumoconiosis in a Georgia mill. In: Wagner WL, Rom WN, Merchant JA, eds. Health issues related to metal and nonmetallic mining. Ann Arbor, MI: Ann Arbor Science,1983:331–348.
34. Kennedy T, Rawlings W, Baser JRM, Tockman M. Pneumoconiosis in Georgia kaolin workers. Am Rev Respir Dis 1983;127:215–220.
35. Lynch KM, McIver FA. Pneumoconiosis from exposure to kaolin dust: kaolinosis. Am J Pathol 1954;30:1117–1122.
36. Ferret J, Moreau P. Mineralogy of talc deposits. In: Bignon J, ed. Health related effects of phyllosilicates. NATO ASI Series, vol G21. Berlin: Springer-Verlag, 1990: 147–158.
37. Canessa PA, Torraca A, Lavecchia MA, et al. Pneumoconiosis (silicosis) in the confectionery industry. Sarcoidosis 1990;7:75–77.
38. Gamble JF, Fellner W, Dimeo MJ. An epidemiologic study of a group of talc workers. Am Rev Respir Dis 1979;119:741–753.
39. Gamble JF, Greife A. Health studies of miners and millers exposed to talc. In: Wagner WL, Rom WN, Merchant JA, eds. Health issues related to metal and nonmetallic mining. Ann Arbor, MI: Ann Arbor Science,1983:277–302.
40. Kleinfield M, Messite J, Shapiro J, Swencicki R. Effect of talc dust inhalation on lung function. Arch Environ Health 1965;10:431.
41. Fine LJ, Peters JM, Burgess WA, DiBerardinis LJ. Studies of respiratory morbidity in rubber workers: 4. Respiratory morbidity in talc workers. Arch Environ Health 1976;31:195–200.
42. Kleinfeld M, Messite J, Zaki MM. Mortality experience among talc workers: a follow-up study. J Occup Med 1974;16:345.

43. Rubino GF, Scansetti G, Piolatto G, Romano CA. Mortality study of talc miners and millers. J Occup Med 1976;18:186–193.
44. Selevan SG, Dement JM, Wagoner JK, Froines JR. Mortality patterns among miners and millers of nonasbestiform talc. In: Lemen R, Dement JM, eds. Dusts and disease. Park Forest South, IL: Pathotox, 1979:379.
45. Thomas TL. Lung cancer mortality among pottery workers in the United States. International Agency for Research on Cancer Publication 97:75–81, 1990.
46. Stille WT, Tabershaw IR. The mortality experience of upstate New York talc workers. J Occup Med 1982;24:480.
47. Gamble JF. A nested case control study of lung cancer among New York talc workers. Int Arch Occup Environ Health 1993;64:449–456.
48. Wagner JC, Chamberlain M, Brown RC, et al. Biological effects of tremolite. Br J Cancer 1982;45:352–360.
49. Amandus HE, Wheeler PE. Morbidity and mortality of vermiculite miners and millers exposed to tremolite-actinolite: 2. Mortality. Am J Ind Med 1987;11:15–26.
50. Slaton ME. Report of fatal and nonfatal illness from a dust disease of the lungs (pneumoconiosis). Pinewood, SC: Mingo Mine, SCAT, August 22, 1978. Mine Safety and Health Administration, Knoxville, TN.
51. Research Committee of the British Thoracic Association and the Medical Research Council Pneumoconiosis Unit. A survey of the long-term effects of talc and kaolin pleurodesis. Br J Dis Chest 197973:285–288.
52. Smith AR. Pleural calcification resulting from exposure to certain dusts. Am J Roentgenol 1952;67:375–382.
53. Kleinfeld M. Pleural calcification as a sign of silicatosis. Am J Med 1966;251: 215–224.
54. Baris YI, Sahin AA, Erkan ML. Clinical and radiographic study in sepiolite workers. Arch Environ Health 1980;35:343–346.
55. Zolov C, Burilkov T, Babadjov L. Pleural asbestos in agricultural workers. Environ Res 1967;1:287–292.
56. Seaton A, Lamb D, Brown WR, et al. Pneumoconiosis of shale miners. Thorax 1981;36:412–418.
57. Shasby DM, Peterson MR, Hodous TK, et al. Respiratory morbidity of workers exposed to wollastonite through mining and milling. In: Lemen R, Dement JM, eds. Dusts and disease. Park Forest South, IL: Pathotox, 1979:251.
58. McDonald JC, McDonald AD, Armstrong B, Sebastien P. Cohort study of mortality of vermiculite miners exposed to tremolite. Br J Ind Med 1986;43:436–444.
59. Amandus HE, Althouse R, Morgan WKC, et al. Morbidity and mortality of vermiculite miners and millers exposed to tremolite-actinolite: 3. Radiographic findings. Am J Ind Med 1987;11:27–37.
60. McDonald JC, Sebastien P, Armstrong B. Radiological survey of past and present vermiculite miners exposed to tremolite. Br J Ind Med 1986;43:445–449.
61. Lockey JE, Brooks SM, Jarabek M, et al. Pulmonary changes after exposure to vermiculite contaminated with fibrous tremolite. Am Rev Respir Dis 1984;129: 952–958.
62. Barrie JH, Gosselin L. Massive pneumoconiosis from a rock dust containing no free silica: nepheline lung. Arch Environ Health 1960;1:109–117.
63. Musk AW, Greville HW, Tribe AE. Pulmonary disease from occupational exposure to an artificial aluminum silicate used for cat litter. Br J Ind Med 1980;37:367–372.
64. Bazas T. Effects of occupational exposure to dust on the respiratory system of cement workers. J Soc Occup Med 1980;30:31–36.
65. Pancheri G, Zanetti E. L'aspetto radiologico della silicon da pomice (liparosi). Rass Med Ind 1963;32:432–445.
66. Atiemo M, Yoshida K, Zoerb GC. Dust measurements in tractor and combine cabs. Trans Am Soci Agric Eng 1980;23:571–576.
67. Green FHY, Yoshida K, Fick G, et al. Characterization of airborne mineral dusts associated with farming activities in rural Alberta, Canada. Int Arch Occup Environ Health 1990;62:423–430.

68. Collan Y, Kosma VM, Anttonen H, Kulju T. Toxicity of richterite in hemolysis test and macrophage cultures. Arch Toxicol Suppl 1986;9:292–295.
69. Hillerdal G. Pleural changes and exposure to fibrous minerals. Scan J Work Environ Health 1984;10(6 Spec No): 473–479.
70. McConnochie K, Simonato L, Mavrides P, et al. Mesothelioma in Cyprus: The role of tremolite. Thorax 1987;4:342–347.
71. Baris YI, Artvinli M, Sahin AA, et al. Diffuse lung fibrosis due to fibrous zeolite (erionite) exposure. Eur J Respir Dis 1987;70:122–125.
72. Casey KR, Shigeoka JW, Rom WN, Moatamed F. Zeolite exposure and associated pneumoconiosis. Chest 1985;87:837–840.
73. Mumpton AF. Natural zeolites: a new industrial mineral commodity. In: Sand LB, Mumpton AF, eds. Natural zeolites, occurrence, properties, use. Oxford, UK: Pergamon Press, 1978:3–27.
74. Weiss B, Boettner EA. Commercial talc and talcosis. Arch Environ Health 1967;14: 304–308.
75. Spain BA, Cummings O, Garcia JGN. Bronchiolitis obliterans in an animal feed worker. Am J Ind Med 1995;28:437–443.
76. Windom H, Griffin J, Goldberg ED. Talc in atmospheric dusts. Environ Sci Technol 1967;1:923.
77. Sherwin RP, Barman ML, Abraham JL. Silicate pneumoconiosis of farm workers. Lab Invest 1979;40:576–582.
78. Gylseth B, Stettler L, Mowe G, et al. A striking deposition of mineral particles in the lungs of a farmer: a case report. Am J Ind Med 1984;6:231–240.
79. Dynnik VI, Khizhniakova LN, Baranenko AA, et al. Silicosis in tractor drivers working on sandy soils on tree farms. Gig Tr Prof Zabol 1981;12:26–28.
80. Fennerty A, Hunter AM, Smith AP, Pooley FD. Silicosis in a Pakistani farmer. Br Med J Clin Res Ed 1983;287:648–649.
81. Sasagawa M, Yamada S, Nakamura O, et al. A case of pulmonary alveolar proteinosis associated with fibrotic changes and alveolitis. Nippon Kyobu Shikkan Gakkai Zasshi 1989;27:1214–1220.
82. Vallyathan V, Kang JH, Van Dyke K, et al. Response of alveolar macrophages to in vitro exposure to freshly fractured versus aged silica dust: the ability of Prosil 28, an organosilane material, to coal silica and reduce its biological reactivity. J Toxicol Environ Health 1991;33:303–315.
83. Wallace E, Keane MJ, Mike PS, et al. Contrasting respirable quartz and kaolin retention of lecithin surfactant and expression of membranolytic activity following phospholipase A2 digestion. J Toxicol Environ Health 1992;37:391–409.
84. Seal S, Krezoski S, Barr TL, et al. Surface chemistry and biological pathogenicity of silicates: an x-ray photoelectron spectroscopic study. Proc R Soc Lond B 1996;263: 943–951.
85. Osornio-Vargas AR, Hernandez-Rodriguez NA, Yanez-Buruel AG, et al. Lung cell toxicity experimentally induced by a mixed dust from Mexicali, Baja California, Mexico. Environ Res 1991;56:31–47.
86. Mann S, Perry CC. Structural aspects of biogenic silica. Ciba Found Symp 1986; 121:40–58.
87. Bhatt TS, Lang S, Sheppard MN. Tumours of mesothelial origin in rats following inoculation with biogenic silica fibres. Carcinogenesis 1991;12:1927–1931.
88. Mulvey JJ, Rothschild H. Sugarcane farming: is there a link with cancer? Ecol Dis 1983;2:267–270.
89. Phoolchund HN. Aspects of occupational health in the sugar cane industry. J Soc Occup Med 1991;41:133–136.
90. Newman R. Association of biogenic silica with disease. Nutr Cancer 1986;8: 217–221.
91. O'Neill C, Jordan P, Bhatt T, Newman R. Silica and oesophageal cancer. Ciba Found Symp 1986;121:214–230.
92. Schoning P, Abraham JL, Burnett BR. Silicate and metal dust in lungs of greyhounds. Am J Vet Res 1996;57:1006–1009.

93. Canfield PJ, Rothwell TLW, Papadimitriou JM, Moore JD. Siliceous pneumoconiosis in two dogs. J Comp Pathol 1989;100:199–202.
94. Roperto F, Samiano S, DeVico G, Galati D. Silicate pneumoconiosis in pigs: optical and scanning electron microscopical investigations with x-ray microanalysis. J Comp Pathol 1994;110:227–236.
95. Evans MG, Slocombe RF, Schwartz LD. Pulmonary silicosis in captive ring-necked pheasants: definitive diagnosis by electron probe x-ray microanalysis. Vet Pathol 1988;25:239–241.
96. Smith BL, Poole WSH, Martinovich D. Pneumoconiosis in the captive New Zealand kiwi. Vet Pathol 1973;10:94–101.
97. Hansen HJ, Jama FM, Nilsson C, et al. Silicate pneumoconiosis in camels (*Camelus dromedarius L*). J Vet Med 1989;36:789–796.
98. Schwartz LW, Knight HD, Whittig LD, et al. Silicate pneumoconiosis and pulmonary fibrosis in horses from the Monterey-Carmel Peninsula. Chest 1981;80: S82-S85.
99. Roperto F, Papparella S, Galati P, et al. Silicate pneumoconiosis in water buffaloes. Note 1: optical and ultrastructural observations. Acta Med Vet 1987;33:307–314.
100. Brambilla C, Abraham J, Brambilla E, et al. Comparative pathology of silicate pneumoconiosis. Am J Pathol 1979;96:149–163.
101. Schenker MB, Pinkerton KE, Green F, et al. Respiratory disease and mineral dust exposure among California farmworkers. Am J Respir Crit Care Med 1997;155: A813.
102. Lapenas D, Gale P, Kennedy T, et al. Kaolin pneumoconiosis. Am Rev Respir Dis 1984;13:282–288.
103. Olscamp G, Herman S, Weisbrod GL. Nepheline rock dust pneumoconiosis. Radiology 1982;142:29–32.
104. Vallyathan V, Craighead JE. Pulmonary pathology in workers exposed to non asbestiform talc. Hum Pathol 1981;12:28–35.
105. Tonning MO. Pneumoconiosis from Fuller's earth. J Ind Hyg Toxicol 1949;31: 41–45.
106. Sakuda A. Pneumoconiosis due to Fuller's earth. Thorax 1961;16:176–179.
107. Churg A, Wright JL. Small airway lesions in patients exposed to nonasbestos mineral dust. Hum Pathol 1983;14:688–693.
108. Davies D, Cotton R. Mica pneumoconiosis. Br J Ind Med 1983;40:22–27.
109. Case records of the Massachusetts General Hospital. Case 35–1982. N Engl J Med 1982;307:605–614.
110. Miller R, Tierstein AS, Bader RE, et al. Talc pneumoconiosis: significance of sublight microscopic mineral particles. Am J Med 1971;50:395–402.
111. Vallyathan V, Green FHY, Mentnech MS, Tucker JH. Pulmonary response to Mt. St. Helens volcanic ash. Environ Res 1983;30:361–371.
112. Sahu AP, Shanker R, Zaidi SH. Pulmonary response to kaolin, mica and talc in mice. Exp Pathol 1978;16:276–282.
113. Seeler AO, Grybostk JS, MacMahon HE. Talc pneumoconiosis. AMA Arch Ind Health 1959;19:392–402.
114. Nam K, Gracey DR. Pulmonary talcosis from cosmetic talcum powder. JAMA 1972;221:492–493.
115. Sepulveda MJ, Vallyathan V, Attfield MD, et al. Pneumoconiosis and lung function in a group of kaolin workers. Am Rev Respir Dis 1983;127:231–235.
116. Wagner JC, Pooley FD, Gibbs A, et al. Inhalation of china stone and china clay dusts: relationship between the mineralogy of dust retained in the lungs and pathological changes. Thorax 1986;41:190–196.
117. Hale LW, Gough J, King EJ, Nagelschmidt G. Pneumoconiosis of kaolin workers. Br J Ind Med 1956;13:251–259.
118. Roub IW, Dekker A, Wagenblast HW, Reece GJ. Pulmonary silicatosis. Am J Clin Pathol 1979;72:871–875.
119. Goldbach PD, Mohsenifar Z, Abraham JL, et al. Talcum powder pneumoconiosis. West J Med 1982;136:439–442.

120. Vestal TF, Winstead JA, Joliet PV. Pneumoconiosis among mica and pegmatite workers. Ind Med 1943;12:11–14.
121. Pare JAP, Fraser RG, Hogg JC, et al. Pulmonary "mainline" granulomatosis: talcosis of intravenous methadone abuse. Medicine 1979;58:229–239.
122. Crouch E, Churg A. Progressive massive fibrosis of the lung secondary to intravenous injection of talc: a pathologic and mineralogic analysis. Am J Clin Pathol 1983;80:520–526.
123. Porro FW, Patton JR, Hobbs AA. Pneumoconiosis in the talc industry. Am J Roentgenol 1983;47:507–524.
124. Feigin DS. Talc: understanding its manifestations in the chest. Am J Roentgenol 1986;146:295–301.
125. Elmes PC, Wagner JC. Fibrosis of lung: an environmental disease? J Clin Pathol 1978;31(Suppl 12):158–164.
126. Tukiainen P, Nichels J, Taskinen E, Nyberg M. Pulmonary granulomatous reaction: talc pneumoconiosis or chronic sarcoidosis? Br J Ind Med 1984;41:84–87.
127. Pimentel JC, Menezes AP. Pulmonary and hepatic granulomatous disorders due to the inhalation of cement and mica dusts. Thorax 1978;33:219–227.
128. Levin JL, Frank Al, Williams MG, et al. Kaolinosis in a cotton mill worker. Am J Ind Med 1996;29:215–221.
129. Sora A, Gaudichet A, Sebastien P, et al. Lung fibrosis after inhalation of fibrous attapulgite. Thorax 1979;34:695 (abstract).
130. Hildrick-Smith GY. The biology of talc. Br J Ind Med 1976;33:217–229.
131. Monso E, Tura JM, Marsal M, et al. Mineralogical microanalysis of idiopathic pulmonary fibrosis. Arch Environ Health 1990;45:185–188.
132. Huuskonen MS, Jarvisalo J, Koskinene H, et al. Preliminary results from a cohort of workers exposed to wollastonite in a Finnish limestone quarry. Scand J Work Environ Health 1983;9:169–175.
133. Liippo KK, Anttila SL, Taikina-Aho O, et al. Hypersensitivity pneumonitis and exposure to zirconium silicate in a young ceramic tile worker. Am Rev Respir Dis 1993;148:1089–1092.
134. Price EW. The association of endemic elephantiasis of the lower legs in East Africa with soil derived from volcanic rocks. Trans R Soc Trop Med Hyg 1976;70: 288–295.
135. Waxweiler RJ, Zumwalde RO, Ness GO, Brown DP. A retrospective cohort mortality study of males mining and milling attapulgite clay. Am J Ind Med 1988;13: 305–15.
136. Phibbs BP, Sundin RE, Mitchell RS. Silicosis in Wyoming bentonite workers. Am Rev Respir Dis 1971;103:1–17.
137. Dreessen WC, Dallavalle JM, Edwards TI, Sayers RR. Pneumoconiosis among mica and pegmatite workers. Washington: Pub Health Bull No. 250, 1940:42.
138. Heinmann H, Moskowitz S, Harihara CR, et al. Silicosis in mica mining in Bihar, India. Arch Ind Hyg Occup Med 1953;8:420–435.
139. McNally WD, Trostler IS. Severe pneumoconiosis caused by the inhalation of fuller's earth. J Ind Hyg 1941;23:118–126.
140. Craighead JE, Emerson RJ, Stanley DE. Slateworker's pneumoconiosis. Hum Pathol 1992;23:1098–1105.
141. Hogue WL, Mallette FS. A study of workers exposed to talc and other dusting compounds in the rubber industry. J Indust Hyg Toxicol 1949;31:359–364.
142. Scansetti G, Rasetti L, Ghemi F. Clinical and radiological evaluation of pneumoconiosis in the talc extracting industry. Med del Lavoro 1963;54:746–749.
143. Delaude A. Talc-related pathology. Bull Acad Natl Med 1977;161:405–409.
144. Messite J, Reddin G, Kleinfield M. Pulmonary talcosis, a clinical and environmental study. Arch Indust Health 1959;20:408–413.

CHAPTER 9

Nonneoplastic Disease Caused by Asbestos

❖ Andrew Churg

INTRODUCTION

Asbestos-induced disease continues to be a major problem. A remarkably large number of individuals, certainly in the millions, have been occupationally exposed to asbestos over the past 50 years. In addition, everyone in the population at large is subject to a much lower exposure from asbestos contamination of ambient air and in some instances from asbestos-insulated buildings; the disease-causing potential of such exposures is a subject of intense debate (1). Personal injury lawsuits against asbestos manufacturers number in the hundreds of thousands, and new cases continue to be filed.

The scientific issues are complex, and although the broad outlines of asbestos-related disease are apparent, many important areas, especially mechanisms of disease induction, are poorly understood. Indeed, something as fundamental as what neoplastic diseases are caused by asbestos is still in dispute. These problems are complicated by differences in biologic effects among asbestos fiber types and by differences in disease incidence for exposure to the same nominal fiber type in different industrial settings (discussed later).

Table 9.1 lists the various diseases known or proposed to be associated with asbestos exposure. This chapter addresses mineralogy of asbestos, uses and exposures, methods of analyzing lung for asbestos content, the findings from such analyses, the effects of asbestos in the general population, and benign pleural and parenchymal conditions. Neoplastic disease is considered separately in Chapter 10.

PHYSICAL, CHEMICAL, AND BIOLOGIC PROPERTIES OF THE ASBESTOS MINERALS

Asbestos is a generic term for a variety of naturally fibrous silicate minerals. Six types of asbestos are recognized: chrysotile, amosite, crocidolite, anthophyllite, tremolite, and actinolite (Table 9.2). These six minerals can be subdivided into two broad mineralogic groups, chrysotile and the amphiboles (amosite, crocidolite, tremolite, actinolite, and anthophyllite).

TABLE 9.1
Diseases Known or Suggested to Be Associated with Asbestos Exposure

DISEASE	ASSOCIATION
Nonneoplastic pleural changes	Established
Pleural effusion	
Pleural fibrosis	
Pleural plaques	
Pleural pseudotumors	
Asbestosis (interstitial fibrosis)	Established
Airway fibrosis (asbestos airways disease)	Established
Carcinoma of the lung in the presence of asbestosis	Established
Malignant mesothelioma of the pleura and peritoneum	Established
Carcinoma of the lung in the absence of asbestosis	Disputed
Gastrointestinal carcinoma	Disputed
Carcinoma of the larynx	Disputed

TABLE 9.2
Chemical and Physical Properties of the Asbestos Minerals

NAME AND CHEMICAL COMPOSITION	RESISTANCE TO ACID	RESISTANCE TO ALKALI	TENSILE STRENGTH (lb/sq in)	SPINNABILITY	MINIMUM TEMP DECOMPOSITION (°C)
Chrysotile $Mg_3(Si_2O_5)(OH)_4$	Poor	Good	80,000–100,000	Very good	450
Amphiboles					
Amosite $(Fe,Mg)_7(Si_8O_{22})(OH)_2$	Fair	Good	16,000–90,000	Fair	600
Crocidolite $Na_2Fe_5(Si_8O_{22})(OH)_2$	Good	Good	100,000–300,000	Fair	400
Tremolite $Ca_2Mg_5(Si_8O_{22})(OH)_2$	Good	Good	1,000–4,000	Poor	950
Actinolite $Ca_2(Mg,Fe)_5(Si_8O_{22})(OH)_2$	Fair	Good	1,000	Poor	620
Anthophyllite $(Mg,Fe)_7(Si_8O_{22})(OH)_2$	Good	Good	4,000	Poor	600

Adapted from Dupres JS, Mustard JF, Uffex RJ. Report of the Royal Commission on Matters of Health and Safety Arising from the Use of Asbestos in Ontario. Toronto: Queen's Printer for Ontario, 1984.

Asbestos minerals are valuable because of their high tensile strength, high heat resistance, relative chemical resistance, and ability to be woven. These properties vary among the types of asbestos (Table 9.2), and the fiber types are to some extent selected for commercial use by these properties. Chrysotile, for example, is fairly flexible and thus relatively easy to weave into textiles but is not useful in acid environments. Amosite is relatively resistant to seawater and was used extensively as insulation and fire retardant in ships. All of the asbestos minerals are stable to about 400 to 500°C.

Asbestos has been used as a heat-resistant material since antiquity, but its current commercial exploitation dates from the end of the last century. In 1981 world production of asbestos was estimated at approximately 5 million metric tons (2), but it has decreased since. Historical details of usage can be found in Selikoff and Lee (3) (Fig. 9.1).

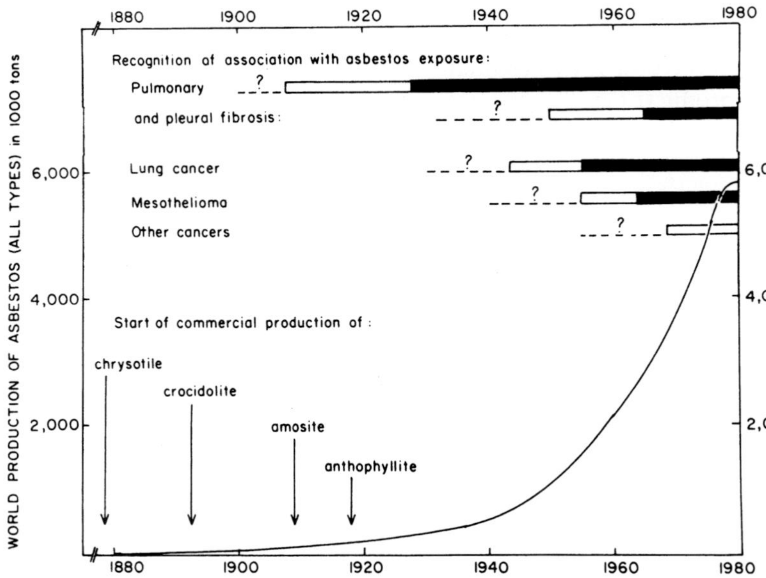

FIGURE 9.1
World production of asbestos and medical recognition of asbestos-induced disease. *Line at bottom,* Yearly production of asbestos. *Arrows,* Start of production of types of asbestos. Various asbestos-induced diseases are listed at the top. *Question mark,* When the association was proposed. *White bar,* When epidemiologic studies investigating the association began to appear. *Black bar,* When the association was generally accepted by the medical community. (Reprinted with permission from Becklake MR. Occupational lung disease: past record and future trend using the asbestos case as an example. Clin Invest Med 1983;6:305–337.)

Most of the asbestos used commercially in the past was chrysotile, which was estimated to account for about 95% of total use in 1977 (4) and accounts for almost 100% of current usage. In North America most chrysotile was obtained from the large mines in Québec, with much smaller amounts from mines in other parts of Canada and the United States. Chrysotile is or has been mined in other parts of the world, including Russia, South Africa, Rhodesia, and Australia. The bulk of amosite and crocidolite used in North America and Europe was imported from South Africa, but considerable crocidolite was also mined locally and used in Australia. It appears that crocidolite was the principal form of amphibole asbestos imported into Great Britain. In North America amosite was much more widely employed, particularly in shipyards (3–5).

The amphiboles anthophyllite, tremolite, and actinolite have seen little commercial exploitation, in part because of their physical and chemical properties but mostly because of the lack of commercially useful deposits. An anthophyllite mine was operated for a number of years in Finland. However, these forms of amphibole asbestos are much more commonly encountered as contaminants of other minerals, particularly vermiculite, talc, chrysotile ore, and probably all forms of processed chrysotile products (2). While tremolite is a natural minor (a few percent) (6) component of the chrysotile from Québec, there are largely anecdotal claims that chrysotile from other areas, such as Zimbabwe and Australia, contains little tremolite and produces little disease.

USES OF ASBESTOS AND OCCUPATIONS AT RISK

In the past it was estimated that asbestos was an ingredient in as many as 3000 products (7). Major historical uses are shown in Table 9.3, but current usage is much more restricted, and at present the bulk of asbestos production goes into the manufacture of cement construction and insulation products. However, because of widespread use in the past, there is the potential for exposure during deliberate or accidental removal of asbestos. Thus asbestos exposure may occur in maintenance of asbestos-containing buildings, in removal of asbestos insulation from pipes and boilers, in the demolition of buildings, and in refitting of ships insulated with asbestos.

In the past and to a lesser extent today not only were persons who worked directly with asbestos exposed to the fiber, but persons working in close proximity might also be exposed, even if they did not normally handle asbestos themselves. The best example of this type of bystander exposure was in ship construction and refitting in World War II, in which a variety of workers in allied trades, such as electricians, welders, plumbers, and sheet metal workers, all received substantial exposure inside small compartments in which asbestos was being installed or removed. Construction work similarly has been a source of potential bystander exposures, albeit at a lower level.

Table 9.3 lists occupations with current or past exposure to asbestos. Although estimates may be inexact, it is clear that in recent times the number of persons exposed to asbestos in an occupational setting is quite large. Nicholson et al. (8) estimated that between 1940 and 1979 some 27 million persons in the United States had occupational contact with asbestos. Of this number only about 7% were engaged in primary mining, milling, and manufacturing of asbestos products, and 4 million were believed to have received exposure in shipyards during World War II.

In evaluating patients who may have asbestos-induced disease, it is important

TABLE 9.3
Uses and Products Containing Asbestos and Occupations with Asbestos Exposure

PROCESS/PRODUCT	USAGE/PRODUCT	OCCUPATIONS	REFERENCE
Mining and milling	Asbestos	Asbestos miners and millers	19
Asbestos cement products	Cement pipes, sheets, other construction materials	Asbestos cement manufacture Construction work	2, 5, 17, 18
Asbestos insulation products	Boiler and pipe insulation Sprayed asbestos insulation	Pipe fitters, boiler makers, asbestos insulators; building demolition; railroad workers; shipyard workers	2, 3, 10, 20
Asbestos friction products	Automotive brake and clutch linings	Friction products manufacture Brake repair	21, 22
Asbestos textiles	Fire-resistant cloth, lagging, curtains	Asbestos textile workers	23, 24
Asbestos floor tiles	Floor tiles	Manufacture and installation	9
Asbestos paper products	Roofing and flooring felts, wall boards and insulating papers	Manufacture and installation	25
Miscellaneous products	Spackling, paints, plastics, fillers	Manufacture and construction	26–28

TABLE 9.4
Occupational and Some Environmental Exposure Levels of Asbestos

STANDARD	LEVEL (F/CC)[a]
USA Occupational Standard 1946[a]	30
USA OHSA occupational standard 1972	5.0
USA OHSA occupational standard 1976	2.0
USA OHSA occupational standard 1986	0.2
USA OHSA occupational standard 1994	0.1
Thetford town ambient air–early 1980s (7)	0.01
Buildings with asbestos insulation (1)	0.0002
Urban ambient air (1)	0.0001

[a] Actually 5 million particles per cubic foot of air, generally thought to be equivalent to 15 to 30 fibers per cubic centimeter.

to be aware not only of typical sources of exposure but also of unusual or occult exposures. For example, floor tile that contains asbestos bound into the matrix ordinarily presents no health hazard, but asbestos-related disease has been reported in floor tile installers who cut the product (9). In some industries asbestos is no longer used; nonetheless, a substantial incidence of asbestos disease may be encountered and appear inexplicable until historical usage is recognized. A good example of this phenomenon is railroad work, since steam locomotives were heavily insulated with asbestos, which is not used in modern diesel locomotives (10).

Disease also occurs in persons with nonoccupational exposures to asbestos. The original report of Wagner et al. (11) showing a link between crocidolite exposure and mesothelioma included individuals who had lived near the mines and played in mine tailings during childhood. There are also well-documented reports of asbestos-related disease developing in women who washed their husband's asbestos-contaminated work clothes (12, 13). These types of exposures, even though not occupational, were not "low level" in any sense, and in fact mineral analysis of lung tissue from some reported cases has indicated that the exposures may have been fairly substantial (13).

Everyone in the population is also exposed to very low levels of asbestos from fibers found in ambient air. This exposure, often called background exposure, has several possible sources. One is commercial asbestos products that have been liberated into the air, either because of deliberate use in an uncontrolled and uncontained setting (for example, spraying asbestos insulation in buildings under construction, a process that is no longer permitted), or because of accidental escape of fibers, for example in demolition of asbestos-containing buildings. While the actual sources are usually not clear, the presence of amosite in both urban air and the lungs of the general population of North America (14–16) indicates unequivocally that atmospheric contamination by commercial fiber must occur on a regular basis, since amosite asbestos is not a naturally occurring mineral in North America.

Another source of background exposure is the use of asbestos insulation (almost entirely chrysotile) in some public buildings. The typical fiber levels in such buildings are extremely low: a recent review by the Health Effects Institute (1) estimated mean building levels at 0.0002 fibers per cubic centimeter, a value only slightly greater than that of typical outdoor urban air (1) (Table 9.4).

A third source of asbestos exposure to the general population is natural air contamination from outcrops of asbestos- bearing soil or rocks. The resulting ambient fiber levels are such that in some countries pleural plaques can be found in inhabitants in local areas where soil contamination is particularly heavy (see section on benign asbestos-induced pleural disease). North America, particularly in the western half of the continent, has fairly extensive areas of asbestiform rock, particularly serpentine (the parent of chrysotile) outcrop.

All of these factors lead to background fiber levels on the order of 0.0001 fibers per cubic centimeter in typical urban areas in North America (1). While this background exposure can readily be detected in lung tissue (15, 16), there is no evidence that it causes disease (discussed later in this chapter and in Chapter 10).

STANDARDS FOR ASBESTOS EXPOSURE

All industrialized countries regulate occupational exposure to asbestos (Table 9.4). The values are based on observations generally derived from fairly heavily exposed cohorts and chosen so that the regulated level in theory will not lead to disease in working populations during a lifetime of exposure. Typically the regulated level applies to an 8-hour time-weighted average, and as a rule the actual determination of exposure level, hence the actual standard, is based on counting only fibers longer than 5 μm using a phase contrast microscope.

With the progressive recognition of asbestos-related disease occurring at exposure levels once thought to be innocuous, there has been a continuing reduction in permitted exposure levels. Table 9.4 shows the regulated levels in the United States over time. Because of the tendency of amphiboles, particularly crocidolite, to induce mesothelioma, most jurisdictions now regulate exposure levels differently for these fiber types. Crocidolite use is banned in some countries, and permitted chrysotile exposure levels are generally higher than amphibole exposure levels. However, in the United States all asbestos fiber types are regulated to the same level.

DEPOSITION AND CLEARANCE OF ASBESTOS FIBERS AND THE RELATION OF FIBER RETENTION TO DISEASE

Ordinary compact (i.e., roughly spherical) particles with aerodynamic diameters greater than about 5 μm may deposit in the bronchial tree but normally do not penetrate into the alveolar parenchyma. Fibers behave quite differently. For straight fibers deposition has been shown to be primarily a function of diameter and much less a function of length (30, 31). Thus fibers with diameters less than about 3 μm but lengths of several hundred micrometers can be found in alveoli (32). However, length is important in that the longer the fiber, the less its statistical chance of penetrating to the alveolar spaces (31, 32).

For insoluble compact particles the major routes of clearance are macrophage phagocytosis and emigration of the macrophages from the lung; transepithelial passage with some fraction of the translocated particles eventually reaching lymph nodes; and transport, either free or in macrophages, up the mucociliary escalator in the large airways, eventually to be coughed up and swallowed. Relatively short fibers of asbestos also appear to be removed from the lung through macrophage phagocytosis and emigration, but there is considerable experimental evidence that amphibole fibers, and to a lesser extent chrysotile fibers, longer than about 20 μm cannot be cleared from the deep lung (32, 33), probably because they are too long for macrophage phagocytosis. As a consequence, the apparent retained fiber length appears to increase with time in experimental animal systems (33–35).

A further complication in regard to asbestos is that the deposition and clearance of chrysotile are considerably different from those of amphiboles. Long fibers of chrysotile are often curled (Fig. 9.2), but in the lung chrysotile fibers are relatively fragile, tending to fragment into straight, short, small fibers or very

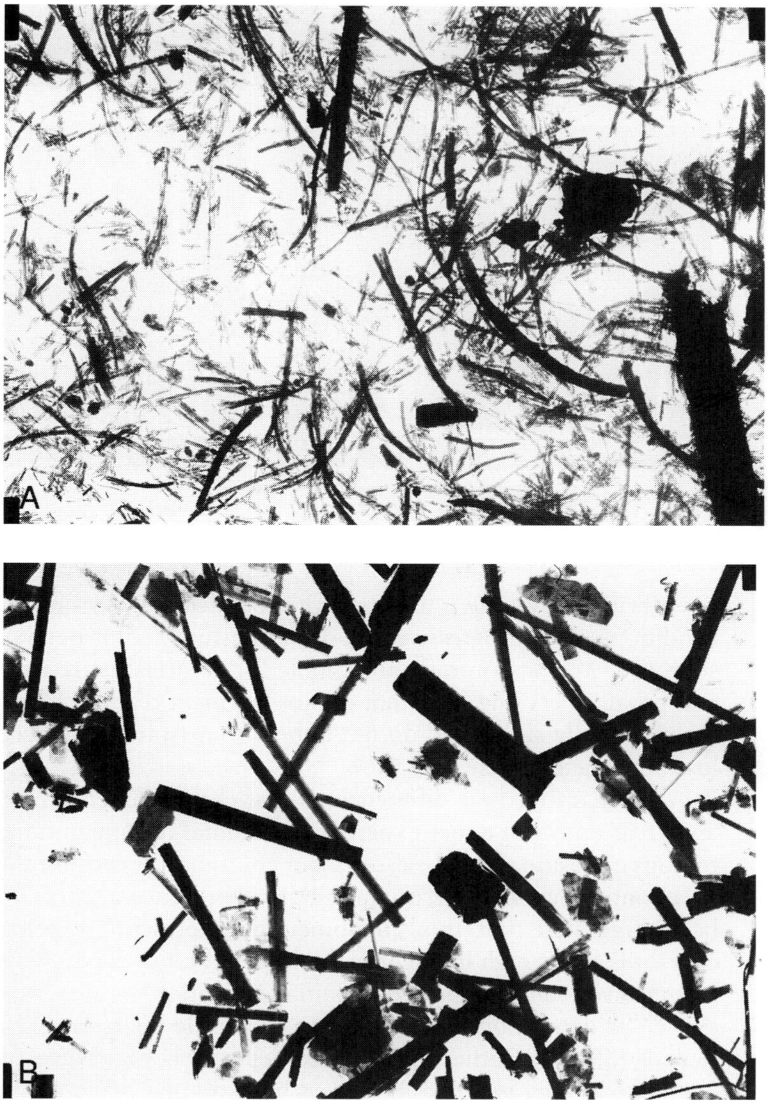

FIGURE 9.2
Identification of asbestos by electron microscopic techniques. **A.** Electron micrograph of chrysotile asbestos. Note the curved longer fibers and the many short fragments. **B.** Electron micrograph of amosite asbestos at the same magnification as **A.** The fibers are broader and straighter, and there are many fewer small fragments. **C** and **D.** Electron diffraction patterns of chrysotile and amosite, respectively. **E** and **F.** Energy-dispersive x-ray spectra of chrysotile and amosite. Each amphibole has a unique composition. With a combination of morphology, energy-dispersive x-ray spectroscopy, and when needed, electron diffraction analysis, it is possible reliably to identify asbestos fibers extracted from lung tissue.

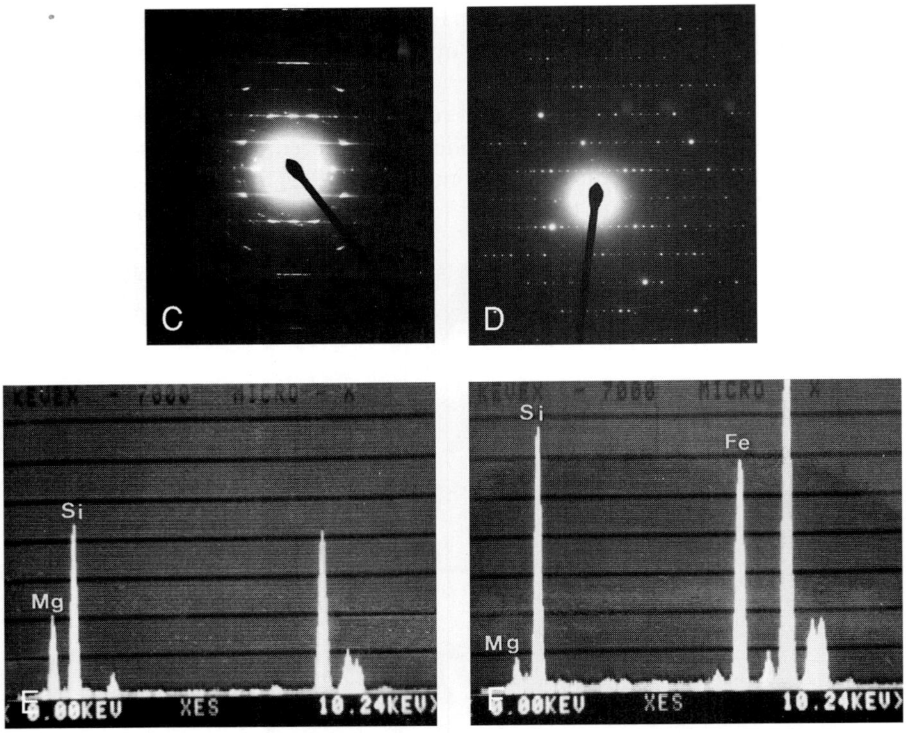

FIGURE 9.2 *(continued)*

fine fibrils. Chrysotile is also believed to be chemically unstable under biologic conditions, with progressive loss of magnesium and/or both silicon and magnesium (36, 37). In contrast, amphibole forms of asbestos are relatively straight and broad fibers (Fig. 9.2) that do not fragment readily. Moreover, amphiboles are chemically stable and do not appear to dissolve or undergo any significant loss of elements in the lung (36).

A corollary of these differences is that chrysotile tends not to accumulate to any great extent in either experimental animal or human lungs, even with continuous exposure (36, 38, 39, 40), but continuous exposure to amphiboles leads to a continuous increase in amphibole fiber concentration (36, 38–40). It has been suggested that this phenomenon reflects interception of long curled chrysotile fibers high in the bronchial tree (41), but experimentally most investigators have found roughly equal initial deposition for chrysotile and amphiboles as well as deposition of equally long chrysotile fibers in central and peripheral regions (33–35). Rather than limited deposition, the failure of chrysotile to accumulate in lung is probably caused by extremely rapid clearance of deposited fibers: if mixtures of chrysotile and amphibole are administered to experimental animals as a single bolus by intratracheal instillation, clearance of chrysotile is found to be much faster than clearance of amphiboles. This effect is demonstrable within a week (42). Whether rapid clearance reflects fiber fragmentation into sizes easily removed by macrophages, or fiber dissolution, or both events, is disputed (36).

Regardless of mechanism, in workers with exposures to chrysotile alone (meaning chrysotile with its natural accompaniment of tremolite) or to mixtures of chrysotile and commercial amosite and crocidolite in which chrysotile was known historically to be the predominant fiber, analysis many years later typically reveals that the amphibole is the major residual fiber, and the chrysotile concentration may be within the limits seen in the general population (14, 15) (Table 9.5). From experimental animal studies and the limited human data that are available, it has been estimated that the clearance half-time of chrysotile is on the order of a few months, whereas the clearance half-time for amphibole fibers is on the order of years to decades (36).

These observations on asbestos fiber deposition and clearance have been used to try to explain some of the pathogenesis of asbestos-induced disease. It is clear that chrysotile asbestos is a very much weaker human mesothelial carcinogen than is amphibole asbestos (see Chapter 10), and it has been proposed that this phenomenon reflects the lack of durability of chrysotile in the lung (36, 41–44). This idea is supported by the observation that low-durability synthetic fibers pose little risk of mesothelioma in experimental animal systems and in human epidemiologic studies (see Chapter 11). Moreover, in experimental systems chrysotile with 90% of the magnesium leached out is less carcinogenic (with reference to mesotheliomas) than native or partially leached chrysotile (45). Lack of durability may also explain the observations that chrysotile appears to be generally less potent as a lung carcinogen (46) and less fibrogenic, fiber for fiber, than are amphiboles (47, 48), although for these diseases fiber type differences are much less marked than for mesothelioma. There is also accumulating evidence that the actual agent of "chrysotile-induced" mesothelioma in man is the tremolite component of the chrysotile ore or product (36, 49), although this issue is not firmly settled (see Chapter 10).

Persistence of long fibers in the lungs is presumed to be related to the distinctly greater fibrogenic and carcinogenic (in terms of mesothelioma) properties of long fibers in experimental animal systems (50–53), but the exact mechanisms behind the greater pathogenicity of long fibers are uncertain. Moreover, the very limited human studies on fiber size and disease have come to generally contradictory conclusions (38, 54) (discussed later in this chapter and in Chapter 10).

Asbestos that reaches lymphatics in the lung may be transported to the pleura or to the hilar nodes, and appropriate digestion techniques fairly commonly turn up asbestos bodies and fibers in hilar nodes (55). Ingested asbestos can penetrate the gut and gain entrance to the lymphatics (56). In those with high exposure,

TABLE 9.5
Relative Proportion of Chrysotile and Amphiboles in Various Exposure Groups (Values as mean and range)

	# REPORTS	AMOSITE, CROCIDOLITE PERCENT (RANGE)	CHRYSOTILE PERCENT (RANGE)	TREMOLITE PERCENT (RANGE)
General population	7	14 (0–46)	72 (31–98)	18 (2–50)
Workers with mixed amphibole and chrysotile exposure	5	58 (9–89)	40 (6–89)	4 (2–5)
Workers in industries using predominantly chrysotile	8	15 (0.3–51)	47 (19–80)	46 (10–81)

Adapted from Churg A. Deposition and clearance of chrysotile. Ann Occup Hyg 1994;38:625–634.

careful search occasionally reveals asbestos fibers or bodies, presumably derived from lymphatic transport, in other organs (57).

ANALYSIS OF ASBESTOS FIBERS AND BODIES IN HUMAN LUNG TISSUE

Asbestos occurs in the lung in two forms. Most of the mineral is bare or uncoated fiber, that is, the form in which it was inhaled. A minority of fibers acquire an iron protein coating in the lung and are then called asbestos bodies (colorplate 2), a specific form of ferruginous body (defined later in this chapter).

A variety of techniques can provide qualitative or quantitative data on the presence and amount of asbestos in human lung tissue (Table 9.6). However, before considering analytical approaches, several points must be mentioned:

1. *Routine gross and microscopic examinations coupled with appropriate clinical and radiographic data are the primary methods of diagnosis in asbestos-related disease.* Analysis of asbestos bodies or fibers are adjunctive methods to be used when necessary, but they are by no means necessary in every case.
2. *No matter how many bodies or fibers are found, by themselves neither fibers nor bodies constitute a disease.* Quantitative data on body or fiber counts provide an estimate of the level of exposure, which may or may not be a guide to the cause of a particular disease. For example, an elevated amosite fiber level or an elevated asbestos body count in a patient with mesothelioma usually implicates asbestos as the agent of the malignancy, but this is not true of carcinoma of the lung. In some instances fiber analysis may reveal evidence of an occult exposure to asbestos that can then be implicated as the cause of the disease in question; however, this scenario is uncommon. Last, fiber analysis may provide information about exposure to or retention of specific types of fibers. This information is useful in understanding the relation between asbestos exposure and disease and sometimes in linking specific exposures to an individual case.
3. *With use of tissue digests, quantitative data are required to show a level of asbestos that is above background, and the laboratory must also state the background level of asbestos in its general population.* Since everyone in the population has asbestos in their lungs, the mere qualitative demonstration of the presence of asbestos fibers or bodies in a tissue digest has no value.
4. *One cannot compare actual numeric values from laboratory to laboratory but must examine each test value with reference to that laboratory's background data.* For reasons that are not entirely clear but that do relate in some part to choice of instrument (such as scanning versus transmission electron microscope), size of fibers counted, counting rules, and other undetermined factors, there are quite marked laboratory-to-laboratory variations in fiber and body counts. This was demonstrated in a formal trial in which samples from the same patient were sent to six laboratories: all reported the high-count specimens as high and the low-count specimens as low, but the absolute magnitude of the counts varied enormously (58). One further complication is that air, water, and even paraffin may be contaminated with chrysotile (59), and such contamination must be taken into account when performing electron optical analysis.

TABLE 9.6
Methods for Quantitative Analysis of Lung Asbestos Content

METHOD	USES	ADVANTAGES AND DISADVANTAGES
Finding asbestos bodies in tissue section	Usually indicates higher than background exposure; required for the diagnosis of asbestosis	Inexpensive and rapid but insensitive; uncoated fibers can be present in large numbers even if bodies are few; bodies from background exposure may occasionally be found; can be done by any laboratory
Counting asbestos bodies from tissue digests with a light microscope	Confirms above background exposure if elevated	Inexpensive and relatively rapid; can be done by any laboratory, but standards for general population must be known; uncoated fibers can be present in large numbers even if bodies are few
Counting uncoated fibers from tissue digests with a phase microscope	Confirms above background exposure if elevated	Inexpensive and relatively rapid; can be done in any laboratory, but standards for general population must be known; limited to fibers of approximately 3–5 μm or longer; misses smaller fibers that are always present in larger numbers; probably misses most chrysotile; no guarantee that observed fibers are really asbestos
Counting and identifying uncoated fibers with a suitably equipped electron microscope	Confirms above background exposure if elevated; only method that allows specific identification of fiber type and measurement of fiber size, which may reveal source of exposure	Slow and expensive; requires special equipment; standards for general population must be known; finds and identifies all asbestos fibers; can be used to identify other minerals

Specific Analytic Methods

Techniques such as polarizing microscopy, dispersion staining, and quantitative x-ray diffraction (60) are suitable for identification of bulk asbestos from specific products or air samples, but they cannot be used in lung tissue. As a rule, fibers that have been in the body for any length of time are not birefringent. Uncoated fibers are usually invisible in tissue sections, and most are below the resolution of the light microscope; even if a fiber is seen, there is no way of determining that it is really asbestos as opposed to the other types of fibers that are common in lung (61).

Asbestos bodies, on the other hand, are readily visible in the light microscope, and as detailed later, are specific markers of asbestos in most populations (62). The simplest, fastest, and least expensive, but also the crudest and least quantifiable, method of determining levels of asbestos in lung is finding or counting asbestos bodies in histologic sections. Because of the small volume of tissue in a

5-μm-thick section, histologic preparations are very insensitive detectors of asbestos bodies. However, this insensitivity is useful: Roggli and Pratt (63) estimate that given the known background level of asbestos bodies in the general population, one should not find an asbestos body from background exposure in more than 1 per 100 carefully screened iron-stained sections, and less frequently if sections are not completely and minutely examined. Thus the observation of even one asbestos body in a 5-μm-thick section usually indicates occupational asbestos exposure.

If asbestos bodies are not easily found in hematoxylin- and eosin-stained sections, iron stains should be used. However, thick (30 to 100 μm) sections or squeeze preparations of lung should be avoided, since they may simply find the bodies that are present in everyone in the population, and there appear to be no numeric data to provide a guideline for occupational versus background numbers of asbestos bodies in these kinds of preparations. Some authors (64) advocate counting the number of asbestos bodies per square centimeter of tissue and using a conversion formula to arrive at the number of uncoated fibers per gram that they believe are in the tissue. Unfortunately, the ratio of asbestos bodies to fibers varies enormously from case to case (65), and as Roggli and Pratt (63) point out, the number of asbestos bodies ones sees in sections also depends on the length of the bodies. Unfortunately, fiber length also varies enormously from case to case. In my opinion attempting to translate asbestos body counts in tissue sections to numbers of uncoated fibers per gram of lung tissue is pure guesswork. Even attempting comparisons between cases by using numbers of asbestos bodies per square centimeter is highly inaccurate. At best counts of asbestos bodies in tissue sections yield a crude estimate of exposure as relatively low versus relatively high.

More accurate quantitative assessment of asbestos content can be performed by digesting the tissue and collecting and counting asbestos bodies or uncoated fibers with a light microscope or by counting uncoated fibers with an electron microscope. As summarized in Table 9.6, each method has advantages and disadvantages. Digestion of lung tissue in bleach followed by collection of the asbestos bodies on a membrane filter and counting of the bodies with a light microscope is quick and inexpensive. A procedure for preparing and counting such filters is detailed in Table 9.7. As is true of all of these methods, it is necessary to know the numbers of bodies to be expected in the local nonexposed population before test data can be interpreted. If high levels are found, occupational exposure is virtually certain. However, some patients and some sizes (short) and types (chrysotile) of fibers appear to form bodies poorly, and this type of analysis may miss real exposure. Observation of asbestos bodies provides no direct information about fiber type, although, as described later, most asbestos bodies are formed on amphibole fibers (62).

Some laboratories digest lungs in bleach or strong base, such as sodium hydroxide, and count uncoated fibers with a white-cell counting chamber or a membrane filter preparation and a phase microscope. This procedure is also relatively quick and inexpensive, but it has a number of disadvantages. Only relatively large fibers (minimum length 3 to 5 μm) can be resolved, so that the majority of fibers go undetected; chrysotile is particularly likely to be missed. There is no way to determine what type of asbestos is present and no guarantee that a given fiber is actually asbestos. If one is certain that substantial amphibole asbestos exposure has occurred, it is probably reasonable to assume that fibers observed in this way are asbestos, but the average lung contains a large number of nonasbestos particulates and fibers (61), and the assumption may be incorrect.

TABLE 9.7
Quantitative Assessment of Asbestos Bodies from Lung Tissue

1. Select piece of nonconsolidated lung tissue approximately 3–5-g for analysis and adjacent piece of lung to be dried to constant weight to determine a wet-to-dry ratio.
2. Cut test sample into small pieces and dissolve in test tube in laundry bleach (30–50 mL) for 24–48 hours.
3. Centrifuge at 1000 g for 20 minutes to sediment asbestos bodies.
4. Aspirate bleach; add 1 : 1 chloroform-to-50% ethanol mixture; shake vigorously. Centrifuge at 120 g 10 minutes. During this time an interface containing most of the carbonaceous debris forms. Aspirate top layer, interface, and all but a few milliliters of lower layer. This step may have to be repeated if lung is exceptionally dirty.
5. Add 25% ethanol to sediment, shake well, and pour solution into collector tube of a Millipore filter or similar membrane filter apparatus. Wash tube twice with 25% ethanol and add to collector tube. A filter pore size of 0.45 μm is adequate to retain all asbestos bodies and gives a reasonable filtration rate. Connect bottom flask to vacuum line and draw solution through filter. Standard type of unit for preparing cytology filters can be used.
6. Allow filter to dry well; mount with Permount or similar mounting medium. Pressure on cover slip while drying helps keep filter flat.
7. To count bodies, filter must be viewed *through* a ×40 objective with condensor racked down; use of a lower-power objective or Koehler illumination hides many bodies.
8. For ordinary lungs, two perpendicular traverses with high dry objective provide a good sample; whole filter need not be examined. If many bodies are present, counting 10 fields with a rectangular grid inserted in eyepiece will suffice.
9. To determine number of bodies per gram of dry lung:
   A. Using a stage micrometer, calculate field of view of high dry objective or area of rectangular eyepiece grid.
   B. Calculate total area of filter actually examined in two perpendicular traverses or 10 fields of rectangular grid. E.g., if field of view of high dry objective is 50 μm and usable filter diameter is 20 mm, 2 perpendicular traverses examine a total area of 2 sq mm.
   C. Calculate ratio of total filter area to area measured in item B (e.g., if filter has a usable diameter of 20 mm and field of view of high dry is 50 μm, ratio of filter area to viewed area is 314:2, or 157).
   D. Multiply this value by number of bodies counted and divide by number of grams of lung dissolved. In this example if 50 bodies are counted and 5 g of lung dissolved, value is 1570 bodies per gram wet lung.
   E. To convert to dry lung, take wet-to-dry weight ratio from separately dried piece of lung and multiply bodies per gram of wet lung by this value. In this example, if wet-to-dry ratio is 8:1, bodies per gram of dry lung are 12,560.

Electron optical analysis is the procedure of choice when it is necessary to determine the total lung burden of asbestos or to obtain information on fiber type and size. Using ultrastructural morphology, chemistry as determined by an x-ray energy spectrometer attached to the microscope, and occasionally electron diffraction, it is possible to definitively identify and measure virtually all asbestos fibers. Chrysotile fibers split longitudinally into very fine fibrils that may be as small as 0.1 × 0.01 μm and that have a distinctive tube shape (Fig. 9.2). Amphibole minerals are much broader and form long, thin, straight fibers (Fig. 9.2), but their appearance is not entirely specific. Chrysotile and amphibole asbestos produce quite different electron diffraction patterns and have different chemical compositions (Fig. 9.2).

However, electron optical analysis is very slow and hence very expensive; the required equipment is also costly, and relatively few laboratories do this type of analysis on a routine basis. The ability to identify fibers by specific type also means that the control population data must be more detailed (Table 9.8). Because there are always more short than long fibers in lung tissue, the apparent fiber level in both the general population and exposed workers changes with the length of fibers counted, and this length varies from laboratory to laboratory, as shown in Table 9.8. Again, each laboratory must supply details of its background values and counting rules.

The choice of specimen type and tissue is important if reliable results are to be obtained. Analysis of tissues other than lung has no value. Tumors, being new growths, contain little or no asbestos. The asbestos content of the pleura does not appear to reflect that of the lung (55, 66), since chrysotile is usually found in the pleura even when amphibole is present in the lung, although a recent report suggests that amphibole fibers do collect in so-called black spots in the parietal pleura (67) (see section on benign pleural disease). It has been claimed that large numbers of very short fibers (fibrils) of chrysotile may be found in various extrapulmonary sites in exposed workers (68), but the fact that fibrils should have very short half-lives (days) in tissue (37) makes this observation suspect. Because very short chrysotile fibers are the typical contaminants of air, water, and paraffin (59), it is likely that the reported analyses reflect contamination rather than asbestos inhaled at the job site.

The problems with analyzing very small specimens such as transbronchial biopsy samples are addressed in Chapter 3; their very small size and the uneven distribution of asbestos within the lung (69, 70) is likely to create huge errors in quantitative analysis. If analysis is to be performed during life, large open biopsy samples or portions of resected specimens should be employed. To minimize site-to-site variations in concentration, I try to use a minimum sample size of 3 to 5 g (inflated wet weight) of lung. The selected area of lung should be as normal as possible.

A few studies report asbestos bodies or fibers in sputum or lavage fluid, with contradictory results (71–76). Roggli et al. (71) suggest a direct correlation be-

TABLE 9.8
Concentration of Asbestos Fibers in the General Population

REPORT, FIBER	MEAN[a]	MEDIAN[a]	95th PERCENTILE[a]
Churg and Wiggs (15) (fibers >0.5 μm)[b]			
Amosite, crocidolite	1,000	0	10,000
Chrysotile	300,000	200,000	1,100,000
Tremolite	400,000	200,000	1,200,000
Case et al. (93) (fibers >5 μm)[c]			
Amosite, crocidolite	10,000		
Chrysotile	62,000		
Tremolite	14,000		

[a] Fibers per gram of dry lung tissue.
[b] General hospital autopsy population.
[c] Accident victims aged 61 or more.

tween numbers of bodies in sputum and tissue concentration but noted that one does not observe asbestos bodies in sputum except at very high tissue levels. Teschler et al. (72) observed a correlation between lavage counts of asbestos bodies or amphibole fibers and tissue concentrations; this did not apply to chrysotile fibers. DeVuyst et al. (73) found higher numbers of bodies in lavage fluid in those with interstitial than with pleural asbestos disease. McClarty et al. (74) also show a correlation between interstitial lung disease and the presence of asbestos bodies in sputa. However, Schwartz et al. (75) conclude that asbestos bodies in lavage fluid are not related to other measures of exposure or disease. It appears that analysis of sputum or lavage may be a useful method of detecting exposure when the history is equivocal, but such analysis is in no way a substitute for a tissue diagnosis. Again, it is necessary to have standards for exposed and nonexposed populations if one wishes to use this type of procedure.

ASBESTOS BODIES AND OTHER TYPES OF FERRUGINOUS BODIES

Ferruginous body is a term coined by Gross et al. (77, 78) to refer to a mineral particle to which pulmonary macrophages have added an iron protein coat. Asbestos bodies are the subset of ferruginous bodies containing an asbestos fiber core. When the core material is something other than asbestos, the type of core material can be used as a specific name, for example, *talc body* or *ferruginous body formed on talc.* Ferruginous bodies with nonasbestos cores have also been called pseudoasbestos bodies, but this term is confusing and should be avoided. The golden yellow coating that covers the mineral core is an iron-containing protein that is probably derived from ferritin or hemosiderin (62). The coat material may be beaded or form a continuous sheath (colorplate 2); illustrations of the numerous shapes the coat material may take are provided by Craighead et al. (79).

Asbestos bodies were first recognized early in this century in the lungs of workers with asbestosis and were called asbestosis bodies (80), but it was soon realized that identical bodies occurred in asbestos-exposed individuals who did not have asbestosis; thus the name was changed to the current *asbestos bodies.* Sundius and Bygden (81) showed in 1938 that the core material was asbestos. Numerous studies using modern electron microscope analytic techniques confirm this finding (81–87) and have established that chrysotile fibers do not form bodies as readily as amphibole fibers. This phenomenon is probably closely related to the observations that chrysotile tends to fragment into short lengths in the lung and that asbestos bodies do not form on short fibers of any type (10 μm is probably the minimal length of fiber that forms a body). For these reasons bodies randomly observed in tissue sections from patients with unknown types of exposure are more likely to be formed on amphiboles than chrysotile; however, with sufficient chrysotile exposure, for example in chrysotile asbestos miners, bodies containing chrysotile are also easily observed (83).

For many years asbestos bodies were viewed as markers of asbestos exposure that were found only in asbestos workers. This belief was challenged by the report of Thomson et al. (88) in 1963, which demonstrated that structures with the appearance of asbestos bodies could be found in a large portion of routine autopsies if smears were prepared from lung tissue. Subsequently numerous studies from North America and Western Europe indicated that virtually everyone in the general population has asbestos bodies in the lungs (62). In the general population asbestos bodies are present in such small numbers that as calculated by Roggli and Pratt (63), one should not observe a body from background asbestos exposure in more than 1 in 100 iron-stained routine-sized paraffin sections, but bodies are easily found if a suitable concentration technique, for example, bleach digestion and collection on a membrane filter, is employed to allow sampling of a large lung volume (62, 89).

The notion that the bodies found in the lungs of the general population were formed on asbestos was challenged by Gross et al. (77, 78), who produced identical structures in the lungs of experimental animals by administration of aluminum silicate whiskers or fibrous glass. Because of these observations, they invented the term *ferruginous body* and proposed that the bodies found in most persons in the population were not formed on asbestos.

Langer et al. (90) and Churg and colleagues (62) isolated more than 600 bodies from the lungs of the general population and exposed workers and showed that bodies with the typical morphology of asbestos bodies did contain asbestos in all instances. The characteristic features of true asbestos-containing bodies (Table 9.9 and colorplate 2) are (*a*) the core material is a colorless, transparent, thin fiber; (*b*) the core and body are usually straight; and (*c*) the body may be branched, reflecting longitudinal splitting of the fiber core. Of the bodies examined in these reports, 98% were found to have amphibole asbestos cores and only 2%, a core of chrysotile asbestos. Thus simple light microscopic observation is adequate to identify asbestos bodies in lung tissue or tissue digests.

However, Gross et al. were correct in concluding that other types of ferruginous bodies do exist in human lungs (colorplate 2). In one region of Turkey, the nonasbestos mineral fiber erionite is present in local rocks and soil, and ferruginous bodies identical to asbestos bodies can be found in the lungs of persons resident in this region (91); however, such bodies have never been reported in North America. All other types of ferruginous bodies are morphologically distinct from asbestos bodies and can often be specifically identified with a light microscope (92) (Table 9.9, colorplate 2). When bodies are formed on sheet silicate such as talc or mica, the cores tend to be irregular plates or very broad fibers with a pale

TABLE 9.9
Types of Ferruginous Bodies

MICROSCOPIC APPEARANCE	NATURE OF MINERAL CORE
Colorless transparent cores, usually straight, sometimes bronched	Asbestos Erionite (reported only from Turkey)
Broad yellow fibers or irregular yellow plates	Sheet silicates such as talc, mica
Black fibers (relatively broad) or plates	Coal, carbon
Fine black fibers	Rutile, silicon carbide, iron (rare)
Black hollow spheres, often with lacy configuration (may be nonferruginated)	Coal fly ash (mullite)
Small irregular solid black particles	Exogenous iron, ? carbon
Ferruginated fragments of elastin	Elastin fibers in conditions of chronic pulmonary hemorrhage (see Chapter 13)

Adapted from Crouch E, Churg A. Ferruginous bodies and the histologic evaluation of dust exposure. Am J Surg Pathol 1984;8:109–116.

yellow color. Bodies with either irregular or fibrous black cores may be formed on carbon fragments, coal, and fibers of iron or silicon carbide. Particulate iron such as that inhaled by hematite miners or condensed iron fume inhaled by welders also becomes ferruginated, but in these instance the cores usually are round or small polygonal forms, and the bodies themselves are round or ovoid.

Identification of asbestos and other types of ferruginous bodies with a light microscope thus provides an extremely simple and economical method for determining the nature of the dust to which a worker was exposed and with application of a proper quantitative method as described in the previous section, can indicate something about the level of exposure.

ASBESTOS BODIES AND FIBERS: CORRELATIONS WITH DISEASE

Numerous published studies examine the asbestos body and fiber content of human lungs and attempt to correlate these findings with the presence or absence of disease. Because of the problems associated with attempting to compare numeric results of such studies from laboratory to laboratory and the problems generated by analysis of quite disparate populations, direct comparison of these studies is difficult. The previous edition of this book (93) provides tabular listings of most of the results published to 1986, and Roggli et al. (89) have generated more extensive and more recent tables. This section summarizes the published findings by extracting what appear to be recurring themes from the results of every laboratory. Additional detail is provided in the various sections of this chapter and Chapter 10 that discuss the different asbestos-related diseases.

The first conclusion to be drawn is that everyone in the population carries a fairly substantial burden of asbestos fibers in their lungs. Table 9.8 shows the actual numeric data for my laboratory and for the group at McGill (89, 93–95). The disparity in values in large part relates to the fact that in my laboratory we count all fibers longer than 0.5 μm, while the McGill group counts only fibers longer than 5 μm; this is a good example of the difficulties inherent in laboratory-to-laboratory comparisons.

Assuming that a pair of dried lungs weighs approximately 40 g, the numbers given in Table 9.8 suggest that one may find as many as 40 million fibers of chrysotile, 40 million of tremolite, and 400,000 fibers of amosite or crocidolite in the lungs of the general population of Vancouver, along with 40,000 asbestos bodies. Even if one follows the McGill protocol and counts only fibers longer than 5 μm on the theory that these are the pathogenic fibers, the total fiber count is still large. Nonetheless, there is no evidence that this fiber burden produces asbestos-related disease in the general population.

A similar conclusion can be drawn from evaluation of the fiber burden of the lungs of long-term residents of the chrysotile mining townships in Eastern Québec (6, 96, 97). The mining and milling operations and the presence of asbestos in the soil have produced ambient atmospheric levels of chrysotile and tremolite several hundred-fold greater than that found in urban areas in North America; the measured levels in the mining townships were on the order of 0.01 fibers per cubic centimeter in early 1980s (6) and reportedly even higher in previous years. Analysis of lung asbestos content indicates that persons living in the townships who have never worked in the mining and milling industry carry a burden of chrysotile and tremolite fivefold to tenfold greater than that of typical urban dwellers in North America (96, 97), but despite these exposures a variety of epidemiologic investigations have failed to show any excess of lung cancer or mesothelioma in these individuals (98). These findings suggest that at least for chrysotile or the short fiber tremolite that contaminates chrysotile, a much greater burden of asbestos than that to which ordinary urban dwellers are ever exposed can be tolerated without the appearance of disease. These data also provide reassurance that the low levels of exposure encountered in the ordinary asbestos-insulated building, which average 0.0002 fibers per cubic centimeter (1), and in urban air (0.0001 fibers per cubic centimeter [1]) have no potential to cause disease.

Despite laboratory-to-laboratory variation in numeric values, a reasonably consistent correlation of fiber burden and disease has emerged from examination of populations with occupational asbestos exposure (54, 38, 89, 95, 99). These correlations are shown in Figure 9.3, which illustrates the fact that disease always appears with fiber burdens considerably greater than those seen in the general population and that different diseases typically appear at different fiber burdens.

Furthermore, this pattern varies from chrysotile to amosite and crocidolite: for amphibole the lowest burdens are seen in members of the general population; those with pleural plaques and mesothelioma have about the same mean burden; and those with asbestosis have a considerably greater burden. For chrysotile exposure the lowest burdens are again seen in persons in various general populations; plaques occur at a higher burden; and cases of mesothelioma and asbestosis occur only at very high and roughly comparable fiber levels. One of the achievements of this type of analysis is to prove that chrysotile does indeed induce mesothelioma in man, a previously disputed point, but at the same time to point out the extraordinary fiber load that is required (38). The latter observation thus reinforces the idea that low-level exposure to chrysotile produces no risk of mesothelioma.

An additional point not made obvious by Figure 9.3 is that a considerably greater burden of chrysotile (with its accompanying tremolite) than of amosite or crocidolite is required to produce any particular disease. An example is provided in Table 9.10 using data from our laboratory generated from the lungs of Québec chrysotile miners and millers and Pacific Northwest shipyard workers and insulators. For example, the mean burden of chrysotile plus tremolite in the lungs of miners and millers with asbestosis is 17 times the amosite burden in the lungs of shipyard workers with asbestosis. Similar differences are seen for pleu-

Increasing fiber burden ⟶

Chrysotile (including tremolite) burden

General population Urban areas	General population Mining townships	Plaques	Asbestosis or mesothelioma

Amosite or crocidolite burden

General population	Plaques Mesothelioma		Asbestosis

FIGURE 9.3
Relation between fiber burden and disease in those with chrysotile or amphibole (amosite or crocidolite) exposure.

TABLE 9.10
Geometric Mean Fiber Concentration by Disease in Workers with Heavy Amosite or Chrysotile Exposure

DISEASE	CHRYSOTILE MINERS AND MILLERS: CHRYSOTILE	CHRYSOTILE MINERS AND MILLERS: TREMOLITE	SHIPYARD WORKERS AND INSULATORS AMOSITE
Asbestosis	30	140	10.0
Airway fibrosis	27	120	4.3
Mesothelioma	34	180	0.9
Pleural plaques	15	75	1.4
Lung cancer	13	49	1.1
No disease	2	9	0.7

Values as millions of fibers per gram of dry lung.

ral plaques. For mesothelioma the difference is even more marked (almost 200-fold). These findings reinforce epidemiologic data indicating that fiber for fiber, chrysotile is a much weaker mesothelial carcinogen and is probably also less fibrogenic in man than are amosite and crocidolite.

Finally, fiber analysis reveals not only the lack of biopersistence of chrysotile (Table 9.5) but also the frequent occurrence of significant amphibole exposure in those with putative chrysotile-induced disease. This amphibole may be tremolite derived from the chrysotile ore itself (Table 9.10) or amosite and crocidolite resulting from the historical use of relatively small amounts of these fibers in various factories and processes that worked mostly with chrysotile. A good example is the chrysotile textile plant at Rochdale, U.K., where crocidolite was used in selected applications; as reported by Wagner et al. (100), analysis of the lungs of workers from this plant revealed quite significant amounts of crocidolite. These findings indicate that some types of "chrysotile-induced" disease may really be tremolite-, amosite-, and crocidolite-induced disease; this is true particularly of mesothelioma (see Chapter 10).

BENIGN ASBESTOS-INDUCED PLEURAL DISEASE

Terminology

Asbestos induces a variety of benign lesions of the pleura (Table 9.1). These conditions have been the subject of more than a little confused nomenclature because of the use by some authors (3) of the term *pleural asbestosis* to refer to pleural instead of parenchymal lung lesions. This is an unfortunate choice of words, since asbestos-associated benign pleural changes are mostly radiographic and pathologic findings that only infrequently have significant symptoms or functional consequences, whereas true asbestosis (i.e., interstitial fibrosis of the parenchyma) is frequently associated with functional impairment as well as with a high incidence of lung cancer. For this reason *pleural lesions should never be called asbestosis* (101).

A less serious problem is the confusion in the literature of pleural plaques and pleural fibrosis, distinctions that are usually but not always evident to the pathologist and can be difficult for the radiologist; this separation has become considerably more obvious at the clinical level with the use of computed tomography (CT) (102). The benign pleural conditions listed in Table 9.1 can occur separately or in any combination and may be found in the presence or absence of any other type of benign or malignant asbestos-related disease (see Fig. 10.1 for some examples). For example, Sargeant et al. (103) observed that of 36 patients with radiographic asbestos disease, 3 had only interstitial parenchymal disease, 4 had both parenchymal and pleural disease, and 29 had only pleural disease.

Pathogenesis

A great deal of speculation has been expended on theories of the pathogenesis of plaques, but our knowledge in this area is still well summarized by Hillerdal (104): "None of the various existing theories on the pathogenesis of pleural plaques is able to explain their peculiarities." Some authors suggest that plaques have a different derivation from effusions and the resulting fibrosis (105); lacking real data on any mechanism, the comments that follow are probably just as applicable to effusions and pleural fibrosis.

Hillerdal (104) summarized the theories of the origin of pleural plaques. They can be divided into two broad groups: (*a*) direct effects of fibers reaching the pleura; and (*b*) remote effects not requiring fibers in the pleura. Remote effects range from normal aging to effects of tuberculous infection to metastatic calcification because of unknown systemic asbestos effects to hypersensitivity reactions. Although it is true that tuberculous infections can produce plaques, it is clear that most patients with asbestos plaques do not have tuberculosis; there is little to recommend the other hypotheses. However, Adamson et al. (106) and Sekhon et al. (107) report that intratracheal instillation of asbestos fibers to mice and rats results in proliferation of pleural mesothelial cells, even though careful analysis reveals that very few fibers actually reach the pleura. These findings suggest that intraparenchymal asbestos fibers induce cytokine production, presumably from macrophages, that can affect both fibrogenic and neoplastic reactions in the pleura and that direct contact of fibers with the pleura may not be necessary for disease to occur.

If plaques and effusions are a direct reaction to fibers reaching the pleura or pleural cavity, it is unclear which pleura is involved and what the mechanisms may be. Most studies of pleural plaques and pleura (55, 66) found largely very short chrysotile fibers even when there was a substantial amphibole concentration in the underlying lung. However, Boutin et al. (67) recently demonstrated that long amphibole fibers do appear to collect in very limited areas of the parietal pleura, possibly around pleural stomata. Asbestos fibers in experimental animals have been shown to redistribute to a subpleural location with time (108), and concentration of particles in the visceral pleura is commonly observed in humans with many types of dust exposure (109) (see Chapter 5). The mechanism of transport is not clear; it has been claimed that asbestos fibers are moved by gravity (110) or lung motion (111, 112), but macrophage transport to collecting lymphatics probably plays the most important role, as it does for mineral dusts in general (see Chapter 5).

Because they are sharp, the notion has been advanced that fibers penetrate the visceral pleura and scratch the parietal pleura, producing small inflammatory reactions or hemorrhages that organize to form plaques (111, 113, 114). Some authors believe that plaques form from the chest wall side (5, 104, 105) and claim that fibers must be transported from visceral pleural to parietal pleural lymphatics, where they exert these mechanical effects, and perhaps stimulate macrophages or fibroblasts to synthesize collagen (104). There is some very indirect evidence for the latter proposition: Kuwahara et al. (114) showed that pleura mesothelial cells in culture will secrete the chemoattractant and matrix protein fibronectin after exposure to asbestos.

There is no good model of pleural plaques, effusions, or pleural fibrosis. Experimental injection of asbestos into the pleura has sometimes been reported to result in calcified plaquelike lesions (115), but the initial response in such preparations was a granulomatous one that has not been observed in human material. Sahn and Antony (105) performed similar experiments using neutropenic or intact animals and claimed that neutropenic animals develop pleural fibrosis and that intact animals form plaques. They suggested that the lack of macrophage response in the neutropenic animals is the important differential mechanism.

A statistical association of pleural disease and cigarette smoking has been proposed (116, 117), but it is controversial (29, 118). As is described in the sections on asbestosis, smoking appears to increase fiber retention in the lung and thus may increase dose to the pleura; however, no direct data address this question.

Plaques occur in workers with exposure to amphiboles and to chrysotile. Studies of fiber burden in such cases consistently show that plaques occur at fiber levels considerably greater than that carried by the general population but much lower than are seen in cases of asbestosis (38, 54, 90, 99) (Fig. 9.3, Table 9.10). The same general conclusion appears to apply to pleural fibrosis (119). These findings emphasize the idea that the pleura is much more sensitive to the effects of asbestos than is the parenchyma. Detailed analysis of fiber size distributions indicates that plaques are associated with fibers with a high aspect ratio and that tremolite rather than chrysotile appears to be responsible for plaque formation in workers with chrysotile exposure (38, 54).

Plaques also occur in populations that are not exposed through work but that live in areas where asbestos or asbestos- sized fibers occur in local soils and rock. The responsible fiber is most often tremolite, but anthophyllite-induced plaques have been reported in Finland (111, 120–127), and erionite, a nonasbestos mineral fiber, also produces such "environmental" plaques in a local area in Turkey (128), implying that a biopersistent fiber of particular dimensions is crucial to the process of plaque formation.

The pathogenesis of asbestos-induced pleural effusions is equally obscure, but histologic observation of human material makes it clear that exudative asbestos effusions can organize into a thick fibrotic pleura (Fig. 9.4), and organization of effusions is most likely the cause of asbestos-induced pleural fibrosis. Epler et al. (129) noted that of some 44 exposed patients with radiographic pleural thickening greater than 5 mm, half had a previous documented asbestos effusion. In a general sense this process is no different from the fibrosing pleurisy seen in other forms of chronic exudative pleural effusion, for example some cases of rheumatoid arthritis and lupus. However, it remains unclear why some patients with asbestos exposure have only fibrosis, some have only plaques, some have both, and what factors influence the peculiar distribution of plaques (discussed later).

Plaquelike structures similar to those seen in the pleural cavity have been reported on the surface of the spleen and liver. They appear to be associated with tuberculosis, cirrhosis, and asbestos exposure (130).

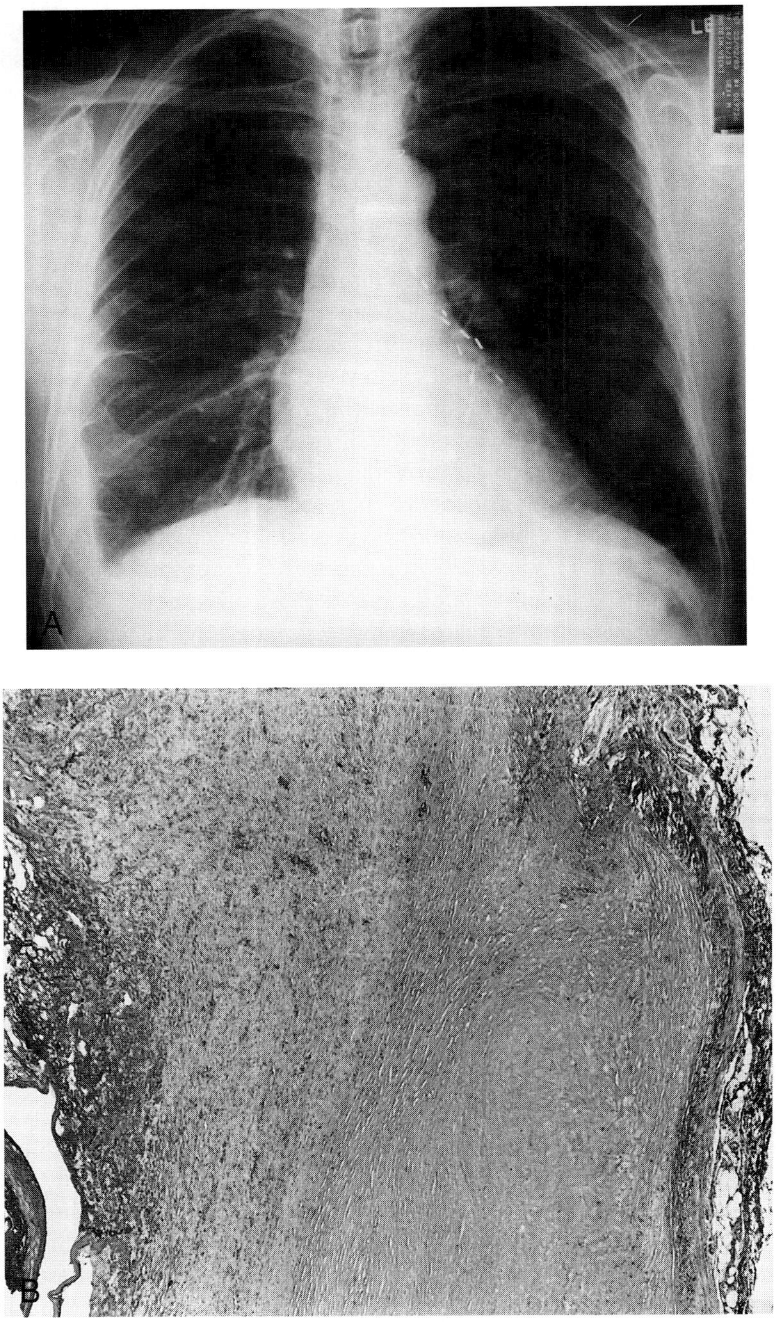

FIGURE 9.4
Asbestos effusion and pleural fibrosis. **A.** Chest radiograph of a man with a long history of asbestos exposure. His chest radiograph at the time of coronary bypass 2 years earlier was normal. He now had a hemorrhagic right-sided effusion and chest pain. This radiograph shows pleural thickening and a small effusion. The clinical impression was malignant mesothelioma. At thoracotomy diffuse pleural thickening was found, but there was no obvious tumor. **B.** Low-power view of the entire thickness of the biopsy specimen. At the left is the pleural cavity with areas of fibrin deposition; at the right, the fat of the chest wall.

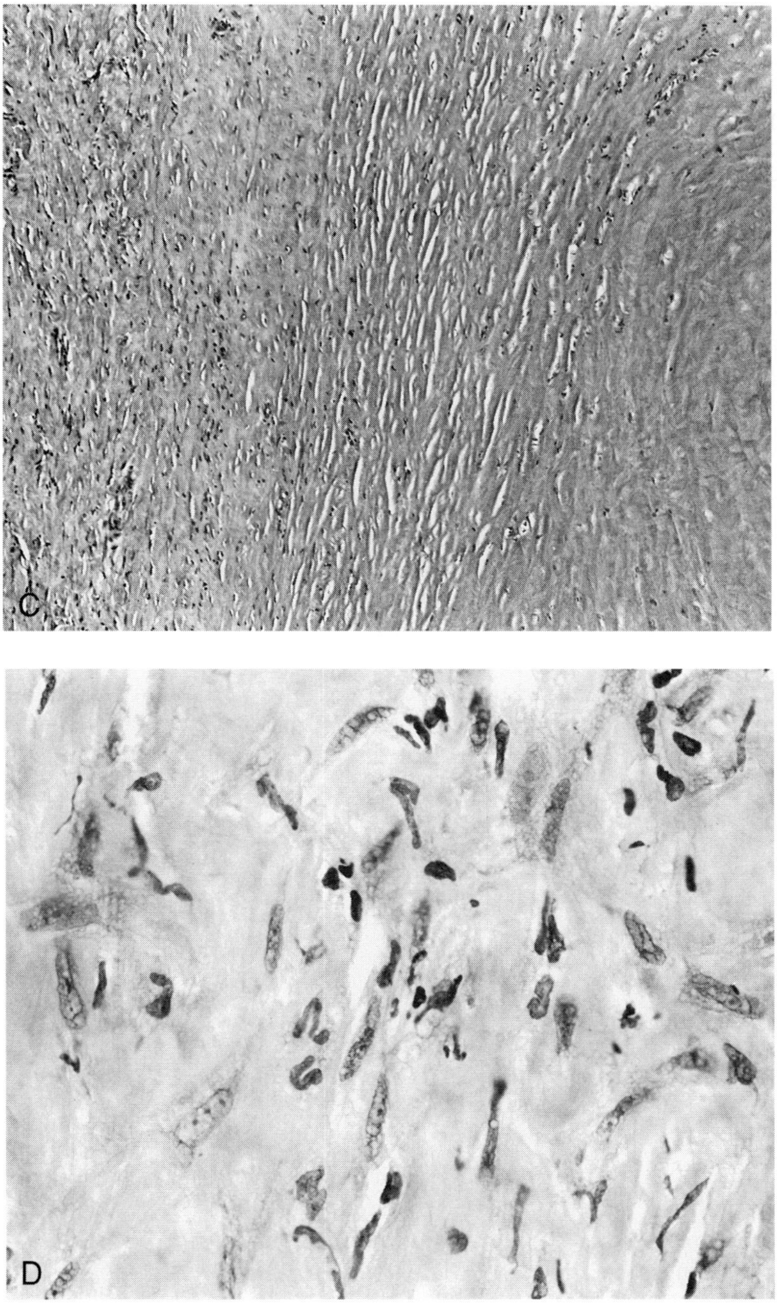

FIGURE 9.4 ***(continued)***

C. Slightly higher-power view showing the apparent sequence of organization of the pleural fibrosis into more and more hyalinized connective tissue. The direction, or sidedness, of the process (inflammation toward the pleural cavity, hyalinization away from the pleural cavity. is evidence for a benign process. Note the inflammatory cells scattered among the mesothelial cells. **D.** High-power view showing extremely bland-looking mesothelial cells and scattered inflammatory cells.

Epidemiologic Features

It has been suggested that benign pleural disease appears in a definite time course (129, 131): effusion is most common within 10 years of first exposure, during which period fibrosis and plaques are rare; thereafter effusion decreases in frequency and fibrosis and plaques increase. This sequence is consistent with the hypothesis that fibrosis and possibly plaques are the residua of old effusions. However, effusions can occur even long after the beginning of exposure. Hillerdal and Ozesmi (132) reported 73 episodes of effusion in 60 patients. The mean latency was 30 years, with a range of 1 to 58 years. The frequency of pleural effusion appears to increase with increasing amount of asbestos exposure. In 1135 current workers, Epler et al. (129) reported a prevalence of 7% in workers with the highest exposure (pipe fitters, asbestos handlers), 3.7% in those with intermediate exposure (e.g., electricians, welders), and 0.2% in those with peripheral exposure.

Pleural fibrosis and plaques occur more frequently with increasing exposure and latency. The prevalence of plaques as detected by plain chest radiographs in populations with known exposure varies considerably, ranging from 5% in some series of asbestos factory workers to 40 to 60% in highly exposed insulators and similar workers (5, 129, 132). Epler et al. (129) showed that the prevalence of plaques increased from about 30% for those with latent periods in the range of 20 to 29 years to 60% for those with latent periods between 40 and 49 years. Rossiter et al. (133) demonstrated that radiographic pleural thickening in chrysotile miners increased from 1.4 to 12.3% between highest and lowest dust exposure categories. It is clear that incidences are higher if lesions are found by pathologic rather than plain film radiographic examination (134–136); Hourihane et al. (135) showed that only 15% of plaques detected at autopsy were visible radiographically, and similar results have been reported by others (134, 136).

Clinical and Radiographic Features

Asbestos effusion is defined by four criteria (129, 131):

1. A history of exposure to asbestos
2. Radiographic or thoracentesis confirmation of effusion
3. No other disease that would produce a pleural effusion
4. No malignant tumor developing within 3 years

Most of these effusions are asymptomatic and are detected only if exposed populations are repeatedly examined by chest radiography. However, some patients present with pleuritic pain, dyspnea, or hemoptysis, and the usual physical findings associated with effusion (e.g., friction rub, dullness) can be seen; clubbing may be present. Radiographically the effusion is usually small to moderate (Fig. 9.4); in a few patients it is bilateral (129, 137). On thoracentesis the effusion is found to be an exudate and is hemorrhagic in as many as 50% of cases (132), raising the possibility of a neoplastic process. Most effusions appear to resolve spontaneously; in the series of Robinson and Musk (137), mean duration to remission was 4 months. Recurrence is seen in about a quarter to a third of cases (129, 137). The major clinical problem in these patients is ruling out other causes of effusion, especially malignancy.

Most patients with pleural plaques and pleural thickening are asymptomatic, and the pleural disease is found incidentally by the pathologist or radiologist.

Details of radiographic diagnosis of these lesions are presented by Sargeant et al. (138) and Staples (102). On plain radiographs plaques appear as linear or elongated opacities, often calcified, along the costal or diaphragmatic margins and rarely on the visceral pleura or mediastinal pleura (139, 140). On CT scan they are usually seen as linear structures along the inner rib margins (Fig. 9.5). Diffuse pleural thickening may vary in manifestation from blunting of the costophrenic angle to widespread thickening surrounding much of the lung; on CT scan shallow extension of the fibrosing process into the underlying lung is sometimes evident (Fig. 9.6). CT scan is considerably more sensitive than plain radiograph as a method of detecting both plaques and pleural thickening (102, 141); for example, Oksa et al. (141) reported that high-resolution CT detected pleural plaques in 90% of asbestos sprayers, compared with a detection rate of 24% on plain radiograph.

It has been suggested that in large-scale population surveys pleural plaques and thickening can be associated with reductions in lung volumes and gas exchange (142, 143), but even here the data may be biased by inclusion of patients with true asbestosis (144). When disease is extremely severe and widespread, it may cause pulmonary insufficiency (145), but this appears to be an unusual event.

Davies et al. (146) reported pericardial effusion and constrictive pericarditis in three asbestos-exposed workers. This phenomenon appears to indicate extension of the pleural effusion and fibrosing process (which was present in all three) to the pericardium.

Pulmonary pseudotumor, also called rounded atelectasis, is an even more uncommon effect of asbestos-induced pleural disease (147–149). These lesions are caused by scarring of the pleura and immediately underlying lung, because of either local pleural fibrosis or an adherent pleural plaque, with retraction of the scar and collapse of a portion of the associated parenchyma. Radiographically

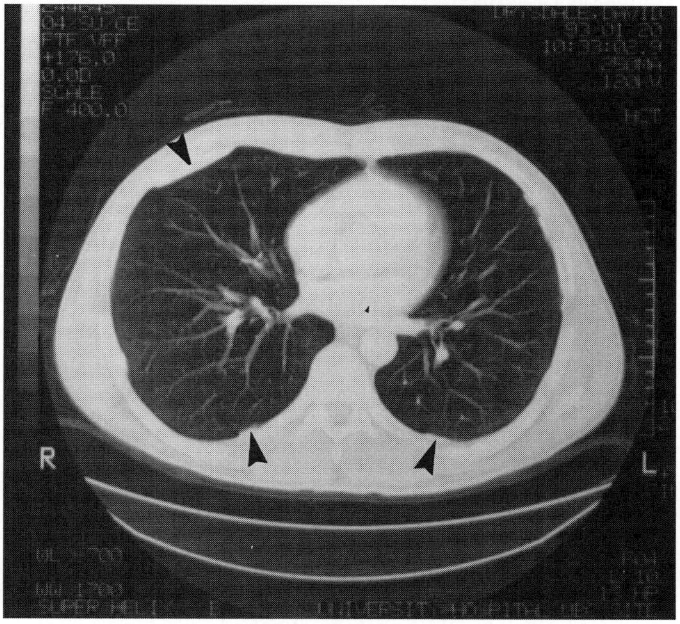

FIGURE 9.5
CT scan showing pleural plaques along the inner rib margins.

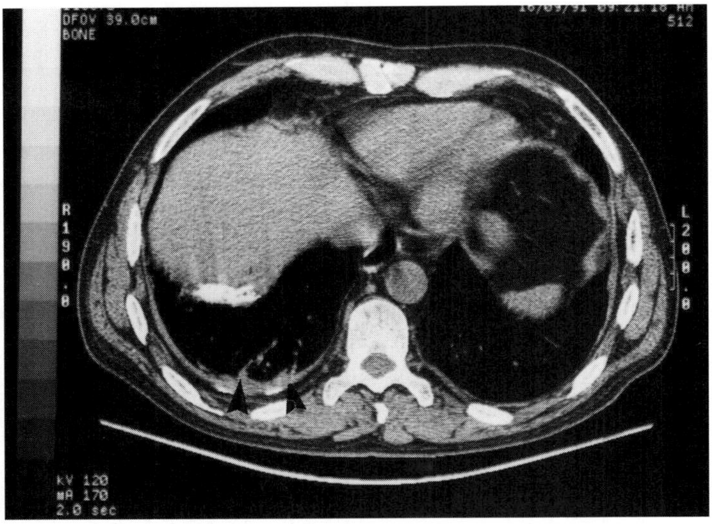

FIGURE 9.6
CT scan showing pleural fibrosis appearing as a linear tissue density along the inner rib margins. Note the focal extension of this process into the underlying lung (*arrows*). This extension is not asbestosis.

they appear to be rounded, sharply marginated mass lesions with a pleural base and surrounding vessels and bronchi that curve into the lesion; they are well seen with CT scan (150, 151) (Fig. 9.7). Although they may be associated with chest pain, they are most often encountered as incidental radiographic findings and resected in the belief that they are neoplasms (147–159).

Pathologic Features

As seen at autopsy, pleural plaques are raised hard yellow to white lesions that are characteristically bilateral, although not symmetric, most typically on the lower portions of the posterior parietal pleurae and diaphragm (135, 152) (Fig. 9.8*A*). Individual lesions may be completely smooth surfaced and flat or composed of small rounded knobs, or both. They can be extensively calcified. The pleural lesions often follow the ribs, and the diaphragmatic lesions tend to lie over the central tendon. Individual plaques, particularly the diaphragmatic ones, may be larger than 10 cm in greatest dimension. As plaques become more extensive, they tend to be found higher and more anterior in the chest. They can virtually encase the lungs but generally spare the apices and costophrenic angles (135, 152). In my experience, when the lesions are very extensive, there are usually diffuse adhesions between the visceral and parietal pleurae, and the distinction between plaques and diffuse pleural fibrosis becomes difficult (Fig. 9.8*B*). On rare occasions a solitary plaque takes on more of a pedunculated appearance (Fig. 9.8*C*) and is mistaken radiographically for a tumor.

Microscopically typical plaques are composed of a basket weave pattern of collagen that can be virtually acellular (Fig. 9.9); any cells that are present appear as slender nuclei with ill-defined cytoplasm lying in the lacunae formed by the collagen fibers. The surface of the plaque may be covered by a single layer of mesothelial cells or may have no apparent covering. The plaque is usually sharply demarcated from the underlying fat of the chest wall. It has been claimed

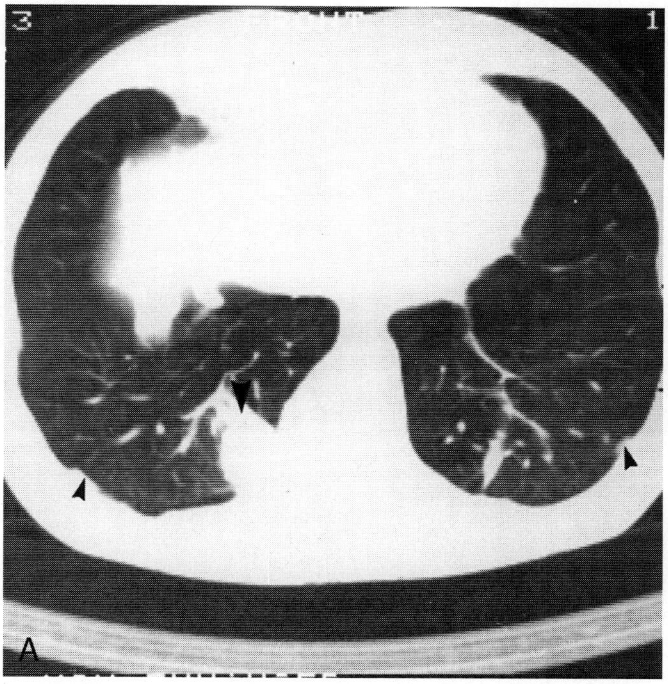

FIGURE 9.7
Asbestos-induced rounded atelectasis. **A.** CT scan showing a pleural-based mass (*arrow*) in a man with a history of foundry work but no known exposure to asbestos. He was a smoker with chest pain; the mass was thought to be a carcinoma. Pleural plaques (*small arrows*) are also present. **B.** Photomicrograph of the surgical specimen. At thoracotomy the surgeon found only pleural scarring under a plaque with infolding of the underlying lung. When the lung was dissected, the mass lesion disappeared. Note scarring associated with the pleura and extending along an interlobular fissure. The remainder of the lung parenchyma is essentially unremarkable. Because of the plaques, this man's work products were investigated, and one was found to contain a large amount of chrysotile asbestos. Analysis of his lung revealed 2.3×10^6 fibers of chrysotile asbestos per gram of dry lung (background expected no more than 1×10^6), indicating the connection between pathologic findings and asbestos. This case illustrates that workers may not know of asbestos exposure. **C.** Gross appearance of rounded atelectasis from another patient. Note the plaque, infolded lung, and retraction of the surrounding tissue.

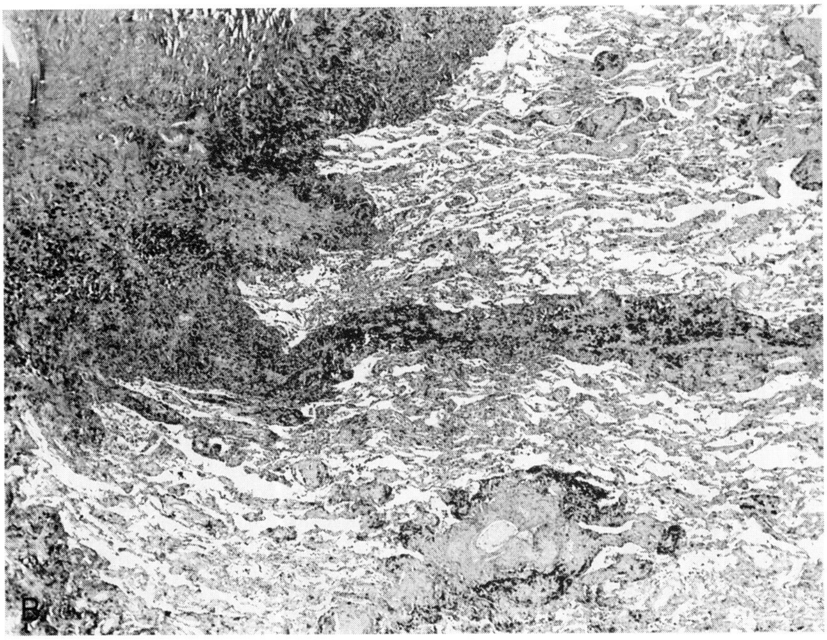

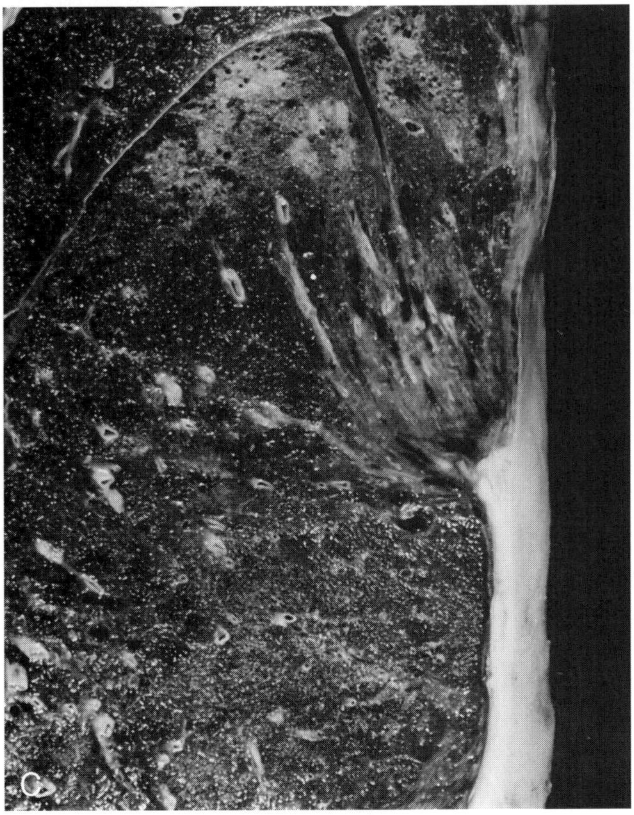

FIGURE 9.7 *(continued)*

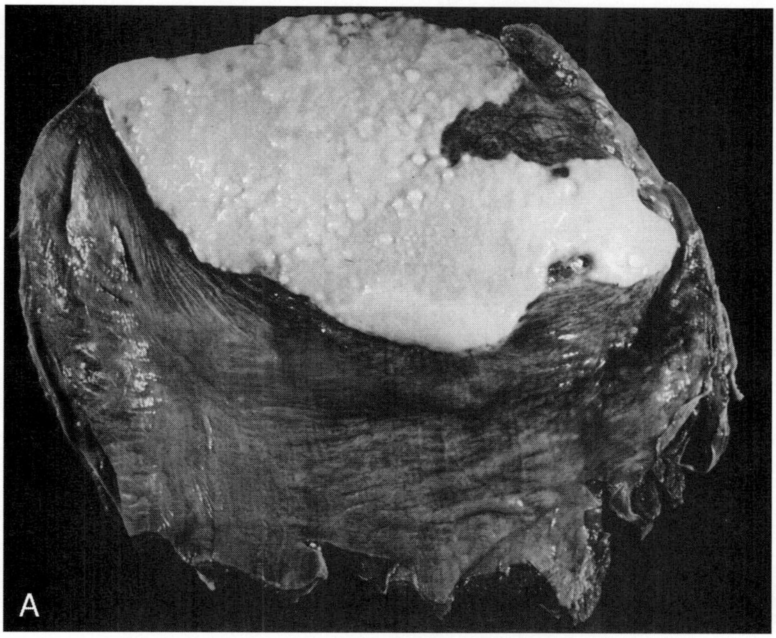

FIGURE 9.8

Appearances of pleural plaque. **A.** Gross appearance of diaphragmatic plaque. Plaques can be smooth-surfaced, knobbly, or as in this instance, both. **B.** Gross appearance of severe pleural plaque with virtual encasement of the lungs. This amount of plaque can cause a restrictive functional impairment. **C.** Low-power micrograph of a pleural plaque that clinically appeared as a nodular pleural-based lesion on radiographic examination. Note the narrow attachment to the chest wall at the left and the rounded appearance. (**B** Courtesy Dr. J. Churg.)

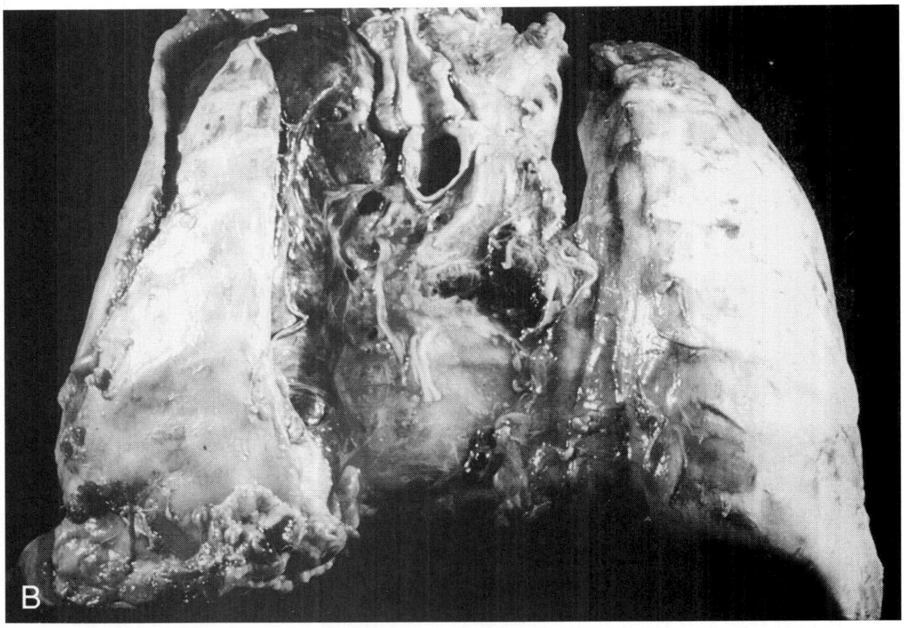

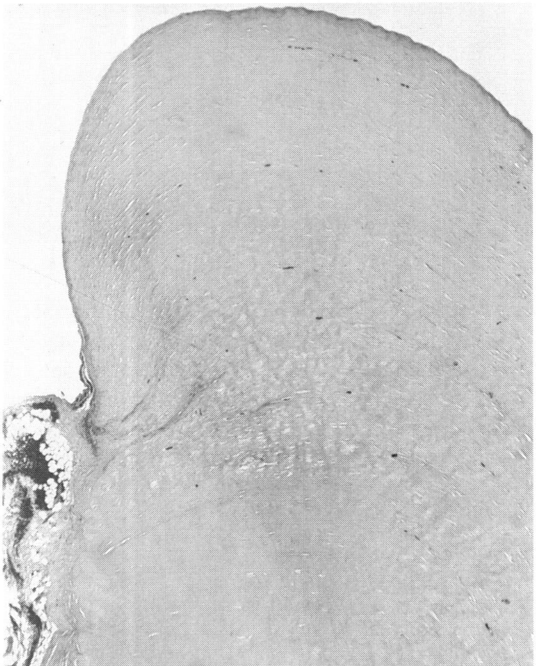

FIGURE 9.8 (*continued*)

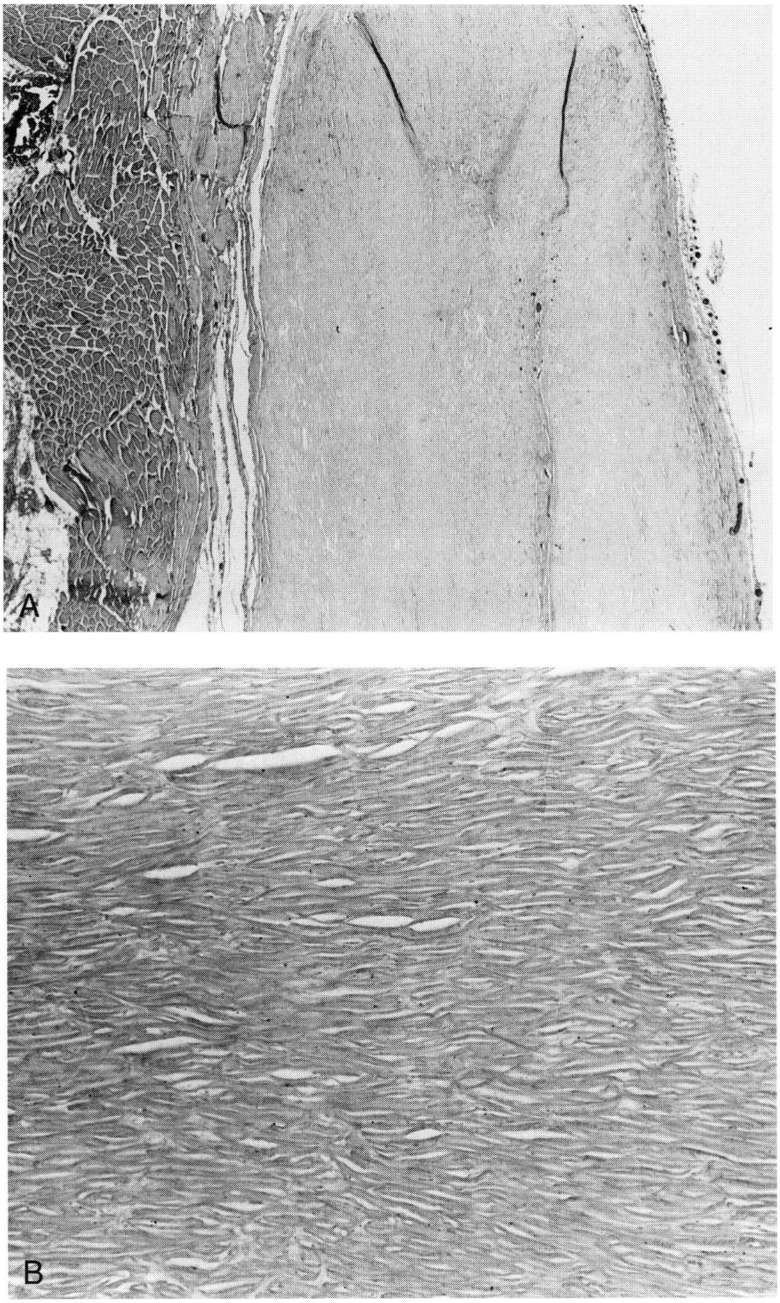

FIGURE 9.9
Microscopic appearances of pleural plaque. **A.** The plaque is sharply demarcated from the underlying muscle of the chest wall, and there is no overlying mesothelial reaction. **B.** The high-power view shows the typical basket weave appearance.

that small collections of inflammatory cells can be found in the fat, hence that plaques must be forming from the chest wall rather than pleural side (110), but I have seen this phenomenon only infrequently.

It is important to remember that the usual basket weave appearance of pleural plaques, although characteristic of lesions associated with asbestos exposure, is not at all specific. Plaque formation appears to be one of the common ways in which the pleura reacts to injury; plaques are formed as a long-term sequel to infection, particularly tuberculosis; trauma (including surgery); and hemopneumothorax (6). The basket weave pattern may be seen in any of these plaques. However, such plaques are typically unilateral and may be found anywhere over the lung, as opposed to the usual distribution of asbestos plaques.

As a rule asbestos bodies are not seen in pleural plaques, although Rosen et al. (153) claim to have extracted a few bodies from some. As mentioned earlier, the asbestos fiber content of plaques and pleurae appears to be quite different from that of the lung, and these sites are not generally useful for analysis to determine asbestos fiber burden.

Grossly, diffuse pleural fibrosis is usually fairly homogeneous and may fuse and distort the edges of the different lobes (Fig. 9.10*A*). Microscopically the appearances vary with the age of the lesion. Old disease appears as a thickened and fibrotic pleura, usually with a fairly minimal infiltrate of chronic inflammatory

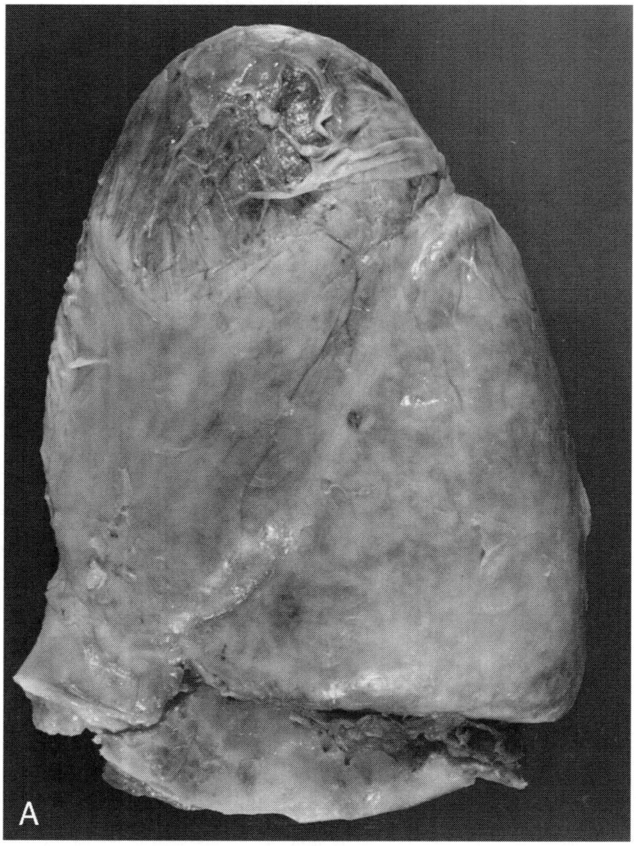

FIGURE 9.10

Asbestos-induced pleural fibrosis. **A.** Gross appearance. The process is severe enough to bridge the fissures and distort the edges of the lobes. This lung also has asbestosis and a carcinoma; the cut section is shown in Figure 10.1*B*.

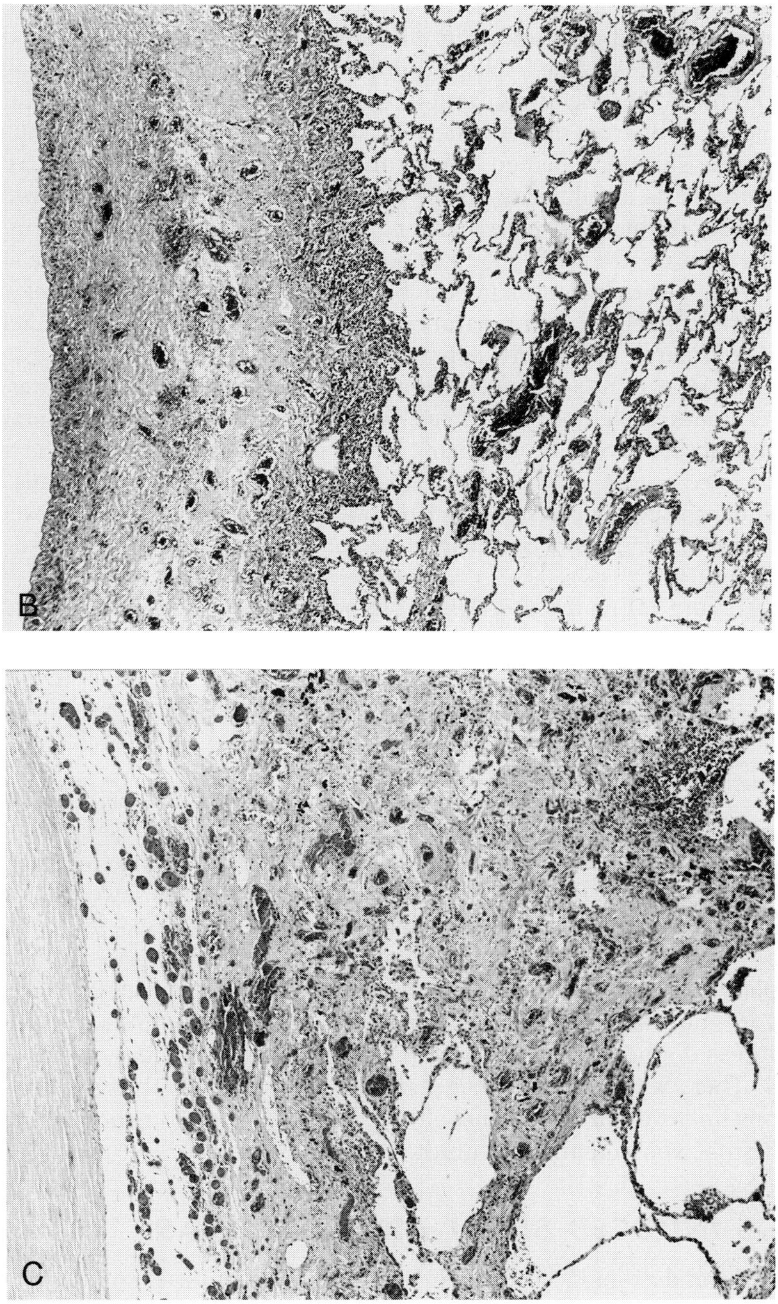

FIGURE 9.10 ***(continued)***
B. Microscopic appearance of typical asbestos-induced pleural fibrosis: the pleura is thickened and shows a mild chronic inflammatory infiltrate without any underlying interstitial fibrosis. **C.** Pleural fibrosis with shallow extension into lung. There is both an overlying plaque at the very left of the field and pleural fibrosis; the pleural space has been obliterated. Interstitial fibrosis underlies the plaque and fibrotic pleura, but this is a purely local phenomenon that does not extend into the lung farther than is shown in the micrograph. This appearance should not be mistaken for asbestosis.

cells (Fig. 9.10*B*). Asbestos bodies may be seen in the underlying lung or occasionally in the fibrotic visceral pleura. When an active effusion is present, the surface immediately under the effusion usually is more cellular and demonstrates proliferating spindled cells, proliferating endothelial cells, inflammatory cells, and fibrin. Distinct organization of the process with decreasing cellularity as one moves away from the pleural cavity side (Fig. 9.4, *B–D*) and an inflammatory infiltrate suggest a benign lesion, and desmoplastic mesotheliomas often show more marked cellularity on the chest wall side and typically have little inflammatory infiltrate. The proliferating spindled cells in the areas of organization of the effusion are usually keratin positive, indicating their mesothelial origin, but keratin positivity is seen in both benign and malignant mesothelial proliferations and is not helpful. The separation of benign and malignant mesothelial reactions is considered further in Chapter 10.

As shown in Figures 9.10, *B* and *C* (see also Figure 9.13*B*, later in the chapter) marked pleural fibrosis can occur with or without diffuse interstitial fibrosis (asbestosis) of the underlying lung. However, pleural fibrosis is frequently associated with a very shallow type of fibrosis of the alveolar walls immediately under the pleura (Figs. 9.6, 9.10C), and extreme care should be exercised before rendering a diagnosis of asbestosis on a superficial biopsy with a thickened pleura.

If surgical material on pseudotumors is obtained, the process appears as a nondescript pleural fibrosis, sometimes associated with overlying adherent plaque (Fig. 9.7, *B* and C). The diagnosis must usually be made from the CT scan or the surgeon's description of the operative findings.

Possible Associations of Plaques with Other Asbestos-Induced Diseases

Although plaques are largely markers of exposure, various reports raise the possibility that patients with plaques have a higher incidence of other asbestos-related diseases, particularly lung cancer. Weiss (154) reviewed 13 studies on this latter question and concluded that the weight of the evidence does not support any independent association of plaques and lung cancer. An association between pleural plaques and carcinoma of the larynx has also been proposed (136, 155, 156), but the association of carcinoma of the larynx itself with asbestos exposure is doubtful (see Chapter 10).

There is no evidence that plaques or diffuse pleural fibrosis are in any way precursors of mesothelioma, although obviously mesothelioma may occur in asbestos-exposed patients with these conditions.

ASBESTOS-INDUCED SMALL AIRWAY DISEASE

Mineral dust–induced small airway disease is discussed and illustrated in Chapter 5 and reviewed by Wright et al. (157). Asbestos is one of the dusts that can produce this type of lesion in the small airways. My colleagues and I have proposed that these lesions be called *asbestos airway disease*. Their significance and diagnostic categorization are disputed (discussed later).

The morphologic features of asbestos-induced small airway lesions are similar to those described for other dusts in Chapter 5; namely, fibrosis of the walls of the membranous and respiratory bronchioles, sometimes with extension into the alveolar ducts (Fig. 9.11). For all practical purposes the changes in the membranous bronchioles are indistinguishable by casual observation from those caused by cigarette smoke (see Chapter 5), but careful grading analysis (158,

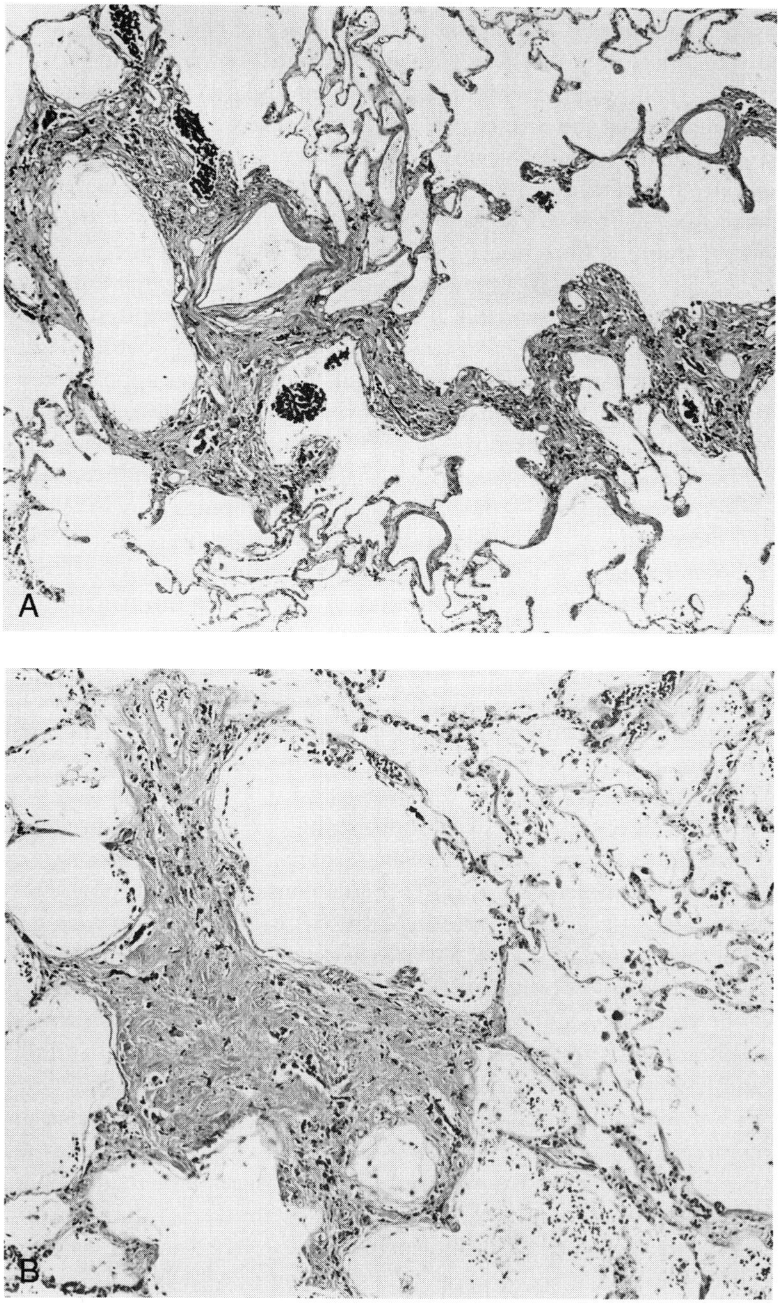

FIGURE 9.11

Asbestos-induced small airway disease. **A.** Micrographs showing a membranous bronchiole cut in cross-section and a respiratory bronchiole cut in longitudinal section. An adjacent respiratory bronchiole is also involved. Note the fibrotic distortion of the airway walls. Compare Figure 5.5. **B.** Cross-section of a respiratory bronchiole showing a severely fibrotic airway wall over part of the circumference. Note the absence of diffuse interstitial fibrosis (asbestosis) in both this and the previous figure. Compare also the images in Figure 5.6. (**A** reprinted with permission from Wright JL, Cagle P, Churg A, et al. State of the art: disease of the small airways. Am Rev Respir Dis 1992;146:240–262.)

159) indicates that the lesions tend to be more severe than those seen in cigarette smokers. However, the lesions in the respiratory bronchioles are morphologically distinct; they consist of fibrosis and distortion of the airway wall, often quite marked, with accompanying pigment and sometimes asbestos bodies. The abnormalities in the alveolar ducts, when these structures are involved, are similar. Somewhat similar lesions can be seen in the respiratory bronchioles of cigarette smokers, although they are uncommon and only rarely demonstrate the severe fibrosis that is frequent in respiratory bronchioles in those with dust exposure; smoking does not appear to affect the alveolar ducts.

Occasional lungs from asbestos-exposed workers show the type of fibrotic small airway with distortion and surrounding focal emphysema that is characteristic of the macular lesions of coal workers' pneumoconiosis and other dusts (see Chapters 5 and 6). These fibrotic macular changes appear to be the ultimate expression of dust-induced airway fibrosis and distortion, but whether the focal emphysema is also caused by asbestos is unclear (discussed later) (157).

The relation of chronic airflow obstruction to dust-induced small airway lesions is discussed in Chapter 5. A number of reports conclude that enough asbestos exposure does indeed produce abnormalities in flow in the small airways; the crucial issue is whether it is clinically significant. Quite marked airflow obstruction can be documented in small animals after intratracheal instillation of asbestos, but these models are known to accentuate the airway effects of asbestos and to produce relatively little true asbestosis (diffuse interstitial fibrosis) (160, 161). Epidemiologic studies using longitudinal data provide increasing evidence that other types of dust can produce clinically apparent airflow obstruction in man (162–164); similar studies are needed to provide a definitive answer to this question in regard to asbestos.

Some believe that asbestos-induced small airway lesions are actually the earliest form of asbestosis (78). However, there are several reasons to regard airway lesions as a completely separate process. Perhaps most important, the idea that these changes actually progress to diffuse fibrosis has never been proven in man, and in fact the lungs of workers with heavy occupational asbestos exposure commonly manifest not only mild but sometimes quite severe and widespread airway lesions with no evidence of diffuse fibrosis (165). Also, as shown in Chapter 5, morphologically identical lesions occur in both humans and animals exposed to a whole variety of dusts that do not produce interstitial fibrosis.

It is also peculiar that the airway lesion is inconstant in human material when unequivocal diffuse fibrosis (asbestosis) is present; if small airway lesions are the earliest form of asbestosis, one would expect them to be invariably present when asbestosis is observed. Furthermore, the distribution of these lesions is quite different from that of true asbestosis. In my experience airway lesions predominate in the upper zones and are much less frequent in the lower zones, whereas true asbestosis is definitely a lower-zone–predominant disease.

Experimental models provide further evidence against the idea that small airway lesions are early asbestosis. It is clear from animal studies that dust settles not only in the small conducting airways but in the alveoli as well (166), and we have noted that asbestos fibers can penetrate directly through airway walls to reach the parenchyma (167). Thus the earliest visible evidence of true interstitial fibrosis may indeed be found *around* the small airways, but this is a different process from that found in the walls of the airways. It is particularly intriguing to note the data of Bégin et al. (167) on the retention of chrysotile fibers in sheep. Those that develop only airway lesions show much less fiber retention than do those that develop diffuse interstitial fibrosis. My colleagues' and my own data on human lungs is similar (Table 9.10); lungs with only airway fibrosis tend to have very high burdens, but less than those seen in asbestosis.

Taken in aggregate, these findings suggest that rather than being a very early form of asbestosis, asbestos-induced small airway lesions are separate stereotypical reactions to mineral particles, entirely analogous to the lesions seen after exposure to other types of mineral dust.

As indicated in Chapters 6 and 7, there is considerable evidence that exposure to coal, silica, and probably other dusts is associated with emphysema, Whether asbestos also induces emphysema has received little attention. Certainly this type of image is morphologically fairly uncommon in asbestos workers, as illustrated by Wright et al. (157), as opposed to its high frequency in coal workers' pneumoconiosis. However, Bégin et al. (168) have reported emphysema detectable on high- resolution CT scans in workers with asbestosis, even in nonsmokers. These observations warrant additional studies to determine whether this is a constant finding.

ASBESTOSIS

Definition

Asbestosis is bilateral diffuse interstitial fibrosis of the lungs caused by the inhalation of asbestos fibers; this is the only condition to which the label *asbestosis* should be applied (101). Some authors include asbestos-related pleural diseases under the heading of asbestosis; this usage is to be avoided, since it lumps together a disparate set of diseases with different epidemiologic, pathogenetic, pathologic, and prognostic features. Harber and Smitherman (169) point out that a number of new diagnostic modalities, such as gallium scanning and high-resolution CT scanning, while providing clinically useful information (see Chapter 1), also produce confusion in regard to nomenclature, since the changes they record may or may not indicate true asbestosis (see section on clinical and radiologic features). Such problems can be avoided by keeping to this strict definition.

Epidemiology

There is general agreement from epidemiologic studies that the development of asbestosis requires heavy exposure to asbestos and that there is a threshold fiber dose below which asbestosis is not seen. A variety of studies suggest that this dose is in the range of 25 to 100 fibers per cubic centimeter–year (2, 29, 170–172). Accordingly, asbestosis is usually observed in individuals who have had many years of high-level exposure, typically asbestos miners and millers, asbestos textile workers, and asbestos insulators. However, asbestosis can be produced by intense exposure of relatively short duration; for example, in shipyard workers employed for a few years inside ship compartments during and after World War II, where exposure levels of hundreds of fibers per cubic centimeter were sometimes reached. Asbestosis has been reported in a worker who operated a carding machine, which creates a very dusty environment, for only 9 months making crocidolite asbestos cigarette filters (173).

The latency period for the appearance of asbestosis is inversely proportional to exposure level. Becklake (4) tabulated the prevalence of radiographic parenchymal disease in six recent reports and one report from 1938; these ranged from 3.8% of a series of 1200 dockyard workers to 16.2% of a series of chrysotile textile workers. The mean years of exposure ranged from 12.6 to 20.2 in the recent series, but in the report from 1938 the average exposure was only 5.2 years, which emphasizes the ideas that asbestosis has an effective dose threshold and that the lower the exposure, the longer it takes to reach this threshold.

Fiber burden studies indicate that the lungs of workers with asbestosis consistently contain the highest fiber levels seen in any of the asbestos-related diseases, with reported ratios of the fiber burden in asbestosis compared with plaque-only cases ranging as high as several hundred-fold (174). In experimental animals (40, 50, 51) and in man all types of asbestos fibers produce asbestosis, but comparison of absolute fiber concentrations as well as direct correlations of fiber burden with degree of fibrosis suggest that fiber for fiber, amosite and crocidolite are more fibrogenic than chrysotile and its accompanying tremolite (38, 54, 47, 48) (Table 9.10). There is general agreement that increasing pathologic grades of severity of asbestosis correlate well with increasing pulmonary fiber load for all types of fiber (47, 48, 95, 99, 174–176).

As well as a fiber type effect in the development of asbestosis, there appears to be an industry- and process-specific effect. Exposure to chrysotile with tremolite asbestos in textile work is associated with a higher incidence of radiographic asbestosis for a given exposure level than is chrysotile mining or milling or chrysotile friction products work (4) (Fig. 9.12). The reason for this is not known; it does not appear to be an artifact of fiber level measurement techniques (177), but it may relate to the use of particularly long fibers in textile work.

Pathogenesis

As in man, development of asbestosis in laboratory animals requires exposure to high concentrations of asbestos for long periods. A large number of experimental data have been collected on possible mechanisms of asbestos-induced fibro-

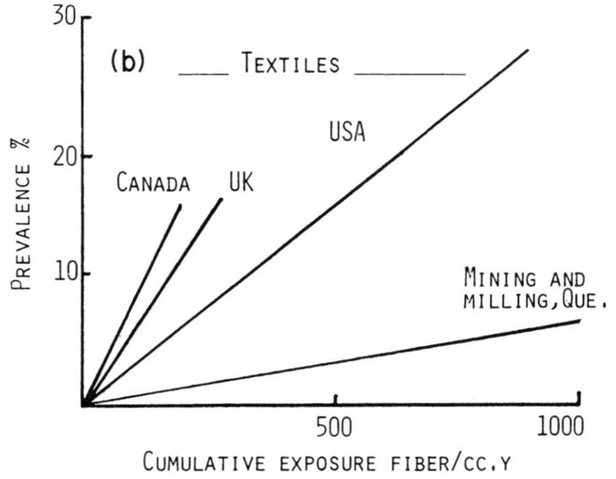

FIGURE 9.12
Prevalence of parenchymal lung changes 1/0 or greater in chest radiographs of workers in chrysotile textile and mining industries. Note the much greater incidence of disease for the same measured exposure in the textile workers. (Reprinted with permission from Becklake MR. Occupational lung disease: past record and future trend using the asbestos case as an example. Clin Invest Med 1983;6:305–337.)

sis; at this point the problem is not to postulate mechanisms but to determine which of the numerous effector substances actually play a role and which are epiphenomena and to understand how the elaboration of mediators leads to the observed pattern of fibrosis.

It is clear that exposure to asbestos, like exposure to any other mineral dust, evokes a marked inflammatory response that varies somewhat with the exact model but in general consists of an initial polymorphonuclear leukocyte influx followed by a macrophage influx (52, 53, 178, 179). Dust appears to activate complement, and this is one mechanism by which macrophages migrate to sites of dust deposition and attempt to phagocytize the fibers (178, 179).

Mossman et al. (43, 44) suggest that the macrophage should be regarded as an effector cell. They postulate that after phagocytizing asbestos fibers, the macrophage secretes a large variety of cytokines and effector substances, including growth factors, interleukins, prostaglandins, fibronectin, plasminogen activator, collagenases and elastases, and active oxygen species such as superoxide anion, hydroxyl radical, and hydrogen peroxide. These substances cause a further influx of inflammatory cells, damage epithelial cells, and stimulate proliferation of epithelial cells and fibroblasts and production of connective tissue matrix proteins.

There is evidence to support this general theory, although interpretation is not entirely straightforward. For example, Brody and colleagues (180–182) have shown that after a short intense exposure to chrysotile asbestos, collections of dust and macrophages can be found at first bifurcations of the alveolar duct. These macrophages produce platelet-derived growth factor (PDGF) and transforming growth factors TGF-α and TGF-β , among other substances. These cytokines are believed to cause fibroblast proliferation and the production of fibronectin and perhaps other connective tissue matrix proteins in the underlying connective tissue. However, the process also appears to resolve completely in a few months (183).

Mossman et al. (43, 44, 184) investigated the role of active oxygen species in the genesis of asbestosis. Active oxygen species are produced both by macrophages that have phagocytized asbestos and by iron-catalyzed reduction of oxygen on the fiber surface itself. Active oxygen species cause direct cell damage, including lipid peroxidation, protein oxidation, and DNA damage, as well as inducing cell proliferation. Particularly notable is that administration of polyethylene glycol-conjugated catalase (catalase is a scavenger of hydrogen peroxide) to rats that have inhaled crocidolite asbestos prevents the inflammatory and fibrotic reaction (185).

A further question is where the crucial reactions take place. Although it is clear that alveolar macrophages do secrete various mediators after asbestos exposure, recent reports raise questions about whether such mediators actually cross epithelia to affect interstitial fibroblasts or whether the interstitial macrophage is the true effector cell (186, 187). In addition to being phagocytized by alveolar macrophages, asbestos fibers tend to enter the airway and alveolar epithelial cells, a process that itself is mediated at least in part by active oxygen species (188). Eventually these fibers completely cross the epithelium to the interstitium, where they are phagocytized by interstitial macrophages. These cells are believed to secrete mediators similar to those produced by alveolar macrophages.

Animal experiments suggest that long fibers are more fibrogenic than short fibers (50–53), although data from human asbestosis cases does not clearly support this idea (47, 48). It has been postulated that the greater pathogenicity of long fibers is related to enhanced production of active oxygen species and possibly other factors by alveolar macrophages. However, Adamson and Bowden (186) have found that in vitro short fibers are just as active as long fibers in eliciting secretion of fibroblast growth factors from macrophages but that short fibers ordinarily cannot cross epithelia, suggesting instead that access of fibers to interstitial macrophages is the crucial issue.

This observation may have considerable importance in humans. My associates and I have demonstrated in experimental animals that cigarette smoke enhances fiber retention in the lung and fiber uptake by epithelial cells and that enhancement of short-fiber uptake is greater than that of long-fiber uptake; also, the combination of smoking and asbestos leads to greater degrees of interstitial fibrosis (161, 189). Furthermore, we have shown that in inflammatory-cell free tracheal explants, active oxygen species such as cigarette smoke lead to greater uptake of fibers by the epithelial cells and cause greater transepithelial migration (188). These findings may explain the apparently greater incidence and progression rate of asbestosis in human cigarette smokers (discussed later).

Equally important is why, cigarette smoking aside, some persons develop disease and others with equal exposure do not. Bégin et al. (190, 191) have shown that when equal doses of asbestos are administered to sheep, radiographic asbestosis as well as lavage evidence of an active alveolitis develops in the sheep that have the lowest fiber clearance and that the differences in fiber clearance precede the appearance of asbestosis. This suggests that in humans, person-to-person variations in fiber retention may be a major determinant of disease induction.

Clinical and Radiographic Features

The clinical features of asbestosis are those of diffuse interstitial fibrosis as described in Chapter 1. In general such patients have shortness of breath and dry cough. Physical examination typically reveals dry rales at the bases on inspiration. Clubbing may be present in advanced disease. Pulmonary function changes correlate in a general way with pathologic and radiographic findings: in the fully developed case, a restrictive pattern of pulmonary function with small lung volumes and decreased diffusing capacity is seen (29, 101, 192–194). However, pathologic examination may reveal mild cases that appear to have no obvious functional defect.

Radiographic examination in well-developed disease shows a lower-zone reticulonodular infiltrate on plain radiograph (Fig. 9.13*A*). Parkes (195) emphasizes the idea that predominantly upper-zone or even mid-zone disease is distinctly against the diagnosis of asbestosis. When asbestosis is well established, the CT features are very similar or identical to those seen in usual interstitial pneumonia, with peripheral bands, lines, thickened interlobular septa, and honeycombing (102, 196), and the disease is clearly most severe at the lung bases.

The clinical, physiologic, and radiologic findings of asbestosis are not in any way specific, and they can be found in diffuse interstitial fibrosis of other causes, particularly usual interstitial pneumonia. However, the presence of calcified pleural plaques on radiographic examination is helpful in suggesting the diagnosis.

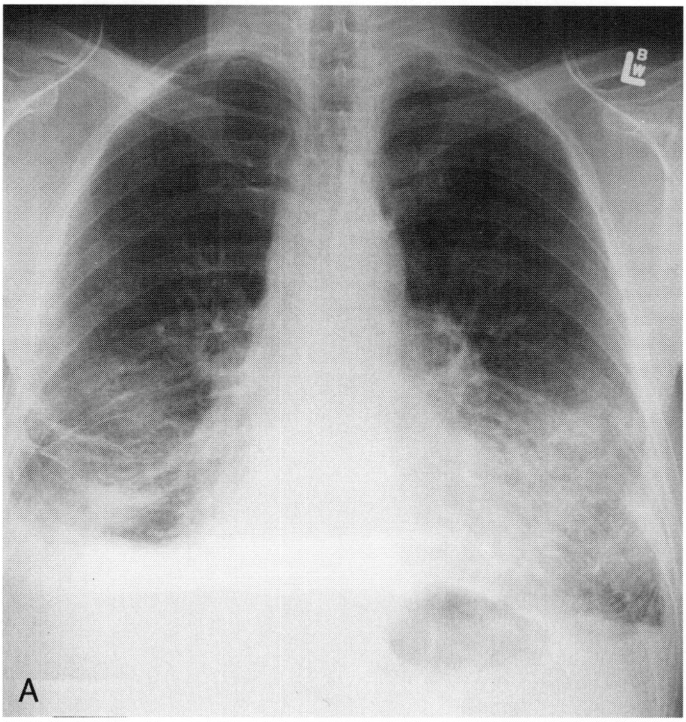

FIGURE 9.13
Asbestosis in a long-time worker in an asbestos processing plant. In 1984 this man died of respiratory failure at age 48. **A.** Chest radiograph shows diffuse lower-zone reticular infiltrates graded as t/t, 3/2; the pattern is typical of asbestosis although nonspecific. **B** and **C.** Gross appearances of asbestosis showing predominantly lower-zone honeycombing and fine fibrosis. Note how the examination of the inflated sliced specimen allows accurate determination of the extent and severity of disease. This lung also shows pleural fibrosis. **D.** Representative low-power micrograph showing patchy interstitial fibrosis alternating with relatively normal alveoli. This is the typical appearance of well-established asbestosis and is not at this power distinguishable from usual interstitial pneumonia. **E.** Higher-power view showing the combination of asbestos bodies and diffuse interstitial fibrosis, the microscopic requirements for the diagnosis of asbestosis. **F.** Varied morphology of asbestos bodies in tissue sections.

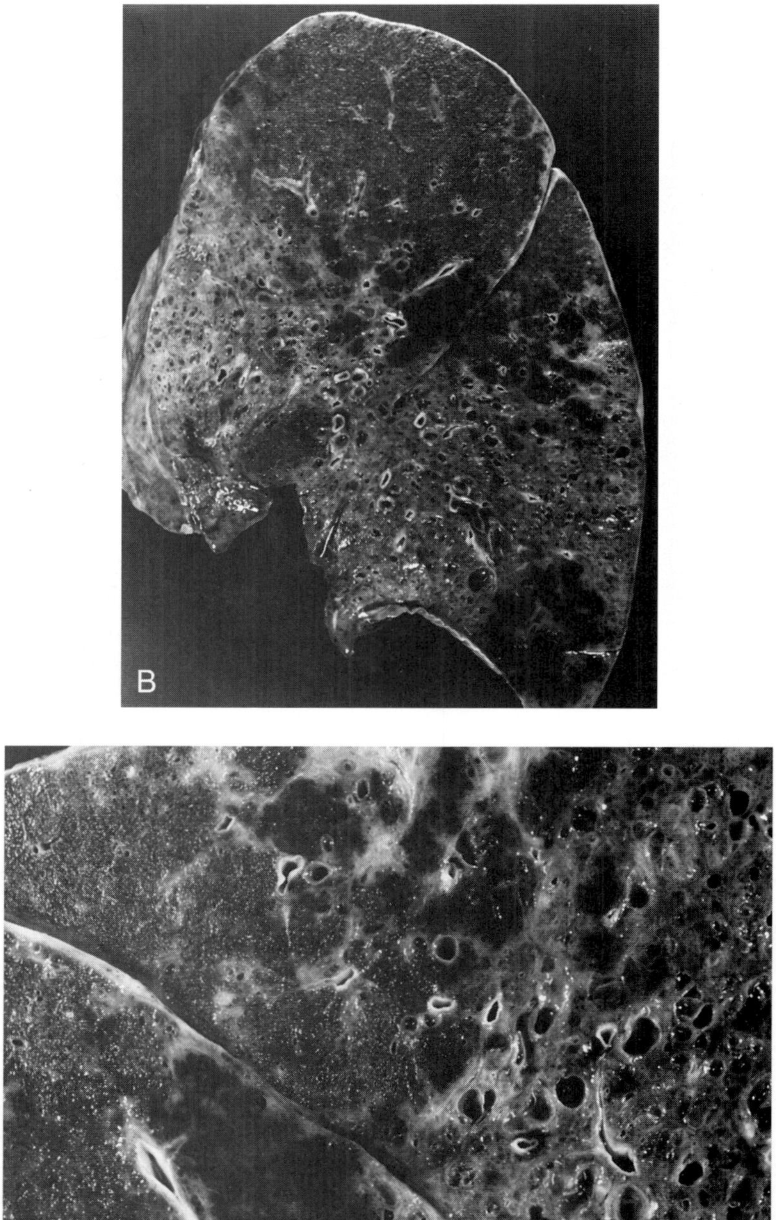

FIGURE 9.13 *(continued)*

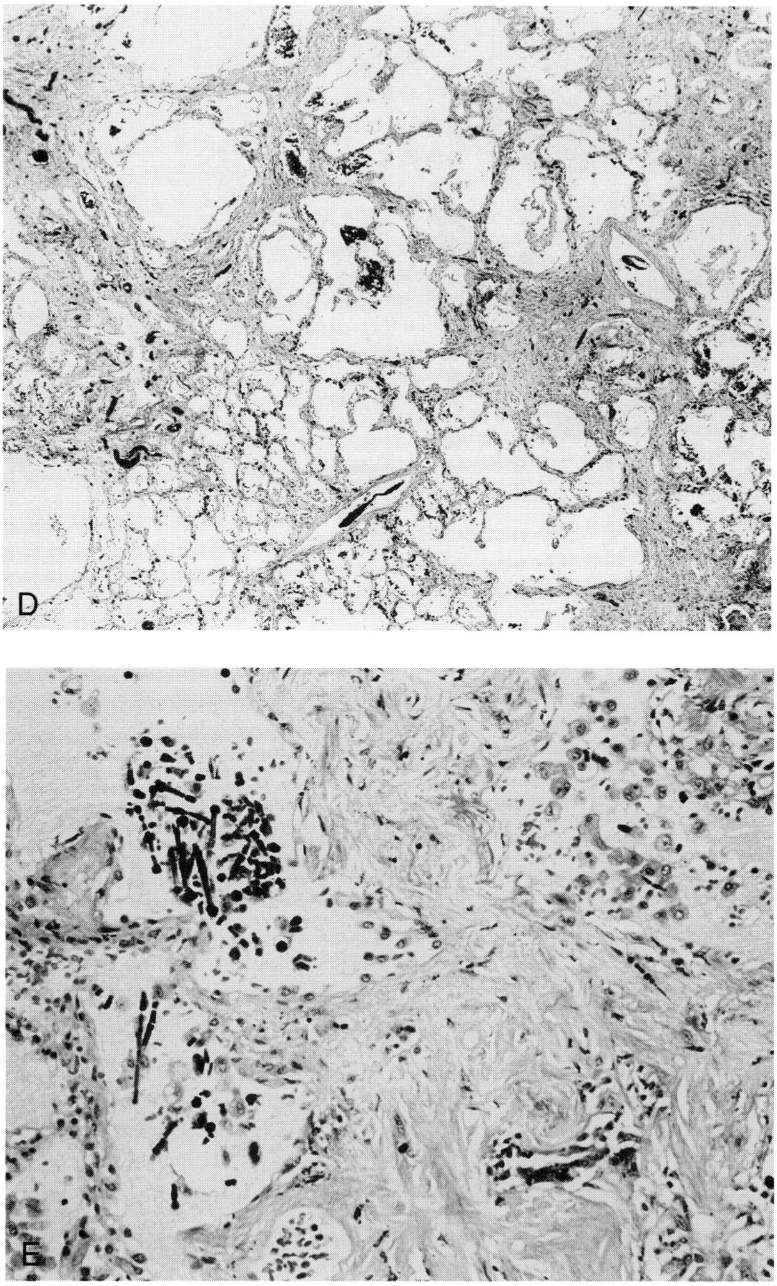

FIGURE 9.13 *(continued)*

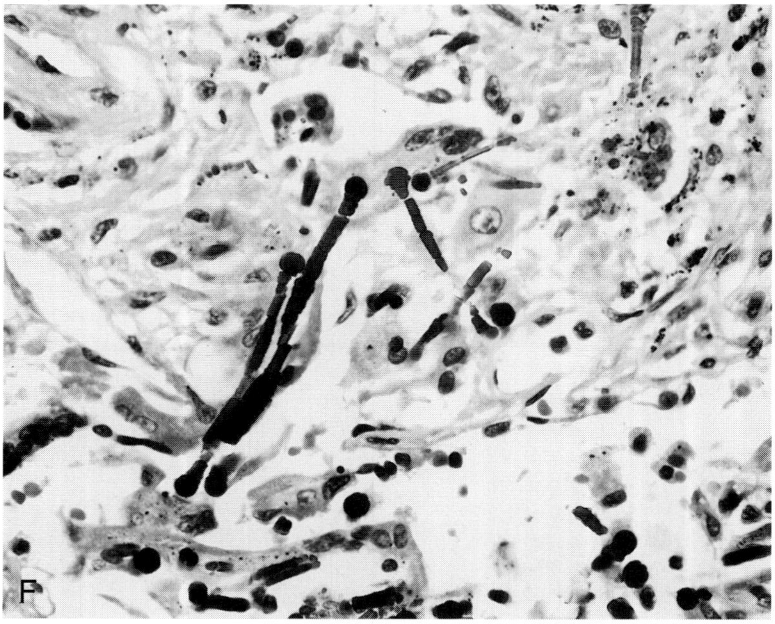

FIGURE 9.13 (*continued*)

There is considerable controversy about very subtle parenchymal CT changes that may be found in asbestos-exposed workers with International Labour Office (ILO) category 0 plain radiographs (i.e., normal chest radiographs). Some claim that they represent early asbestosis (197); others believe the findings are nonspecific (198). This issue is beyond the scope of this book; suffice it to say the claimed changes have no very clear pathologic correlations. Moreover, as noted in the discussion of benign pleural disease, visceral pleural fibrosis can show shallow extension into the underlying parenchyma (Figs. 9.6 and 9.10C), and it is likely that at least some of what is being called early asbestosis on CT scan may really be pleural fibrosis.

Various sets of specific criteria for the diagnosis of asbestosis have been published. For example, Murphy et al. (192) proposed that the combination of a history of exposure, bibasilar fine rales, forced vital capacity (FVC) less than 80% predicted or single breath diffusing capacity of less than 80% predicted, and ILO category 2/1 or greater reticulonodular opacities established the diagnosis. The American Thoracic Society (101) has suggested that the combination of a history of exposure, ILO category greater than or equal to 1/1, and FVC and diffusing capacity less than the lower limit of normal be used. Harber and Smitherman (169) present a detailed listing of other proposed criteria.

When there is a history of heavy exposure to asbestos and the features just listed are present, biopsy is generally not necessary. Lung biopsy should be reserved for cases in which the history of exposure is unclear or the clinical features are not typical of asbestosis. In these circumstances biopsy may be very important to determining whether there is instead a treatable condition that is not asbestosis; it should not be forgotten that asbestos-exposed workers develop all of the types of interstitial lung disease seen in the general population (195, 199) (see section on diagnostic pitfalls).

Pathologic Features

Gross Examination. Gross examination of lungs with asbestosis often reveals a fibrotic visceral pleural (Fig. 9.10A, 9.13*B*, and Fig. 10.1); however, the pleural disease is *not* asbestosis but rather asbestos-induced pleural fibrosis, as described earlier. Some cases of asbestosis do not demonstrate pleural fibrosis. In other cases there are both pleural fibrosis and pleural plaques, and the plaques may adhere to the lung.

On cut section the typical case of asbestosis shows diffuse interstitial fibrosis most marked in the lower zones, with the worst disease generally seen closest to the pleura and with relative sparing of the central portions of the lung (Fig. 9.13, *C* and *D*, and Fig. 10.1) (200, 201). Involvement is always bilateral and generally roughly equal in extent. Honeycombing with small cysts is fairly common in advanced disease. The severely honeycombed areas and areas of confluent fibrosis are easy to see with the naked eye, but examination with a hand lens and palpation often reveals much more extensive areas of fine fibrosis.

There are no set rules for grading the extent of involvement. Hinson et al. (201) suggest that the gross changes be recorded as covering 0 to 25% of the parenchyma, 25 to 50%, and so on, but a good gross description serves the purpose equally well. *The critical issue for the pathologist is to document in some fashion the fact that fibrosis is diffuse*, not just a local scar or local reaction around a tumor. Furthermore, there is nothing specific about the gross appearance of the parenchymal fibrosis in asbestosis that allows it to be separated from other conditions such as usual interstitial pneumonia that produce predominantly lower-zone disease.

A basic requirement for accurate gross assessment of fibrosis is a well-inflated specimen. Resected lobes and whole lungs are easily inflated through the bronchus with a tank of formalin placed on a shelf; the inflation pressure and time are not critical, but I usually leave specimens inflated overnight if there is no compelling reason (such as a large tumor mass that will not fix) to cut them. The fixed inflated lung can then be sliced in a sagittal (Fig. 9.13, *B* and *C*), frontal, or CT plane for accurate assessment of the parenchyma. Open biopsy specimens can also be inflated with a formalin-filled syringe (202), and such specimens should be examined grossly for fibrosis, a point that is often overlooked.

There are also no set rules for tissue sampling. In general an attempt should be made to show the grossly worst and best areas to sample peripheral and central portions of all lobes, and to show that scarring is more than just a local phenomenon. In many instances a gross photograph is more informative than a large number of tissue blocks, particularly in regard to documenting the extent of fibrosis.

Microscopic Examination. The microscopic requirements for the diagnosis of asbestosis are (*a*) *diffuse interstitial fibrosis* and (*b*) *asbestos bodies in ordinary* 5-μm paraffin sections (79, 200, 201). In well-established disease the interstitial process appears as dense interstitial fibrosis with a chronic inflammatory infiltrate that is usually mild (Figs. 9.13, *D* and *E*, and 9.14). Metaplastic bronchiolar or hyperplastic type II epithelium may cover scarred foci. The interstitial disease is typically patchy (Figs. 9.13, *D* and *E*, and 9.14), much in the pattern of usual interstitial pneumonia, which it greatly resembles. Honeycombed areas may show much more severe inflammation, extensive fibrosis, and inflammatory cells, including neutrophils, presumably reflecting local infection. Asbestos bod-

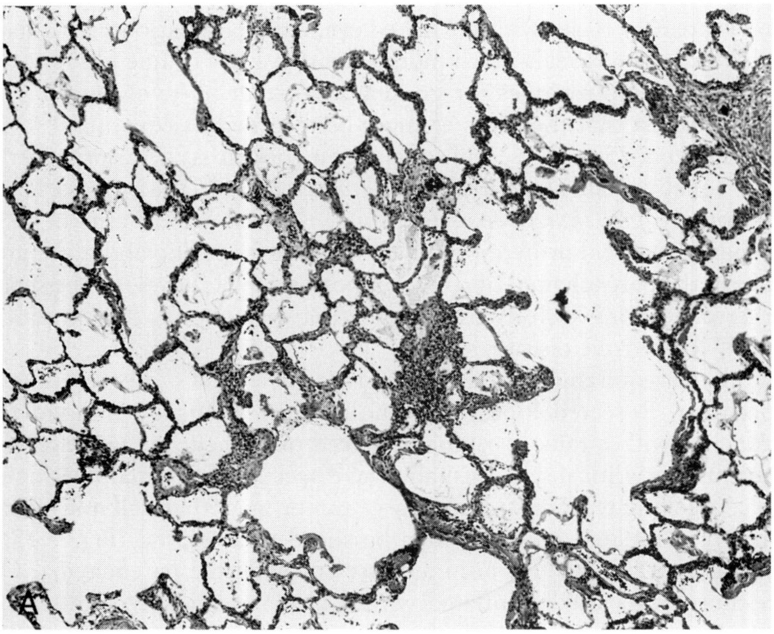

FIGURE 9.14
Microscopic appearance of asbestosis in a long-time textile worker. Note variability of the patterns, which range from severe scarring with honeycombing (**B**) to diffuse but mild fibrosis (**A**). Asbestos bodies were scanty and were much better seen with iron stain (**C**).

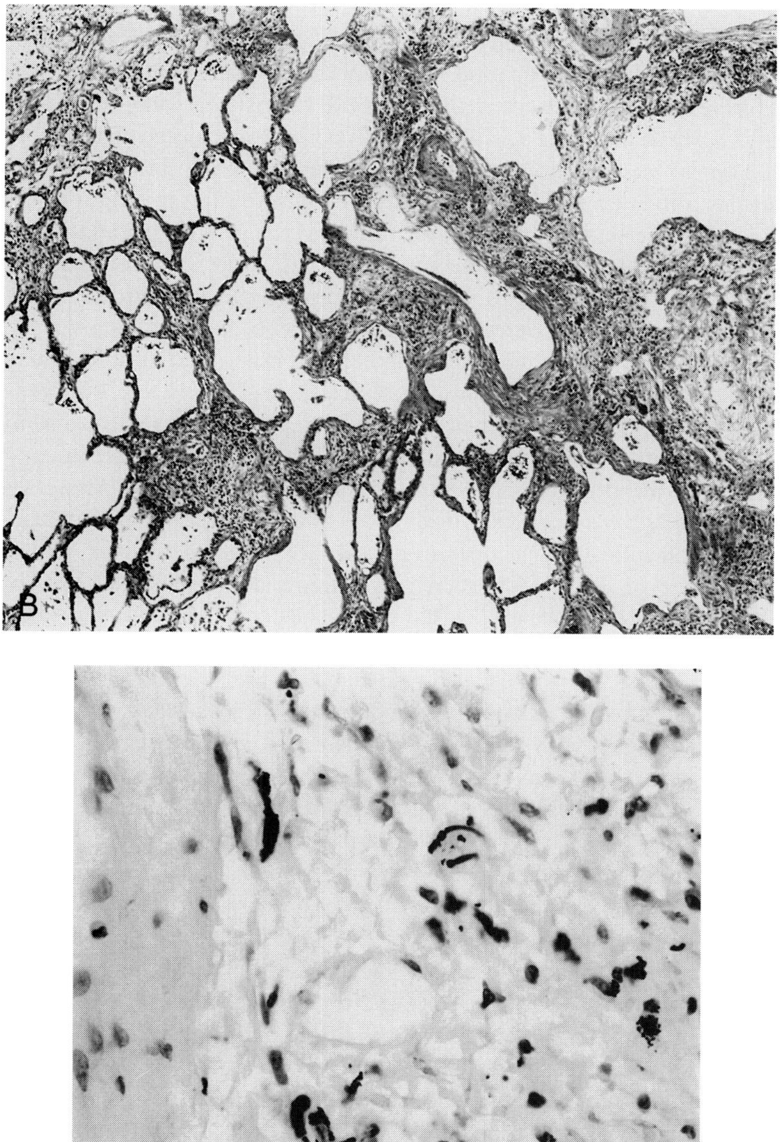

FIGURE 9.14 *(continued)*

ies are described and are illustrated in the colorplates. In asbestosis, asbestos bodies may be seen in airspaces, in the interstitium, and sometimes in isolated giant cells.

A document on diagnostic criteria (79) suggested that one should observe at least two asbestos bodies in tissue sections before rendering a diagnosis of asbestosis. This precaution was meant to avoid the possibility that an asbestos body created by background atmospheric exposure would lead to overdiagnosis of asbestosis in a patient with interstitial fibrosis on some other basis. However, as described previously, Roggli and Pratt (63) calculated that the chance of finding an asbestos body from background exposure in an ordinary iron-stained tissue section is extremely low, about 1%. Combining this figure with the general rarity of interstitial fibrosis of all causes in the general population, the chance of overdiagnosing asbestosis seems very small indeed. Thus, the requirement for two asbestos bodies is probably overcautious; the problem is more theoretic than real, and in my experience once one body is found, others always turn up. Iron stains are extremely helpful in detecting bodies and should always be used if bodies are not visible in routine preparations.

A variety of grading schemes have been proposed to allow a semiquantitative microscopic assessment of asbestosis (79, 201). There are meant as research tools and are not necessary in a diagnostic setting, where the terms *mild*, *moderate*, and *severe* (based on both gross and microscopic examination) suffice.

Cytoplasmic hyaline resembling Mallory bodies of liver cells has been observed in type II cells in the lungs of patients with asbestosis; although they were initially thought to be associated with asbestosis (203), later studies suggest that hyaline may be seen in a variety of conditions and has no diagnostic specificity (204).

Although asbestosis has been examined microscopically for at least 80 years, there are still areas of dispute about criteria for diagnosis. One major problem is early disease and the concept of spread of disease. Some authors view asbestosis as a process that begins in the small airways and progresses by airway-to-airway extension of interstitial fibrosis (79). Airway lesions are described and illustrated earlier in this chapter, and the reasons for not regarding them as asbestosis are discussed. It is likely that asbestosis does actually start around (but not in) small airways, and in some specimens one can see interstitial fibrosis that does appear to be most severe around airways (Fig. 9.15). But in many perfectly acceptable cases this pattern is not obvious and the disease is for all practical purposes microscopically identical to usual interstitial pneumonia except for the presence of asbestos bodies.

Another problem arises when the diagnosis of asbestosis has been suggested on historical or clinical grounds but asbestos bodies cannot be readily found in tissue sections. Gaensler et al. (199) recently examined this issue by looking at a series of patients with interstitial lung disease and known historical asbestos exposure levels. They found that in those with a history of heavy, prolonged exposure and clinical features of asbestosis, asbestos bodies were readily found in tissue sections and the uncoated fiber burden determined by electron microscopy was also high. Conversely, when the history indicated lower exposure, asbestos bodies were not found in tissue sections and the uncoated fiber count was similar to that of a series of unexposed controls.

Roggli (205) similarly analyzed a series of asbestos body–negative cases of diffuse interstitial fibrosis of unknown etiology, and a series of unequivocal asbestosis cases; The fiber burden in all of the cases of unknown etiology was be-

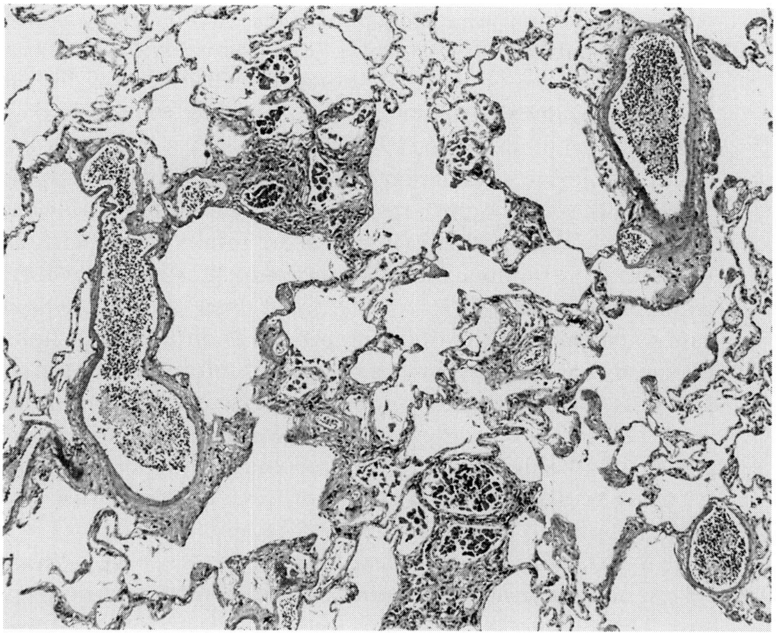

FIGURE 9.15
Early asbestosis in an insulator showing both fibrosis of the airways (asbestos-induced small airway disease) and fine interstitial fibrosis around the airways. The latter is true asbestosis.

low the 95% confidence interval for the burdens in the asbestosis cases. Thus the absence of asbestos bodies in tissue section makes it highly unlikely that the patient has asbestosis, and examination of multiple sections with iron stains to detect asbestos bodies remains the fastest and most economical method of proving the diagnosis.

There are, nonetheless, a few reported cases in which mineral analysis does show large numbers of fibers despite the apparent absence of asbestos bodies in tissue sections (206–208). At least one of these, that of Miller et al. (208), in which innumerable short chrysotile fibers and no other fibers were found, probably reflects specimen contamination, but others may indeed be unusual variants of asbestosis.

Diagnostic Pitfalls. As pointed out by Gaensler et al. (199), there is a tendency for clinicians and pathologists to regard any diffuse interstitial lung disease in those with a history of asbestos exposure as asbestosis. However, all the other types of interstitial lung disease seen in the general population occur in asbestos-exposed workers. This phenomenon is increasing in importance as progressive lowering of exposure standards greatly reduces the incidence of asbestosis (195, 199). Some other disease should be suspected when the history does not indicate heavy exposure, the clinical features are atypical for asbestosis, no asbestos bodies can be seen on iron stains in tissue sections, or the disease process is morphologically another interstitial lesion.

While the statement about morphology may appear unnecessary, it is quite common in my experience for pathologists to refer cases in consultation with a label of asbestosis when an asbestos body is seen or there is a history of exposure, even though another type of distinctly different disease, for example bronchiolitis obliterans organizing pneumonia (BOOP) or even sarcoid, is clearly present. In a patient with a history of asbestos exposure that is not particularly heavy and a lung biopsy that shows diffuse interstitial fibrosis but no asbestos bodies on iron stains, it is perfectly acceptable to make a diagnosis of usual interstitial pneumonia (195, 199) (Fig. 9.16).

If pathologic examination is needed for the diagnosis of asbestosis, an open biopsy, a thoracoscopic biopsy, or a whole lobe (preferably a lower lobe) or lung is required. Transbronchial biopsies are totally inadequate, as they are in usual interstitial pneumonia and other morphologically similar forms of diffuse interstitial lung disease (209). Even with an open biopsy, the pathologist must take care to ensure that the fibrosing process is diffuse, since nonspecific local scars may mimic asbestosis; for this reason consultation with the clinician or radiologist to assess the presence of diffuse disease is important. Furthermore, asbestosis is bilateral and predominantly lower zonal, with worse fibrosis in the periphery. Radiologic evidence of predominantly upper-zone or unilateral disease is strong evidence for some other process, even if diffuse fibrosis and asbestos bodies appear to be present microscopically.

It must again be emphasized that the presence of asbestos bodies by themselves, no matter how numerous, do not constitute asbestosis or any other disease. Diffuse interstitial fibrosis must also be present to allow a diagnosis of asbestosis.

Last, the light microscopic diagnosis of asbestosis by definition is based on the detection of asbestos bodies in 5-μm tissue sections. Thick (30 to 50 μm) sections should not be used because there are no standards to indicate how many bodies one should see in such preparations to make a diagnosis of asbestosis, and these techniques greatly increase the chance of finding asbestos bodies created by background exposure. Electron microscopic fiber counts must be accompanied by data from the laboratory that performed the count indicating their established levels for definite asbestosis.

Role of Cigarette Smoke

Considerable evidence suggests that cigarette smoking increases the incidence of asbestosis and its rate of progression. As described earlier, experiments in small laboratory animals and tracheal explants show that smoke increases asbestos retention, the rate of particle transport into pulmonary epithelial cells, and the degree of asbestos-induced fibrosis (161, 188, 189). Analysis of the asbestos content of human lung parenchyma has generally not shown an effect of smoking (38, 54), but we have demonstrated that smoking dramatically enhances retention of fibers of all types in the airway mucosa (210). Schwartz et al. (211) made the interesting point that a substantial portion of the increased cellularity seen in lavage in cigarette smokers with asbestosis appears to be attributable to the smoke and suggested from these observations that smoke might be important in the pathogenesis of asbestosis.

The issue of smoking and asbestos has generally been assessed by examination of chest radiographs. This approach may be confounded by the ability of cigarette smoke to produce so-called dirty lungs on plain chest radiographs. Nonetheless, Weiss (212) reviewed 21 studies up to 1983 and concluded that the majority favored an interaction between cigarette smoke and asbestos exposure in producing asbestosis. Browne (29) summarizes later reports in detail and also concludes that smoking is a major risk factor for progression.

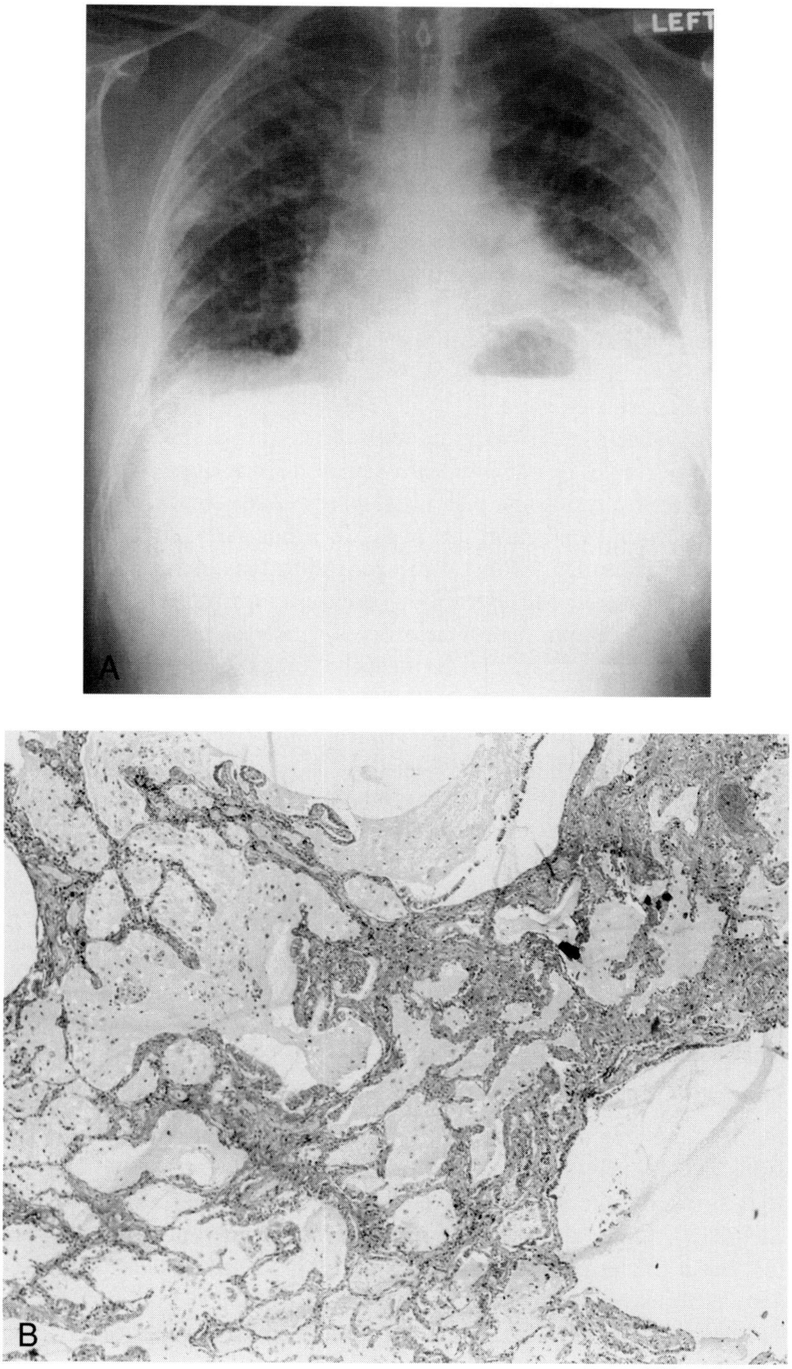

FIGURE 9.16
Usual interstitial pneumonia mimicking asbestosis. This patient had a poorly defined history of asbestos exposure thought to have occurred in a steel mill. He developed diffuse interstitial fibrosis, as seen in his chest radiograph (**A**) and histologically (**B**). However, asbestos bodies were not found in any section, and analysis of his lung tissue failed to reveal any more asbestos than would be expected from background exposure to the general population, indicating that this was indeed not asbestosis.

Progression, Therapy, Prognosis, and Complications

Whether established asbestosis always progresses has been debated in the literature and is reviewed by Browne (29). The older literature, which dealt with very heavily exposed patients, implied that progression was the rule, but recent studies suggest that progression is by no means inevitable. Progression correlates positively with cumulative exposure, age, and smoking and negatively with interval between first exposure and the appearance of radiographic disease. Interestingly, workers with amphibole exposures are much more likely to progress than are workers with pure chrysotile exposures; in chrysotile exposure those with initial films of category less than 1/1 are unlikely to progress. This phenomenon probably reflects rapid clearance of chrysotile but prolonged retention of amphibole in the lung (36). Asbestosis can first appear considerably after cessation of exposure (29, 171, 213, 214).

Severe asbestosis is associated with shortening of life (194, 215, 216). The loss of life expectancy in patients with severe disease appears to be proportional to the degree of physiologic disability. Berry (216), reporting on patients granted disability, found that mortality was 2.6 times as much as was expected. In the study of Huuskonen (194) overall mortality was about 2.5 times expectations, and smokers faired considerably worse than nonsmokers. Patients with asbestosis may die of the parenchymal process, either of respiratory failure or cor pulmonale or of lung cancers or mesotheliomas. Among Huuskonen's workers (194) 42% died of asbestosis; 32%, of lung cancer; and 6%, of other cancers; the ratio of observed to expected risk of lung cancer was 9. Berry (216) reported deaths primarily from asbestosis in 20% of 295 workers with asbestosis and from lung cancer in 38% of these same workers. The lung cancer deaths were a 9.1-fold increase over expected mortality. Lung cancer as a complication of asbestosis is discussed in Chapter 10.

There is no therapy for asbestosis. Steroids and cyclophosphamide appear to be ineffective.

MISCELLANEOUS BENIGN CONDITIONS

Massive fibrosis has occasionally been reported in asbestos workers, largely those engaged in mining asbestos ores in quartz-bearing rock (217). Similarly, lesions of Caplan's type are occasionally seen in asbestos-exposed individuals, but it is unclear whether they are dust-related or real rheumatoid nodules (5, 217–219). Older descriptions of asbestosis sometimes mention bronchiectasis (6), but if the lesions were not just ectatic bronchi caused by honeycombing, the association was undoubtedly fortuitous.

Hammar and Hallman (220) reported a small number of cases of BOOP and a granulomatous process that is histologically identical to sarcoid in patients with known asbestos exposure. Asbestos bodies were visible in the tissue sections and in the granulomas. The paper implies that asbestos is the causative agent of both lesions. However, in my opinion this association amounts to nothing more than documenting the fact that all of the forms of interstitial lung disease that occur in the general population also occur in those with asbestos exposure, and the study design definitely does not allow one to ascribe these lesions to asbestos exposure.

REFERENCES

1. Health Effect Institute, Asbestos Research: Asbestos in public and commercial buildings: a literature review and synthesis of current knowledge. Cambridge, MA: Health Effects Institute, 1991.
2. Dupres JS, Mustard JF, Uffen RJ. Report of the Royal Commission on Matters of Health and Safety Arising from the Use of Asbestos in Ontario. Toronto: Queen's Printer for Ontario, 1984.
3. Selikoff IJ, Lee DHK. Asbestos and Disease. New York: Academic Press, 1978.
4. Becklake MR. Occupational lung disease: past record and future trend using the asbestos case as an example. Clin Invest Med 1983;6:305–337.
5. Parkes WR. Silicates and lung disease. In: Parkes WR, ed. Occupational lung disorders, 2nd ed. London: Butterworths, 1982:233–332.
6. Sebastien P, Plourde M, Robb R, et al. Ambient air asbestos survey in Quebec mining towns: 2. Main study. Environment Canada Report 5/AP/RQ-2E. Ottawa: Environment Canada, 1986.
7. Hendry NW. The geology, occurrences, and major uses of asbestos. Ann N Y Acad Sci 1965;135:12–22.
8. Nicholson WJ, Perkel G, Selikoff IJ. Occupational exposure to asbestos: population at risk and projected mortality—1980–2030. Am J Indust Med 1982;3:259–311.
9. Murphy RL, Levine BW, Al Bazzaz FJ, et al. Floor tile installation as a source of asbestos exposure. Am Rev Respir Dis 1971;104:576–580.
10. Mancuso TF. Mesothelioma among machinists in railroad and other industries. Am J Indust Med 1983;4:501–513.
11. Wagner JC, Sleggs CA, Marchand P. Diffuse pleural mesothelioma and asbestos exposure in the North Western Cape Province. Br J Indust Med 1960;17:260–271.
12. Anderson HA, Lilis R, Daum SM, et al. Household contact asbestos neoplastic risk. Ann N Y Acad Sci 1976;271:310–323.
13. Roggli VL, Long WE. Mineral fiber content of lung tissue in patients with environmental exposures: household contacts vs building occupants. In: Landrigan PJ, Kazemi H, eds. The third wave of asbestos disease: exposure to asbestos in place. New York: New York Academy of Sciences, 1991:511–518.
14. Churg A, Warnock ML. Asbestos fibers in the general population. Am Rev Respir Dis 1980;122:669–678.
15. Churg A, Wiggs B. Fiber size and number in users of processed chrysotile ore, chrysotile miners, and members of the general population. Am J Indust Med 1986; 9:143–152.
16. Weill H, Hughes J, Waggenspack C. Influence of dose and fiber type on respiratory malignancy risk in asbestos cement manufacturing. Am Rev Respir Dis 1979;120: 345–354.
17. Finkelstein MM. Asbestosis in long-term employees of an Ontario asbestos-cement factory. Am Rev Respir Dis 1982;125:496–501.
18. Selikoff IJ, Lilis R, Nicholson WJ. Asbestos disease in United States shipyards. Ann N Y Acad Sci 1979;330:295–312.
19. McDonald JC, Liddell FDK, McDonald AD. The 1891–1920 birth cohort of Quebec chrysotile miners and millers: mortality 1987–1988. Br J Indust Med 1993;50: 1073–1081.
20. Blot WJ, Harrington M, Toledo A, et al. Lung cancer after employment in shipyards during World War II. N Engl J Med 1978;299:620–624.
21. McDonald AD, Fry JS, Woolley AJ, McDonald JC. Dust exposure and mortality in an American chrysotile asbestos friction products plant. Br J Indust Med 1984;41: 151–157.
22. Rohl AN, Langer AN, Wolff MS, Weisman T. Asbestos exposure during brake maintenance and repair. Environ Res 1976;12:110–128.
23. Dement JM, Harris RL, Symons MJ, Shy C. Estimates of dose-response for respiratory cancer among asbestos textile workers. Ann Occup Hyg 1982;26:869–887.

24. McDonald AD, Fry JS, Woolley AJ, McDonald JC. Dust exposure and mortality in an American chrysotile asbestos textile plant. Br J Indust Med 1983;40:361–367.
25. Fischbein A, Rohl AN, Langer AM, Selikoff IJ. Drywall construction and asbestos exposure. Am Indust Hyg Assoc J 1979;40:402–407.
26. Nicholson WJ, Maggiore CJ, Selikoff IJ. Asbestos contamination of parenteral drugs. Science 1972;177:171–173.
27. Cunningham HM, Pontefract R. Asbestos fibers in beverages and drinking water. Nature 1971;232:332–333.
28. Rohl AN, Langer AM, Selikoff IJ, Nicholson WJ. Exposure to asbestos in the use of consumer spackling, patching, and taping compounds. Science 1975;189:551–554.
29. Browne K. Asbestos-related disorders. In: Parkes WR, ed. Occupational lung disorders, 2nd ed. London: Butterworths, 1982:411–504.
30. Timbrell V. Deposition and retention of fibres in the human lung. Ann Occup Hyg 1982;26:347–369.
31. Ashgarian B, Yu CP. Deposition of inhaled fibrous particles in the human lung. J Aerosol Med 1988;1:37–50.
32. Morgan A. Effect of length on the clearance of fibres from the lung and on body formation. In: Wagner JC, ed. Biological effects of mineral fibers. Lyon: International Agency for Research on Cancer, 1980:329–336.
33. Coin PG, Roggli VL, Brody AR. Deposition, clearance, and translocation of chrysotile asbestos from peripheral and central regions of the lung. Environ Res 1992;58:97–116.
34. Roggli VL, Brody AR. Changes in numbers and dimensions of chrysotile asbestos fibers in lungs of rats following short- term exposure. Exp Lung Res 1984;7: 133–147.
35. Roggli VL, George MH, Brody AR. Clearance and dimensional changes of crocidolite asbestos isolated from lungs of rats following short-term exposure. Environ Res 1987;42, 94–105.
36. Churg A. Deposition and clearance of chrysotile. Ann Occup Hyg 1994;38: 625–634.
37. Hume LA, Rimstidt JD. The biodurability of chrysotile asbestos. Am Mineralogist 1992;77:1125–1128.
38. Churg A, Wright JL, Vedal S. Fiber burden and patterns of disease in chrysotile miners and millers. Am Rev Respir Dis 1993;148:25–31.
39. Sebastien P, Begin R, Case BW, McDonald JC. Inhalation of chrysotile dust. In: Wagner JC, ed. The biological effects of chrysotile. Philadelphia: JB Lippincott, 1986:19–29.
40. Wagner JC, Berry G, Skimore JW, Timbrell V. The effects of the inhalation of asbestos in rats. Br J Cancer 1974;29:252–269.
41. McDonald JC, McDonald AD. Epidemiology of malignant mesothelioma. In: Antman K, Aisner J, eds. Asbestos-related malignancy. New York: Grune & Stratton, 1986:57–79.
42. Churg A, Wright JL, Gilks B, DePaoli L. Rapid short term clearance of chrysotile compared to amosite asbestos in the guinea pig. Am Rev Respir Dis 1989;139: 885–890.
43. Mossman BT, Gee JBL. Asbestos-related diseases. N Engl J Med 1989;320: 1721–1730.
44. Mossman BT, Bignon J, Corn M, et al. Asbestos: scientific developments and implications for public policy. Science 1990;294–300.
45. Morgan A, Davies P, Wagner JC, et al. The biological effects of magnesium-leached chrysotile asbestos. Br J Exp Pathol 1977;58:465–473.
46. McDonald JC. Cancer risks due to asbestos and man-made fibres. Recent Results Cancer Res 1990;120:122–133.
47. Churg A, Wright JL, DePaoli L, Wiggs B. Mineralogic correlates of fibrosis in chrysotile miners and millers. Am Rev Respir Dis 1989;139:891–896.

48. Churg A, Wright J, Wiggs B, DePaoli L. Mineralogic parameters related to amosite asbestos–induced fibrosis in man. Am Rev Respir Dis 1990;142:1331–1336.
49. McDonald AD, McDonald JC, Liddell FDK, et al. Mesothelioma in Québec chrysotile miners and millers: epidemiology and etiology. Ann Occup Hyg (in press).
50. Davis JMG, Addison J, Bolton RE, et al. The pathogenicity of long versus short fibre samples of amosite asbestos administered to rats by inhalation and intraperitoneal injection. Br J Exp Pathol 1986;67:415–430.
51. Davis JMG, Jones AF. Comparison of the pathogenicity of long and short fibres of chrysotile asbestos in rats. Br J Exp Pathol 1988;69:717–737.
52. Adamson IYR, Bowden DH. Response of mouse lung to crocidolite asbestos: 1. Mineral fibrosis reaction to short fibres. J Pathol 1987;152:99–107.
53. Adamson IYR, Bowden DH. Response of mouse lung to crocidolite asbestos: 2. Pulmonary fibrosis after long fibres. J Pathol 1987;152:109–117.
54. Churg A, Vedal S. Fiber burden and patterns of asbestos-related disease in workers with heavy mixed amosite and chrysotile exposure. Am J Respir Crit Care Med 1994;150:663–669.
55. Dodson RF, Williams MG, Corn CJ, et al. Asbestos content of lung tissue, lymph nodes, and pleural plaques from former shipyard workers. Am Rev Respir Dis 1990;142:843–847.
56. Sebastien P, Masse R, Bignon J. Recovery of ingested asbestos fibers from the gastrointestinal lymph in rats. Environ Res 1980;22:201–216.
57. Auerbach O, Conston AS, Garfinkel L, et al. Presence of asbestos bodies in organs other than the lung. Chest 1980;77:133–137.
58. Gylseth B, Churg A, Davis JMG, et al. Analysis of asbestos fibers and asbestos bodies in human lung tissue samples: an international laboratory trial. Scand J Work Environ Health 1985;11:107–110.
59. Lee RJ, Florida RG, Stewart IM. Asbestos contamination in paraffin tissue blocks. Arch Pathol Lab Med 1995;119:528–532.
60. Champress PE, Cliff G, Lorimer GW. The identification of asbestos. J Micros 1976; 108:231–249.
61. Churg A, Wiggs B. Types, numbers, and sizes of mineral particles in the lungs of urban male smokers. Environ Res 1987;42:121–129.
62. Churg A, Warnock ML. Asbestos and other ferruginous bodies. Am J Pathol 1981; 102:447–456.
63. Roggli VL, Pratt PC. Numbers of asbestos bodies on iron-stained sections in relation to asbestos body counts in lung tissue digests. Hum Pathol 1983;14:355–361.
64. Warnock ML, Wolery G. Asbestos bodies or fiber and the diagnosis of asbestosis. Environ Res 1987;44:29–44.
65. Sebastien T. Possibilités actuelles de la biometrologie et poussières sur eschantillons de liquide de lavage bronchoalveolaire. Ann Biol Clin 1982;40:279–283.
66. Sebastien P, Janson X, Gaudichet A, et al. Asbestos retention in human respiratory tissues: comparative measurements in lung parenchyma and in parietal pleura. In: Wagner JC, ed. Biological effects of mineral fibers. Lyon: International Agency for Research on Cancer, 1980:237–246.
67. Boutin C, Dumortier P, Rey F, et al. Black spots concentrate oncogenic asbestos fibers in the parietal pleura. Am J Respir Crit Care Med 1996;153:444–449.
68. Suzuki Y, Kohyama N. Translocation of inhaled asbestos fibers from the lung to other tissues. Am J Indust Med 1991;19:701–704.
69. Churg A, Wood P. Observations on the distribution of asbestos fibers in human lungs. Environ Res 1983;31:374–380.
70. Morgan A, Holmes A. Distribution and characteristics of amphibole asbestos fibres, measured with the light microscope, in the left lung of an insulation worker. Br J Indust Med 1983;40:45–50.
71. Roggli VL, Greenberg SD, McLarty JW, et al. Comparison of sputum and lung as-

bestos body counts in former asbestos workers. Am Rev Respir Dis 1980;122: 941–945.
72. Teschler H, Friedrichs KH, Hoheisel GB, et al. Asbestos fibers in broncho alveolar lavage and lung tissue of former asbestos workers. Am J Respir Crit Care Med 1994;149:641–645.
73. DeVuyst P, Jedwab J, Dumortier P, et al. Asbestos bodies in bronchoalveolar lavage. Am Rev Respir Dis 1982;126:972–976.
74. McClarty JW, Greenberg SD, Hurst GA, et al. The clinical significance of ferruginous bodies in sputa. J Occup Med 1980;22:92–96.
75. DiMenza L, Hirsch A, Sebastien P, et al. Assessment of post asbestos exposure in patients: occupational questionnaire versus monitoring in broncho-alveolar lavage. In: Wagner JC, ed. Biological effects of mineral fibers. Lyon: International Agency for Research on Cancer, 1980:609–614.
76. Schwartz DA, Galvin JR, Burmeister LF, et al. The clinical utility and reliability of asbestos bodies in bronchoalveolar lavage fluid. Am Rev Respir Dis 1991;144: 684–688.
77. Gross P, Cralley LJ, De Treveille RTP. "Asbestos" bodies: their nonspecificity. Am Indust Hyg Assoc J 1967;28:541–542.
78. Gross P, deTreville RTP, Haller MN. Pulmonary ferruginous bodies in city dwellers: a study of their central fiber. Arch Environ Health 1969;19:186–188.
79. Craighead JE, Abraham JL, Churg A, et al. The pathology of asbestos-associated diseases of the lungs and pleural cavities: diagnostic criteria and proposed grading schema. Arch Pathol Lab Med 1982;106:544–596.
80. Stewart MJ, Haddow AC. Demonstration of the peculiar bodies of pulmonary asbestosis ("asbestosis bodies") in material obtained by lung puncture and in the sputum. J Pathol Bacteriol 1929;32:172.
81. Sundius N, Bygden A. Der Staubinhalt einer Asbestosis-lunge und die Beschaffenheit der sogenannten Asbestosiskorperchen. Arch Gewerbepathol Gewerbehyg 1938;8:26–70.
82. Pooley FD. Asbestos bodies: their formation, composition, and character. Environ Res 1972;5:363–379.
83. Holden J, Churg A. Asbestos bodies and the diagnosis of asbestosis in chrysotile miners. Environ Res 1986;39:232–236.
84. Suzuki Y, Churg J. Structure and development of the asbestos body. Am J Pathol 1969;55:79–107.
85. Davis JMG. Further observations on the ultrastructure and chemistry of the formation of asbestos bodies. Exp Molec Pathol 1970;13:346–358.
86. Botham SK, Holt PF. Development of asbestos bodies on amosite, chrysotile, and crocidolite fibres in guinea pig lungs. J Pathol 1971;105:159–167.
87. Holmes A, Morgan A. Clearance of anthophyllite fibers from the rat lung and the formation of asbestos bodies. Environ Res 1980;22:13–21.
88. Thomson JG, Kaschula ROC, MacDonald RR. Asbestos as a modern urban hazard. S Afr Med J 1963;37:77–81.
89. Roggli VL, Greenberg SD, Pratt PC. Pathology of asbestos-associated diseases. Boston: Little Brown, 1992.
90. Langer AM, Rubin IB, Selikoff IJ. Chemical characterization of asbestos body cores by electron microprobe analysis. J Histochem Cytochem 1972;20:723–734.
91. Sebastien P, Gaudichet A, Bignon J, Baris YI. Zeolite bodies in human lung from Turkey. Lab Invest 1981;44:420–426
92. Crouch E, Churg A. Ferruginous bodies and the histologic evaluation of dust exposure. Am J Surg Pathol 1984;8:109–116.
93. Case BW, Sebastien P, McDonald JC. Lung fiber analysis in accident victims: a biological assessment of general environmental exposure. Arch Environ Health 1988; 43:178–179.
94. Churg A. Nonneoplastic disease caused by asbestos. In: Churg A, Green FHY, eds. Pathology of occupational lung disease. New York: Igaku-Shoin, 1988:213–278.

95. Roggli VL. Human disease consequences of fiber exposures: a review of human lung pathology and fiber burden data. Environ Health Perspect 1990;88:295–303.
96. Case BW, Sebastien P. Fibre levels in lung and correlation with air samples. In: Bignon J, Peto J, Saracci R, eds. Nonoccupational exposure to mineral fibres. Lyon: International Agency for Research on Cancer, 1989:207–219.
97. Churg A. Lung asbestos content in long-term residents of a chrysotile mining town. Am Rev Respir Dis 1986;134:125–127.
98. McDonald JC. Health implications of environmental exposure to asbestos. Environ Health Perspect 1985;62:329–328.
99. Wagner JC, Newhouse ML, Corrin B, et al. Correlation between fibre content of the lung and disease in East London factory workers. Br J Indust Med 1988, 45: 305–308.
100. Wagner JC, Berry G, Pooley FD. Mesotheliomas and asbestos type in asbestos textile workers. Br Med J 1982;285:603–606.
101. American Thoracic Society. Diagnosis of nonmalignant diseases related to asbestos. Am Rev Respir Dis 1986;134:363–368.
102. Staples CA. Computed tomography in the evaluation of benign asbestos-related disease. Radiol Clin North Am 1992;30:1191–1207.
103. Sargeant EN, Gordonson J, Jacobson G, et al. Bilateral pleural thickening: a manifestation of asbestos dust exposure. Am J Roentgenol 1978;131:579–585.
104. Hillerdal G. The pathogenesis of pleural plaques and pulmonary asbestosis: possibilities and impossibilities. Eur J Respir Dis 1980;61:129–138.
105. Sahn SA, Antony VB. Pathogenesis of pleural plaques: relationship of early cellular response and pathology. Am Rev Respir Dis 1984;130:884–887.
106. Adamson IYR, Bakowska J, Bowden DH. Mesothelial cell proliferation: a nonspecific response to lung injury associated with fibrosis. Am J Respir Cell Molec Biol 1994;10, 253–258.
107. Sekhon H, Wright J, Churg A. Effects of cigarette smoke and asbestos on airway, vascular, and mesothelial cell proliferation. Int J Exp Pathol 1995;76:411–418.
108. Morgan A, Evans JC, Holmes A. Deposition and clearance of inhaled fibrous minerals in the rat: studies using radioactive tracer techniques. In:Walton WH, McGovern B, eds. Inhaled particles 4, part 2. New York: Pergamon Press, 1977: 259–274.
109. Gaensler EA, Carrington CB, Coutu RE, et al. Pathological, physiological, and radiological correlations in the pneumoconioses. Ann N Y Acad Sci 1972;200: 574–607.
110. Thomson JG. The pathogenesis of pleural plaques. In: Shapiro HA, ed. Pneumoconiosis. Proceedings of the International Conference, Johannesburg. London: Oxford University Press, 1970:138–141.
111. Meurman L. Asbestos bodies and pleural plaques in a Finnish series of autopsy cases. Acta Pathol Micro Scand 1966; 181(Suppl):1–107.
112. Ulrich P. Pathologische Anatomie der hyalinen Pleuraplatten. Pneumonol 1971; 146:159–177.
113. Kiviluoto R. Pleural calcification as a roentgenographic sign of nonoccupational endemic anthophyllite-asbestosis. Acta Radiol 1960; 194(Suppl):1–67.
114. Kuwahara M, Kuwahara M, Verma K, et al. Asbestos exposure stimulates pleural mesothelial cells to secrete the fibroblast chemoattractant, fibronectin. Am J Respir Cell Mol Biol 1994;10:167–176.
115. Davis JMG. Asbestos dust as a nucleation center in the calcification of old fibrous tissue lesions and the possible association of this process to the formation of asbestos bodies. Exp Mol Pathol 1970;12:133–147.
116. Weiss W, Levin R, Goodman L. Pleural plaques and cigarette smoking in asbestos workers. J Occup Med 1981;23:427–430.
117. Andrion A, Pira E, Mollo F. Pleural plaques at autopsy, smoking habits, and asbestos exposure. Eur J Respir Dis 1984;65:125–130.

118. Yano E, Tanaka K, Funaki M, et al. Effect of smoking on pleural thickening in asbestos workers. Br J Indust Med 1993;50:898–901.
119. Gibbs AR, Stephens M, Griffiths DM, et al. Fibre distribution in the lungs and pleura of subjects with asbestos related diffuse pleural fibrosis. Br J Indust Med 1991;48:762–770.
120. Voisin C, Marin I, Brochard P, Pairon JC. Environmental airborne tremolite asbestos pollution and pleural plaques in Afghanistan. Chest 1994;106:974–976.
121. Churg A, DePaoli L. Environmental pleural plaques in residents of a Québec chrysotile mining town. Chest 1988;94:58–60.
122. Hillerdal G. Endemic pleural plaques. Eur J Respir Dis 1986;69:1–3.
123. Boutin C, Viallat JR, Steinbauer J, et al. Bilateral pleural plaques in Corsica: a nonoccupational asbestos exposure marker. Eur J Respir Dis 1986;69:4–9.
124. Burilkov T, Michailova L. Asbestos content of the soil and endemic pleural asbestosis. Environ Res 1979;3:443–451.
125. Constantopoulos SH, Malamou-Mitsi VD, Goudevenos JA, et al. High incidence of malignant pleural mesothelioma in neighboring villages of Northwestern Greece. Respiration 1987;51:266–271.
126. Yazicioglu S, Ilcayto R, Balci K, et al. Pleural calcification, pleural mesotheliomas, and bronchial cancers caused by tremolite dust. Thorax 1980;35:564–569.
127. Kiviluoto R. Pleural calcification as a roentgenologic sign of nonoccupational endemic anthophyllite asbestosis. Acta Radiol 1960(Suppl)194:1–67.
128. Artvinli M, Baris YI. Environmental fiber-induced pleuro-pulmonary disease in an Anatolian village: an epidemiological study. Arch Environ Health 1982;37: 177–181.
129. Epler GR, McLoud TC, Gaensler EA. Prevalence and incidence of benign asbestos pleural effusion in a working population. JAMA 1982;247:617–622.
130. Mollo F, Bekkus D, Magnani C, et al. Hyaline splenic and hepatic plaques: correlation with cirrhosis, pulmonary tuberculosis, and asbestos exposure. Arch Pathol Lab Med 1993;117:1017–1021.
131. Gaensler EA, Kaplan AI. Asbestos pleural effusion. Ann Intern Med 1971;74: 178–191.
132. Hillerdal G, Ozesmi M. Benign asbestos pleural effusion:73 exudates in 60 patients. Eur J Repsir Dis 1987;71:113–121.
133. Rossiter CE, Bristol LJ, Cariter PH, et al. Radiographic changes in chrysotile asbestos workers. Arch Environ Health 1972;24:388–394.
134. Jones JSP, Sheers G. Pleural plaques. In: Bogovoski P, Gilson JC, Timbrell V, Wagner JC, eds. Biological effects of asbestos. Lyon: International Agency for Research on Cancer, 1973:243–248.
135. Hourihane D, Lessof L, Richarson PC. Hyaline and calcified pleural plaques as an index of exposure to asbestos. Br Med J 1966;1:1069–1072.
136. Wain SL, Roggli WL, Foster WL. Parietal pleural plaques, asbestos bodies, and neoplasia. Chest 1984;86:707–722.
137. Robinson BWS, Musk AW. Benign asbestos pleural effusion: diagnosis and course. Thorax 1981;36:896–900.
138. Sargeant EN, Jacobson G, Gordonson JS. Pleural plaques: a signpost of asbestos dust inhalation. Semin Roentgenol 1977;12:287–297.
139. Solomon A, Sluis-Cremer GK, Boldstein B. Visceral pleural plaque formation in asbestosis. Environ Res 1979;19:258–264.
140. Solomon A, Sluis-Cremer GK, Thomas RG, Wright VMF. Calcified plaques on mediastinal pleural reflections associated with asbestos dust exposure: four case reports. Am J Indust Med 1984;6:53–57.
141. Oksa P, Suoranta H, Koskinen H, et al. High resolution computed tomography in the early detection of asbestosis. Int Arch Occup Environ Health 1994;65:299–304.
142. Lilis R, Miller A, Godbold J, et al. Pulmonary function and pleural fibrosis. Am J Indust Med 1991;20:145–161.

143. Schwartz DA, Galvin JR, Dayton CS, et al. Determinants of restrictive lung function in asbestos-induced pleural fibrosis. J Appl Physiol 1990;68:1932–1937.
144. Shih JF, Wilson JS, Broderick A, et al. Asbestos-induced pleural fibrosis and impaired exercise physiology. Chest 1994;105:1370–1376.
145. Miller A, Tierstein AS, Selikoff IJ. Ventilatory failure due to asbestos pleurisy. Am J Med 1983;75:911–919.
146. Davies D, Andrew MIJ, Jones JSP. Asbestos-induced pericardial effusion and constrictive pericarditis. Thorax 1991;46:429–432.
147. Mintzer RA, Cugell DW. The association of asbestos-induced pleural disease and rounded atelectasis. Chest 1982;81:457–460.
148. Hillerdal G, Hemmingsson A. Pulmonary pseudotumours and asbestos. Acta Radiol Diagn 1980;21:615–620.
149. Hillerdal G. Rounded atelectasis: clinical experience with 74 patients. Chest 1989; 95:836–841.
150. Lynch DA, Gamsu G, Ray CS, Aberle DR. Asbestos-related focal lung masses: manifestations on conventional and high- resolution CT scans. Radiology ;169: 603–607.
151. Voisin C, Fisekci F, Voisinsaltiel S, et al. Asbestos related rounded atelectasis: radiologic and mineralogic data in 23 cases. Chest 1995;107:477–481.
152. Roberts GH. The pathology of parietal pleural plaques. J Clin Pathol 1971;24: 348–353.
153. Rosen P, Gordon P, Savino A, Melamed M. Ferruginous bodies in benign fibrous pleural plaques. Am J Clin Pathol 1973;60:608–612.
154. Weiss W. Asbestos-related pleural plaques and lung cancer. Chest 1993;103: 1854–1859.
155. Hillerdal G, Lindholm CE. Laryngeal cancer and asbestos. J Otol Relat Spec 1980; 42:233–241.
156. Mollo F, Andrion A, Colombo A, et al. Pleural plaques and risk of cancer in Turin, northwestern Italy. Cancer 1984;54:1418–1422.
157. Wright JL, Cagle P, Churg A, et al. State of the art: disease of the small airways. Am Rev Respir Dis 1992;146:240–262.
158. Wright JL, Churg A. Morphology of small airways disease induced by asbestos exposure. Hum Pathol 1984;15:68–74.
159. Wright JL, Churg A. Severe diffuse small airways disease in long term chrysotile miners. Br J Indust Med 1985;42:556–559.
160. Bégin R, Masse S, Bureau MA. Morphologic features and function of the airways in early asbestosis in the sheep model. Am Rev Respir Dis 1982;126:870–876.
161. Tron V, Wright JL, Harrison N, et al. Cigarette smoke makes airway and early parenchymal asbestos-induced lung disease worse in the guinea pig. Am Rev Respir Dis 1987;136:271–275.
162. Becklake MR. Chronic airflow limitation: its relationship to work in dusty occupations. Chest 1985;88:608–617.
163. Becklake MR. Occupational exposures: evidence for a causal association with chronic obstructive pulmonary disease. Am Rev Respir Dis 1989;140:S85–S91.
164. Oxman AD, Mujir DCF, Shannon HS, et al. Occupational dust exposure and chronic obstructive pulmonary disease: a systematic overview of the evidence. Am Rev Respir Dis 1993;148:38–48.
165. Wright JL, Churg A. Severe diffuse small airways disease in long term chrysotile miners. Br J Indust Med 1985;42:556–559.
166. Filipenko D, Wright JL, Churg A. Pathologic changes in the small airways of the guinea pig after amosite asbestos exposure. Am J Pathol 1985;119:273–279.
167. Bégin R, Masse S, Sebastien P, et al. Asbestos exposure and retention as determinants of airway disease and asbestos alveolitis. Am Rev Respir Dis 1988;134: 1176–1181.
168. Bégin R, Filion R, Ostiguy G. Emphysema in silica- and asbestos-exposed workers seeking compensation. Chest 1995;108:647–653.

169. Harber P, Smitherman J. Asbestosis: diagnostic dilution. J Occup Med 1991;33 786–793.
170. Weill H. Asbestos cement manufacturing. Ann Occup Hyg 1994;38:533–538.
171. Jacobsson K, Stromberg U, Albin M, et al. Radiological changes in asbestos cement workers. Occup Environ Med 1995;52:20–27.
172. Cookson W, de Klerk N, Musk A, et al. The natural history of asbestosis in former crocidolite workers of Wittenoom. Am Rev Respir Dis 1986;133:994–998.
173. Goff AM, Gaensler EA. Asbestosis following brief exposure in cigarette filter manufacture. Respiration 1972;29:83–93.
174. Roggli VL, Pratt PC, Brody AR. Asbestos content of lung tissue in asbestos associated disease: a study of 110 cases. Br J Indust Med 1986;43:18–29.
175. Ashcroft T, Heppleston AG. The optical and electron microscope determination of pulmonary asbestos fibre concentrations and its relation to the human pathological reaction. J Clin Pathol 1973;26:224–234.
176. Whitwell F, Scott J, Grimshaw M. Relationship between occupations and asbestos-fibre content of the lungs in patients with pleural mesothelioma, lung cancer, and other diseases. Thorax 1977;32:377–386.
177. Sebastien P, Mcdonald JC, McDonald AD, et al. Respiratory cancer in chrysotile textile and mining industries: exposure inferences from lung analysis. Br J Indust Med 1989;46:180–187.
178. Rom WN, Travis WD, Brody AR. Cellular and molecular basis of the asbestos-related disease. Am Rev Respir Dis 1991;143:408–422.
179. Warheit DB, Chang LY, Hill LH, et al. Pulmonary macrophage accumulation and asbestos-induced lesions at sites of fiber deposition. Am Rev Respir Dis 1984;129: 301–310.
180. Perdue TD, Brody AR. Distribution of transforming growth factor-B1, fibronectin, and smooth muscle actin in asbestos- induced pulmonary fibrosis in rats. J Histochem Cytochem 1994;42:1061–1070.
181. Liu JY, Morris GF, Lei WH, et al. Up-regulated expression of transforming growth factor-alpha in the bronchioloalveolar duct regions of asbestos exposed rats. Am J Pathol 1996;149:205–217.
182. Bonner JC, Goddell AL, Coin PG, Brody AR. Chrysotile asbestos upregulates gene expression and production of alpha- receptors for platelet derived growth factor (PDGF-AA) on rat lung fibroblasts. J Clin Invest 1993;92:425–430.
183. Pinkerton KE, Elliot A, Frame SR, Warheit DB. Reversibility of fibrotic lesions in rats inhaling size-separated chrysotile asbestos for 2 weeks. Inhaled particles 8 (in press).
184. Mossman BT, Marsh JP. Evidence supporting a role for active oxygen species in asbestos-induced toxicity and lung disease. Environ Health Perspect 1989;81:91–94.
185. Mossman BT, Marsh JP, Sesko A, et al. Inhibition of lung injury, inflammation, and interstitial pulmonary fibrosis by polyethylene glycol-conjugated catalase in a rapid inhalation model of asbestosis. Am Rev Respir Dis 1990;141:1266–1271.
186. Adamson ITR, Bowden DH. Pulmonary reaction to long and short asbestos fibers is independent of fibroblast growth factor production by alveolar macrophages. Am J Pathol 1990;137, 523–529.
187. Adamson IYR, Letourneau HL, Bowden DH. Comparison of alveolar and interstitial macrophages in fibroblast stimulation after silica and long or short asbestos. Lab Invest 1991;64:339–344.
188. Churg A. The uptake of mineral particles by pulmonary epithelial cells. Am J Respir Crit Care Med 1996;154:124–1140
189. McFadden D, Wright J, Wiggs B, Churg A. Smoking increases the penetration of asbestos fibers into airway walls. Am J Pathol 1986;123:95–99.
190. Bégin R, Sebastien P. Excessive accumulation of asbestos fibre in the bronchoalveolar space may be a marker of individual susceptibility to developing asbestosis: experimental evidence. Br J Indust Med 1989;46:853–855.
191. Bégin R, Cantin A, Sebastien P. Chrysotile asbestos exposures can produce an alve-

olitis with limited fibrosing activity in a subset of high fibre retainer sheep. Eur Respir J 1990;3:81–90.
192. Murphy RLJ, Gaensler EA, Ferris BG, et al. Diagnosis of "asbestosis": observations from a longitudinal survey of shipyard pipe coverers. Am J Med 1978;65:488–498.
193. Medical Advisory Panel to the Asbestos International Association. Criteria for the diagnosis of asbestosis and considerations in the attribution of lung cancer and mesothelioma to asbestos exposure. Int Arch Occup Environ Health 1982;49: 357–361.
194. Huuskonen MS. Clinical features, mortality and survival of patients with asbestosis. Scand J Work Environ Health 1978;4:265–274.
195. Parkes WR. An approach to the differential diagnosis of asbestosis and nonoccupational diffuse interstitial pulmonary fibrosis. In: Parkes WR III, ed. Occupational lung disorders. 3rd ed. London: Butterworths, 1994:505–535.
196. Muller NL, Miller RR. Computed tomography of chronic diffuse infiltrative lung disease. Am Rev Respir Dis 1990;142:1206–1215, 1440–1448.
197. Staples Ca, Gamsu G, Ray CS, Webb WR. High resolution computed tomography and lung function in asbestos-exposed workers with normal chest radiographs. Am Rev Respir Dis 1989;139:891–896.
198. Bergin CJ, Castellino RA, Blank N, Moses L. Specificity of high-resolution CT findings in pulmonary asbestosis: do patients scanned for other indications have similar findings. Am J Roentgenol 1994;163:551–555.
199. Gaensler EA, Jederlinic PJ, Churg A. Idiopathic pulmonary fibrosis in asbestos-exposed workers. Am Rev Respir Dis 1991;144:689–696.
200. Hourihane DO'B, McCaughey WTE. Pathological aspects of asbestosis. Postgrad Med 1966;42:613–622.
201. Hinson KFW, Otto H, Webster I, Rossiter CE. Criteria for the diagnosis and grading of asbestosis. In: Bogovski P et al., eds. Biological effects of asbestos. Oxford, UK: Pergamon Press, 1973:54–57.
202. Churg A. A procedure for inflation of lung biopsies. Am J Surg Pathol 1983;7: 69–72.
203. Kuhn C, Kuo TT. Cytoplasmic hyalin in asbestosis: a reaction of injured alveolar epithelium. Arch Pathol 1973;95:190–194.
204. Warnock ML, Press M, Churg A. Further observations on cytoplasmic hyaline in the lung. Hum Pathol 1980;11:59–66.
205. Roggli VL. Scanning electron microscopic analysis of mineral fiber content of lung tissue in the evaluation of diffuse pulmonary fibrosis. Scan Micros 1991;5:71–83.
206. Dodson R, Williams MG, O'Sullivan MF, et al. A comparison of the ferruginous and uncoated fiber content in the lungs of former asbestos workers. Am Rev Respir Dis 1985;132:143–147.
207. Seal RME. Current views on pathological aspects of asbestosis: the unresolved questions and problems. In: Wagner JC, ed. Biological effects of mineral fibers. Lyon: International Agency for Research on Cancer, 1980:217–235.
208. Miller A, Langer AM, Tierstein AS, Selikoff IJ. "Nonspecific" interstitial pulmonary fibrosis: association with asbestos fibers detected by electron microscopy. N Engl J Med 1975;292:91–94.
209. Wall CP, Gaensler EA, Carrington CB, Hayes JA. Comparison of transbronchial and open biopsies in chronic infiltrative lung disease. Am Rev Respir Dis 1981;123: 280–285.
210. Churg A, Stevens B. Enhanced retention of asbestos fibers in the airways of human smokers. Am J Respir Crit Care Med 1995;151:1409–1413.
211. Schwartz DA, Galvin JR, Merchant RK, et al. Influence of cigarette smoking on bronchoalveolar lavage cellularity in asbestos-induced lung disease. Am Rev Respir Dis 1992;145:400–405.
212. Weiss W. Cigarette smoke, asbestos, and small irregular opacities. Am Rev Respir Dis 1984;130:293–301.
213. Viallat JR, Boutin C, Pietri JF, Fondarai J. Late progression of radiographic changes

in Canari chrysotile mine and mill exworkers. Arch Environ Health 1983;38: 54–58.
214. Cookson M, de Klerk N, Musk WA, et al. Natural history of asbestosis in former crocidolite workers of Wittenoom Gorge. Am Rev Respir Dis 1986;133:994–998.
215. Coutts II, Turner-Warwick M. Factors predicting outcome in intrapulmonary fibrosis associated with asbestos exposure (asbestosis). In: Gee JBL, Morgan WKC, eds. Occupational lung disease. New York: Raven Press, 1984:208–209.
216. Berry G. Mortality of workers certified by pneumoconiosis medical panels as having asbestosis. Br J Indust Med 1981;38:130–137.
217. Solomon A, Goldstein B, Webster I, Sluis-Cremer GK. Massive fibrosis in asbestosis. Environ Res 1971;4:430–439.
218. Greaves IA. Rheumatoid pneumoconiosis (Caplans syndrome) in an asbestos worker: a 17 years' follow-up. Thorax 1979;34:404–405.
219. Mattson SB. Caplan's syndrome in association with asbestosis. Scand J Respir Dis 1971;52:153–161.
220. Hammar SP, Hallman KO. Localized inflammatory pulmonary disease in subjects occupationally exposed to asbestos. Chest 1993;103:1792–1799.

CHAPTER 10

Neoplastic Asbestos-Induced Disease

❖ Andrew Churg

INTRODUCTION

As indicated in Chapter 9, progressive lowering of standards for permitted occupational exposure to asbestos has markedly decreased the incidence and severity of asbestosis. Benign pleural disease, particularly plaque, is still seen with considerable frequency, but it generally has little or no functional import. On the other hand, neoplasms, whether actually caused by asbestos or merely claimed to be caused by it, have become the area of greatest concern in the field of asbestos-related disease.

There are major gaps and problems in our understanding of asbestos-related neoplasms. A fundamental problem is the lack of understanding of the mechanisms by which asbestos produces tumors and why this process appears to be different for lung cancers and mesotheliomas. Another equally important question is exactly what tumors are associated with asbestos exposure. Although there is no doubt of the association of carcinoma of the lung with asbestosis and malignant mesothelioma of the pleura and peritoneum, the situation for other tumors is disputed. A related question is whether the low asbestos levels to which the general population is exposed are potentially dangerous. Last, both fiber type and industrial process or product appear to affect the type and incidence of asbestos-induced malignancies in complicated ways that are not entirely clear.

CARCINOMA OF THE LUNG

Epidemiologic and Related Data

Epidemiologic studies show a definite association between heavy occupational exposure to asbestos and an excess risk of lung cancer (1–5). However, essentially all of the (positive) data on the relation between asbestos exposure and lung cancer were derived from studies of workers exposed at what would today be considered quite high levels, and where information exists, many of these workers turn out to have asbestosis (discussed later). Thus the oft-repeated statement that "asbestos causes lung cancer" is an oversimplification. In fact the questions of the amount of exposure required to produce an excess lung cancer risk and whether the risk is increased only in the presence of asbestosis are greatly disputed. These issues are important for understanding how asbestos induces disease, for setting exposure standards, and for compensation of workers.

McDonald (4), reviewing a large number of series, concluded that lung cancer accounted for up to 26% of deaths in some groups of asbestos workers, whereas in men in the United States and Britain during the same period it accounted for about 5 to 9% of deaths. When an excess risk is observed, this is not apparent until about 10 years from exposure, and there appears to be a peak in incidence at about 30 years from first exposure (3, 4, 6).

At high occupational exposure levels there is a dose–response relation between exposure and lung cancer incidence, and at these levels this relation is more or less linear (3, 4, 7). However, as was noted in the discussion of asbestosis in Chapter 9, there are quite marked differences in lung cancer incidence, and thus in the slope of the exposure–incidence relation, by type of industry. The chrysotile mining and milling industry and the chrysotile friction products industry have relatively low risks of lung cancer. The cement and mixed-products industries have a somewhat greater risk, and by far the highest risk is seen in chrysotile textile workers (1, 3).

Why the risk varies among industries is unclear. In part it may reflect the use of amphiboles (amosite and crocidolite) as compared with chrysotile. McDonald (1, 4) summarized data from 42 cohorts in the literature and noted that the excess lung cancer mortality in those with exposure to amphiboles was 6.3%, whereas in those with exposure only to chrysotile it was 1.8%. It is likely that there are also process-specific effects. It has been postulated that the fibers encountered by textile workers are longer and thus in theory more pathogenic than those encountered by chrysotile miners and millers (8), but two studies examined this question and came to opposite conclusions (9, 10). It has also been suggested that oils sprayed on the fibers in the textile industry may be carcinogenic (3, 11). However, a much simpler explanation for the increased risk of lung cancer in textile workers is that they are at increased risk for asbestosis (8) (compare the asbestosis risks by industry in Figure 9.12; the lung cancer incidence data show a remarkably similar pattern).

An additional important factor is the role of cigarette smoking. It was initially believed that an increased risk of asbestos-associated lung cancers was seen only in cigarette smokers, but subsequent studies suggest an excess risk for nonsmokers as well (4, 12, 13). However, the number of nonsmokers on which these estimates are based is quite small. It is generally agreed that in those with heavy exposure the combination of cigarette smoke and asbestos produces a more than additive risk; that is, the incidence of lung cancer in asbestos-exposed smokers is greater than would be expected from simply adding the two separate risks. Whether the risks are multiplicative, as in Table 10.1, or less than multiplicative but more than additive (Table 10.2) is debated (3). In all probability the pattern varies from cohort to cohort.

While these data are more or less agreed on, prevailing opinions on the exact relation of occupational asbestos exposure and lung cancer are quite discrepant. These opinions can be divided into three broad groups: (*a*) Any exposure to asbestos increases the risk of lung cancer. (*b*) Only relatively heavy exposure (probably sufficient to produce asbestosis) increases risk. (*c*) Only the actual presence of asbestosis increases risk (14–17).

TABLE 10.1
Relative Risk of Dying of Lung Cancer in Asbestos Insulation Workers

GROUP	RELATIVE RISK
Nonsmokers, no asbestos exposure	1.00
Nonsmokers with asbestos exposure	5.17
Smokers, no asbestos exposure	10.85
Smokers with asbestos exposure	53.24

Adapted with permission from Hammond EC, Selikoff IJ, Seidman H. Asbestos exposure, cigarette smoking, and death rates. Ann N Y Acad Sci 1979;330:473–491.

TABLE 10.2
Risk of Dying of Lung Cancer for Workers in the Québec Chrysotile Industry

	ASBESTOS EXPOSURE CATEGORY		
SMOKING CATEGORY	LOW	MODERATE	HIGH
Nonsmokers	1.0	2.0	6.9
Moderate smokers	6.3	7.5	12.8
Heavy smokers	11.8	13.3	25.0

Adapted with permission from McDonald JC, Liddell FDK, Gibbs GW, et al. Dust exposure and mortality in chrysotile mining, 1910–1975. Br J Indust Med 1980;37:11–24.

The idea that any exposure to asbestos, no matter how small, leads to an increase in lung cancer risk is unsupported by any direct epidemiologic evidence (in fact it is contradicted by a great deal of evidence, as discussed later); it depends in large part on extrapolations of dose–response curves from high-exposure conditions over several orders of magnitude to much lower-exposure conditions, even down to the levels of ambient asbestos encountered by the general population (Chapter 9). The scientific validity of such extrapolations is at best dubious (8, 18, 19).

The other basis of this theory stems from observations in tissue culture systems, in which under certain conditions asbestos damages DNA or affects cell proliferation. There are quite marked differences in the responses of different cell types to asbestos fibers: tracheobronchial epithelial cells are relatively resistant to the effects of asbestos, but mesothelial cells are highly sensitive (see section on pathogenesis). More to the point, positive tissue culture experiments in the face of negative epidemiologic findings must raise doubts about the significance of the in vitro data rather than the other way around.

The notion that only relatively high level exposure increases risk can be summarized thus: asbestos-induced lung cancers do not appear until a threshold cumulative exposure has been reached, and this threshold is in the range of the cumulative exposure required to produce asbestosis.

The evidence for a threshold effect is quite strong (8). Various epidemiologic and fiber burden studies have been carried out on residents of the chrysotile mining townships of Québec who never worked in the mining and milling industry. This population has had lifelong ambient asbestos exposures much higher than those of ordinary urban dwellers (20) (see Table 9.4). As described in Chapter 9, fiber burden studies show that they carry a considerably greater fiber load than do residents of urban areas of North America. Nonetheless, once those employed in the mining and milling industry are excluded, epidemiologic investigations fail to demonstrate an increased lung cancer risk in the mining townships (18).

A number of studies describe cohorts of workers with relatively low-level exposure (in the range of one to five fibers per cubic centimeter) and also fail to show any increased risk of lung cancer (21–23). Examining workers with still higher exposure, Browne reviewed a number of older epidemiologic studies and noted that every report showed a threshold for increased lung cancer risk; several subsequent investigations (5, 24, 25) came to the same conclusion. The threshold level of exposure at which an increased risk is seen in this whole group of studies is in the range reported to produce asbestosis (see Chapter 9).

These data thus set relatively high exposure as a necessary condition for an increased lung cancer risk, but both animal and human studies suggest that it is specifically asbestosis that confers the risk. Davis and Cowie (26) reviewed the published data on induction of asbestosis in laboratory animals. While they pointed out that none of these investigations was actually designed to examine the question of lung cancer, it was nonetheless found that where cancers did occur, the tumors appeared to be spatially associated with the fibrosing process and that overall the incidence of cancers paralleled the degree of fibrosis.

There is no doubt that in workers receiving compensation for asbestosis the incidence of lung cancer is very high, ranging up to 50% of deaths in some series and averaging about 30% of deaths (27–31). Most epidemiologic studies do not provide data on the presence or absence of asbestosis, but those that do strongly support the association of lung cancer and asbestosis. The original report of Doll (32) described 11 lung cancer deaths, all associated with asbestosis, versus 0.8 expected. In those without asbestosis no lung cancers were found. Bohlig et al. (33), using chest radiographs, found a rate of 8 lung cancers per 1000 in workers with severe asbestosis, 1 per 1000 workers in those with minimal asbestosis, and 0.4 per 1000 in those without asbestosis. The last figure is equivalent to the rate seen in the general population. Liddell and McDonald (34) examined chest radiographs of chrysotile miners and millers and found a standard mortality ratio for lung cancer of 3.5 in those with evidence of asbestosis but only 1.08 (statistically not elevated) in those without.

Two retrospective pathologic studies also lend weight to the idea that lung cancer risk is specifically linked to asbestosis. Kipen et al. (35) and Newhouse et al. (36) examined the lungs of heavily exposed workers selected because they had lung cancer; they reported asbestosis in 100 and 90%, respectively, of the histologic sections. These numbers suggest that all of the excess lung cancer incidence in heavily exposed workers is accounted for by asbestosis.

This issue has also been examined in two prospective studies containing data on both asbestosis and cumulative exposure. Hughes and Weill (37) investigated the incidence of lung cancer as a function of radiographic asbestosis in asbestos cement workers, and Sluis-Cremer and Bezuidenhout (38) performed a similar study using autopsy lungs from amosite miners. In both studies an increased rate of lung cancer was found only in the presence of asbestosis (Table 10.3). Both studies provided data on measured cumulative exposure, and in neither did cumulative exposure explain the presence of lung cancer, although Sluis-Cremer and Bezuidenhout (38) found a weak association with years of exposure. Overall these studies provide strong support for the notion that asbestosis is crucial to the development of asbestos-associated lung cancers.

This idea has considerable biologic plausibility, since diffuse interstitial fibrosis of any origin increases lung cancer risk. Quite markedly elevated lung cancer rates have been reported in large series of cases of idiopathic interstitial fibrosis by Turner-Warwick et al. (39) and by Nagai et al. (40). In the latter study lung cancer occurred in 11% of the nonsmokers and 38% of the smokers.

All of the reports described thus far specifically examined cohorts of asbestos-exposed workers. Several recent epidemiologic studies attempt to refute the specific association of asbestosis and lung cancer using retrospective analyses of hospitalized lung cancer patients (41), analyses of lung cancer incidence by postal code (42), and what are best described as theoretic arguments based on expected ratios of lung cancers to mesotheliomas (43). None of these studies used worker groups with documented asbestos exposure; none provides any real information about measured exposure or about asbestosis; and none of them in my opinion succeeds in denying the association. The details of these reports are beyond the scope of this book, but the interested reader is referred to the commentary by Jones et al. (44).

Some authors have attempted to approach this question by examining fiber burden. Warnock and Isenberg (45), in a study that is very difficult to understand, quantified fiber burden in 62 smokers with a history of asbestos exposure. It appears from their descriptions that at least 50 of these patients had asbestosis and that the more severe the asbestosis, the higher the fiber burden found. As discussed in Chapter 9, this latter observation has been made many times; however, nothing in the Warnock and Isenberg paper sheds any light on whether lung cancer risk is increased in the absence of asbestosis.

More recently, Karjalainen et al. (46) examined the risk of lung cancer as a function of fiber burden in a series of 113 surgical lung cancer patients and 297 autopsy controls. Although the abstract to the paper indicates that risk of lung cancer increased as asbestos fiber burden increased, and that the risk was greater for adenocarcinoma than for squamous cell carcinoma, in fact the correct statistical interpretation is that over all cases the risk was not increased for squamous carcinoma. More important, when the authors removed the patients with asbestosis from their analysis, the association of increased fiber burden and lung cancer risk disappeared. Thus these data actually support the specific association of lung cancer and asbestosis.

TABLE 10.3
Relation of Asbestosis to Lung Cancer in Two Recent Studies

REPORT	ASBESTOSIS	SMR	SIGNIFICANT INCREASE?
Hughes and Weill (37)	None	1.06	No
Chest radiograph, asbestos cement workers	Present	4.32	Yes
Sluis-Cremer and Bezuidenhout (38)	None	0.89	No
Autopsy pathology, amosite asbestos miners	Mild	4.17	Yes
	Moderate to severe	5.65	Yes

SMR = standardized mortality ratio.

Pathogenesis

As was described for the pathogenesis of asbestosis in Chapter 9, an enormous variety of observations concerning possible mechanisms of asbestos-induced carcinogenesis have been published; the problems are to determine which are relevant and to differentiate mechanisms that apply to the genesis of lung cancer as opposed to mesothelioma.

Asbestos is unusual in that unlike all other accepted human carcinogens except conjugated estrogens, it is not active in the commonly employed bacterial mutation assays or rodent bone marrow assays for detection of chromosomal aberrations and micronucleated erythrocytes (47, 48). However, more sophisticated approaches using hamster–human hybrid cell lines reveal that asbestos does induce a variety of deletion mutations (49, 50). These effects appear to be mediated through the fiber-catalyzed formation of active oxygen species (51, 52). In mesothelial cell lines asbestos produces chromosomal abnormalities and aneuploidy, in part by penetration into the cell and direct interference with the mitotic apparatus (53, 54), and in part through oxidant-mediated mechanisms, but tracheobronchial epithelial cells appear to be relatively resistant to these effects (52).

While asbestos appears to behave as a complete carcinogen for mesothelial cells, the effects of asbestos on the bronchial epithelium are in many respects like those of classic tumor promotors: long but not short asbestos fibers lead to dose-dependent induction of ornithine decarboxylase as well as protein kinase C, both markers of cell proliferation, and characteristic findings with chemical tumor promotors (55, 56). More recent data suggest that asbestos fibers can activate the proto-oncogenes c-fos and c-jun, which encode transcription factors intrinsic to initiation of DNA synthesis (52, 57). Again, the effects are more marked in mesothelial than in tracheal epithelial cells. Asbestos also causes induction of NF-κB–dependent gene expression in tracheal epithelial cells (58); these genes, which include interleukins, nitric oxide synthetase, and the proto-oncogene c-myc, are important in cell proliferation and inflammation.

Asbestos fibers can also interact with other carcinogens in ways that may be very important in explaining the role of cigarette smoke. As noted in Chapter 9, one of the effects of cigarette smoke is to increase fiber retention in the lung and fiber penetration into tissues. In experimental systems asbestos fibers adsorb and enhance the transport of carcinogens such as benzo(a)pyrene into cells (59), and this observation is probably also true of the numerous other carcinogenic components of cigarette smoke. Once in the cells, asbestos fibers may enhance the generation of the active carcinogenic metabolites of substances such as benzo(a) pyrene (52). Thus the effect of smoke may be to increase the total dose of adsorbed carcinogen delivered to target tissues.

The mechanistic reasons for the association of lung cancer with asbestosis are as yet unclear. However, as several groups have noted and as has been described in Chapter 9 in regard to the development of asbestosis, in experimental animals treated with asbestos there is an association of chronic inflammation, oxidant production, cytokine production, fibrosis, and chronic cell proliferation; and chronic cell proliferation in general is associated with the appearance of malignancies (52, 60) (see Chapter 9).

Clinical Features

The clinical features of carcinoma in asbestos workers, apart from manifestations of asbestosis and benign pleural disease, are no different from those seen in individuals without asbestos exposure.

Pathologic Features

For the pathologist the basic question regarding asbestos-induced lung cancers is whether any features other than the concomitant presence of asbestosis (Figs. 9.13 and 10.1) allow one to determine whether a particular tumor is caused by asbestos. Two features are frequently cited when this problem arises: tumor site and histologic subtype.

As shown in Table 10.4, the majority of ordinary cigarette smoke–induced lung tumors arise in the upper lobes (upper to lower lobe ratio approximately 2:1). By contrast, in some studies of asbestos workers carcinomas are more frequent in the lower lobes; Kannerstein and Churg (62) found a ratio of approximately 1:1.5 for upper to lower lobes; Whitwell et al. (63), a ratio of approximately 1:3.5; Hourihane and McCaughey (64), a ratio of 1:2; and Karjalainen et al. (67), a ratio of approximately 1:2. However, Auerbach et al. (65) observed that two-thirds of the tumors in asbestos insulation workers were in the upper lobes, and Johanssen et al. (66) reported similar findings in asbestos cement workers. It has also sometimes been claimed that the asbestos tumors are peripheral (63, 66), but Kannerstein and Churg (62) were unable to show any differences in peripheral versus central tumor distribution between tumors in asbestos workers and in controls.

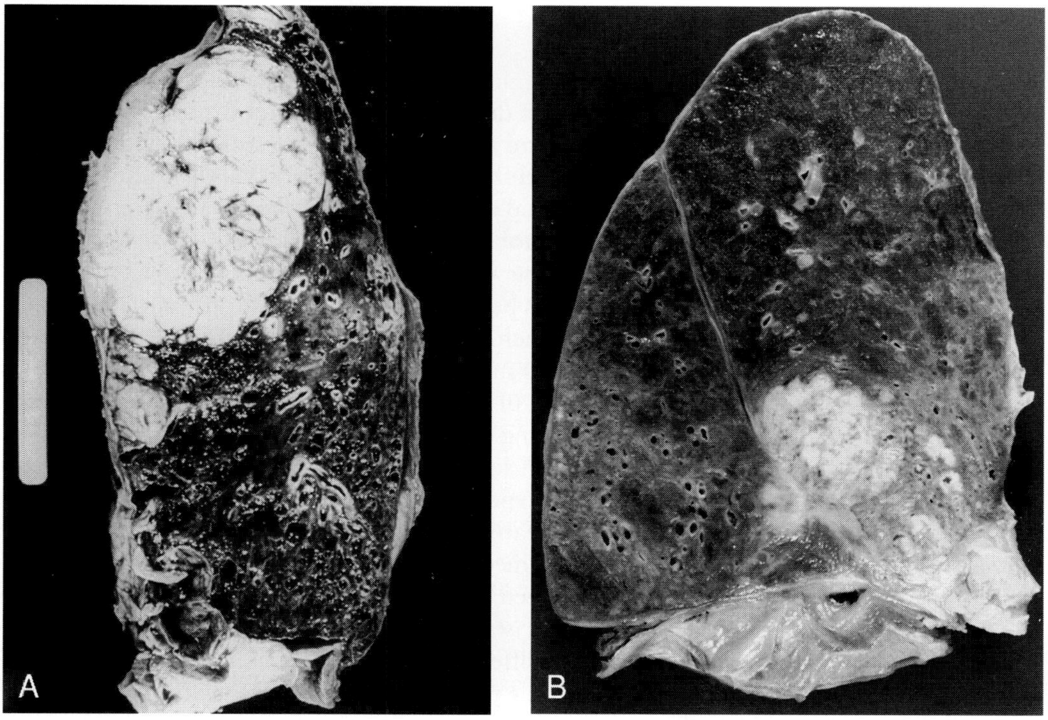

FIGURE 10.1

A. A carcinoma of the lung in a worker with asbestosis. This man worked in an asbestos processing plant for many years. This particular tumor violates all of the "rules" some have promulgated regarding asbestos-related tumors: it occurs in the upper lobe and is an oat cell carcinoma. In practice asbestos-related carcinomas can have any histologic type and any location in the lung. In this instance the association with asbestosis, seen as marked honeycombing in the lower lobe, indicates that asbestos caused the tumor. **B.** An adenocarcinoma in the lower lobe in a different patient who also has asbestosis. Asbestos-induced pleural fibrosis is also present.

TABLE 10.4
Ratios of Upper to Lower Lobe Lung Cancers in Patients with and without Asbestos Exposure

REPORT	UPPER LOBE[a]	LOWER LOBE
Control		
Garland et al. (61)	64%	36%
Control		
Kannerstein and Churg (62)	71	29
Exposed		
Kannerstein and Churg (62)	41	59
Exposed		
Whitwell et al. (63)	22	78
Exposed		
Hourihane and McCaughey (64)	35	65
Exposed		
Auerbach et al. (65)	66	34
Exposed		
Johanssen et al. (66)	66	34
Exposed		
Karjalainen et al. (67)	39	61

[a] Ignoring middle-lobe tumors.

A great deal of effort has been devoted in the literature to the propositions that specific types of carcinoma are associated with asbestos and with other occupational exposures (68, 69) and that such information can be useful in determining the association of individual cases of lung cancer with asbestos exposure. However, the importance of intraobserver variations in the histologic typing of lung cancer, differences in frequency of histologic types between biopsy and resection specimens, and differences between surgical and autopsy specimens have largely been ignored in making such assertions. Another issue that has not been generally appreciated is the secular increase in the frequency of adenocarcinomas and the decrease in the frequency of squamous carcinomas; the former are now the most frequent single type of lung cancer in the United States in non–asbestos-exposed cigarette smokers of both sexes (68, 69). Last, there may be differences in the frequency of different cell types in Europe and North America.

In practice these problems mean that basing data in regard to lung cancer types on unreviewed diagnoses in medical records or death certificates must have a huge inherent error and that even when cases have been reviewed and classified by a single pathologist, there is a good chance that another equally competent pathologist could arrive at different results. These considerations have led two reviewers (68, 69) to conclude that aside from the association of small cell carcinoma with radiation and with chloromethyl ether exposure, there are no specific associations of lung cancer cell type and particular occupational exposures.

Nonetheless, assertions about histologic cell type and asbestos exposure abound in the literature. It is commonly stated that adenocarcinoma is the cell type most frequently seen in asbestos-related cancers (70, 71), but the data to support this claim are dubious. The report most frequently cited as demonstrating a high frequency of adenocarcinoma is that of Whitwell et al. (63). In that study 35% of lung cancers (counting both men and women) were adenocarcinoma. It is true that this was the highest value of any histologic subtype, but it is scarcely an overwhelming percentage. Moreover, comparison of asbestos-exposed and control cases, using those necropsy values, shows no statistical difference between exposed and control groups. In the other four series in Table 10.5 that have internal control groups there is a preponderance of squamous carcinomas in three reports and a roughly even distribution in one; in fact, only the relatively recent report of Johannsen et al. (66) shows any apparent increase in adenocarcinoma. It is true that Hourihane and McCaughey (64) found that 46% of cases and Hasan et al. (73), that 50% of carcinomas in documented series of asbestosis cases were adenocarcinomas. However, the series were very small (26 and 12 cases, respectively) and contained a large proportion of women, in whom adenocarcinomas were much more common in the past (68, 69), and no control data were presented.

More recently Raffin et al. (74) examined lung cancer by histologic type in Danish asbestos cement workers and found an elevated risk of both adenocarcinoma and squamous carcinoma, with a greater elevation for adenocarcinoma. However, Karjalainen et al. (67) found no differences between exposed and control populations in regard to histologic type, although they claimed in a subsequent study (46) that increasing asbestos fiber burden was associated with an increased risk of adenocarcinoma. However, their results appear to depend entirely on the presence of asbestosis.

There is also a persisting belief that carcinomas arising in patients with asbestosis should be adenocarcinomas because adenocarcinomas are said to be more common in idiopathic or collagen disease–associated interstitial fibrosis (16). In fact two large series reporting lung cancer in patients with idiopathic

TABLE 10.5

Comparison of Cell Types in Series of Lung Cancers from Patients with Asbestos Exposure and Internal Control Cases

REPORT			SQUAMOUS	SMALL CELL	ADENO-CARCINOMA	LARGE CELL
Kannerstein and Churg (62)	Exposed	N = 39	28%	28%	28%	15%
	Control	N = 43	28	33	21	19
Whitwell et al. (63)	Exposed	N = 93	23	28	35	14
	Control	N = 96	18	40	30	13
Martischnig et al. (72)	Exposed	N = 49	53	45	2	0
	Control	N = 112	69	24	7	0
Auerbach et al. (65)	Exposed	N = 193	50	25	15	10
	Control	N = 648	52	16	19	14
Blot (cited by Ives [68])	Exposed	N = 36	67	19	14	0
	Control	N = 161	64	17	19	0
Johanssen et al. (66)	Exposed	N = 29	37	17	31%	14
	Control	N = 87	48	26	15%	10

interstitial fibrosis documented all of the usual histologic types seen in cigarette smokers (39, 40).

The practical lessons I draw from these observations are these: (*a*) There is no consistent evidence that tumors associated with asbestos exposure have different sites of origin from those without asbestos exposure. (b) Asbestos-related tumors can occur in any lobe. (*c*) The data on cell type indicate that all of the types of carcinomas that occur in cigarette smokers occur in asbestos workers. Thus *cell type has no value in determining whether a given case was or was not caused by exposure to asbestos.*

How can these observations be applied to the individual case in which the pathologist is asked to determine whether a given tumor is associated with asbestos exposure? I follow a very simple scheme: If asbestosis is present pathologically or by good radiographic evidence (Fig. 10.1), the carcinoma should be ascribed to asbestos exposure; this practice is entirely consistent with the existing data. Small airway disease caused by asbestos (Chapter 9), which some believe is the earliest form of asbestosis, also involves tissue scarring and probably should be treated as if it were asbestosis for this purpose. If the patient is or was a smoker, smoking also contributed to causation. If asbestosis is not present by clinical or pathologic criteria, the tumor should not be ascribed to asbestos exposure; the usual causative agent in such cases is cigarette smoke.

MALIGNANT MESOTHELIOMA

The very existence of tumors originating in the pleura has been a matter of considerable historical controversy. In the 1930s Klemperer and Rabin (75) popularized the term *mesothelioma* for primary pleural tumors and suggested the division of such neoplasms into local and diffuse forms. Nonetheless, the existence of primary mesothelial tumors was still questioned in standard textbooks as late as the 1960s (76). It was proposed that all such tumors were metastases, lesions arising from endothelial cells, or lesions arising from embryonic rests of lung (77). While these theories have primarily historical interest, they do emphasize the fact that the diagnosis of mesothelioma can be difficult. The work of Stout and Murray (77), who showed that cultured mesothelial cells could grow in both epithelial and spindled forms, helped explain the varied appearances of tumors claimed to be primary in the pleura. Cases of what are in retrospect clearly mesotheliomas were described during the first half of this century (78), but it was not until Wagner et al. (79) reported the association of crocidolite asbestos exposure and the development of mesothelioma in 1960 that real interest was generated in both the epidemiologic associations and pathologic features of these tumors.

The only type of mesothelioma proved to be associated with asbestos exposure is diffuse malignant mesothelioma of the pleura and peritoneum. Nomenclature is confusing in this area because the term *mesothelioma* is or has been applied to other types of pleural tumor that are not associated with asbestos exposure. These entities, including solitary fibrous tumor (fibrous mesothelioma), localized malignant mesothelioma, well-differentiated papillary mesothelioma, and so-called pseudomesotheliomatous carcinoma, are briefly discussed in the section on separation of diffuse malignant mesothelioma from other primary pleural tumors. Battifora and McCaughey (78) and McCaughey et al. (80) provide illustrations and a detailed discussion. Whenever the term *mesothelioma* is used in this chapter, it explicitly refers to diffuse malignant mesothelioma, except as noted.

Epidemiologic and Related Data

The accepted causes of mesothelioma in man are listed in Table 10.6. The proportion of mesotheliomas associated with asbestos exposure varies considerably with study design and population examined. Rubino et al. (81) summarized 16 studies from the literature: histories of exposure varied from 11% to 91% of subjects. By contrast, in 70 cases from South Africa reported by Cochrane and Webster (82), 99% of the patients had been exposed. McDonald (83) concluded that by 1980 the overall proportion of male patients with exposure was 80%, and that of female patients was quite low, only about 5%. More recently Spirtas et al. (84) re-examined this issue using data accumulated between 1975 and 1980 from Los Angeles, New York, and 39 large Veterans Administration hospitals. They concluded that in men the attributable risk of pleural mesothelioma was 88% and peritoneal mesothelioma, 58%. In women, for whom much smaller numbers of cases were diagnosed, the overall attributable risk was 23%. Recent data from the United States (85) suggest an overall ratio of pleural to peritoneal tumors of about 9:1 in men and 2:1 in women. The latter is probably the ratio for idiopathic tumors. By contrast, in Britain the ratio for women is about 5:1, reflecting a much greater proportion of exposed subjects (11). A few heavily exposed cohorts have shown a predominance of peritoneal tumors (discussed later).

A high incidence of mesothelioma has also been clearly shown after exposure to erionite, a durable mineral fiber with dimensions comparable to those of amphibole asbestos. However, this phenomenon has been reported only from a very small area of Turkey (86, 87). There are also 30 or so published cases of mesothelioma following irradiation (88, 89) and another handful of cases associated with marked pleural scarring, generally from previous plombage therapy, induced pneumothorax for tuberculosis, or chronic empyema (90). Last, as these data indicate, some proportion of cases (in fact the bulk of cases in women) have no defined cause, and there is nothing to suggest that such cases are associated with asbestos exposure. A detailed review of malignant mesotheliomas not related to asbestos is provided by Peterson et al. (91).

In the general population the incidence of pleural mesothelioma in North America is in the range of 2 to 3 cases per million persons per year (11, 83, 85, 92, 93); these are the numbers seen in women, few of whom have been exposed to asbestos. In men the rate is much higher, reaching 15 to 20 cases per million persons per year for the United States as a whole by the early 1990s (93). There is considerable variation by geographic area, with coastal regions that had large shipbuilding industries in World War II having particularly high rates (94). Studies of secular trends make it clear that rates in men have increased dramatically over the past 20 years, largely reflecting occupational exposure to asbestos,

TABLE 10.6
Accepted Causes of Malignant Mesothelioma

Asbestos
Erionite (only in parts of Turkey)
Therapeutic radiation
Severe pleural scarring
Idiopathic

whereas the rates in women are statistically unchanged (11, 83, 85, 88, 93). An estimated 1600 cases occurred in the United States in 1980 (94), and there has been an increase since that time (95). The numbers of cases seen in different countries varies in a way that appears to parallel the use of amphiboles (amosite and particularly crocidolite). For example, in Great Britain, with a population only about one-fifth that of the United States, more than 1000 mesotheliomas are diagnosed each year (8). Equivalently high incidences are seen in Australia.

Modeling of rates from exposed cohorts suggests that the incidence of the disease is exponentially related to latency (time since first exposure) (96). However, whether there is a clear dose response is disputed. Peto et al. (96) suggest that mesothelioma incidence is linearly related to dose, but Browne (11) argues that the effect of dose is to reduce latency. However, this argument mostly applies to cumulative dose, since it is hard to argue with the observation that most mesotheliomas are seen in persons with substantial occupational exposure. An additional conclusion that arises from these epidemiologic studies is that unlike carcinoma of the lung, asbestos-induced mesothelioma is not associated with cigarette smoking (92).

The latency period for asbestos-induced mesothelioma is long, with a mean value of 30 to 40 years (110). Lanphear and Buncher (98) reviewed latencies in 1105 cases with confirmed diagnoses and clearly documented exposures; 99% had a latency period longer than 15 years and 96%, a latency period longer than 20 years. This is true even in workforces with very heavy amphibole exposure, such as asbestos insulators (92, 97). Thus when latencies shorter than 15 years are claimed in an individual case, evidence of more remote exposures should be found before attributing the case to asbestos exposure. Also, as exposure level decreases, the latency period increases (11). Thus the lower the exposure, the less likely it is that a case with a marginal latency is caused by asbestos.

Although the association of asbestos exposure with diffuse malignant mesothelioma is well established, it has become increasingly clear that there are very marked differences in disease potential between chrysotile and the commercial amphiboles amosite and crocidolite (11, 17, 105). This is shown in Table 10.7, which documents the percentage of deaths due to mesothelioma in various occupationally exposed populations. The table was constructed by listing death rates in increasing order. It becomes obvious in reading from top to bottom that chrysotile is associated with a much lower mesothelioma rate than either amosite or crocidolite. Indeed, some chrysotile-exposed populations show no death rate from mesothelioma, and in none does it exceed 0.5%. In contrast, in cohorts with heavy exposure to pure crocidolite as many as 18% of deaths have been caused by mesothelioma. The result of these differences between amphiboles and chrysotile in terms of mesothelioma induction is that the greatest numbers of mesotheliomas are seen in persons who worked as asbestos insulators, in asbestos production and manufacture, and in shipbuilding or repair, particularly before and during World War II and through the 1960s (92). This was because heavy amphibole exposure was common in these trades during these periods. By contrast, mesotheliomas are rare in chrysotile-exposed workforces engaged in mining and milling, textile work (despite the high incidence of asbestosis and lung cancer in textile work), and friction products manufacture, in which amphibole was not used or was used in very limited amounts for specific purposes. There is also no epidemiologic evidence of an increased risk for garage mechanics despite exposure to chrysotile brake dust (92).

These observations have raised the issue whether chrysotile asbestos produces

TABLE 10.7
Percentage of Deaths from Mesothelioma in Various Asbestos-Exposed Populations

EXPOSURE GROUP	DEATHS (%)
Chrysotile cement plant (22)	0.0
Chrysotile friction plant (99)	0.0
Chrysotile friction plant (24)	0.0
Chrysotile cement plant (101)	0.05
Chrysotile textile factory workers (100)	0.3
Canadian chrysotile miners and millers (5)	0.5
Balangero chrysotile mine (102)	0.5
Crocidolite and chrysotile friction materials factory workers (103)	0.6
Anthophyllite miners (104)	0.8
Chrysotile and amphibole textile factory workers (105)	1.3
Australian crocidolite miners (106)	3.3
Amosite factory workers (107)	4.6
Insulation workers (amosite and chrysotile exposure (108)	9.0
UK crocidolite-containing gas mask assemblers (109)	10.0
Canadian crocidolite-containing gas mask assemblers (110)	16.0
Workers manufacturing crocidolite cigarette filters (111)	18.0

mesothelioma in man at all. It is generally accepted on the basis of epidemiologic investigations that asbestos-induced peritoneal mesothelioma is associated only with heavy exposure to amosite and crocidolite and is not caused by chrysotile exposure (1, 8, 11, 112), and my associates and I (113) found only pleural mesotheliomas in a sequential series of 300 autopsies of chrysotile miners and millers with extremely heavy occupational exposure.

The data on pleural tumors are confusing because many factories that supposedly used only chrysotile turned out on closer examination to use small amounts of amosite and crocidolite as well, and in some instances mineralogic analysis of the lungs of workers from such plants indicates that exposure of the workforce to the amphibole was widespread (114–116). Thus the few reported mesotheliomas from these plants were probably caused by amphiboles. But detailed mineralogic analysis of the lungs of workers with mesothelioma from the chrysotile mining townships of eastern Québec, the cohort with the highest reported incidence of chrysotile-induced mesotheliomas, reveals that most patients were exposed only to chrysotile and its natural contaminant, the amphibole tremolite (113, 117, 118).

These observations leave no doubt that enough exposure to chrysotile ore can produce mesothelioma in man. Even in this group, however, the absolute number of cases is small; a recent review suggests that out of more than 8000 deaths, only 38 were caused by mesothelioma, and of these no more than 26 were attributable to chrysotile ore exposure (112). Equally important, in today's terms the exposure levels encountered by these workers were extraordinary, probably on the order of 50 fibers per cubic centimeter (9) for periods upward of 20 years (112). This exposure is reflected quite clearly in analyses of lung fiber burden. As shown in Table 9.11, chrysotile-induced mesotheliomas in these workers appear at a fiber burden comparable with that seen in asbestosis, in contrast to the situation in workers with amosite or crocidolite exposure, in whom mesotheliomas appear at a burden much lower than that found in cases of asbestosis

(113, 119–122) (see Chapter 9). There is also increasing evidence that the actual agent of mesothelioma in these workers is the tremolite component of the ore (112, 123).

These observations have considerable practical application, since they imply that any regulatory standard for chrysotile exposure that avoids the development of asbestosis will also protect against mesothelioma and that chrysotile-induced mesothelioma is only a historical problem. In fact, the notion of a threshold for chrysotile-induced mesothelioma has been accepted in a recent review of fiber toxicology by the British Health and Safety Executive (8). If one accepts the argument that lung cancer is also directly related to asbestosis, the same conclusion applies.

These data apply to populations with occupational exposure to asbestos. In the United States there is considerable controversy about the possible effects of very low level asbestos exposure in public buildings in which asbestos has been used for insulation and fireproofing. As discussed in Chapter 9, these exposures are usually only to chrysotile and are on the order of 0.0002 fibers per cubic centimeter (2). This level is about twice the average of urban ambient air and is only one-thousandth to one ten-thousandth of the occupational standard used in different countries. It is also four to five orders of magnitude lower than the exposures that have been documented to lead to asbestosis, carcinoma of the lung, and mesothelioma in occupationally exposed cohorts.

A careful review of the evidence suggests that such low-level exposure poses no real risk (1, 2, 83, 105). As with workers with occupational chrysotile exposure, it appears that induction of both mesothelioma and carcinoma of the lung requires exposures sufficient to produce asbestosis (i.e., on the order of at least 25 to 100 fibers per cubic centimeter–years), and it is clear that it is impossible even to begin to accumulate such exposures at ambient levels of 0.0002 fibers per cubic centimeter.

Additional evidence for the absence of risk of mesothelioma after low-level exposure to chrysotile comes from the failure to find an increase in mesothelioma rates in women in the general population over the past 20 years (1, 83, 85, 92) despite the widespread use of asbestos insulation in buildings in the past 30 years. Similarly, the observation that lifetime residents of the chrysotile mining townships of Québec who never worked in the industry apparently do not have an increased incidence of mesothelioma, although they are continuously exposed to ambient air levels several hundred times those of North American cities (83, 124), argue against a mesothelioma risk from building exposures.

One can nonetheless calculate theoretic risks by extrapolating incidence data from high-level occupational exposure to the levels of asbestos found in buildings. Such calculations produce lifetime mesothelioma risks on the order of 4 per million persons, which translates to an excess of 10 mesothelioma deaths per year in the United States (2). These theoretic risks are far below established real risks, such as smoking, driving to work, bicycling, and even eating peanut butter, which may contain small amounts of the carcinogen aflatoxin (2, 125). Thus there is little evidence to support the idea that very low level exposure to asbestos poses any real risk to health.

Pathogenesis

Some possible molecular and physical mechanisms by which asbestos induces both carcinoma of the lung and mesothelioma were discussed earlier. There are definite differences between the bronchial epithelium and the mesothelium; in particular, the mesothelium is much more sensitive to the effects of asbestos, and asbestos appears to function as a complete carcinogen for mesothelial cells (126).

There has been extensive investigation of the relation of mesothelioma induction and fiber size in experimental models. Using intrapleural inoculation of different types of fibers with different size distributions, Stanton et al. (127) concluded that long, thin (i.e., high aspect ratio) fibers were much more powerful mesothelial carcinogens than were short, thick fibers and that fiber type was less important. The exact size of fiber that qualifies as long and thin is unclear: fibers lengths longer than 8 μm and widths narrower than 1.5 μm are usually cited from Stanton's work, but the same experiments showed that fibers with lengths greater than 4 μm and widths less than 0.25 μm were also effective carcinogens. The Stanton hypothesis has been supported by animal inhalation experiments using size-separated fibers: few mesotheliomas were found with either amosite or chrysotile prepared to contain few fibers longer than 5 μm (128, 129).

Human data on the question of fiber length and mesothelioma are equivocal. The tremolite found as a natural constituent of chrysotile ore is a relatively short, thick fiber compared with commercial amosite or crocidolite (113, 122), and if one attributes "chrysotile-induced" mesotheliomas in man to the tremolite component, the differences in mesothelioma by fiber type do correlate with fiber size. However, attempts to prove this proposition directly have produced equivocal results. McDonald et al. (130) and Rogers et al. (131) both compared the types and sizes of fibers found in the lungs of mesothelioma patients with those of general population control cases. McDonald et al. concluded that the number of fibers longer than 8 μm explained most mesotheliomas and that chrysotile played no role. However, Rogers et al. found that fibers both longer and shorter than 10 μm, including chrysotile fibers, played a role, although long fibers were generally more important. The problem with both of these studies is that most patients with mesothelioma have had occupational asbestos exposure, and fibers in lungs from those with occupational exposure are always longer than fibers in the general population (132); thus the same result would have been obtained if the test group were exposed but had no disease or some disease other than mesothelioma. My colleagues and I (113) have attempted to circumvent this problem by comparing fiber sizes in a chrysotile mining and milling cohort and a cohort with heavy amosite exposure (122), using exposed workers with no disease as the control group. In neither cohort could we show that fibers in mesothelioma cases were significantly longer and thinner than those in the other disease categories or even in the disease-free workers.

Another factor that is believed to be important in the pathogenesis of mesothelioma is durability of fibers. Fibers such as chrysotile and fibrous glass, which are rapidly cleared from lung tissue, are either weakly carcinogenic (in the case of chrysotile) or noncarcinogenic (fibrous glass) in man; amphiboles, which are cleared very slowly (123) are potent mesothelial carcinogens. Intraperitoneal inoculation experiments, which must be viewed with extreme caution because of the enormous doses and nonphysiologic routes of administration employed, do suggest that fibers of any type of sufficiently low durability are less potent mesothelial carcinogens than more durable fibers (see Chapter 11). However, these types of experiments and even some inhalation experiments are oversensitive, since they implicate fibrous glass, chrysotile, and crocidolite as essentially equally effective mesothelial carcinogens (127, 133) (see Chapter 11).

The foregoing discussion makes the implicit assumption that mesothelioma is induced by fibers reaching the pleural or peritoneal cavities. Although this idea makes intuitive sense, attempts to demonstrate fibers in the pleural cavity in man have been largely unsuccessful or have mostly shown short fibers of chrysotile; the one exception is the very recent report of Boutin et al. (134) (see Chapter 9). Adamson et al. (135) report that mesothelial proliferation can also be induced by intratracheal administration of crocidolite asbestos or any agent that produces intrapulmonary fibrosis, and Sekhon et al. (136) confirm that in this type of experiment very few fibers reach even a subpleural location and that there is no correlation between the local mesothelial mitotic index and the local concentration of subpleural fibers. These observations suggest that the intrapulmonary generation of mitogenic cytokines may influence mesothelioma induction.

Other possible mechanisms of mesothelioma induction have also been proposed. Gan et al. (137) found that asbestos fibers could act as adsorptive agents to translocate plasmid DNA into mesothelial cells in culture. Whether this occurs in vivo in man is unknown. The effect appears to be nonspecific, since calcium phosphate, a common mineral in the body, is even more effective than asbestos. Carbone et al. (138) reported simian virus 40–like DNA sequences in 60% of human mesotheliomas studied but not in the matching lung samples. They suggested that the virus may be acting as an independent carcinogen or a cocarcinogen with asbestos.

Clinical Features

In most series the median age at presentation is approximately 60, and few cases are seen in men under age 30; however, peritoneal mesotheliomas are more common in young women. Clinically and histologically typical mesotheliomas have been reported in children and adolescents (139, 140).

The typical presenting complaints for patients with pleural mesothelioma are dyspnea and chest pain; peritoneal tumors may cause ascites, pain, weight loss, and a palpable mass. Hypertrophic osteoarthropathy, clubbing, and hypoglycemia may also be seen in malignant mesothelioma but less commonly than in solitary fibrous tumor. Initial physical examination of patients with pleural mesothelioma usually reveals little except dullness over the affected hemothorax, but late in the disease contraction of the chest wall is also observed. Bowel obstruction is generally a late complication of peritoneal mesothelioma. Tumor may grow along needle biopsy tracks or surgical incisions; this phenomenon is typical of mesothelioma and uncommon with other types of tumor. Conversely, the finding of clinically evident metastatic disease at the time of presentation favors a diagnosis of carcinoma, although rare patients presenting with metastatic mesothelioma have been reported (141).

Radiographic examination may show any of several patterns. Effusion is almost invariable, and its absence makes the diagnosis much less likely. Once the effusion is drained, the pleura may appear diffusely thickened or nodular, and tumor can often be seen to surround the lung (Fig. 10.2). Occasionally an apparently solitary circumscribed mass mimics an intrapulmonary process (139, 142–144). Putative pleural mesotheliomas that appear as radiographic solitary circumscribed masses also must be carefully differentiated from solitary fibrous tumors, localized malignant mesotheliomas, and localized pleural sarcomas (see section on separation of diffuse malignant mesothelioma from other primary pleural tumors). Other radiographic features of asbestos exposure may or may

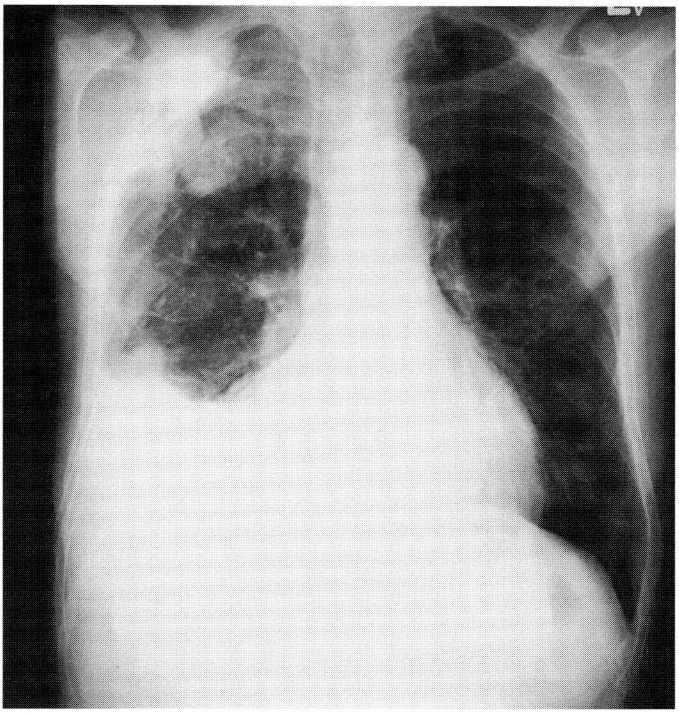

FIGURE 10.2
Chest radiograph of a worker with malignant mesothelioma. Note the pleural effusion and bulky tumor masses, which are all pleural and in many areas can be seen to surround the lung.

not be present. Most patients with pleural mesothelioma induced by occupational asbestos exposure do not show evidence of asbestosis, although pleural plaques are common. Evidence of asbestosis is much more common in cases of peritoneal mesothelioma, an observation that correlates with the idea that peritoneal mesothelioma tends to occur in patients with very heavy asbestos exposure (145). The pleural effusion is serosanguinous or overtly bloody in 25 to 50% of cases (139, 142) and may occasionally be quite gelatinous, which reflects the presence of large quantities of glycosaminoglycan, especially hyaluronic acid, secreted by mesothelial cells.

Pathologic Features

Extensive descriptions of the pathologic features of malignant mesothelioma can be found in several reports (78, 80, 145–148).

The diagnosis of malignant mesothelioma presents two major problems. First is to arrive at the diagnosis on the basis of pathologic evidence. Second is to separate mesotheliomas from carcinomas and sarcomas metastatic to the pleura or peritoneum and from sarcomas arising in the chest wall. All of these tumors can closely mimic the gross and microscopic appearance of mesothelioma (see Fig. 10.14, later in the chapter). Separation from localized primary pleural tumors is occasionally a diagnostic problem (discussed later).

Although the older literature suggests that one cannot be sure of the diagnosis of mesothelioma without an autopsy (145, 149), most mesotheliomas, like most other human tumors, show characteristic gross, microscopic, and histochemical or immunohistochemical patterns, and open surgical biopsies or large thoracoscopic biopsies usually prove adequate for the purpose (150). Cutting needle biopsies are sometimes diagnostic but much less often than video-directed thoracoscopic biopsies. The reliability of the diagnosis of mesothelioma on the basis of pleural or ascitic fluid cytology remains a controversial and difficult issue.

Gross Appearances. The gross appearance of mesothelioma is characteristic but not by itself diagnostic. By definition diffuse malignant mesotheliomas do not originate in a solid organ; rather they tend to surround viscera, particularly in the thorax, where one lung is commonly encased by hard white tumor at autopsy (Fig. 10.3*A*). Often, particularly at an earlier stage of disease, the tumor appears as multiple nodules studded over the pleura and diaphragm. Occasionally a diffuse malignant mesothelioma appears grossly as a dominant circumscribed mass (Fig. 10.3*C*), and careful examination may be required to demonstrate diffuse pleural involvement. As a rule, by the time of diagnosis tumor is present on both parietal and visceral pleurae, but there is some evidence that tumor may first develop on the parietal surface (149).

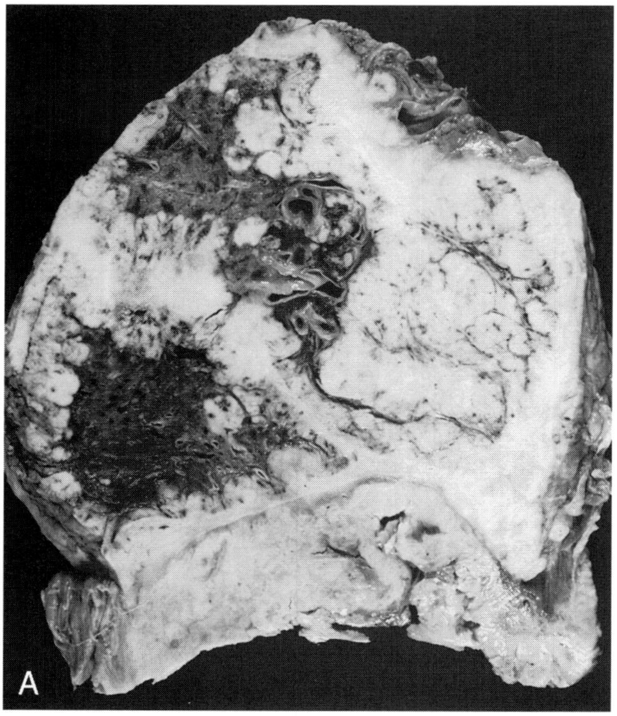

FIGURE 10.3
Gross appearance of mesothelioma. **A.** Typical mesothelioma with extensive tumor surrounding the lung and growing into the lung from the pleural surface. Notice the extension along the interlobar fissure and through the diaphragm. **B.** Metastases in opposite lung from this tumor. Metastatic disease is common in mesothelioma and is not evidence against the diagnosis. **C.** A mesothelioma with a large bulky mass that appears to be intrapulmonary and that mimics a carcinoma.

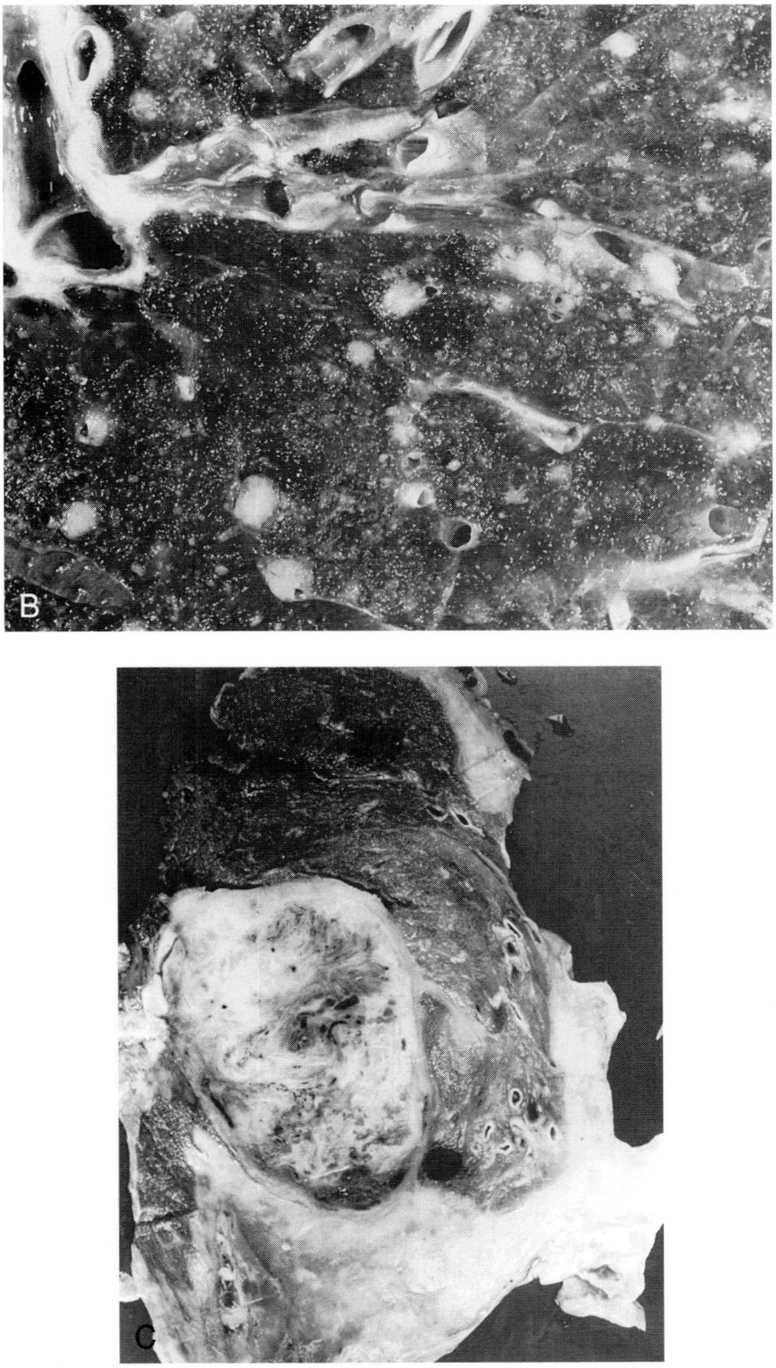

FIGURE 10.3 *(continued)*

Pleural tumors may show extensive growth into the mediastinum with compression of the vascular structures. As well, they usually spread along the fissures and also into the underlying lung, typically by growing along interlobular septa, through lymphatics (Fig. 10.4) from the pleural surface, and sometimes even invading the bronchial tree (Fig. 10.4). Spread through the diaphragm and into the chest wall, especially along needle or surgical tracks, is also common. But it should be kept in mind that peripheral carcinomas of the lung can also grow by encasement (151) (see Fig. 10.14, later in the chapter), and lymphomas and sarcomas, including sarcomas of the chest wall, sometimes produce diffuse tumor on the pleura surface.

Peritoneal malignant mesotheliomas have similar gross features, appearing either as diffuse nodules over the peritoneum simulating disseminated carcinoma or as plaques or massive aggregates of tumor encasing abdominal organs (145). Such tumors may also form a dominant mass, particularly in the pelvis.

Microscopic Appearances. Table 10.8 shows a scheme for subclassifying malignant mesothelioma by microscopic appearance. Mesotheliomas can be broadly divided into epithelial, sarcomatous, and mixed types. Legha and Muggia (139) summarized data on pleural tumors from 382 patients in 9 reports and found that 55% were epithelial; 22%, sarcomatous; and 24%, mixed. Kannerstein and Churg (145) examined 82 cases of peritoneal mesothelioma; of these 75% were epithelial; 24%, mixed; and only 1%, purely sarcomatous. The microscopic patterns of pleural and peritoneal tumors are identical.

Although pure forms do occur, many epithelial mesotheliomas display several

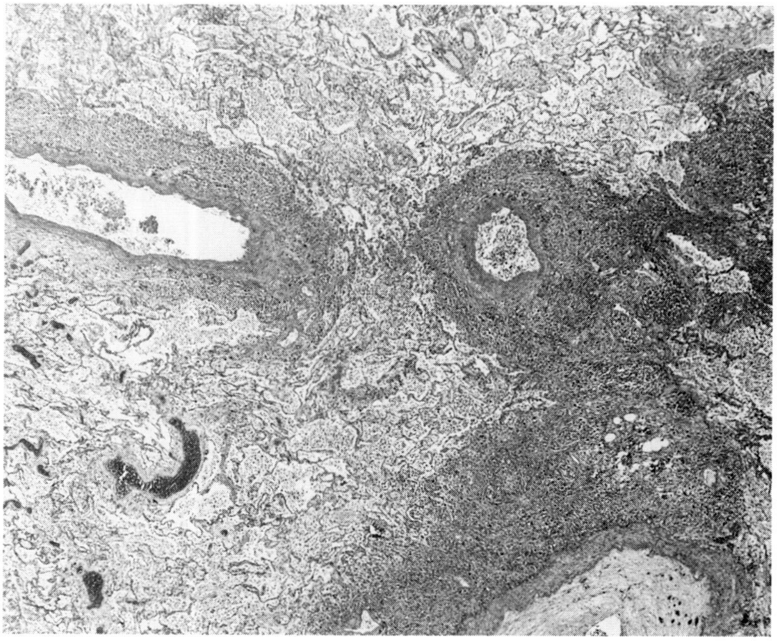

FIGURE 10.4
Lymphangitic spread of mesothelioma within the lung. *Lower right,* Involvement of the wall of an airway. This common finding should not be taken as evidence against the diagnosis of mesothelioma.

of the patterns listed in Table 10.8. The most characteristic form is the tubulopapillary variant (Fig. 10.5, *A* and *B*) in which the tumor forms branching tubules and papillae covered by flattened to cuboidal cells, usually intermixed with glands lined by very flattened cells. Columnar cells can be seen in mesothelioma but are more characteristic of adenocarcinoma. Psammoma bodies are distinctly uncommon, and their presence in large numbers in a peritoneal tumor should raise a question of an ovarian primary tumor or a primary serous carcinoma of the peritoneum (146, 148, 152).

Another common form of epithelial mesothelioma is composed of large cells with copious eosinophilic cytoplasm and distinct cell borders, in Table 10.8 called epithelioid or mesothelial cell-like (Figs. 10.5 *C* and *D* and 10.6, *A* and *B*). Sometimes these cells are arranged in pavementlike sheets, and in other instances they resemble aggregates of large polygonal mesothelial cells of the type commonly found in reactive pleural effusions.

The cytoplasm in epithelial mesotheliomas may be vacuolated, but the vacuoles do not stain with stains for neutral mucin, for example with digested periodic acid-Schiff (PAS) stain. This is diagnostically helpful. However, PAS stains may reveal basement membrane–like material surrounding tumor cells or even forming small droplets in the centers of cell aggregates, and care must be taken to distinguish staining of basement membrane material from mucin.

Another variant of epithelial mesotheliomas is the so-called adenomatoid pattern in which glandlike spaces formed by extremely attenuated cells contain lakes of pale blue staining hyaluronic acid (Fig. 10.7). These tumors may be mistaken for benign adenomatoid tumors, but their diffuse pattern of growth and frequent admixture with other forms of mesothelioma usually make the distinction obvious. As far as I know, benign adenomatoid tumors do not occur in the pleura.

In general epithelial mesotheliomas are composed of relatively large cells, but Mayall and Gibbs (153) recently reported 13 examples of tumors in which a component of small cells somewhat resembling small-cell carcinoma of the lung was found. In all of these cases areas showing other readily diagnosed forms of epithelial mesothelioma were present.

Sarcomatous mesotheliomas also occur in several patterns. The most common is composed of spindled cells that resemble fibroblasts, arranged either in dense fascicles resembling fibrosarcoma or in a storiform pattern (Fig. 10.8) indistinguishable on ordinary stains from malignant fibrous histiocytoma (78, 80,

TABLE 10.8
Histologic Patterns of Malignant Mesothelioma

Epithelial
Tubulopapillary
Epithelioid (mesothelial cell-like)
Adenomatoid
Desmoplastic
Sarcomatous
Resembling fibrosarcoma or malignant fibrous histiocytoma
With heterologous elements resembling chondrosarcoma or osteosarcoma
Desmoplastic
Mixed Epithelial and Sarcomatous

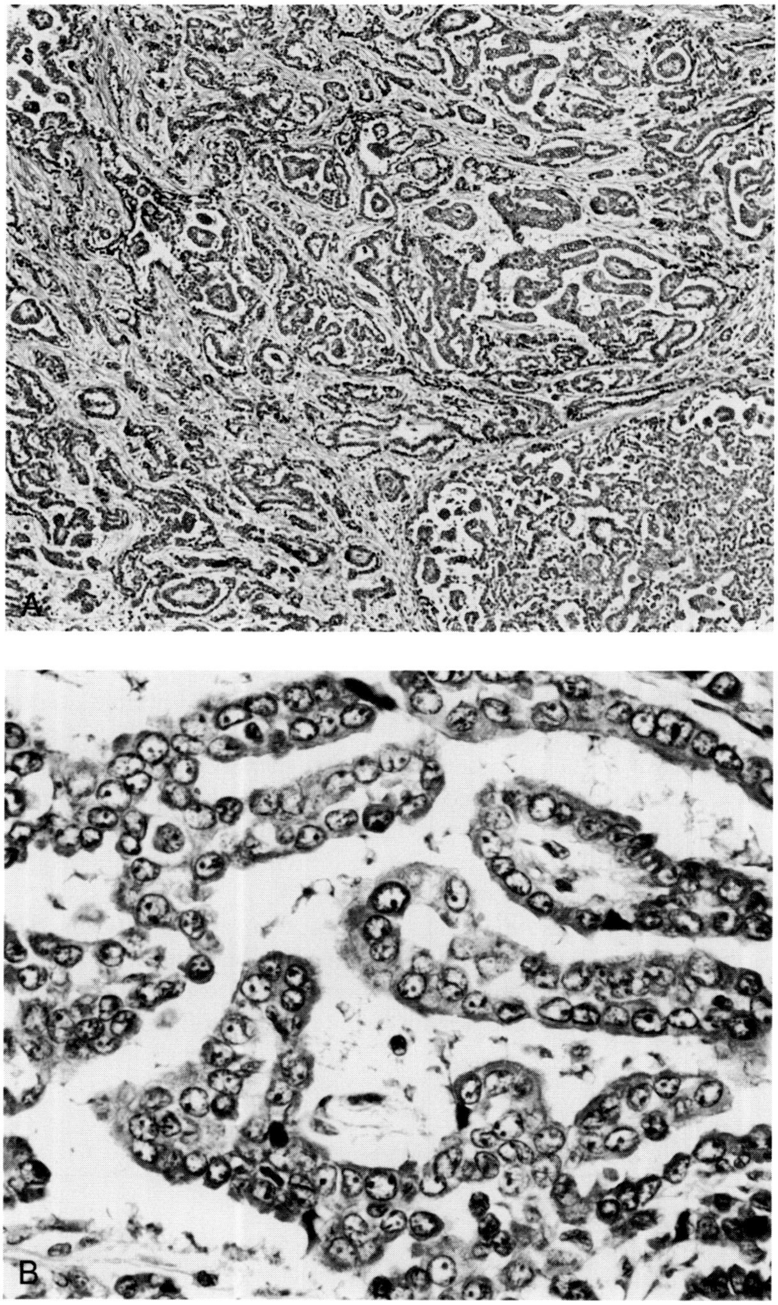

FIGURE 10.5

Epithelial malignant mesothelioma. **A** and **B.** Typical tubulopapillary pattern forming papillae and branching tubules lined by cuboidal to columnar cells. **C** and **D.** Epitheloid or mesothelial cell-like pattern in the same tumor. Note the vacuole in one of the tumor cells in **D.** Vacuoles such as this may give the initial impression of a carcinoma, but PAS stain fails to demonstrate any mucin, whereas colloidal iron or Alcian blue stain often shows hyaluronic acid in the vacuoles.

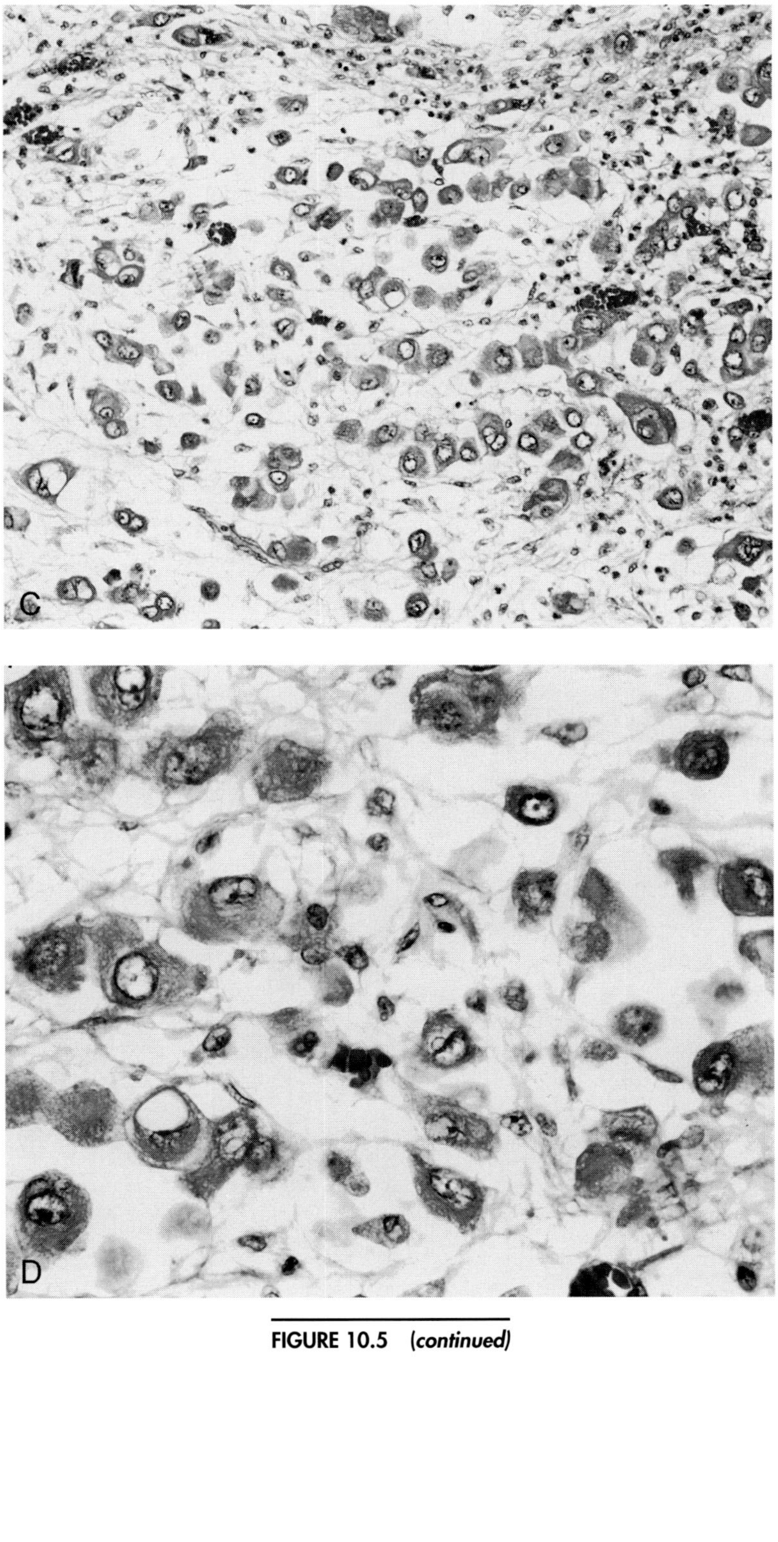

FIGURE 10.5 ***(continued)***

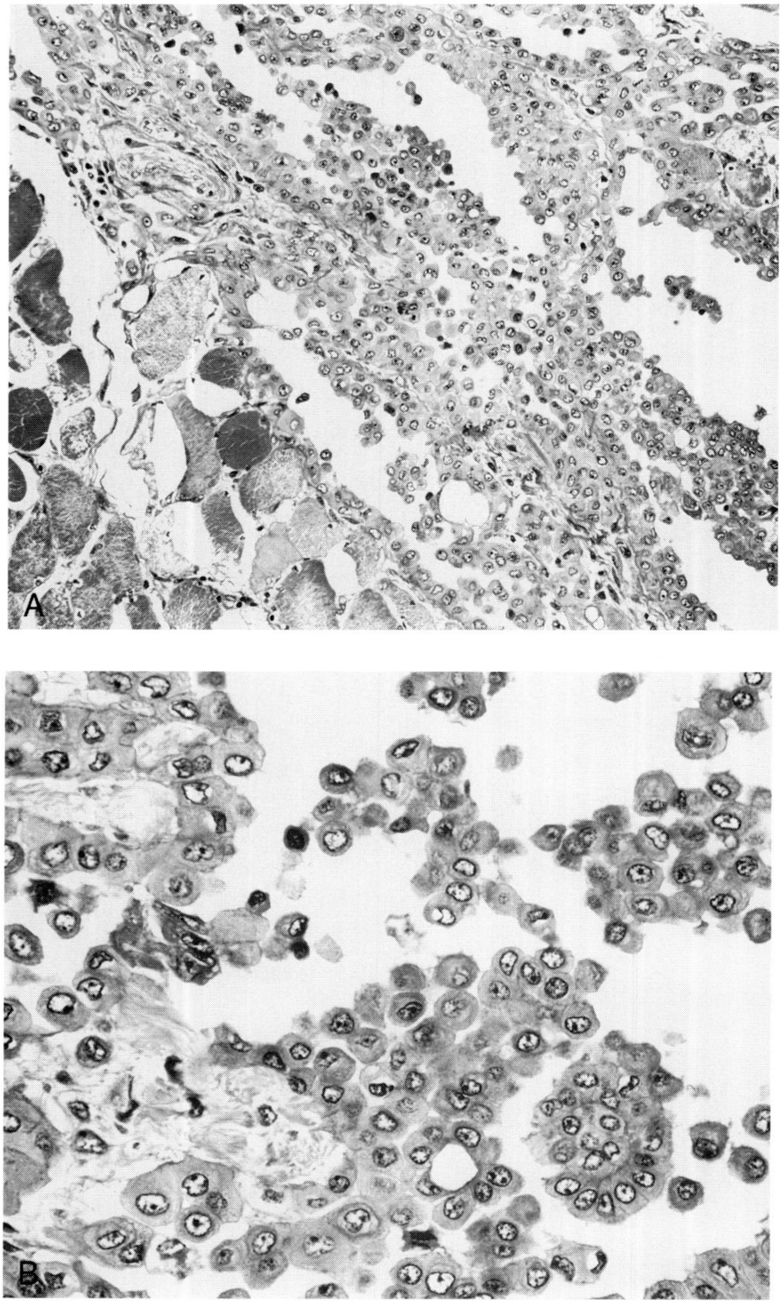

FIGURE 10.6

Epitheloid or mesothelial cell-like mesothelioma. **A** and **B.** Cells resembling the mesothelial cells seen in effusions invade the muscle of the chest wall. **C.** Colloidal iron stain demonstrating a droplet of hyaluronic acid in the cell cytoplasm (proved by predigesting another slide with hyaluronidase).

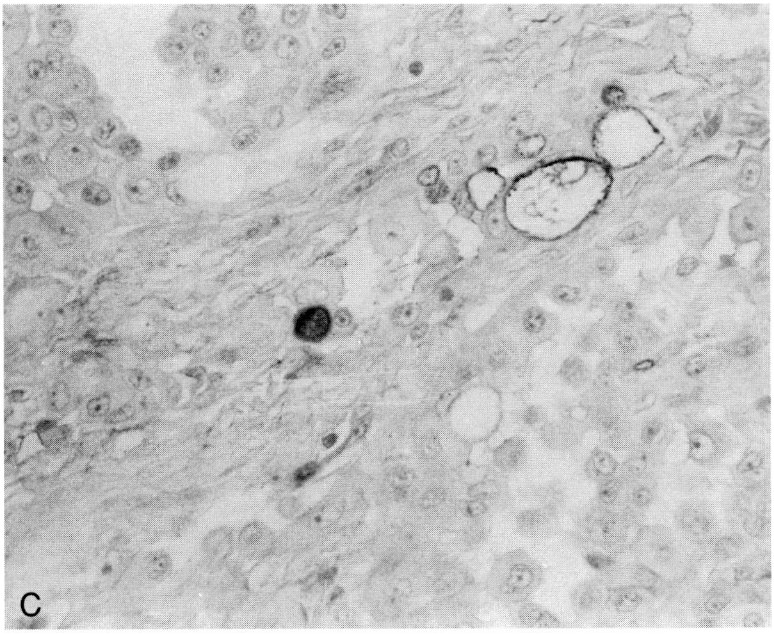

FIGURE 10.6 *(continued)*

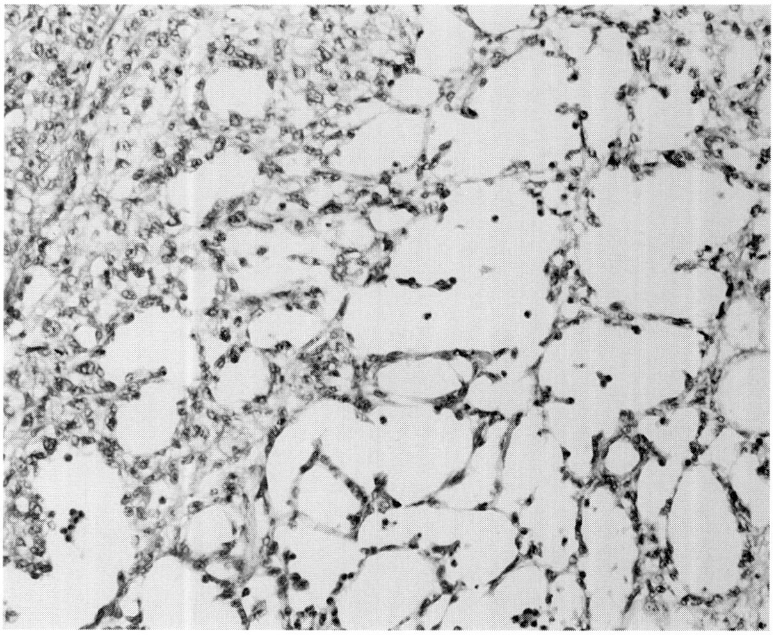

FIGURE 10.7
So-called adenomatoid variant of epithelial mesothelioma. This type of growth pattern is associated with lakes of hyaluronic acid in the large extracellular spaces.

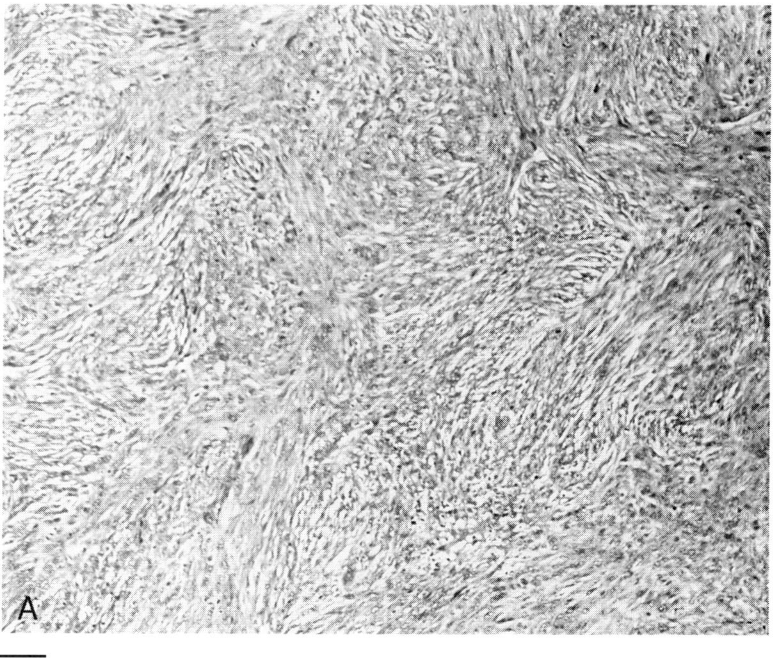

FIGURE 10.8
Sarcomatous mesothelioma mimicking malignant fibrous histocytoma. **A** and **B.** Low- and medium high–power views showing spindled cells forming storiform patterns. Despite the storiform pattern, this is not a desmoplastic mesothelioma because it is highly cellular. **C.** Immunochemical staining for cytokeratin is diffusely positive, indicating that this is not sarcoma.

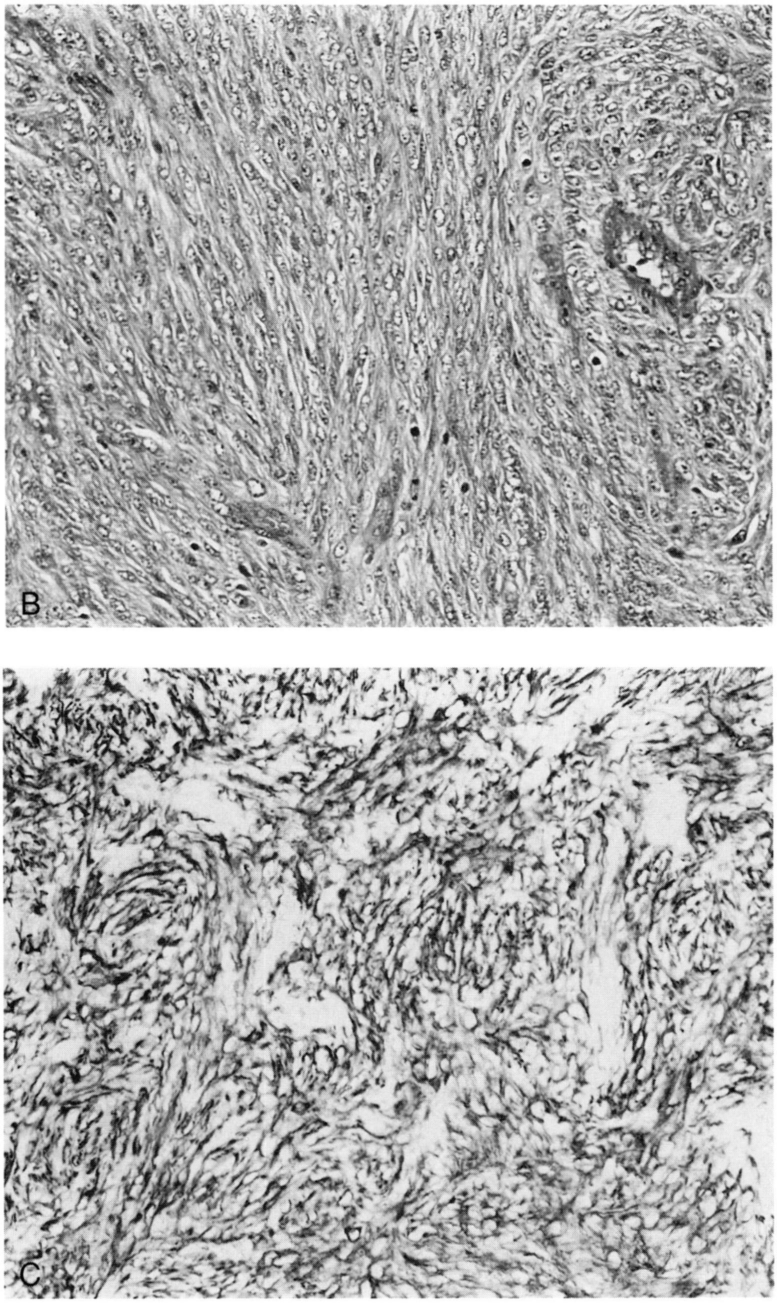

FIGURE 10.8 *(continued)*

154). Another pattern is desmoplastic mesothelioma (Figs. 10.9 and 10.10), in which the collagenous stroma makes up almost the whole of the tumor mass, with the cellular component represented by single entrapped cytologically atypical cells (147, 155). Desmoplastic mesotheliomas can be extremely difficult to separate from benign fibrotic pleural reactions (fibrosing pleurisy). Mangano et al. (156) suggest that the combination of a storiform pattern of growth or alternatively, a pattern like that of the haphazard arrangement of collagen and cells seen in solitary fibrous tumor (so-called patternless pattern), along with bland necrosis, stromal invasion, or clear foci of sarcomatous differentiation, support the diagnosis. This topic is considered further in the section on separation of benign and malignant mesothelial reactions. Occasionally epithelial mesotheliomas also show desmoplastic foci (155) (Fig. 10.11).

Sarcomatous mesotheliomas can also display cartilaginous and osseous differentiation (157) (Fig. 10.12C). An additional unusual variant, which they called lymphohistiocytoid mesothelioma, has recently been described by Hendersen et al. (158). These are predominantly sarcomatous mesotheliomas with a very intense lymphoid infiltrate and tumor cells that resemble large atypical histiocytes. Immunohistochemical staining for keratin is extremely valuable in demonstrating that all of these unusual forms are actually mesotheliomas and not sarcomas (discussed later).

Mixed epithelial and sarcomatous mesotheliomas (Fig. 10.12) demonstrate combinations of typical epithelial and mesenchymal elements. In some instances the two components are sharply separated, and in others they transform gradually from one to the other.

Histochemical Reactions. Histochemical staining for mucins can be helpful in the separation of mesothelioma from carcinomas metastatic to the pleura and peritoneum (Table 10.9). Tumors that form PAS-positive mucins by definition are adenocarcinomas (148–150, 159) (see Fig. 10.14, later in the chapter). Mesotheliomas produce hyaluronic acid that stains with Alcian blue or colloidal iron and can be removed by predigestion with hyaluronidase (Fig. 10.6C).

A number of cautions and caveats must be applied to the interpretation of these reactions. The PAS reaction must stain droplets of mucin (see Fig. 10.14, later in the chapter) and not merely granular debris in the cytoplasm or basement membrane material. Colloidal iron or Alcian blue must also stain droplets (Fig. 10.6C) in the cytoplasm and not just stroma, since the stroma of all tumors contains hyaluronic acid. Meyer's mucicarmine stain can be misleading, because hyaluronic acid may show a variable reaction depending on the exact technique used (159, 160). Hammar et al. (161) recently reported 10 epithelial mesotheliomas that were both mucicarmine and PAS positive, but the staining could be

TABLE 10.9
Usual Histochemical Staining Reactions of Mesotheliomas and Carcinomas

STAIN	MESOTHELIOMA	ADENOCARCINOMA
Colloidal iron or Alcian blue	Positive	Positive or negative
Colloidal iron or Alcian blue predigested with hyaluronidase	Negative	If positive before digestion, remains positive
PAS (diastase digested) or mucicarmine	Negative	Positive

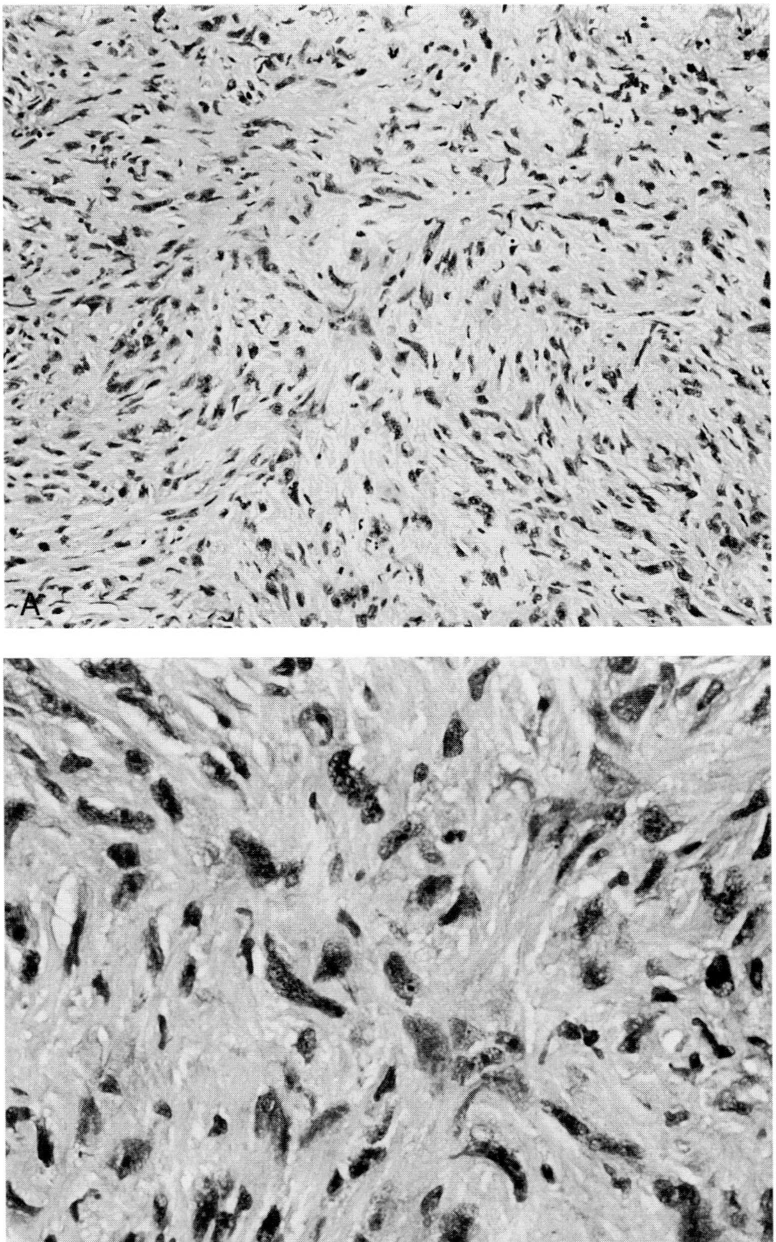

FIGURE 10.9
Sarcomatous (desmoplastic) mesothelioma. **A.** Low-power view showing scattered tumor cells, which might make one think of a reactive pleural process such as is shown in Figure 9.4. However, the cellularity is higher than would be expected in a benign reaction, and the high-power view (**B**) shows cytologically atypical cells. This tumor could be classified as a desmoplastic mesothelioma.

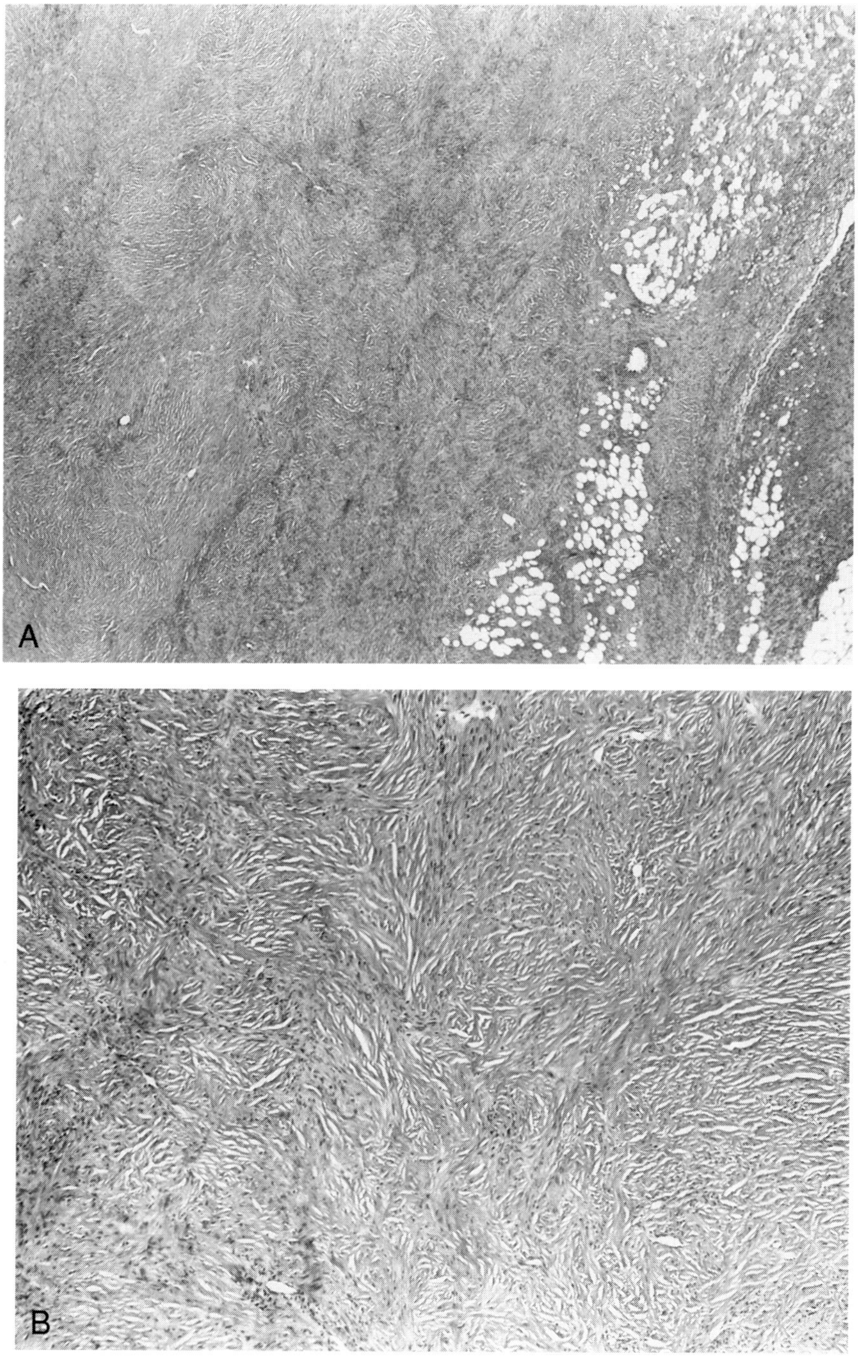

FIGURE 10.10

Desmoplastic mesothelioma. **A.** Low-power view showing infiltration of the fat of the chest wall at the bottom of the field. **B.** Higher-power view showing paucicellular patternless pattern. **C.** High-power view showing infiltration of fat by cytologically atypical tumor cells.

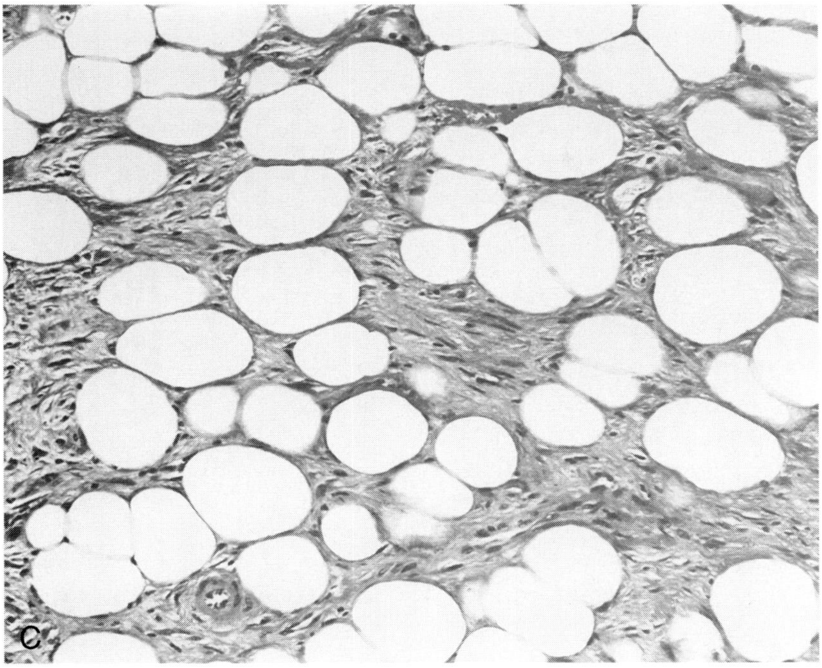

FIGURE 10.10 *(continued)*

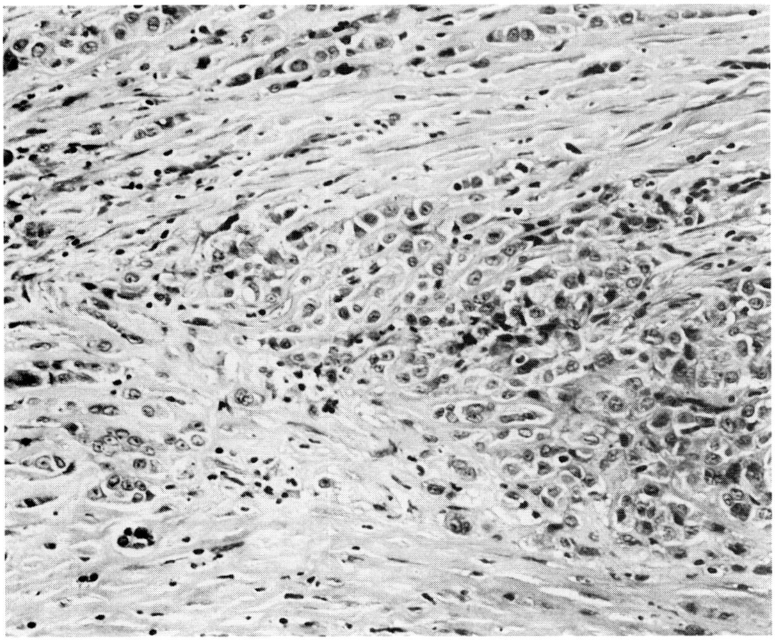

FIGURE 10.11

Desmoplastic variant of epithelial mesothelioma. At the right of the field the tumor forms solid masses of cells of epithelial type, but at the left individual cells are surrounded by dense bundles of collagen.

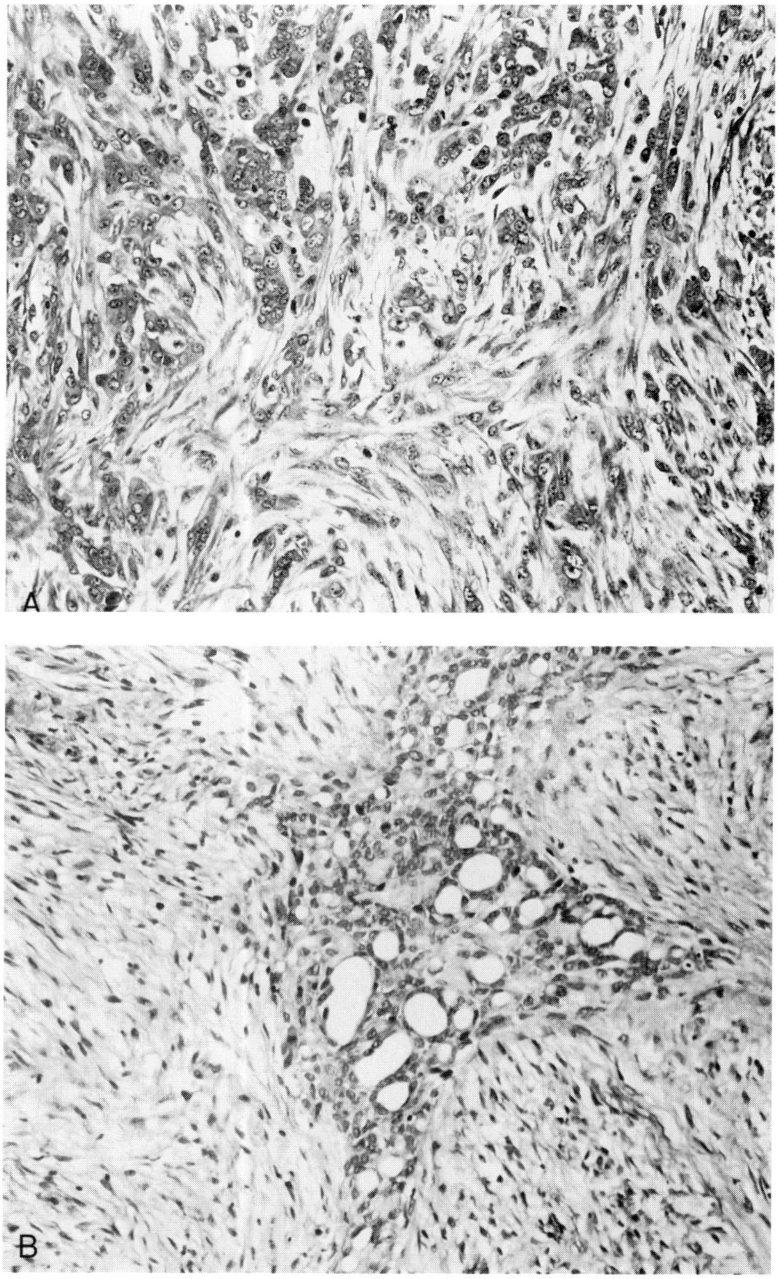

FIGURE 10.12
Mixed epithelial and sarcomatous mesotheliomas. **A.** A tumor with spindled and epitheloid cells and blending of one pattern into the other. **B.** A tumor in which the epithelial and sarcomatous patterns form discrete areas. **C.** A tumor showing a combination of tubulopapillary mesothelioma at the right of the field and sarcomatous mesothelioma with osteosarcomatous differentiation at the left. All components were keratin positive.

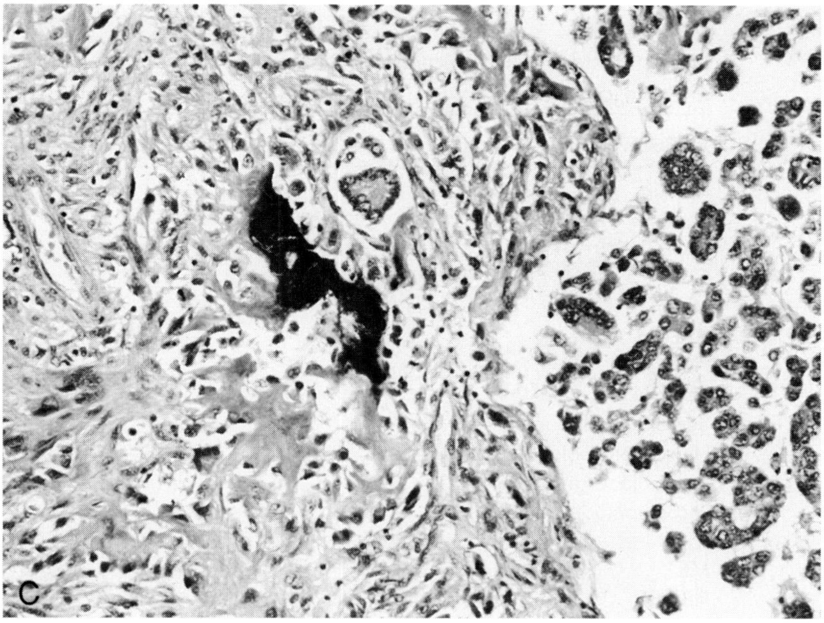

FIGURE 10.12 *(continued)*

removed by digestion with hyaluronidase. Such tumors are, however, relatively rare.

Mucin staining definitely misses some carcinomas: in a recent review of results from the U.S.–Canadian Mesothelioma Reference Panel (150), PAS stain was positive for mucin in only about half of the tumors considered by a majority of the panel to be carcinomas. Staining for hyaluronic acid also has limited utility, since hyaluronic acid is very water labile and often leaches out of tissue sections. It has been claimed that such stains are positive in 50% of otherwise acceptable cases of epithelial mesothelioma (148, 149, 159). Histochemical stains offer the advantages of simplicity of technique and low cost but in general are not as sensitive as a battery of immunohistochemical stains.

Immunohistochemical Reactions. Wang et al. (162) were the first to suggest that an immunohistochemical reaction, namely staining of carcinomas but not mesotheliomas for carcinoembryonic antigen (CEA), could be used to separate these two types of tumor (see Fig. 10.14, later in the chapter). Since that time an intense effort has been devoted to finding additional immunochemical markers for this purpose. The results of this effort can be summarized succinctly by stating that at present a variety of markers are generally positive in carcinomas and generally negative in mesotheliomas; a few markers are claimed to show the opposite reaction, but few are applicable to paraffin sections; and cross-reactions are sufficiently common that great care must be taken in interpretation of results.

These problems notwithstanding, immunohistochemical staining is a valuable adjunct to the diagnosis of mesotheliomas. Table 10.10 presents a consensus of the literature. Despite the large number of antibodies that mark carcinomas, most laboratories use CEA, B72.3, LeuM1, BEREP4, or a combination of thereof, so there is reasonably good data regarding their specificity. Many of the other markers shown in Table 10.8 are documented in only one or two series and

TABLE 10.10
Immunohistochemical Staining Patterns in Carcinomas and Mesotheliomas

ANTIGEN	MESOTHELIOMA	CARCINOMA
Keratin	+	+
Vimentin	+	+
EMA	+	+
CEA	−	+
Leu M1	−	+
B72.3	−	+
HMFG	+[a]	+[a]
BER-EP4	+/−	+
Secretory component	−	+
Human placental lactogen	−	+
Lewis blood group antigens	−	+
Thrombomodulin	+	+
K1	+	−
ME1	+	+
HBME1	+[a]	+[a]
Calretinin	+	−

Principal staining reactions. Most of the antibodies that stain primarily carcinomas also occasionally stain mesotheliomas and vice versa.
[a] Cytoplasmic staining seen only in carcinomas; heavy membrane staining seen in mesotheliomas.

their reliability is uncertain. It is crucial to remember that the occasional mesothelioma will stain with any of the carcinoma markers, albeit generally not very strongly, and some proportion of carcinomas also stain with the few mesothelioma markers (162–183). Some antibodies are less useful because their staining reactions may be difficult to interpret; for example, antibodies to milk fat globule protein (HMFG) commonly stain both mesotheliomas and carcinomas, but in mesotheliomas staining is confined to cell membranes, where it typically makes a very thick line, and in carcinomas it is seen in both membranes and cytoplasm (78, 171, 172). One particularly helpful approach is to use several of the carcinoma markers; statistical analysis suggests that two or more positive reactions greatly increase the probability of carcinoma, with claimed specificities from about 75 to 95% (167, 173, 180). Hammar et al. (161) suggest that some of the false-positive reactions of carcinoma markers in documented mesotheliomas are due to nonspecific staining of hyaluronic acid; this does appear to be true in the occasional case, but their own data suggest that it is not a very common phenomenon.

Both mesotheliomas and carcinomas stain for epithelial membrane antigen (EMA), and contrary to some initial hopes, EMA does not appear to reliably separate benign from malignant mesothelial proliferations. The observation that mesotheliomas are often both keratin and vimentin positive has lost much of its diagnostic specificity because a large proportion of carcinomas show the same staining reactions (184, 187–189). It was also claimed in the past that mesotheliomas but not carcinomas were strongly keratin positive (162, 185, 186, 190), but it is now clear that both types of tumor are strongly and diffusely positive with the common commercial broad-spectrum antikeratins (175). There is some evidence that the keratins of mesotheliomas and carcinomas do differ (166, 175,

171, 184), but thus far these differences are not diagnostically useful. Keratin staining is thus of no help in separating epithelial mesotheliomas and carcinomas. However, sarcomatous mesotheliomas, including the forms with chondrosarcomatous and osteosarcomatous features, are almost invariably keratin positive. Therefore keratin staining is extremely valuable for confirming that a sarcomatous pleural or peritoneal tumor is a mesothelioma and not a sarcoma (184, 191, 192).

Table 10.10 also lists some antibodies that are claimed to stain mesotheliomas. K1 (178) may be specific, but it works only on frozen sections, as does ME1. The latter also stains carcinomas (177, 179). HBME1 (193) does work on paraffin sections but stains about 50% of adenocarcinomas, although the mesotheliomas typically show a membranous rather than cytoplasmic staining pattern (78) and staining of carcinomas appears to be greatly decreased with high antibody dilution. Collins et al. (176) reported that antibodies to thrombomodulin stained mesotheliomas and very few carcinomas, but a later report (183) claims that thrombomodulin staining in adenocarcinomas is common. Doglioni et al. (179) very recently reported that antibodies to calretinin, a calcium-binding protein, stained 100% of mesotheliomas and only about 10% of carcinomas in paraffin section. Thus it is clear that none of these antibodies provides a magic bullet, and immunostaining reactions must be considered in the context of gross and routine microscopic information.

Ultrastructure. The ultrastructure of mesotheliomas has been reviewed (161, 194). Despite claims to the contrary (194–197), most of the ultrastructural features of malignant mesothelioma are nonspecific, reflecting differentiation toward a secretory type of epithelial cell or a fibroblastic mesenchymal cell and various intermediate and/or poorly differentiated variants (194). The surfaces of the epithelial forms and sometimes the surfaces of the spindled forms demonstrate microvilli that may be quite numerous and long (194) (Fig. 10.13). Inter-

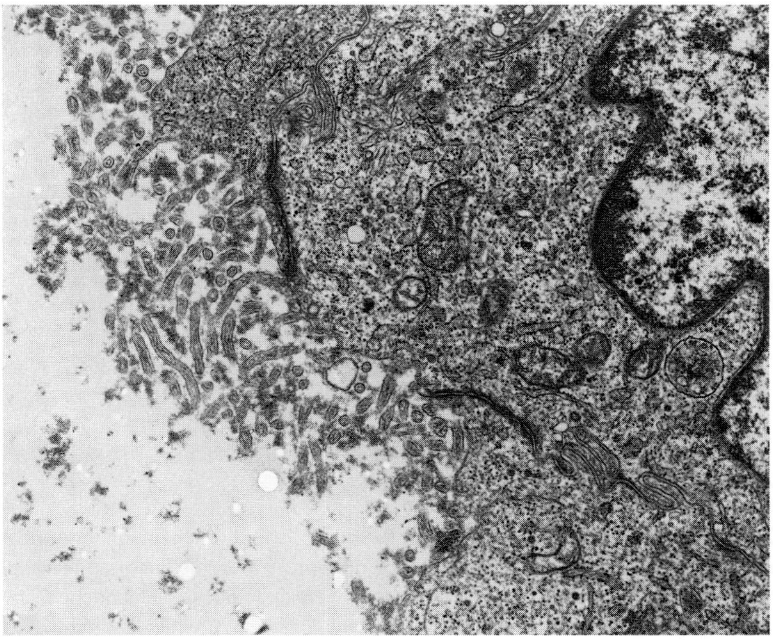

FIGURE 10.13
Electron micrograph of an epithelial mesothelioma demonstrating numerous microvilli.

cellular and intracellular lumina are common. In epithelial mesotheliomas the cells are linked by numerous well-formed desmosomes; some cells have large numbers of tonofilament bundles in the cytoplasm.

The aspect (length to width) ratio of the microvilli has been proposed as the ultrastructural feature that is most useful in separating mesotheliomas from carcinomas (78, 194, 198–201), with high ratios said to be characteristic of mesothelioma and low ratios characteristic of adenocarcinomas. Although this is true in a statistical sense, there tends to be so much overlap in the values obtained for these two types of tumor that only values at the upper extreme are likely to have any diagnostic use (198). It is also claimed that the microvilli of adenocarcinomas are covered by a glycocalyx and those of mesotheliomas are not, but as the recent report of Hammar et al. (161) makes clear, this is by no means always true. Microvilli interdigitating with collagen along the basal poles of tumor cells and perinuclear aggregates of tonofilaments have also been proposed as findings that favor a diagnosis of mesothelioma (194, 198), but even these authors agree that in poorly differentiated tumors, that is, when one really needs diagnostic help, many of these features are not present. Overall, I believe that ultrastructural examination is far inferior to the faster and considerably less expensive histochemical and immunohistochemical stains (Fig. 10.14).

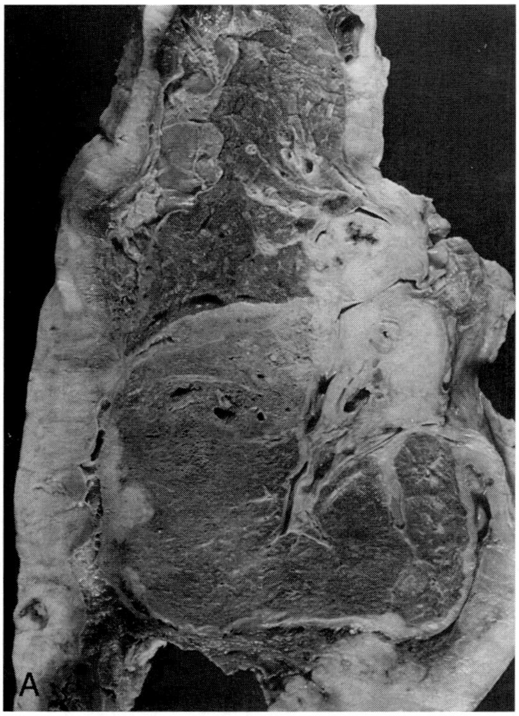

FIGURE 10.14

Carcinoma mimicking mesothelioma. **A.** Gross appearance of an adenocarcinoma completely surrounding lung. **B.** Microscopic appearance of this tumor showing polygonal cells that may be an epitheloid type of malignant mesothelioma. **C.** Immunochemical stain for CEA showing strong diffuse positivity throughout the tumor cells, which is diagnostic of carcinoma. This tumor also had numerous cells with PAS-positive mucin droplets. **D** and **E.** Photomicrographs of a diffuse abdominal tumor from a man. Histologically this resembles mesothelioma, but the PAS stain (**E**) shows unequivocal mucin droplets (*arrow*).

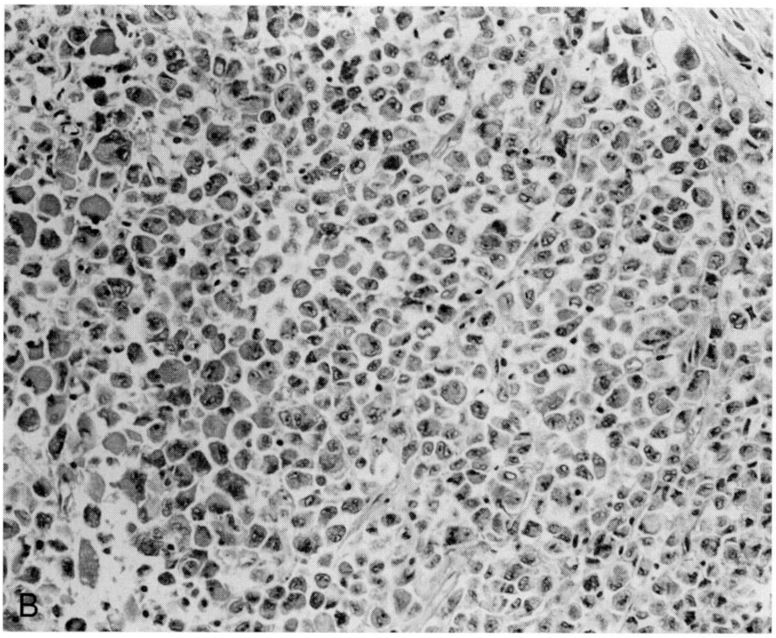

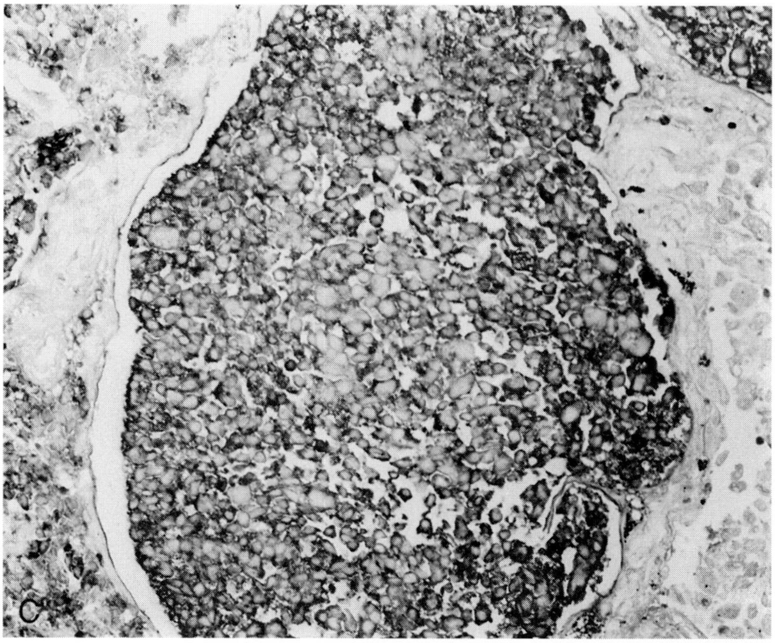

FIGURE 10.14 *(continued)*

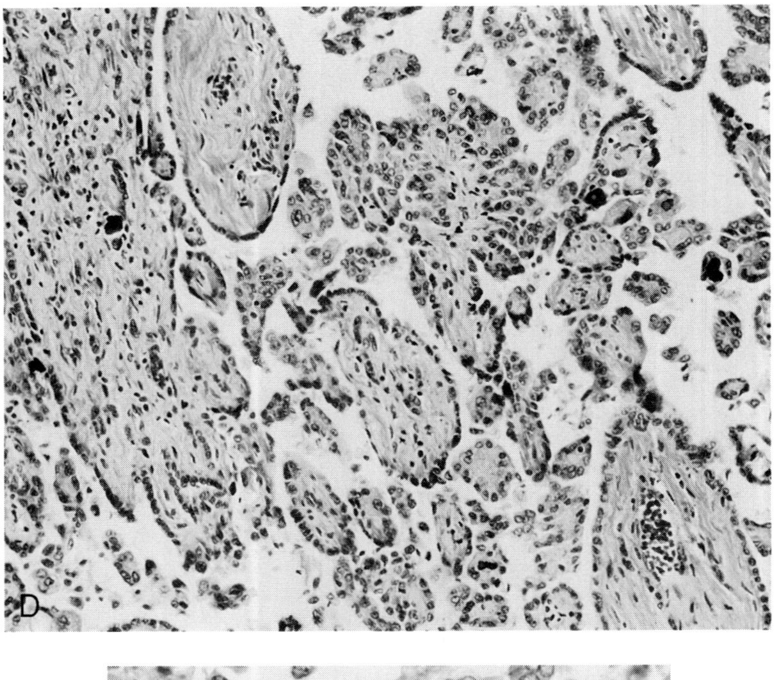

FIGURE 10.14 *(continued)*

Separation of Mesotheliomas from Reactive Mesothelial Proliferations. Sometimes the question posed by histologic examination is not the mesothelial origin of a proliferative process but whether it is neoplastic or inflammatory (Table 10.11). The commonly used criteria of malignancy, namely necrosis, cytologic atypia, and high mitotic rate, are less useful than might be presumed because many mesotheliomas appear remarkably innocuous and many reactive proliferations are cytologically quite atypical and sometimes show numerous mitoses.

A number of features are helpful in this situation. A good rule of thumb is that benign mesothelial reactions do not invade the stroma, and *in the pleura* the finding of mesothelial cells deep to free surfaces (for example, invading the fat of the chest wall) indicates malignancy, no matter how bland the cells appear (Fig. 10.15). Great care must be taken when applying this principle to small biopsies, in which en face cuts of the surface mesothelium can mimic invasion. Invasion of mesenteric fat is usually a reliable sign of mesothelial malignancy in the peritoneal cavity as well, but some inflammatory reactions, particularly around the ovary and adnexa, can trap mesothelial cells, again giving a false impression of invasion (202, 203). One helpful finding in this situation is that the apparently invasive mesothelial cells are arranged in linear arrays (202, 203), whereas true mesothelial malignancies show random patterns of invasion.

Probably the area of greatest concern is the separation of organizing pleural effusions from desmoplastic mesotheliomas (Figs. 10.9 and 10.10). The combination of a storiform or patternless pattern with bland necrosis; areas of cellular, frank sarcoma; or definite stromal invasion by tumor cells favors the diag-

TABLE 10.11
Separation of Benign and Malignant Mesothelial Proliferations

	BENIGN REACTIONS	MESOTHELIOMAS
True stromal invasion	Not seen in benign reactions	Strong evidence of malignancy
Cellularity	Low except under effusion	High except in desmoplastic tumors
Sidedness of cell proliferation	More cellular toward effusion; less cellular away from effusion	Cellularity may be high anywhere
Necrosis	Rare	Uncommon
Capillaries	Often long, with perpendicular orientation to surface	Inconspicuous in tumor
Cytologic atypia	Benign reactions can be atypical, particularly in the pleural space	Useful when marked, but many mesotheliomas appear relatively monotonous and bland
Mitoses	Common in reactive proliferations	Uncommon in most mesotheliomas
Immunohistochemistry	p53 may be positive in benign conditions Keratin positive	p 53 may be positive or negative Keratin positive

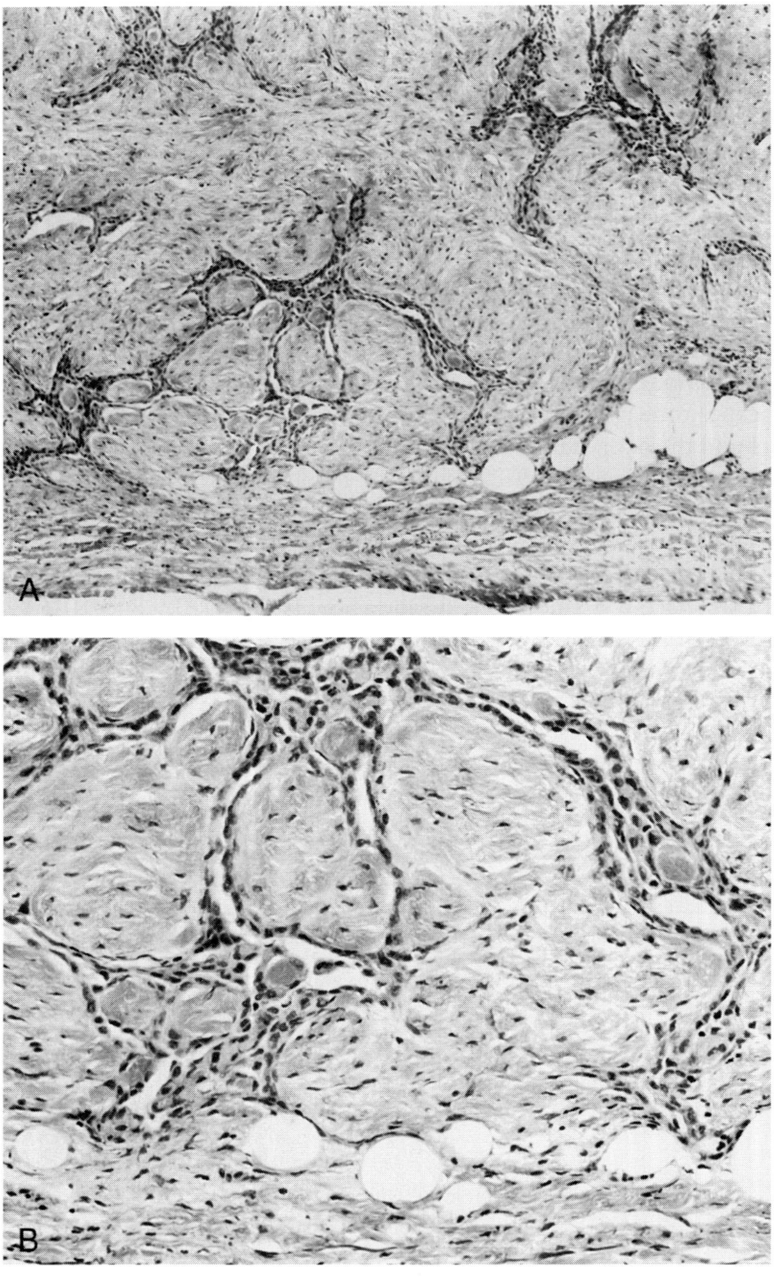

FIGURE 10.15

Epithelial mesothelioma showing bland features that might be mistaken for a reactive process. **A.** Glands lined by flattened cells extend through a greatly thickened pleura. **B.** The tumor cells are flattened and appear innocuous. However, it is clear from both photographs that the process is invading deep into the pleura and extending into the subcutaneous fat of the chest wall, findings that always indicate malignancy.

nosis of mesothelioma. Benign reactions may appear quite cellular and sometimes cytologically atypical immediately under the fibrinous effusion, but they become more and more sclerotic as one moves toward the chest wall (see Fig. 9.4). By contrast, sarcomatous mesotheliomas often have a homogeneous cellularity or are more cellular away from the fibrin layer. Suspect cases should always be completely blocked and sectioned, since areas of high cellularity or stromal invasion can be very focal. Roggli et al. (204) have pointed out that long, thin capillaries oriented perpendicular to the pleural surface are often seen in benign pleural fibrotic reactions.

Immunohistochemical stains for intermediate filaments are unfortunately not useful in this context, since proliferating mesothelial cells, whether benign or malignant, are typically both keratin and vimentin positive (191, 192, 205, 206), and benign keratin-positive spindled mesothelial cells can be found even in plaques and pleural scars. However, keratin stains often do give a better indication of the presence and distribution of mesothelial cells than hematoxylin and eosin stains, and this is sometimes helpful in assessing invasion.

Ramael et al. (207, 208) have claimed that mesotheliomas express immunoreactivity for the B-chain of platelet-derived growth factor and for a specific glycoprotein (P-170) and reactive mesothelial proliferations do not; whether this distinction will prove useful in sorting out benign and malignant proliferations remains to be seen. Mayall et al. (209) reported that mesotheliomas express p53 and that this expression is not seen in reactive processes. However, Walts et al. (210) reported that p53 staining could be found in benign mesothelial cells in effusions. My own experience is not only that p53 expression in mesotheliomas is inconstant but that interobserver variation in interpretation of positivity is so great that this test is not reliable (156).

Separation of Diffuse Malignant Mesothelioma from Other Primary Pleural Tumors. Diffuse malignant mesothelioma is the only *primary* pleural tumor to encase the lung or show numerous tumor nodules. Thus in general the separation from other types of primary pleural tumors is straightforward. Solitary fibrous tumors (submesothelial fibromas) are circumscribed pleural-based lesions that are histologically distinctive (211, 212); the major area of diagnostic confusion is the continued use of the term *fibrous mesothelioma* for these tumors. Recent studies indicate that morphologically identical tumors occur in a variety places outside the thorax, indicating clearly that the tumors do not arise in the mesothelium (213, 214). The occasional malignant variants may appear as rather nondescript spindle cell sarcomas but are nonetheless local tumors. Both benign and malignant solitary fibrous tumors are keratin negative and CD34 positive (213, 214), in sharp contrast to malignant mesotheliomas.

Well-differentiated papillary mesotheliomas are composed of prominent broad fibrovascular cores covered by very thin to cuboidal mesothelial cells. They are usually incidental findings in the peritoneal cavity, but rarely they occur in the pleural cavity and sometimes are multiple (78, 80, 215, 216). They generally are benign.

More troublesome from the morphologic point of view is the newly described entity of localized malignant mesothelioma (217). These tumors are histologically identical to diffuse malignant mesotheliomas; they occur in epithelial, sarcomatous, and mixed forms and show similar immunostaining and ultrastructural features. However, they are always sharply circumscribed pleural-based nodules. They can both recur locally and spread by metastasis, but even when they recur, they do not spread over the pleural surface. Various defined sarcomas, such as angiosarcomas (218), do occur as primary pleural and peritoneal tumors. These lesions are extremely rare and are not related to mesotheliomas.

Although not referring to a primary pleural tumor, the term *pseudomesotheliomatous carcinoma* has sometimes been applied to peripheral carcinomas of the lung that grow by spreading over the pleural surface (151) (Fig. 10.14*A*). Histologically these lesions are usually adenocarcinomas, but other cell types are occasionally seen. There is no evidence that these tumors have any particular relation to asbestos exposure, and the term *pseudomesotheliomatous carcinoma* should probably be dropped, since it tends to sow both diagnostic and etiologic confusion. Illustrations of all these entities can be found in various reports (78, 80, 217). None is associated with asbestos exposure.

Patterns of Spread. Mesotheliomas spread by contiguous growth into adjoining viscera and body walls or by hematogenous and lymphatic metastases. In the past it was believed that metastases militated against the diagnosis of mesothelioma, and this is still generally true when considering clinically evident metastases at presentation. However, it is now clear that metastases are present in at least half of the cases of both pleural and peritoneal mesothelioma at autopsy (219–222), and as described previously, metastatic lesions are occasionally a presenting sign (141). The most common site of metastases are lymph nodes within the thoracic or abdominal cavities; pleural tumors may also metastasize to supraclavicular or cervical nodes and abdominal tumors, to inguinal nodes. Common sites of visceral metastases include lungs, liver, pleura, bone, adrenal glands, and heart.

Therapy and Prognosis. The course of disease in most patients with malignant mesothelioma is rapid progression. Legha and Muggia (139) summarized 267 patients from eight series; mean survival was 12.5 months from the onset of symptoms, and 75% of the patients were dead within a year of diagnosis. In a more recent series of nearly 1500 patients, Spirtas et al. (223) found a median survival of 7 months, and Ribak and Selikoff (224) reported similar data for 457 asbestos insulators.

Some patients do survive longer. Antman (225) summarized 5 series of 331 patients whose disease was sufficiently local to permit surgical resection; survivals were 47% at l year, 28% at 2 years, and 8% at 5 years. Spirtas et al. (223) observed that patients below age 50 fared considerably better than the group as a whole, and this observation has also been made by Antman et al. (226); this is particularly true of women with peritoneal tumors.

There is a correlation between prognosis and histologic pattern (142, 155). Elmes and Simpson (142) found that those whose tumors showed a purely epithelial pattern had a mean survival of 18 months; those with a mixed pattern, a survival of 11 months; and those with a purely sarcomatous pattern, a survival of 8 months. Sarcomatous tumors of the desmoplastic type appear to be particularly aggressive (155).

Radiation therapy and chemotherapy have been applied to mesothelioma with very limited success. Doxorubicin (Adriamycin) containing regimens seem to be most effective, with claimed response rates up to 40%. However, even with a response, survival is still extremely poor. Antman et al. (227) recorded a median survival of 15 months for those treated with chemotherapy and 8.5 months for those not treated. Similar results were reported by Yap et al. (228). Occasional patients do have prolonged survivals, sometimes exceeding 5 years, even without chemotherapy (229, 230).

OTHER TUMORS CLAIMED TO BE ASSOCIATED WITH ASBESTOS EXPOSURE

At various times claims that laryngeal, esophageal, gastric, and colorectal carcinomas are associated with occupational asbestos exposure have been advanced (11, 231–239). These are purely epidemiologic issues, since even if an association were demonstrated, no specific pathologic findings would allow attribution of causation in a specific case. All of these tumors are common in the general population and have various well-documented causes, including smoking (larynx, esophagus), alcohol (larynx, esophagus), diet (stomach, colorectal), and social class (10, 231). Recent summaries have concluded that there is no consistent evidence for an elevated risk of any of these tumors in asbestos-exposed cohorts, nor is there evidence for a dose response (232–239). Claims regarding a possible association between asbestos exposure and lymphoproliferative malignancies (240) have similarly not been borne out on further study (11, 241).

REFERENCES

1. McDonald JC. Cancer risks due to asbestos and man-made fibres. Recent Results Cancer Res 1990;120:122–133.
2. Health Effects Institute—Asbestos Research. Asbestos in public and commercial buildings: a literature review and synthesis of current knowledge. Cambridge, MA: Health Effects Institute, 1991.
3. McDonald JC, McDonald AD. Epidemiology of asbestos-related lung cancer. In: Antman K, Aisner J, eds. Asbestos-related malignancy. New York: Grune & Stratton, 1986:57–79.
4. McDonald JC. Asbestos and lung cancer: has the case been proven? Chest 1980;78: 374–376.
5. McDonald JC, Liddell FRDK, Dufresne A, McDonald AD. The 1891–1920 birth cohort of Quebec chrysotile miners and millers: mortality 1976–1988. Br J Ind Med 1993;50:1073–1081.
6. Selikoff IJ, Hammond EC, Seidman H. Latency of asbestos disease among insulation workers in the United States and Canada. Cancer 1980;46:2736–2740.
7. Huuskonen MS. Asbestos and cancer. Eur J Respir Dis 1982;63 (Suppl 123): 145–152.
8. Health and Safety Executive. Review of fiber toxicology. Sudbury, UK: HSE Books, 1996.
9. Sebastien P, McDonald JC, McDonald AD, Case B, Harley R. Respiratory cancer in chrysotile textile and mining industries: exposure inferences from lung analysis. Br J Ind Med 1989;46:180–187.
10. Dement JM. Carcinogenicity of chrysotile asbestos: evidence from cohort studies. Ann N Y Acad Sci 1991;643:15–23.
11. Browne K. Asbestos-related disorders. In: Parkes WR, ed. Occupational lung disorders. 3rd ed. London: Butterworths, 1994:411–504.
12. Hammond EC, Selikoff IJ, Seidman H. Asbestos exposure, cigarette smoking, and death rates. Ann N Y Acad Sci 1979;330:473–491.
13. McDonald JC, Liddell FDK, Gibbs GW, et al. Dust exposure and mortality in chrysotile mining, l910–l975. Br J Ind Med 1980;37:11–24.
14. Browne K. A threshold for asbestos related lung cancer. Br J Ind Med 1986;43: 556–558.

15. Browne K. Is asbestos or asbestosis the cause of the increased risk of lung cancer in asbestos workers. Br J Ind Med 1986;43:145–149.
16. Churg A. Asbestos, asbestosis, and lung cancer. Mod Pathol 1993;6:509–511.
17. Roggli VL, Hammar SP, Practt PC, et al. Does asbestos or asbestosis cause carcinoma of the lung. Am J Ind Med 1994;26:835–838.
18. McDonald JC. Health implications of environmental exposure to asbestos. Environ Health Perspect 1985;62:329–328.
19. Tubiana M. The carcinogenic effect of exposures to low doses of carcinogens. Br J Ind Med 1992;49:601–605.
20. Sebastien P, Plourde M, Robb R, et al. Ambient air asbestos survey in Quebec mining towns: 2. Main study. Environment Canada Report 5/AP/RQ-2E, 1986.
21. Berry G, Newhouse ML. Mortality of workers manufacturing friction materials using asbestos. Br J Ind Med 1983;40:1–7.
22. Gardner MJ, Winter PD, Pannett B, Powell CA. Follow up study of workers manufacturing chrysotile asbestos cement products. Br J Ind Med 1986;43:726–732.
23. Neuberger M, Kundi M. Individual asbestos exposure, smoking and mortality: a cohort study in the asbestos cement industry. Br J Ind Med 1990;47:615–620.
24. Newhouse ML, Sullivan KR. A mortality study of workers manufacturing friction materials, 1941–86. Br J Ind Med 1989;46:176–179.
25. de Klerk NH, Armstrong BK, Musk AW, Hobbs MST. Cancer mortality in relation to measures of occupational exposure to crocidolite at Wittenoom Gorge. Br J Ind Med 1989;46:529–536.
26. Davis JMG, Cowie HA. The relationship between fibrosis and cancer in experimental animals exposed to asbestos and other fibers. Environ Health Perspect 1990; 88:305–309.
27. Huuskonen MS. Clinical features, mortality and survival of patients with asbestosis. Scand J Work Environ Health 1978;4:265–274.
28. Coutts II, Turner-Warwick M. Factors predicting outcome in intrapulmonary fibrosis associated with asbestos exposure (asbestosis). In: Gee JBL, Morgan WKC, eds. Occupational lung disease. New York: Raven Press, 1984:208–209.
29. Berry G. Mortality of workers certified by pneumoconiosis medical panels as having asbestosis. Br J Ind Med 1981;38:130–137.
30. Chief Inspector of Factories. Annual Report for 1947. London: His Majesty's Stationery Office, 1947:79–81.
31. Buchanan WD. Asbestosis and primary intrathoracic neoplasms. Ann N Y Acad Sci 1965;132:507–518.
32. Doll R. Mortality from lung cancer in asbestos workers. Br J Ind Med 1955;12: 81–86.
33. Bohlig H, Jacob G, Muller H. Die Asbestose der Lunger. Suttgart: Georg Thieme, 1960:60.
34. Liddell FDK, McDonald JC. Radiological findings as predictors of mortality in Quebec asbestos workers. Br J Ind Med 1980;37:256–267.
35. Kipen HM, Lilis R, Suzuki Y, et al. Pulmonary fibrosis in asbestos insulation workers with lung cancer: a radiological and histopathological evaluation. Br J Ind Med 1987;44:96–100.
36. Newhouse ML, Berry G, Wagner JC. Mortality of factory workers in east London 1933–80. Br J Ind Med 1985;42:4–11.
37. Hughes JR, Weill H. Asbestosis as a precursor of asbestos related lung cancer. Br J Ind Med 1991;48:229–233.
38. Sluis-Cremer GK, Bezuidenhout BN. Relation between asbestosis and bronchial cancer in amphibole asbestos miners. Br J Ind Med 1989;46:537–540.
39. Turner-Warwick M, Lebowitz M, Burrows B, Johnson A. Cryptogenic fibrosing alveolitis and lung cancer. Thorax 1980;35:496–499.
40. Nagai A, Chiyotani A, Nakadate T, Konno K. Lung cancer in patients with idiopathic pulmonary fibrosis. Tohoku J Exp Med 1992;167:231–237.

41. Wilkinson P, Hansell DM, Janssens J, et al. Is lung cancer associated with asbestos exposure when there are no small opacities on the chest radiograph? Lancet 1995; 345:1074–1078.
42. Irvine H, Lamont DW, Hole DJ, Gillis CR. Asbestos and lung cancer in Glasgow and the West of Scotland, BMJ 1993;306:1503–1506.
43. Barroetavena MC, Teschke K, Bates DV. Unrecognized asbestos-induced disease. Am J Ind Med 1996;29:183–185.
44. Jones RN, Hughes JM, Weill H. Asbestos exposure, asbestosis, and asbestos-attributable lung cancer. Thorax 1996;51(Suppl 2):S9–S15.
45. Warnock ML, Isenberg W. Asbestos burden and the pathology of lung cancer. Chest 1986;89:20–26.
46. Karjalainen A, Anttila S, Vanhala E, Vainio H. Asbestos exposure and the risk of lung cancer in a general urban population. Scand J Work Environ Health 1994;20: 243–250.
47. Chamberlin M, Tarmy EM. Asbestos and glass fibers in bacterial mutation tests. Mutat Res 1977;43:159–164.
48. Shelby MD. The genetic toxicity of human carcinogens and its implications. Mutat Res 1988;204:3–15.
49. Hei TK, Piao CQ, He ZY, et al. Chrysotile fiber is a strong mutagen in mammalian cells. Cancer Res 1992;52:6305–6309.
50. Hei TK. Oncogenic transformation by asbestos fibers and radon-stimulated alpha particles. In: Mossman BT, Bégin RO, eds. Berlin: Springer-Verlag, 1989:389–398.
51. Hei TK, He ZY, Suzuki K. Effects of antioxidants on fiber mutagenesis. Carcinogenesis 1995;16:1573–1578.
52. Mossman BT, Kamp DW, Weitzman SA. Mechanisms of carcinogenesis and clinical features of asbestos-associated cancers. Cancer Invest 1996;14:464–478.
53. Hesterberg TW, Barrett JC. Induction by asbestos fibers of anaphase abnormalities: mechanism for aneuploidy induction and possibly carcinogenesis. Carcinogenesis 1985; 6:473–475.
54. Wang NS, Jaurand MC, Magne L, et al. The interactions between asbestos fibers and metaphase chromosomes of rat pleural mesothelial cells in cultures. Am J Pathol 1987;126:343–349.
55. Marsh JP, Mossman BT. Mechanisms of induction of ornithine decarboxylase activity in tracheal epithelialal cells by asbestiform minerals. Cancer Res 1988;48: 709–714.
56. Perderiset M, Marsch JP, Mossman BT. Activation of protein kinase C by crocidolite asbestos in hamster tracheal epithelial cells. Carcinogenesis 1991;12: 1499–1502.
57. Heintz NH, Janssen YM, Mossman BT. Persistent induction of c-fos and c-jun expression by asbestos. Proc Natl Acad Sci U S A 1993;90:3299–3303.
58. Janssen YMW, Barchowsky A, Treadwell M, et al. Asbestos induces nuclear factor kB (NF-kB) DNA-binding activity and NF-kB-dependent gene expression in tracheal epithelial cells. Proc Natl Acad Sci U S A 1995;92:8458–8462.
59. Reiss B, Tong C, Telang S, Williams GM. Enhancement of benzo[a]pyrene mutagenicity by chrysotile asbestos in rat liver epithelial cells. Environ Res 1983;31: 100–104.
60. Quinlan TR, Berube KA, Marsh JP, et al. Patterns of inflammation, cell proliferation, and related gene expression in lung after inhalation of chrysotile asbestos. Am J Pathol 1995;147:728–739.
61. Garland LH, Beier RL, Coulson W, et al. The apparent sites of origin of carcinomas of the lung. Radiology 1962;78:1–11.
62. Kannerstein M, Churg J. Pathology of carcinoma of the lung associated with asbestos exposure. Cancer 1972;30:14–21.
63. Whitwell F, Newhouse MD, Bennett DR. A study of the histological cell types of lung cancer in workers suffering from asbestosis. Br J Ind Med 1974;31:298–303.

64. Hourihane DO'B, McCaughey WTE. Pathological aspects of asbestosis. Postgrad Med J 1966;42:613–622.
65. Auerbach O, Garfinkel VA, Joubert L. Histologic type of lung cancer and asbestos exposure. Cancer 1984;54:3017–3021.
66. Johannson L, Albin M, Jakobsson K, Mikoczy Z. Histological type of lung carcinoma in asbestos cement workers and matched controls. Br J Ind Med 1992;49: 626–630.
67. Karjalainen A, Anttila S, Heikkila L, et al. Lobe of origin of lung cancer among asbestos exposed patients with or without diffuse interstitial fibrosis. Scan J Work Environ Health 1993;19:102–107.
68. Ives JC, Buffler PA, Greenberg D. Environmental associations and histopathologic patterns of carcinoma of the lung. Am Rev Respir Dis 1983;128:195–209.
69. Churg A. Lung cancer cell type and occupational exposure. In: Samet JM, ed. Epidemiology of lung cancer. New York: Marcel Dekker, 1994:413–436.
70. Becklake MR. Occupational lung disease: past record and future trend using the asbestos case as an example. Clin Invest Med 1983;6:305–317.
71. Parkes WR. Silicates and lung disease. In: Parkes WR, ed. Occupational lung disorders. 2nd ed. London: Butterworths, 1982:233–332.
72. Martischnig KM, Newell DJ, Barnsley WC, et al. Unsuspected exposure to asbestos and bronchogenic carcinoma. Br Med J 1977;1:746–749.
73. Hasan FM, Nash G, Kazemi H. Asbestos exposure and related neoplasia. Am J Med 1978;65:649–654.
74. Raffin E, Lynge E, Korsgaard B. Incidence of lung cancer by histologic type among asbestos cement workers in Denmark. Br J Ind Med 1993;50:85–89.
75. Klemperer P, Rabin CB. Primary neoplasms of the pleura. Arch Pathol 1931;11: 385–401.
76. Willis RA. Pathology of Tumors. 4th ed. London: Butterworths, 1967.
77. Stout AP, Murray MR. Localized pleural mesothelioma. Arch Pathol 1942;34: 951–961.
78. Battifora H, McCaughey WTE. Tumors of the serosal membranes. Washington: Armed Forces Institute of Pathology, 1994.
79. Wagner JC, Sleggs CA, Marchand P. Diffuse pleural mesothelioma and asbestos exposure in the North Western Cape Province. Br J Ind Med. 1960;17:260–269.
80. McCaughey WTE, Kannerstein M, Churg J. Tumors of the serosal membranes. Washington: Armed Forces Institute of Pathology, 1985.
81. Rubino GF, Scansetti G, Donna A, Palestro G. Epidemiology of pleural mesothelioma in northwestern Italy (Piedmont). Br J Ind Med 1972;29:436–442.
82. Cochrane JC, Webster I. Mesothelioma in relation to asbestos fiber exposure. South Afr Med J 1978;78:279–281.
83. McDonald JC. Health implications of environmental exposure to asbestos. Environ Health Perspect 1985;62:319–328.
84. Spirtas R, Heineman EF, Bernstein L, et al. Malignant mesothelioma: attributable risk of asbestos exposure. Occup Environ Med 1994;51:804–811.
85. Spirtas R, Beebe GW, Connelly RR, et al. Recent trends in mesothelioma incidence in the United States. Am J Ind Med 1986;9:397–407.
86. Artvinli M, Baris YI. Malignant mesotheliomas in a small village in the Anatolian region of Turkey: an epidemiologic study. J Natl Cancer Inst 1979;63:17–24.
87. Artvinli M, Baris YI, Sahin AA. Environmental mesothelioma in Turkey. Ann N Y Acad Sci 1979;330:423–432.
88. Gilks B, Hegedus C, Freeman H, et al. Malignant peritoneal mesothelioma after remote abdominal radiation. Cancer 1988;61:2019–2021.
89. Maurer R, Egloff B. Malignant peritoneal mesothelioma after cholangiography with thorotrast. Cancer 1975;36:1381–1385.
90. Hillerdal G, Berg J. Malignant mesothelioma secondary to chronic inflammation and old scars: two new cases and review of the literature. Cancer 1985;55: 1968–1972.

91. Peterson JT, Greenberg SD, Buffler PA. Non-asbestos-related malignant mesothelioma. Cancer 1984;54:501–513.
92. McDonald AD, McDonald JC. Epidemiology of malignant mesothelioma. In: Antman K, Aisner J, eds. Asbestos-related malignancy. New York: Grune and Stratton, 1986:31–55.
93. National Cancer Institute. SEER Cancer Statistics Review 1973–1993.Bethesda: National Cancer Institute, 1996.
94. National Research Council. Nonoccupational health risks of asbestiform fibers. Washington: National Academy Press, 1984.
95. Connelly RR, Spirtas R, Myers MH, et al. Demographic patterns for mesothelioma in the United States. J Natl Cancer Inst 1987;78:1053–1060.
96. Peto J, Seidman H, Selikoff IJ. Mesothelioma mortality in asbestos workers: implications for models of carcinogenesis and risk assessment. Br J Cancer 1982;45: 124–135.
97. Selikoff IJ, Hammond EC, Seidman H. Latency of asbestos disease among insulation workers in the United States and Canada. Cancer 1980;46:2736–2740.
98. Lanphear BP, Buncher CR. Latent period for malignant mesothelioma of occupational origin. J Occup Med 1992;34:718–721.
99. McDonald AF, Fry JS, Woolley AJ, McDonald JC. Dust exposure and mortality in an American chrysotile friction products plant. Br J Ind Med 1984;41:151–157.
100. Dement JM, Brown RP, Okun A. Followup study of chrysotile textile asbestos workers. Am J Ind Med 1994;26:431–437.
101. Hughes JM, Weill H, Hammad YY. Mortality of workers employed in two asbestos cement manufacturing plants. Br J Ind Med 1987;44:161–174.
102. Piolatto G, Negri E, La Vecchia C, et al. An update of cancer mortality among chrysotile asbestos miners in Balangero, northern Italy. Br J Ind Med 1990;47: 810–814.
103. Berry G, Newhouse MI. Mortality of workers manufacturing friction materials using asbestos. Br J Ind Med 1983;40:1–7.
104. Karjalainen A, Meurman LO, Pukkala E. Four cases of mesothelioma among Finnish anthophyllite miners. Occup Environ Med 1994;51:212–215.
105. McDonald AF, Fry JS, Woolley AJ, McDonald JC. Dust exposure and mortality in an American factory using chrysotile, amosite, and crocidolite in mainly textile manufacture. Br J Ind Med 1983;40:368–374.
106. Hobbs MST, Woodward SD, Murphy B, et al. The incidence of pneumoconiosis, mesothelioma, and other respiratory cancer in men engaged in mining and milling crocidolite in western Australia. In: Wagner JC et al., eds. Biological effects of mineral fibres, vol 2. Lyon: International Agency for Research on Cancer, 1980: 615–625.
107. Selikoff IJ, Seidman H, Hammond ED. Mortality effects of cigarette smoking among amosite asbestos factory workers. J Natl Cancer Inst 1980;65:507–513.
108. Selioff IJ, Seidman H. Asbestos-associated deaths among insulation workers in the United States and Canada 1967–1987. Ann N Y Acad Sci 1991;643:1–44.
109. Jones JSP, Smith PG, Pooley FD, et al. The consequences of exposure to asbestos dust in a wartime gas-mask factory. In: Wagner JC et al., eds. Biological effects of mineral fibres, vol 2. Lyon: International Agency for Research on Cancer, 1980: 187–189.
110. McDonald AD, McDonald JC. Mesothelioma after crocidolite exposure during gas mask manufacture. Environ Res 1978;17:340–347.
111. Talcott JA, Thurber WA, Kantor AF, et al. Asbestos-associated diseases in a cohort of cigarette-filter workers. N Engl J Med 1989;321:1220–1223.
112. McDonald AD, McDonald JC, Liddell FDK, et al. Mesothelioma in Québec chrysotile miners and millers: epidemiology and etiology. Ann Occup Hyg (in press).
113. Churg A, Wright JL, Vedal S. Fiber burden and patterns of disease in long-term chrysotile miners and millers. Am Rev Respir Dis 1993;148:25–31.

114. Churg A. Chrysotile, tremolite, and mesothelioma in man. Chest 1988;93:621–628.
115. Wagner JC, Berry G, Pooley FD. Mesotheliomas and asbestos type in asbestos textile workers: a study of lung contents. Br Med J 1982;285:603–606.
116. Green FHY, Harley R, Vallyathan V, et al. Pulmonary fibrosis and asbestos exposure in chrysotile asbestos textile workers: preliminary results. Accomplishments Oncol 1986;1:59–68.
117. Churg A, DiPaoli L, Kempe B, Stevens B. Lung asbestos content in chrysotile workers with mesothelioma. Am Rev Respir Dis 1984;130:1042–1045.
118. Dufresne A, Bégin R, Churg A, Masse S. Mineral fibre content of lungs in mesothelioma cases seeking compensation in Québec. Am J Respir Crit Care Med 1996; 153:711–718.
119. Churg A. Analysis of lung asbestos content. Br J Ind Med 1991;48:649–652.
120. Roggli VL, Pratt PC, Brody AR. Asbestos content of lung tissue in asbestos associated disease: a study of 110 cases. Br J Ind Med 1986;43:18–29.
121. Wagner JC, Newhouse ML, Corrin B, et al. Correlation between fibre content of the lung and disease in East London asbestos factory workers. Br J Ind Med 1988; 45:305–308.
122. Churg A, Vedal S. Fiber burden and patterns of asbestos-related disease in workers with heavy mixed amosite and chrysotile exposure. Am J Respir Crit Care Med 1994;150:663–669.
123. Churg A. Deposition and clearance of chrysotile asbestos. Ann Occup Hyg 1994; 38:625–634.
124. Semiatycki J. Health effects on the general population: mortality in the general population in asbestos mining areas. In: Proceeding of the world symposium on asbestos. Montreal: Canadian Asbestos Information Centre, 1982:337–348.
125. Weill H, Hughes JM. Asbestos as a public health risk: disease and policy. Ann Rev Public Health 1986;7:171–192.
126. Mossman BT, Bignon J, Corn M, et al. Asbestos: scientific developments and implications for public policy. Science 1990;247:294–301.
127. Stanton MF, Layard M, Tegeris A, et al. Relation of particle dimension to carcinogenicity in amphibole asbestoses and other fibrous minerals. J Natl Cancer Inst 1981;67:965–975.
128. Davis JMG, Addison J, Bolton RE, et al. The pathogenicity of long vs short fibre samples of amosite asbestos administered to rats by inhalation and intraperitoneal injection. Br J Exp Pathol 1986;67:415–430.
129. Davis JMG, Jones AD. Comparisons of the pathogenicity of long and short fibre chrysotile asbestos in rats. Br J Exp Pathol 1986;69:717–737.
130. McDonald JC, Armstrong B, Case B, et al. Mesothelioma and asbestos fiber type: evidence from lung tissue analysis. Cancer 1989;63:1544–1547.
131. Rogers AJ, Leigh J, Berry G, et al. Relationship between lung asbestos fiber type and concentration and relative risk of mesothelioma. Cancer 1991;67:1912–1920.
132. Churg A, Wiggs B. Fiber size and number in users of processed chrysotile ore, chrysotile miners, and members of the general population. Am J Ind Med 1986;9: 143–152.
133. Wagner JC, Berry G, Timbrell V. Mesotheliomas in rats after innoculation with asbestos and other materials. Br J Cancer 1973;28:173–185.
134. Boutin C, Dumortier P, Rey F, et al. Black spots concentrate oncogenic asbestos fibers in the parietal pleura. Am J Respir Crit Care Med 1996;153:444–449.
135. Adamson IYR, Bakowska J, Bowden DH. Mesothelial cell proliferation: a nonspecific response to lung injury associated with fibrosis. Am J Respir Cell Mol Biol 1994;10:253–258.
136. Sekhon H, Wright J, Churg A. Effects of cigarette smoke and asbestos on airway, vascular, and mesothelial cell proliferation. Int J Exp Pathol 1995;76:411–418.
137. Gan L, Savransky EF, Fasy TM, Johnson EM. Transfection of human mesothelial cells mediated by different asbestos fiber types. Environ Res 1993;62:28–42.
138. Carbone M, Pass HI, Rizzo P, et al. Simian virus 40-like DNA sequences in human pleural mesotheliomas. Oncogene 1994;9:1781–1790.

139. Legha SS, Muggia FM. Pleural mesothelioma: Clinical features and therapeutic implications. Ann Intern Med 1977;87:613–620.
140. Grundy GW, Miller RW. Malignant mesothelioma in childhood. Cancer 1972;30:1216–1221.
141. Sussman J, Rosai J. Lymph node metastases as the initial manifestation of malignant mesothelioma. Am J Surg Pathol 1990;14:819–828.
142. Elmes PC, Simpson MJC. The clinical aspects of mesothelioma. Q J Med 1976;45:427–441.
143. Ellis K, Wolff M. Mesotheliomas and secondary tumors of the pleura. Semin Roentgenol 1977;12:303–312.
144. Abele DR. High-resolution computed tomography of asbestos-related disease. Semin Roentgenol 1991;26:118–131.
145. Kannerstein M, Churg J. Peritoneal mesothelioma. Hum Pathol 1977;8:83–93.
146. McCaughey WTE. Criteria for diagnosis of diffuse mesothelial tumors. Ann N Y Acad Sci 1965;32:603–612.
147. Kannerstein M, Churg J. Desmoplastic diffuse malignant mesothelioma. Prog Surg Pathol 1980;1:19–27.
148. Kannerstein M, McCaughey WTE, Churg J, Selikoff IJ. A critique of the criteria for the diagnosis of diffuse malignancy mesothelioma. Mt Sinai J Med 1977;44:485–491.
149. Churg J, Selikoff IJ. Geographic pathology of pleural mesothelioma. In: Liebow AA, ed. The lung. Baltimore: Williams & Wilkins, 1968:284.
150. McCaughey WTE, Colby TV, Battifora H, et al. Diagnosis of diffuse malignant mesothelioma: Experience of a US/Canadian mesothelioma panel. Mod Pathol 1991;4:342–353.
151. Koss M, Travis W, Moran C, Hochholzer L. Pseudomesotheliomatous adenocarcinoma: a reappraisal. Semin Diagn Pathol 1992;9:117–123.
152. Raji U, Fine G, Greenawald KA, Ohorodnik JM. Primary papillary serous neoplasia of the peritoneum. Hum Pathol 1989;20:426–436.
153. Mayall FG, Gibbs AR. The histology and immunohistochemistry of small cell mesotheliomas. Histopathol 1992;20:47–51.
154. Adams VI, Unni KK. Diffuse malignant mesothelioma of pleura. Am J Clin Pathol 1984;82:15–23.
155. Cantin R, Al-Jabi M, McCaughey WTE. Desmoplastic diffuse mesothelioma. Am J Surg Pathol 1982;6:215–221.
156. Mangano WD, Cagle PT, Churg A, et al. The diagnosis of desmoplastic malignant mesothelioma and its distinction from fibrous pleurisy. Am J Clin Pathol (in press).
157. Yousem SA, Hochholzer L. Malignant mesothelioma with osseous and cartilaginous differentiation. Arch Pathol Lab Med 1987;111:62–66.
158. Henderson DW, Attwood HD, Constance J, et al. Lymphohistiocytoid mesothelioma: a rare lymphomatoid variant of predominantly sarcomatoid mesothelioma. Ultrastruct Pathol 1988;12:367–384.
159. Kannerstein M, Churg J, Magner D. Histochemical studies in the diagnosis of mesothelioma. In: Bogovski P, Gilson JC, Timbrell V, Wagner JC, eds. Biological effects of asbestos. Lyon: IARC Scientific Publications, No. 8, 1973:62.
160. Whitwell P, Rawcliffe RM. Diffuse malignant pleural mesothelioma and asbestos exposure. Thorax 1971;26:6–13.
161. Hammar SP, Bockus DE, Remington FL, Rohrback KA. Mucin positive epithelial mesotheliomas: a histochemical, immunohistochemical, and ultrastructural comparison with mucin-producing pulmonary adenocarcinomas. Ultrastruct Pathol 1996;20:293–325.
162. Wang NS, Huang SN, Gold P. Absence of carcinoembryonic antigen-like material in mesothelioma. Cancer 1979;44:937–943.
163. Corson JM, Pinkus JS. Mesothelioma: Profile of keratin proteins and carcinoembryonic antigen. Am J Pathol. 1982;108:80–86.

164. Dewar A, Valente M, Ring NP, Corrin B. Pleural mesothelioma of epithelial type and pulmonary adenocarcinoma: An ultrastructural and cytochemical comparison. J Pathol 1987;152:309–316.
165. Sheibani K, Battifora H, Burke JS. Antigenic phenotype of malignant mesotheliomas and pulmonary adenocarcinomas. Am J Pathol 1986;123: 212–219.
166. Ordonez NG. The immunochemical diagnosis of mesothelioma. Am J Surg Pathol 1989;13:276–291.
167. Wick MR, Loy T, Mills SE, et al. Malignant epithelioid pleural mesothelioma versus peripheral pulmonary adenocarcinoma. Hum Pathol 1990;21:759–766.
168. Noguichi M, Nakajima T, Hirohashi S, et al. Immunohistochemical distinction of malignant mesothelioma from pulmonary adenocarcinoma with anti-surfactant apoprotein, anti-Lewis[a], and anti-Tn antibodies. Hum Pathol 1989;20:53–57.
169. Jordon D, Jagirdar J, Kaneko M. Blood group antigens, Lewis[x] and Lewis[y] in the diagnostic discrimination of malignant mesothelioma versus adenocarcinoma. Am J Pathol 1989;135:931–937.
170. Whitaker D, Sterrett GF, Shilkin KB. Detection of tissue CEA-like substance as an aid in the differential diagnosis of malignant mesothelioma. Pathology 1982;14: 255–262.
171. Otis CN, Carter DC, Cole S, Battifora H. Immunohistochemical evaluation of pleural mesothelioma and pulmonary adenocarcinoma. Am J Surg Pathol 1987;11: 445–456.
172. Tron V, Wright JL, Churg A. Carcinoembryonic antigen and milk-fat globule protein staining of malignant mesothelioma and adenocarcinoma of the lung. Arch Pathol Lab Med 1987;111:291–293.
173. Brown RW, Clark GM, Tandon AK, Allred DC. Multiple-marker immunohistochemical phenotypes distinguishing malignant pleural mesothelioma from pulmonary adenocarcinoma. Hum Pathol 1993;24:347–354.
174. Gaffey MJ, Mills SE, Swanson PE, et al. Immunoreactivity for BER-EP4 in adenocarcinomas, adenomatoid tumors, and malignant mesotheliomas. Am J Surg Pathol 1992;16:593–599.
175. Sheibaini K, Esteban JM, Bailey A, et al. Immunopathologic and molecular studies as an aid to the diagnosis of malignant mesothelioma. Hum Pathol 1992;23: 107–116.
176. Collins CL, Ordonez NG, Schaefer R, et al. Thrombomodulin expression in malignant pleural mesothelioma and pulmonary adenocarcinoma. Am J Pathol 1992; 141:827–833.
177. O'Hara CJ, Corson JM, Pinkus GS, Stahel RA. ME1: A monoclonal antibody that distinguishes epithelial-type malignant mesothelioma from pulmonary adenocarcinoma and extrapulmonary metastases. Am J Pathol 1990;136:421–428.
178. Chang K, Pai LH, Pass H, et al. Monoclonal antibody K1 reacts with epithelial mesothelioma but not with lung adenocarcinoma. Am J Surg Pathol 1992;16: 259–268.
179. Doglioni C, Tos APD, Laurino L, et al. Calretinin: a novel immunocytochemical marker for mesothelioma. Am J Surg Pathol 1996;20:1037–1046.
180. Frisman DM, McCarthy WF, Schleiff P, et al. Immunocytochemistry in the differential diagnosis of effusions: use of logistic regression to select a panel of antibodies to distinguish adenocarcinomas from mesothelial proliferations. Mod Pathol 1993;6:179–185.
181. Wick MR, Mills SE, Swanson PE. Expression of myelomonocytic antigens in mesotheliomas and adenocarcinomas involving the serosal surfaces. Am J Clin Pathol 1990;94:18–26.
182. Sheibani K, Shin SS, KezirianJ, Weiss LM. BER-EP4 antibody as a discriminant in the differential diagnosis of malignanrt mesothelioma vs adenocarcinoma. Am J Surg Pathol 1991;15:779–784.
183. Ascoli V, Carnovlae S, Taccogna S, Nardi F. The diagnostic value of thrombomod-

ulin immunolocalization in serous effusins. Arch Pathol Lab Med 1995;119: 1136–1140.
184. Blobel GA, Moll R, Franke WW, et al. The intermediate filament cytoskeleton of malignant mesotheliomas and its diagnostic significance. Am J Pathol 1985;121: 235–247.
185. Said JW, Nash G, Tepper G, Banks-Schlegel S. Keratin proteins and carcinoembryonic antigen in lung carcinoma. Hum Pathol 1983;14:70–76.
186. Bejui-Thivolet F, Patricot LM, Vauzelle JL. Keratins in malignant mesotheliomas and pleural adenocarcinomas. Pathol Res Pract 1984;179:67–73.
187. Jasani B, Edwards RE, Thomas ND, Gibbs AR. The use of vimentin antibodies in the diagnosis of malignant mesothelioma. Virchows Arch Pathol Anat 1985;406: 441–448.
188. Upton MP, Kirohashi S, Tome Y, et al. Expression of vimentin in surgically resected adenocarcinomas and large cell carcinomas of the lung. Am J Surg Pathol 1986;10: 560–567.
189. Azumi N, Battifora H. The distribution of vimentin and keratin in epithelial and nonepithelial neoplasms. Am J Clin Pathol 1987;88:286–296.
190. Szpak CA, Johnston WW, Roggle V, et al. The diagnostic distinction between malignant mesothelioma of the pleura and adenocarcinoma of the lung as defined by a monoclonal antibody (B72. 3). Am J Pathol 1986;122:252–260.
191. Montag AG, Pinkus GS, Corson JM. Keratin protein immunoreactivity of sarcomatoid and mixed types of diffuse malignant mesothelioma. Hum Pathol 1988;19: 336–342.
192. Cagle PT, Truong LD, Roggli VL, Greenberg SD. Immunohistochemical differentiation of sarcomatoid mesotheliomas from other spindle cell neoplasms. Am J Clin Pathol 1989;92:566–571.
193. Miettinin M, Kovatich AJ. HBME-1 a monocloncal antibody useful in the differential diagnosis of mesothelioma, adenocarcinoma, and soft-tissue and bone tumors. Appl Immunohistochem 1995;3:115–122.
194. Coleman M, Henderson DW, Mukherjee TM. The ultrastructural pathology of malignant pleural mesothelioma. Pathol Ann 1989;24:303–353.
195. Davis JMG. Ultrastructure of human mesotheliomas. J Natl Cancer Inst 1974;52: 1715–1723.
196. MacKay B, Osbourne BM, Wilson RA. Ultrastructure of lung neoplasms. In: Straus MJ, ed. Lung cancer: clinical diagnosis and treatment. New York: Grune & Stratton, 1977:71.
197. Suzuki Y, Churg J, Kannerstein M. Ultrastructure of human malignant diffuse mesothelioma. Am J Pathol 1976;85:241-250.
198. Warhol MJ, Corson JM. An ultrastructural comparison of mesotheliomas and adenocarcinomas of the lung and breast. Hum Pathol 1985;16:50–55.
199. Burns TR, Greenberg SD, Mace ML, Johnson EH. Ultrastructural diagnosis of epithelial malignant mesothelioma. Cancer 1985;56:2036–2041.
200. Roggli VL, Kolbeck J, Sanfilippo F, Shelburne JD. Pathology of human mesothelioma. Pathol Ann 1987;22(Part 2):91–131.
201. Warhol MJ, Hickey WF, Corson JM. Malignant mesothelioma: ultrastructural distinction from adenocarcinoma. Am J Surg Pathol 1982;6:307–314.
202. McFadden DE, Clement PB. Peritoneal inclusions cysts with mural mesothelial proliferation. Am J Surg Pathol 1986;10:844–854.
203. Clement PB, Young RH. Florid mesothelial hyperplasia associated with ovarian tumors. Int J Gynecol Pathol 1993;12:51–58.
204. Roggli VR, Sanfillip F, Shelburne JD. Mesothelioma. In: Roggli VL, Greenberg SD, Pratt PC, eds. Pathology of asbestos-associated diseases. Boston: Little Brown, 1992:109–264.
205. Ghosh AK, Gatter KC, Dunnill MS, Mason DY. Immunohistological staining of reactive mesothelioma, mesothelioma, and lung carcinoma with a panel of monoclonal antibodies. J Clin Pathol 1987;40:19–25.

206. Brockman M, Brockman I, Fischer M, Muller KM. Reaction lesions of the pleura: immunohistochemical characterization. Pathol Res Pract 1990;186:238–246.
207. Ramael M, Buysse C, van den Bossche J, et al. Immunoreactivity for the B chain of the platelet-derived growth factor receptor in malignant mesothelioma and non-neoplastic mesothelium. J Pathol 1992;167:1–4.
208. Ramael M, van den Bossche J, Buysse C, et al. Immunoreactivity for P-170 glycoprotein in malignant mesothelioma and in non-neoplastic mesothelium of the pleura using the murine monoclonal antibody JSB-1. J Pathol 1992;167:5–8.
209. Mayall FG, Goddard H, Gibbs AR. p53 immunostaining in the distinction between benign and malignant mesothelial proliferations using formalin-fixed paraffin sections. J Pathol 1992;168:377–381.
210. Walts A, Said JW, Koeffler HP. Is immunoreactivity for p53 useful in distinguishing benign from malignant effusions? localization of p53 gene product in benign mesothelial and adenocarcinoma cells. Mod Pathol 1994;7:462–466.
211. England DM, Hochholzer L, McCarthy MJ. Localized benign and malignant fibrous tumors of the pleura. Am J Surg Path 1989;13:640–658.
212. Briselli M, Mark EJ, Dicersin GR. Solitary fibrous tumors of the pleura. Cancer 1981;47:2678–2689.
213. van de Rijn M, Lombard CM, Rouse RV. Expression of CD34 by solitary fibrous tumors of the pleura, mediastinum, and lung. Am J Surg Path 1994;18:814–820.
214. Westra WH, Gerald WL, Rosai J. Solitary fibrous tumor: consistent CD34 immunoreactivity and occurrence in the orbit. Am J Surg Path 1994;18:992–998.
215. Daya D, McCaughey WTE. Well differentiated papillary mesothelioma of the peritoneum. Cancer 1990;65:292–296.
216. Yesner R, Hurwitz A. Localized pleural mesothelioma of epithelial type. J Thorac Surg 1952;26:325–329.
217. Crotty TB, Myers JL, Katzenstein ALA, et al. Localized malignant mesothelioma. Am J Surg Path 1994;18:357–363.
218. Lin BTY, Colby T, Gown AM, et al. Malignant vascular tumors of the serious membranes mimicking mesothelioma. Am J Surg Pathol 1996;220:1431–1439.
219. Kannerstein M, Churg J, McCaughey WTE. Asbestos and mesothelioma: a review. Pathol Ann l978;(Part 1):8l-129.
220. Roberts GH. Distant visceral mestastases in pleural mesothelioma. Br J Dis Chest l976;70:246–249.
221. Wanebo JH, Martini N, Melamed MR, et al. Pleural mesothelioma. Cancer l976; 38:248l–2490.
222. Law MR, Hodson ME, Heard BE. Malignant mesothelioma of the pleura: relation between histological type and clinical behaviour. Thorax 1982;37:810–816.
223. Spirtas R, Connelly RR, Tucker MA. Survival patterns for malignant mesothelioma: the SEER experience. Int J Cancer 1988;41:525–530.
224. Ribak J, Selikoff IJ. Survival of asbestos insulation workers with mesothelioma. Br J Ind Med 1992;49:732–735.
225. Antman KH. Malignant mesothelioma. N Engl J Med l980;303:200–205.
226. Antman KH, Osteen RT, Klegar KL, et al. Early peritoneal mesothelioma: a treatable malignancy. Lancet 1985;2:977–981.
227. Antmann KH, Blum RH, Greenberger JS, et al. Multimodality therapy for malignant mesothelioma based on a study of natural history. Am J Med l980;68: 356–361.
228. Yap BH, Benjamin RS, Burgess MA, Bodey GP. The value of Adriamycin in the treatment of diffuse malignant pleural mesothelioma. Cancer l978;42:l692–1697.
229. Chahinian AP, Suzuki Y, Mandel EM, Holland JF. Diffuse pulmonary malignant mesothelioma: response to doxorubicin and 5-Azacytidine. Cancer l978;42: l687–1692.
230. Fischbein A, Suzuki Y, Selikoff IJ, Bekesi JG. Unexpected longevity of a patient with malignant pleural mesothelioma. Cancer l978;42:l999–2003.
231. Doll R, Peto R. The causes of cancer: quantitative estimates of avoidable risks of cancer in the United States today. J Natl Cancer Inst 1981;66:1192–1308.

232. Homas DM, Garabrant DH, Gillespie BW. A meta-analysis of colorectal cancer and asbestos exposure. Am J Epidmiol 1994;139:1210–1222.
233. Gamble J. Asbestos and colon cancer: a weight of the evidence review. Environ Health Perspect 1994;102:1038–1050.
234. Weiss W. Asbestos and colorectal cancer. Gastroenterology 1990;99:876–884.
235. Edelman DA. Exposure to asbestos and the risk of gastrointestinal cancer. Br J Ind Med 1988;45:75–82.
236. Wortley P, Vaughn TL, Davis S, et al. A case-control study of occupational risk factors for laryngeal cancer. Br J Ind Med 1992;49:837–844.
237. Chan CK, Gee JBL. Asbestos exposure and laryngeal cancer. J Occup Med 1988; 30:23–27.
238. Edelman DA. Laryngeal cancer and occupational exposure to asbestos. Int Arch Occup Environ Health 1989;6:223–227.
239. Liddell FDK. Laryngeal cancer and asbestos. Br J Ind Med 1990;47:289–291.
240. Kagan E, Jacobson RJ. Lymphoid and plasma cell malignancies: asbestos-related disorders of long latency. Am J Clin Pathol 1980;80:14–20.
241. Bengtsson N, Hardell L, Eriksson M. Asbestos exposure and malignant lymphoma. Lancet 1982;2:1463.

CHAPTER 11

Diseases Due to Synthetic Fibers

- A. R. Gibbs
- J. C. Wagner
- Andrew Churg

INTRODUCTION

Synthetic fibers can be classified into two major groups: (*a*) inorganic ones, which are usually called synthetic or man-made vitreous fibers (MMVF) and (*b*) organic ones, which include carbon, aramid, and polyolefin fibers. The first group are produced in much greater amounts than the second. Generally consumption and production of synthetic fibers are increasing and for asbestos they are decreasing.

The first successful commercial manufacture of MMVF in the United States occurred in the late nineteenth century, although it is probable that glass fiber manufacture by humans dates to 4000 years ago (1). In 1985 the estimated world production of MMVF was 6 million tons. These synthetic fibers can be inhaled and deposited in the respiratory tract and may have toxicologic and biologic properties similar to those of asbestos. Over the past 2 decades a considerable number of in vitro, in vivo, and epidemiologic studies of the health effects of these fibers have been carried out.

MINERALOGY

MMVF are amorphous (noncrystalline) glassy silicates that are less chemically resistant than asbestos fibers. Also, because they are not crystalline, they do not have planes of cleavage predisposing them to split longitudinally; they tend to fracture transversely. MMVF, which comprise inorganic fibers made from rock, clay, slag, and glass (Fig. 11.1), can be divided into four main groups: slag wools, derived from industrial slag; rock wools, produced from molten rock; glass wools; and filaments (2). All synthetic vitreous fibers are made from a high-temperature (1000 to 1500°C) liquid melt of mined or quarried material, manufactured chemicals, or byproduct materials. However, their length and diameter

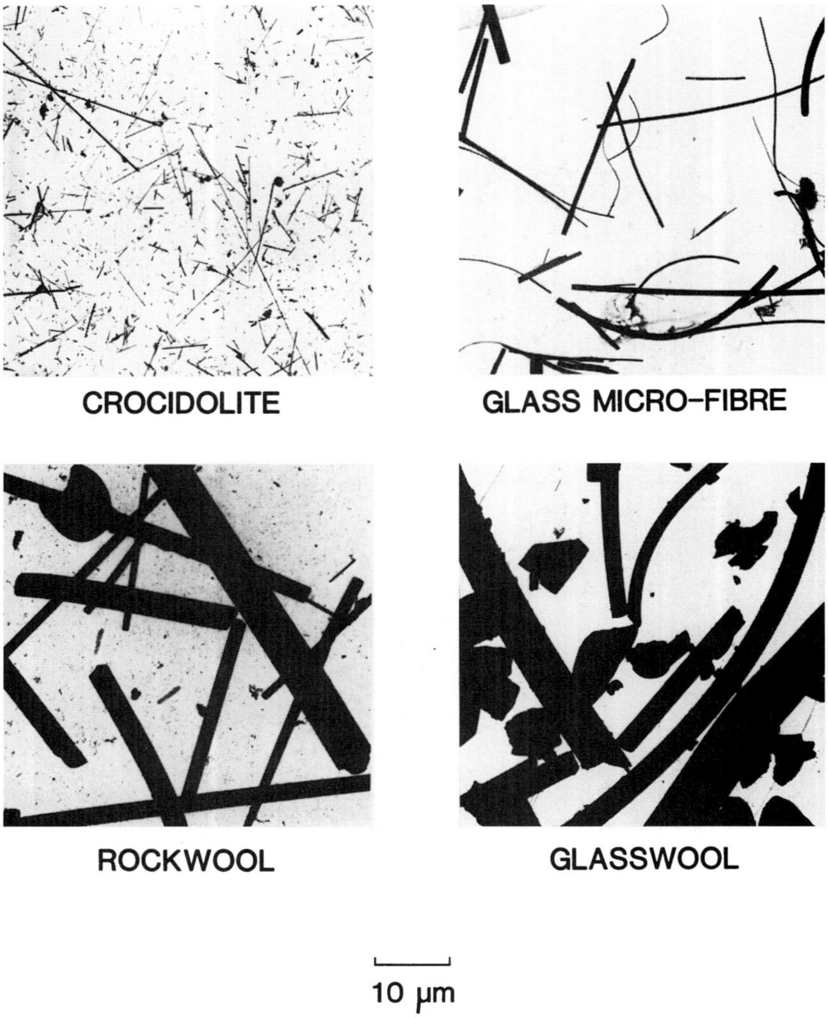

FIGURE 11.1
Electron microscopic appearances of various types of man-made mineral fibers. Crocidolite asbestos, a naturally occurring fiber, is included for comparison.

distributions vary according to the production method and their chemical composition, which in turn forms the basis for their desired commercial properties. MMVF fall into four broad categories:

1. Textile (continuous filament) fiberglass products, which first appeared commercially in the late 1930s, are incorporated into plastics, cement, paper, roofing, and woven materials. Their average diameter varies from 3 to 25 μm, and the majority are greater than 8 μm.
2. Insulation and tile wools are used in insulation, ceiling tile, and horticultural products. Produced by spinning or blowing, they contain fibers nominally between 1 and 6 μm in diameter, but there is a wide variation around the nominal diameter, and fibers can be as small as 0.2 μm in diameter.
3. Refractory ceramic fibers, which are used primarily for high-temperature insulation, comprise only about 1 to 2% of world production; production

did not reach a significant level until the 1970s. They are used for high-temperature furnace insulation and in paper, board, felts, textiles, gaskets, and filters. They should not be confused with ceramic crystalline synthetic fibers such as silicon carbide and silicon nitride. Refractory ceramic fibers are usually composed of relatively high percentages of aluminosilicate. The diameter of the fibers usually shows a mean between 2 and 4 μm, but there is a wide range, and many are within the respirable range.

4. Most special-purpose fibers are aluminoborosilicates, which have smaller diameters, generally less than 3 μm and sometimes less than 1 μm. They are used in aircraft, spacecraft, and special filters. They form a very small percentage of production.

MMVF are usually coated with binding compounds to produce fabricated shapes and forms. The insulation wool binders historically included bitumen, urea, and phenol–formaldehyde resins, but new binding agents are continually being introduced.

ORGANIC FIBERS

Organic fibers include polyvinyl alcohol, polyacrylonitrile, polyolefins, aramid fibers, graphite, and other carbon fibers. They have been used most in the fiber cement industries, but they have diverse applications, including textiles, paper sizing, paper coating, surgical prostheses, furniture, carpets, protective clothing, gaskets, brake pads, and cables (3).

Most organic fibers have diameters above the respirable range. However, production of aramid and graphite or other carbon fibers may result in respirable-size fibers, and low levels have been measured in the workplace (4).

EXPERIMENTAL STUDIES

Synthetic Vitreous Fibers

Largely because of the known pathogenic effects of asbestos, an enormous amount of work has gone into studies of the effects of MMVF in animals and in vitro experimental systems. Such studies often contradict each other, and their interpretation depends to a great extent on decisions about what test method or methods are appropriate to evaluate disease risks in man. This section briefly summarizes results of these various types of studies, which are detailed in recent reviews (5–10).

In Vitro Studies. Numerous experiments have been performed in which MMVF and other types of fibers are applied to monolayer cultures. A variety of cell types, many of them not related to the lung or pleura, are used in such studies. A general summary of the results is that any long, thin fiber is taken up by the cell and can physically interfere with the mitotic spindle and with cytokinesis. These effects appear to depend primarily on fiber length and little or not at all on fiber type (11). In vitro assays thus imply that all types of MMVF, as well as virtually all other fibers, are potentially carcinogenic. However, given the existing human epidemiologic data and the long-term animal inhalation data, these results indicate that in vitro tests are useful in examining mechanisms but have little predictive value in determining whether specific types of MMVF are carcinogenic in man.

Intraperitoneal and Intrapleural Inoculation Studies. Some investigators have adopted the technique, originally used by Stanton et al. (12), of instilling fibers into the peritoneal or pleural cavities of experimental animals and observing tumor incidence. The most extensive studies were done by Pott et al. (13, 14) using intraperitoneal instillation of fibers in rats.

The results of such studies are in a general sense similar to those seen with in vitro monolayer cultures. Virtually all fibers produce mesothelioma. The effect depends on dose and to a certain extent fiber length. Only fibers that are extremely soluble fail to produce tumors. Fibers that on the basis of human epidemiologic studies are thought to produce quite different tumor incidences—for example, chrysotile and amosite or crocidolite asbestos—produce essentially the same tumor incidence by intraperitoneal inoculation.

Although intrapleural and particularly intraperitoneal inoculation tests form the basis for the classification of glass fibers as possible human carcinogens (15, 16), they are extremely controversial and have been the subject of considerable criticism (5–10, 17). The intraperitoneal test in particular appears to depend on a marked and very nonspecific sensitivity of the rat peritoneum to foreign materials. This sensitivity is so extreme that even instillation of saline has been shown to produce a 6% incidence of mesotheliomas (5), compared with large control series of untreated rats in which the incidence of peritoneal mesothelioma is less than 1% (18). Other fibrous and nonfibrous particulates that have never been suggested to be mesothelial carcinogens in man, for example calcium–sodium metaphosphate, gypsum, sepiolite, basalt, silicon carbide, and even iron oxide, also produce increased incidences of mesothelioma in this system (14).

Use of inoculation tests also bypasses normal fiber defense mechanisms, which prevent most fibers, particularly relatively soluble fibers such as glass, from ever reaching the pleura. These tests also allow extremely long fibers, which may be highly carcinogenic, to reach the pleura by a totally nonphysiologic route, whereas such fibers could never reach the pleura or even the lung parenchyma by inhalation. Moreover, the doses used in inoculation tests often are massive. Last, inoculation tests by definition produce only mesotheliomas, and although some claim that this indicates the potential of the fibers to cause carcinomas (13, 14), carcinoma of the lung has numerous other well defined etiologies, and probably is associated (at least in the rat) with parenchymal fibrosis. There is no rational mechanistic basis for using mesothelioma incidence by intraperitoneal inoculation to predict the parenchymal carcinogenicity of fibers. For these reasons most reviewers (5–10, 17) have concluded that inoculation tests are not suitable for predicting the carcinogenicity of fibers in man.

Inhalation and Intratracheal Instillation Tests. There are numerous in vivo studies on MMVF, most using long-term inhalation and a few using intratracheal instillation. Much of this material has been reviewed recently (7, 8, 19). The most extensive and carefully designed studies are those summarized by Bunn et al. (19) and described in more detail in Hesterberg et al. (20) and others (21–23). In these experiments rats were exposed by inhalation to glass fibers, slag wool, rock wool, and refractory ceramic fibers at concentrations up to about 250 fibers per cubic centimeter for periods up to 24 months. Of note are the facts that the MMVF fiber sizes and exposure levels in these studies were roughly the same and that analysis of lung content revealed high burdens, indicating plainly that the fibers were respirable.

Table 11.1 summarizes fibrogenicity and carcinogenicity of the various MMVF fiber types as determined from these and other published experiments.

For fibrous glass and slag wool no significant fibrosis was seen in any study, nor was there an excess incidence of either cancers or mesotheliomas over that of the control group. For rock wool slight fibrosis was found at the highest doses, but there was no evidence of excess lung cancers. In contrast, refractory ceramic fibers produced pulmonary fibrosis, an increased incidence of carcinoma of the lung, and mesotheliomas. The mesotheliomas appeared to have some species specificity, since they were mostly found in hamsters: in one experiment (23) 42% of hamsters inhaling a kaolin-based refractory ceramic fiber developed mesothelioma. Fibrosis and lung cancers largely occurred in rats, although mesotheliomas were also seen in the rats. These and other studies have led to the general notion that refractory ceramic fibers are likely to be human carcinogens. However, the mesotheliomas were microscopic and not associated with mortality and are the subject of further histopathologic review (24).

Thus there is general agreement that the animal inhalation data on glass wool, slag wool, and rock wool are negative, but for refractory ceramic fibers the data are positive for both fibrosis and malignancies. The findings from the other types of dust administration are still the subject of controversy. The details of these arguments, which in large measure revolve around the significance of inoculation tests, are beyond the scope of this book, but the interested reader is referred to other reviews (5–10, 13, 14, 17, 25). Controversy notwithstanding, the consensus from animal inhalation studies appears to be that glass wool and slag wool certainly and rock wool probably carry no risk of pulmonary fibrosis or malignancies.

Organic Fibers

No effects on animals have been shown with polyvinyl alcohol, polyacrylonitrile, or polyolefin fibers (3). Chronic inhalation studies have been carried out with para-aramid fibers. The inhaled fibers undergo biodegradation in the lungs of rats, with the median length of retained fibers progressively reducing from 11 to 4 μm over 18 months (26). Acute inhalation studies demonstrate transient pulmonary inflammatory and cell labeling responses (27). In the chronic inhalation studies some of the rats developed squamous lesions, which have been des-

TABLE 11.1
Summary of Experiment Results with MMVF

TEST	CARCINOGENICITY	FIBROGENICITY
In vitro (monolayer culture)	All fibers positive; evidence of DNA damage	NA
Intraperitoneal inoculation	Virtually all fibers positive except for some highly soluble types of glass fiber	NA
Long-term high-dose inhalation	Glass, slag wool, rock wool negative; RCF positive both carcinomas and mesotheliomas	Glass and slag wool definitely negative; Rock wool mildly fibrogenic; RCF definitely fibrogenic

ignated by an international panel of pathologists as a proliferative keratin cyst, a lesion not encountered in humans (28, 29). It was thought to be a form of squamous metaplasia. Apart from one study using intratracheal instillation, animal inhalation studies with graphite and other carbon fibers have been negative for lung fibrosis and tumors (3).

HUMAN STUDIES

Man-Made Vitreous Fibers

There have been a number of epidemiologic studies of workers exposed to slag wool, rock wool, and glass fibers; glass fibers have been the most extensively studied. These studies have recently been reviewed (30). As has been pointed out in a recent editorial (31), many of the studies suffer from deficiencies in methodology, including lack of control for smoking, comparison of death rates with national rather than local rates, misclassification of potential confounders, and short-term worker bias.

Six studies specifically examined rock wool and slag wool workers; three reported a significantly increased risk of respiratory system cancer and three did not (30). However, two of the three positive studies did not control for cigarette smoking, and the increased risk did not appear to be related to increasing cumulative exposure, latency, or duration of employment. It has been suggested that the excess risk associated with some slag wool plants may have been due to arsenic or polycyclic aromatic hydrocarbons exposures that were present in significant amounts in slag during the early technologic phase (32).

At least 4 case-control and 10 cohort studies examined respiratory cancer in relation to glass fiber or mixed synthetic vitreous fiber (30). Generally the studies report no association between exposure to glass fiber and respiratory system cancer. However, an increased lung cancer statistical mortality review (SMR) was reported for a U.S. (TIMA) cohort of glass fiber workers in 1986 compared with national white men's mortality rates (33). A significant proportion of that U.S. TIMA cohort (38%) were the fibrous glass workers from the Owens-Corning factory in Newark, Ohio. A case control study of this Newark cohort was conducted to determine whether the risk of lung cancer was related to working in a particular area of the plant, production process, calendar time, cigarette smoking, or other known carcinogens. This study showed that some of the excess of lung cancer could be accounted for by differences in the prevalence of smoking between Newark and the United States as a whole, which was higher in the former (34). A more recent paper by Chiazze et al. (35) examined the data further and found that if the confounding effect of cigarette smoking was adjusted for, the lung cancer SMR for this Newark cohort could be reduced to an insignificant level.

In summary, it appears that exposure to glass fibers does not increase the risk of respiratory tract cancer. The increased SMR for lung cancer found in some cohorts of slag wool workers might well have been due to exposures to other carcinogenic agents during the early technologic phase of production that were not present in the later production processes.

To date there has been no evidence of an increased incidence of mesothelioma in these industries, but in view of its long latency, surveillance of these industries is still necessary.

Cross-sectional studies of glass wool, slag wool, and rock wool workers generally have not demonstrated a relation between exposure and either the prevalence of small irregular opacities on chest radiographs (36, 37) or pleural changes (38). The study by Kilburn et al. (39), which reported a 15% prevalence of "pneumoconiosis" among workers exposed to fine fibrous glass, can be criticized on the basis of the diagnosis of pneumoconiosis and the presence of numerous confounders (40). Most studies have not shown an increase of nonmalignant respiratory disease, such as obstructive airway disease, emphysema, and asthma, with exposures to glass and rock wool in the production industry (40). The fiber content of lung tissue samples from 112 U.S. MMVF workers taken at autopsy were examined; siliceous fibers were noted in only 28 of them, and only in very small quantities (41).

Refractory Ceramic Fibers

A recent study administered by questionnaire, lung function tests, and chest radiographs examined the respiratory health of 628 current employees of seven European factories manufacturing refractory ceramic fibers (42, 43). Concurrent surveys of levels of airborne fibers within the factories by optical microscopy of personal samplers were made. Exposure varied from 0 to 22.94 f/ml-years with a mean of 3.84. Nasal stuffiness and eye and skin irritation were frequent in all plants and increased with current exposure. After adjustment for several confounders, including smoking and past exposure to other respiratory hazards, the studies found a significant decrease in both forced expiratory volume in 1 second (FEV_1) and forced midexpiratory flow for current smokers and FEV_1 for ex-smokers, but not for nonsmokers. The findings were related to increasing cumulative exposure of respirable fibers (43). These results are in contrast to those found in glass fiber workers, in whom no effect has been found (36, 44). The conclusion was that cumulative exposure to respirable ceramic fibers promoted the obstruction of airways by cigarette smoke. Small opacities were found in 13% of the chest radiographs, but these were unrelated to cumulative exposure, and in this group there was a high prevalence of potential confounding exposures.

A small number of workers with pleural disease were identified, and these individuals appeared likely not to have been exposed to asbestos, but the numbers were insufficient to investigate dose–response relationships. Lemasters et al. (45), in a longitudinal study of pulmonary morbidity in U.S. refractory ceramic workers, found pleural plaques in 2.4% but no evidence of pulmonary fibrosis, no excess of lung cancers, and no mesotheliomas. Further studies are required to assess the significance of the finding of pleural plaques. Thus far there is no evidence of an increased incidence of malignancies.

Lung tissues from three refractory ceramic workers have been examined (46); substantial numbers of fibers found in each contained aluminium and silica in a ratio consistent with refractory ceramic fibers. Also, a study of fibers in the bronchoalveolar lavage fluids from seven healthy workers employed at a refractory ceramic fiber production plant revealed fibers with chemistries consistent with RCFs in all but one of the subjects (47).

Organic Fibers

No deleterious pulmonary effects on humans have been associated with workplace exposures to polyvinyl alcohol, polyacrylonitrile, polyolefin, aramid, graphite, or other carbon fibers.

SUMMARY

At present there appears to be little evidence of pulmonary and pleural disease in humans caused by exposures to synthetic vitreous or organic fibers. In view of the long latency of fiber-related diseases and the data on carcinogenicity of refractory ceramic fibers, continued vigilance is necessary.

REFERENCES

1. Peters GA, Peters BJ. Sourcebook on asbestos diseases: medical, legal and engineering aspects, vol. 2. New York: Garland Law Publishing, 1986.
2. Nomenclature Committee of TIMA Inc. Man-made vitreous fibres: nomenclature, chemical and physical Properties. Stanford, CT: TIMA, 1991.
3. Gruber UF. Alternatives to mineral fibres. In: Liddell D, Miller K, eds. Mineral fibres and health. Boca Raton: CRC Press, 1991:347–360.
4. Warheit DB. A review of inhalation toxicology studies with para-aramid fibres. Ann Occup Hyg 1995;39:691–697.
5. Bignon J, Brochard P, Brown R, et al. 1994. Final Report: Assessment of toxicity of man made fibres. Ann Occup Hyg 1995;39:89–106.
6. Brown RC, Davis JMG, Douglas D, et al. Carcinogenicity of the insulation wools: reassessment of the IARC evaluation. Regul Toxicol Pharmacol 1991;14:12–23.
7. McClellan RO, Miller FJ, Hesterberg TW, et al. Approaches to evaluating the toxicity and carcinogenicity of man-made fibers: summary of a workshop held November 11–13 1991, Durham, NC. Regul Toxicol Pharmacol 1992;16:321–364.
8. Government of Canada. Mineral fibres (man-made vitreous fibres). Ottawa: Communication Group-Publishing, Catalog En40–215/30E. 1994.
9. World Health Organization. Validity of methods for assessing the carcinogenicity of man-made fibres. Copenhagen: WHO Regional Office for Europe. 1992.
10. World Health Organization. Validity of methods for assessment of carcinogenicity of fibres. WHO European Regional Office. 1994.
11. Hart GA, Kathman LM, Hesterberg TW. In vitro cytotoxicity of asbestos and man-made vitreous fibers: roles of fiber length, diameter, and composition. Carcinogenesis 1994;15: 971–977.
12. Stanton JF, Layard M, Tegeris A, et al. Relation of particle dimension to carcinogenicity in amphibole asbestoses and other fibrous minerals. J Natl Cancer Inst 1981; 67:965–975.
13. Pott F, Ziem U, Reiffer F, et al. Carcinogenicity studies on fibres, metal compounds and some other dusts in rats. Exp Pathol 1987;32:129–152.
14. Pott F, Roller M, Rippe RM, et al. Tumours by the intraperitoneal and intrapleural routes and their significance for the classification of mineral fibres. in: brown RC, ed. mechanisms in fibre carcinogenesis. New York: Plenum Press, 1991:547–563.
15. International Agency for Research on Cancer. IARC Monograph on the evaluation of carcinogenic risks to human man made mineral fibers and radon, vol 43. Lyon: IARC, 1988.
16. National Toxicology Program, US Department of Health and Human Services. Seventh Annual Report on Carcinogens, 1994.
17. Bernstein DM. An evaluation of the use of an inhalation model versus intraperitoneal injection model for the assessment in rats of the carcinogenicity of natural and man-made vitreous fibres. Zentralbl Arbeitsmed 1993;43:120–128.
18. Haseman JK, Arnold J, Eustis SL. Tumor incidence in Fischer 344 rats: NTP historical data. In: Pathology of the Fischer rat: reference and atlas. New York: Academic Press, 1990:555–564.
19. Bunn WB, Bender JR, Hesterberg TW, et al. Recent studies of man-made vitreous fibers: chronic animal inhalation studies. J Occup Med 1993;35:101–113.
20. Hesterberg TW, Miller WC, McConnell EE, et al. Chronic inhalation toxicity of size-separated glass fibers in Fischer 344 rats. Fundam Appl Toxicol 1993;20:464–476.

21. McConnell EE, Kamtrup O, Musselman R, et al. Chronic inhalation study of size-separated rock and slag wool insulation fibers in Fischer 344/N rats. Inhal Toxicol 1994;6:571–614.
22. McConnell EE, Mast RW, Hesterberg TW, et al. Chronic inhalation toxicity of a kaolin-based refractory ceramic fiber in Syrian golden hamsters. Inhal Toxicol 1995; 7:503–532.
23. Mast RW, McConnell EE, Anderson R, et al. Studies on the chronic toxicity (inhalation) of four types of refractory ceramic fiber in male Fischer 344 rats. Inhal Toxicol 1995;7:425–467.
24. Glass LR, Brown RC, Hoskins JA. Health effects of refractory ceramic fibres: scientific issues and policy considerations. Occup Environ Med 1995;52:433–440.
25. Infante PF, Schuman LD, Dement J, Huff J. Fibrous glass and cancer. Am J Ind Med 1994;26:559–584.
26. Kelly DP, Merriman EA, Kennedy GL, Lee KP. Deposition, clearance and shortening of Kevlar para-aramid fibrils in acute, subchronic and chronic inhalation studies in rats. Fundam Appl Toxicol 1993;21:345–354.
27. Warheit DB, Kellar KA, Hartsky MA. Pulmonary cellular effects in rats following aerosol exposures to ultrafine Kevlar aramid fibrils: evidence for biodegradability of inhaled fibrils. Toxicol Appl Pharmacol 1992;116:225–239.
28. Carlton WW. "Proliferative keratin cyst", a lesion in the lungs of rats following chronic exposure to para-aramid fibrils: report of a pathology workshop. Fundam Appl Toxicol 1994;23:304–307.
29. Levy LS. Squamous lung lesions associated with chronic exposure by inhalation of rats to p-aramid fibrils (fine fibre dust) and to titanium dioxide: findings of a pathology workshop. In: Mohr U, Dungworth DL, Mauderly JL, Oberdorster G, eds. Toxic and carcinogenic effects of solid particles in the respiratory tract. Washington: ILSI Press, 1994:473–478.
30. Lee IM, Hennekens CH, Trichopoulos D, Buring JE. Man-made vitreous fibres and risk of respiratory system cancer: a review of the epidemiologic evidence. JOM 1995; 37:725–738.
31. Bender JR, Bunn W III, Rossiter CE, Fayerweather WE. Epidemiologic studies of fibreglass: methods, findings and implications. JOM 1995;37:653–655.
32. Simonato L, Fletcher AC, Cherrie JW, et al. International Agency for Research on Cancer historical cohort study of MMMF production workers in seven European countries: extension of the follow up. Ann Occup Hyg 1987;31:603–623.
33. Enterline PE, Marsh GM, Henderson V, Callahan C. Mortality update of a cohort of U.S. man-made mineral fibre workers. Ann Occup Hyg 1987;31:625–656.
34. Chiazze L, Watkins DK, Fryar C. A case control study of malignant and non-malignant respiratory disease among employees of a fibreglass manufacturing facility. Br J Ind Med 1992;49:326–333.
35. Chiazze L, Watkins DK, Fryar C. Adjustment for the confounding effect of cigarette smoking in an historical cohort mortality study of workers in a fibreglass manufacturing facility. JOM 1995;37:744–748.
36. Hill JW, Rossiter CE, Foden DW. A pilot respiratory morbidity study of workers in a MMMF plant in the United Kingdom. In: Biological effects of man-made mineral fibres: proceedings of a WHO/IARC Conference, Copenhagen 1982. World Health Organization 1984;1:413–426.
37. Hughes J, Jones R, Glindmeyer H, et al. Follow-up study of workers exposed to man-made mineral fibres. Br J Ind Med 1993;50:658–667.
38. Weill H, Hughes J, Hammad Y, et al. Respiratory health in workers exposed to man-made vitreous fibres. Am Rev Respir Dis 1983;128:104–112.
39. Kilburn K, Powers D, Warshaw R. Pulmonary effects of exposure to fine fibreglass: irregular opacities and small airways obstruction. Br J Ind Med 1992;49:714–720.
40. De Vuyst P, Dumortier P, Swaen GMH, et al. Respiratory health effects of man-made vitreous (mineral) fibres. Eur Respir J 1995;8:2149–2173.
41. McDonald JC, Case BW, Enterline PE, et al. Lung dust analysis in the assessment of

past exposure to man-made mineral fibre workers. Ann Occup Hyg 1990;34: 427–441.
42. Trethowan WN, Burge PS, Rossiter CE, et al. Study of the respiratory health of employees in seven European plants that manufacture ceramic fibres. Occup Environ Med 1995;52:97–104.
43. Burge PS, Calvert IA, Trethowan WN, Harrington JM. Are the respiratory health effects found in manufacturers of ceramic fibres due to the dust rather than the exposure to fibres? Occup Environ Med 1995;52:105–109.
44. Hill JW, Whitehead WS, Cameron JD, Hedgecock GA. Glass fibres: absence of pulmonary hazard in production workers. Br J Ind Med 1973;30:174–9.
45. Lemasters
46. Roggli VL. Rare pneumoconiosis: metalloconiosis. In: Saldana MS, ed. Pathology of pulmonary disease. Philadelphia: Lippincott, 1994:411–422.
47. Sebastien P, Vergnon JM, Blachard O, et al. Durability of ceramic fibres in the human lung: preliminary results. Ann Occup Hyg 1994;38 (Suppl 1):723–730.

CHAPTER 12

Occupational Asthma, Byssinosis, Extrinsic Allergic Alveolitis and Related Conditions

❖ Francis H. Y. Green
❖ Andrew Churg

INTRODUCTION

Exposure to organic dusts in the workplace can result in a variety of pulmonary diseases. These include occupational asthma, reactive airways dysfunction syndrome (RADS), byssinosis, organic dust toxic syndrome, and extrinsic allergic alveolitis (EAA). Although these diseases can be clinically distinct, many cases show overlapping clinical and pathologic features, which indicates a spectrum of diseases in this general category (1). The major clinical and pathologic characteristics of these diseases are given in Table 12.1.

OCCUPATIONAL ASTHMA

Occupational asthma is similar in most respects to nonoccupational asthma but also has unique features. It is "variable airflow limitation and/or airway hyperresponsiveness due to causes and conditions attributable to a particular occupational environment and not to stimuli encountered outside the workplace" (2). Two major types can be distinguished. The more common type entails sensitization to a high- or low-molecular-weight agent and a variable latency period followed by a long period of bronchoreactivity to the agent. This type is described as occupational asthma with prior sensitization. The exposure concentration of the agent during sensitization does not appear critical. The second type has no latency period and is initiated by a single exposure to a high concentration of an irritant vapor, fume, or smoke (3). This is variously described as RADS or irritant-induced asthma.

OCCUPATIONAL ASTHMA WITH PRIOR SENSITIZATION

Clinical Features

The symptoms of occupational asthma with prior sensitization to a substance in the workplace are similar to those of nonoccupational asthma. Nasal and ocu-

TABLE 12.1
Major Clinical and Pathologic Features of Organic Dust–Induced Lung Disease

DISEASE	CLINICAL FEATURES	PATHOLOGIC FEATURES
OA with prior sensitization	History of atopy, latency period, specific antibodies (IgE and/or IgG); cough, shortness of breath, chest tightness, wheezing on challenge	Classic features of asthma (basement membrane thickening, eosinophilic infiltrates, mucous cell hyperplasia, bronchial smooth muscle hypertrophy)
Reactive airways dysfunction syndrome	Sudden onset following exposure to high concentration of an irritant substance; nonimmune mechanisms; symptoms may be similar to OA	Poorly documented; nonspecific epithelial cell changes and chronic inflammation; failure to adequately repair acutely injured mucosa
Byssinosis	Across-shift decline in FEV_1; symptoms worse at beginning of work week; nonimmune mechanisms	No distinctive features
Organic dust toxic syndrome	Acute lung injury with systemic symptoms following massive exposure to organic dusts containing fungal and bacterial elements	Acute lung injury (alveolar duct hyaline membranes, neutrophils)
Extrinsic allergic alveolitis	Acute, subacute, and chronic interstitial lung disease in response to inhalation of organic dusts; type III and type IV immune mechanisms	Chronic interstitial pneumonia with granulomas, giant cells and bronchiolitis obliterans

OA, occupational asthma.

lar signs and symptoms, which may precede or coexist with the chest symptoms of asthma, include lacrimation, itching or burning of the eyes, sneezing, rhinorrhea, and nasal congestion. The classic respiratory signs and symptoms are cough usually accompanied by shortness of breath, chest tightness, and wheezing.

Three major patterns of response have been identified: (*a*) an isolated early response developing within minutes of exposure and lasting for 1.5 to 2 hours; (*b*) an isolated late response developing after 4 hours from exposure and persisting for 12 hours or more; and (*c*) a dual response with characteristics of both the immediate and delayed responses. A nocturnal reaction in which symptoms develop in the early hours of the morning following exposure at work the previous day has also been identified. The isolated early response and the dual response are characteristic of an immunoglobulin (Ig) E–mediated response (4) and are the most common types in association with exposure to high-molecular-weight sensitizing agents. The isolated late response is more commonly associated with low-molecular-weight agents and may not involve IgE-mediated mechanisms.

The dose and length of exposure required to induce occupational asthma are highly variable. However, onset is usually within 1 or 2 years of first exposure.

The latency period may be shorter for low-molecular-weight agents (5). Once a person is sensitized, concentrations as low as one part per billion may be enough to initiate an asthmatic response (6). These levels may be several orders of magnitude below the exposure limits recommended for protection of the "average" worker, which makes the regulatory and engineering problems posed by allergenic substances in the workplace immense.

The natural history of occupational asthma is shown in Figure 12.1. If subjects remain in the same workplace, their symptoms persist and their pulmonary function generally deteriorates. Removal from exposure may result in improvement, but a significant minority of former workers develop persistent asthma (7). Others develop long-standing bronchial hyperreactivity (5). Inhaled corticosteroids have been shown to be helpful when combined with removal from further exposure (8).

Although occupational and nonoccupational forms of asthma are similar in many respects, some features may be helpful in making the distinction between the two (9) (Table 12.2). However, there is much overlap between the conditions, and it is possible for one person to have both occupational and nonoccupational asthma.

Population at Risk and Prevalence

The National Institute for Occupational Safety and Health (NIOSH), using data from the National Exposure Survey Database, has estimated the number of male and female persons in the United States who may be exposed to sensitizing agents in the workplace at just over 11 million (10, 11).

With the possible exception of asbestos-related lung disease, occupational asthma is the most frequently reported cause of occupational lung disease (12). In the United States 37.7% of occupational lung diseases reported to the NIOSH surveillance database were for occupational asthma (11). In the United Kingdom a figure of 26% was reported in the surveillance of work-related and occupational respiratory disease (SWORD) program for occupational lung diseases

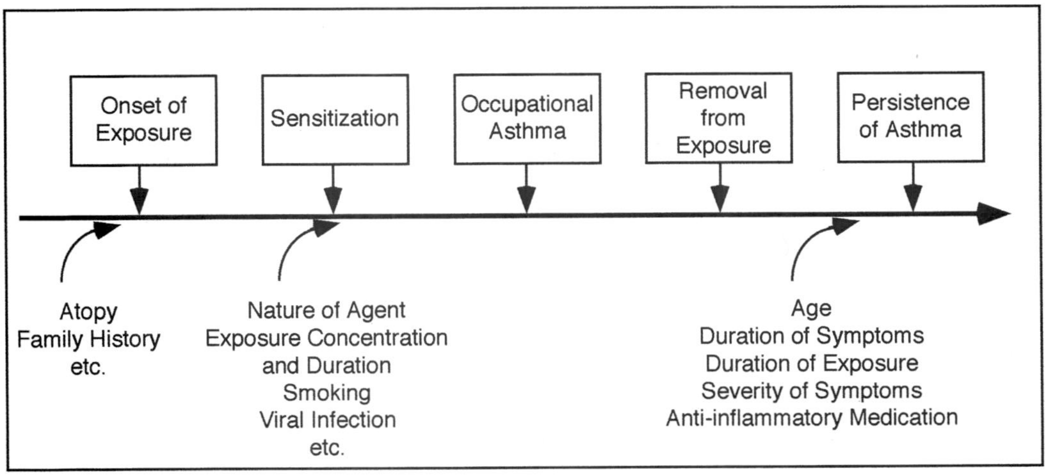

FIGURE 12.1
The natural history of occupational asthma. (Adapted from Chan-Yeung M, Malo JL. Natural history of occupational asthma. In: Bernstein IL, Chen-Yeung M, Malo JL, Bernstein DI, eds. Asthma in the workplace. New York: Marcel Dekker, 1993:299–322.)

TABLE 12.2
Contrasting Features of Occupational and Nonoccupational Asthma

FEATURE	NONOCCUPATIONAL ASTHMA	OCCUPATIONAL ASTHMA
Agent	Usually molecular weight >1000 d	Both high and low (<1000 d) molecular weight substances
Mechanism	Usually IgE mediated	Multiple mechanisms
Family history of asthma	Common	Less common
History of atopy	Great majority	Many cases without
Age of onset	Childhood	Adult
Gender	Males = females	Males predominate
Asthma episodes		
Seasonal variation in symptoms	Yes	No
Improvement on weekends and holidays	Variable	Yes
Worsening at work	Variable	Yes
Response to skin testing and/or challenge	Usually multiple positive response to environmental agents	Usually restricted to agent found in workplace

Adapted from Axon EJ, Beach JR, Burge PS. A comparison of some of the characteristics of patients with occupational and nonoccupational asthma. J Occup Med 1995;45:109–111.

(13). In Québec asthma accounts for most recognized workers' compensation claims for lung disease (14).

Information on the prevalence of occupational asthma is derived from three sources: the general population, community studies, and selected workforces. In the United States asthma is estimated to affect 3 to 10% of the general population. Approximately 2 to 15% of these cases are occupational (15). This finding is supported by large community studies in which a majority have shown a significant relation between the symptoms of asthma and exposure to dusts, fumes, and/or gases in the workplace (16). The prevalence of asthma in workforces exposed to both high- and low-molecular-weight asthmagens has been reviewed by Becklake (16). Among workers exposed to high-molecular-weight agents the prevalence of asthma ranged from approximately 10% of those who work with laboratory animals to 50% in workers manufacturing enzyme detergents. The average prevalence of asthma in 10 studies was 23.5%. Review of the 12 studies of workers exposed to low-molecular-weight agents revealed asthma prevalences ranging from 3 to 8% in workers exposed to western red cedar to 54% in platinum refinery workers. The average prevalence of asthma in the group exposed to low-molecular-weight agents was 17.9%.

Causes of Occupational Asthma

Sensitizing agents occur in a wide range of industries. They are most prevalent in the chemical and metal industries, followed by forest products, textiles, food industry, pharmaceuticals, medical biologic products, agriculture, and others (10). Office building–related asthma has also been reported (17). A listing of sensitizing agents and the associated industries and occupations are given in Table 12.3. They have been subdivided into high- and low-molecular-weight agents.

TABLE 12.3
Causes of Occupational Asthma

MAJOR CLASS	SUBCATEGORIES	OCCUPATION OR INDUSTRY
High molecular weight sensitizing agents		
Animal-derived products	Laboratory animals	Veterinarian, medical research
	Chicken	Poultry workers, agriculture
	Prawns	Fish processing
	Bat guano	Mining, fertilizer manufacturer
	Egg protein	Egg producers
Insects	Grain mite	Laboratory workers
	Honeybee	Honey processors
	Fowl mite	Poultry workers
Plants	Grain dust	Farmers, grain elevator operators
	Wheat, rye, soy flour	Bakers, millers
	Castor bean	Oil industry
	Tobacco leaf	Tobacco manufacture
	Hops	Brewery
	Henna	Hairdressers
Biologic Enzymes	*Bacillus Subtilis*	Detergent industry
	Trypsin	Plastic industry
	Papain, pepsin	Pharmaceutical industry
	Fungal amylase	Bakers
Vegetable Gums	Acacia	Printers
	Karaya	Hairdressers
	Guar	Carpet manufacturing
Low molecular weight sensitizing agents		
Aliphatic amines	Ethylene diamine	Shellac manufacture, photography
	Aminoethylethonolamine	Soldering
	Dimethylethylolamine	Spray paint
Fluxes	Colophony	Electronics industry
	Zinc chloride and ammonium chloride flux	Metal jointing
Wood dust	Western red cedar	Sawmills, carpentry
	Mahogany, oak, African maple, others	Woodcarving
Diisocyanates	Toluene diisocyanate	Plastics, paints, varnish
	Diphenyl methane diisocyanate	Foundry work
	Combinations of isocyanates	Paint shops
Anhydrides	Phthalic anhydride	Plastics, resins
	Trimellitic anhydride	Epoxy resins, plastics
	Pyromellitic dianhydride	Epoxy adhesive
	Himic anhydride	Flame retardants
Metals	Platinum, nickel, cobalt, zinc, tungsten, chromium	Metal refining, soldering, welding, metal plating, tanning, printing, machining
Drugs	Penicillins, cephalosporins, Psyllium, methyl dopa, salbutamol, tetracyclines, hydralazine, cimetidine, ipecac	Pharmaceutical industry, nurses, hospital workers
Chemicals	Polyvinyl chloride	Meat wrappers
	Persulphate salts and henna	Hairdressers
	Azodicarbonamide	Plastics, rubber
	Formaldehyde	Hospital staff, diverse industries
	Reactive dyes	Dye manufacture
	Gluteraldehyde	Electron microscopy technicians, endoscopy units
	Methyl methacrylate	Adhesive manufacture
	Latex	Glove manufacturers, hospital staff

Adapted from Chan-Yeung M, Malo JL. Compendium I: table of the major inducers of occupational asthma. In: Berstein IL, Chan-Yeung M, Malo JL, Bernstein DI, eds. Asthma in the Workplace. New York: Marcel Dekker, 1993: 595–623.

PATHOGENESIS

Asthma is a remarkably diverse disease with many precipitating agents and mechanisms of progression. The underlying cause is not known. Why one worker responds to an inhaled agent with an allergic immune response and another responds with a protective (or no) immune response and remains symptom free on re-exposure remains a mystery. The mechanisms whereby asthma is induced by a sensitizing agent are also poorly understood. There is a much greater understanding of the ways in which agents incite or trigger asthma once the disease is established.

Most cases of asthma in the general population are induced by high-molecular-weight agents that initiate IgE-dependent responses in atopic individuals, but many of the sensitizing agents in the workplace are low-molecular-weight compounds that can initiate airway inflammation and bronchoconstriction through both immune and nonimmune pathways. Many agents that cause occupational asthma operate through more than one mechanism.

As with most occupational lung diseases, smoking is an important confounder. Smoking increases the risk of developing occupational asthma and reduces the latency period between first exposure and development of symptoms (19). The mechanism or mechanisms for this are not fully understood; however, smoking has been shown to enhance IgE-specific responses (20, 21), possibly by increasing airway permeability to antigenic materia1 (22).

A family history of atopy (eczema, hay fever, urticaria, asthma, and anaphylaxis) is associated with a greater risk of developing both occupational and nonoccupational asthma (23, 24). This observation suggests a strong genetic influence; however, the inheritance does not appear to follow the classical Mendelian patterns for single-gene diseases (24, 25). Methods for identifying disease genes include linkage analysis, sibling pair analysis, association studies, and analysis of quantitative phenotypes. Candidate genes or loci identified to date include the high-affinity receptor for IgE interleukin (IL) 4, β_2-adrenergic receptor, T-cell antigen receptor, human leukocyte antigen (HLA) class II antigens, α_1-antitrypsin gene variants, and tumor necrosis factor (TNF) α (25).

Evidence for the heritability of asthma is shown by the high concordance of asthma in monozygotic twins and by segregation analysis (25). Although segregation analysis of the IgE and other phenotypes confirms the genetic basis of the allergic disorders, it has not revealed a consistent model of inheritance. This may be because the various components of the asthma phenotype (e.g., high IgE, bronchial hyperresponsiveness, airway wall remodeling) have different genetic bases. For example, although there is a strong association between bronchial hyperresponsiveness and atopy, family and twin studies indicate that they are separate hereditary traits (26, 27).

Genetic factors have been investigated in nonatopic occupational asthma. Asthma induced by isothiocyanates has been associated with the HLA-DQB1*0503 allele and the allelic combination DQB1*0201/0301 (28, 29).

An intrinsic abnormality in airway smooth muscle has been considered in the pathogenesis of asthma. Decreased β_2-adrenergic responsiveness has been observed in airway smooth muscle taken from patients with fatal asthma (30); however, no such findings were reported in smooth muscle obtained from surgically resected lungs from persons with mild asthma (31). Genetic studies have associated a variant of the β-adrenergic receptor gene with severe asthma (32) and with nocturnal asthma (33). Changes in bronchial smooth muscle contractility as a result of inflammation or recruitment of functionally different smooth muscle phenotypes have also been considered in the pathogenesis of the airway hyperresponsiveness in asthma (34).

The role of viral infections in the pathogenesis of asthma has received considerable attention. There is good evidence that acute viral respiratory infections can trigger or exacerbate asthma (35, 36). The roles of viral infections in early infancy and of latent viral infection in asthma pathogenesis are as yet unknown (37–39).

Acute and chronic inflammation of the airways are primary characteristics of the asthmatic response. During acute asthma there is a rapid increase in mucosal blood flow, increased vascular permeability, and exudation of fluid and plasma proteins, resulting in mucosal congestion and edema. This is followed by up-regulation of adhesion molecules in capillary endothelial cells (40), emigration of eosinophils and to a lesser extent neutrophils (41), release of proinflammatory mediators from eosinophils and mast cells (42), and shedding of the airway epithelium (43, 44). The inflammatory reaction and/or neural reflexes trigger the cough, bronchoconstriction, and massive secretion of mucus characteristic of an acute attack (45).

Eosinophils are considered central to the inflammatory response in asthma (46). Activated eosinophils release cytotoxic factors such as major basic protein, eosinophil chemotactic protein, eosinophilic cationic protein, eosinophil-derived neurotoxin, and eosinophil peroxidase (47–51), which induce epithelial shedding, fibroblast activation, and thickening of the basement membrane (44). The role of the thickened basement membrane in the pathogenesis of the disease is not known. Recently it has been shown that bronchial myofibroblasts secrete cytokines that prolong eosinophil survival in vitro (52).

Mast cells are also increased in the mucosa of asthmatic airways and are degranulated during an acute attack (43, 53). Mast cell degranulation occurs in response to antigen-specific IgE as well as to complement components (C3a, C5a), cytokines, and neuropeptides (42). Mast cells release preformed mediators such as histamine, heparin, and tryptase as well as cytokines (IL-4, IL-5, and IL-6) and lipid mediators (leukotriene B_4, leukotriene C_4, prostaglandin D_2, and platelet activating factor) (42). Mediators released from mast cells play an important role in capillary permeability and edema, smooth muscle contraction, mucous secretion, and recruitment of other inflammatory cells into the airway. Histamine also induces smooth muscle proliferation (54) and thus may contribute to the smooth muscle hyperplasia characteristic of the disease. T lymphocytes also play a central role in asthma, and their numbers are greatly increased in the airways of asthmatics (48, 49). A failure of tissue macrophage T-cell regulation has been proposed as a mechanism for bronchial hyperresponsiveness and asthma (55). Autoimmunity has also been considered as a factor in the pathogenesis of asthma but has not been conclusively demonstrated (56).

Although all forms of asthma appear to have an inflammatory basis, evidence is accumulating for different mechanisms in atopic and nonatopic forms. Atopic asthma is associated with the activation of CD-4–positive T lymphocytes in the bronchial mucosa (57). Studies in the mouse indicate that CD-4 lymphocytes may differentiate into two major phenotypes, Th1 and Th2, according to the pattern of lymphokines they secrete. The Th1 cells secrete TNF-β and interferon-γ (42, 57, 58). Th2 CD-4 lymphocytes secrete IL-4 and IL-5. Both Th1 and Th2 CD-4 lymphocytes secrete IL-3 and granulocyte-macrophage colony-stimulating factor. The cytokines produced by Th2 lymphocytes favor the recruitment and activation of mast cells and eosinophils (IL-5) and the production of IgE antibody (IL-4), and Th1 clones tend to suppress these effects (57, 59). The pathogenesis of atopic asthmatic inflammation can be viewed as a tendency to favor CD-4 Th2 lymphocyte clonal expansion after antigen challenge. The exogenous factors that influence Th1 and Th2 differentiation are unknown.

By contrast, nonatopic asthma, including most cases of toluene di-isocyanate (TDI) induced asthma, may be mediated by a different immune mechanism. It is associated with an expansion of CD8+ T-cell clones in the bronchial mucosa, IL-5 secretion (but not IL-4), and eosinophilia (60–63).

PATHOLOGY OF ASTHMA

Asthma affects all levels of the conducting airways from trachea to respiratory bronchioles and all components of the wall. The mesenchymal components affected by asthma include basement membrane, airway smooth muscle, longitudinal elastic and collagen bundles, cartilage, and the bronchial vasculature. It is not known whether these changes result from the inflammatory response in asthma, altered mechanics of the airways, or both. Together these changes are responsible for the airway wall remodeling seen in asthma (64). The major physiologic effect, however, appears to be in the terminal bronchioles, and this is the region that limits airflow most (65–67).

FATAL ASTHMA (STATUS ASTHMATICUS)

Gross Appearance

In fatal asthma it is common for the lungs to bulge out of the thoracic cavity at autopsy. Examination of these hyperinflated lungs reveals extensive areas of atelectasis, which in some cases may be the predominant gross finding (Fig. 12.2). Pneumothorax is a rare spontaneous event in asthma but is more common in asthmatics who have been resuscitated and artificially ventilated. The lungs may prove difficult or impossible to inflate with fixative because of extensive and tenacious mucous plugs in the airways. The mucous plugs are pale gray and are firmly fixed to the airway wall. Silicone rubber casts show blunting of the airways as a result of the mucous plugs, and the airway profile is irregular and distorted by extensive airway wall remodeling (Fig. 12.3). The cut surface of the fixed lung may be unremarkable. Areas of atelectasis may be seen. Mucous plugs are usually present, and the airway walls may appear red and thick. Emphysema is not a prominent feature of asthma, but it may be seen in older individuals who smoke.

Microscopic Appearance

Because asthma involves almost all structures in the airways, no one histologic feature is diagnostic. The pathologic diagnosis is best made on the presence of

FIGURE 12.3

A. Negative pressure injection silicone rubber casts of airways from normal nonasthmatic, showing segmental bronchus and divisions down to the respiratory bronchiole. The normal airway shows a dichotomous branching pattern with smooth parallel walls. **B.** By contrast, a cast from the same segment from a patient with fatal asthma shows truncation of the airways by mucous plugs, marked distortion of the airway profile with horizontal constrictions (smooth muscle hypertrophy), longitudinal banding (elastic fiber hypertrophy), and extensive pits in the wall (mucous gland ectasia).

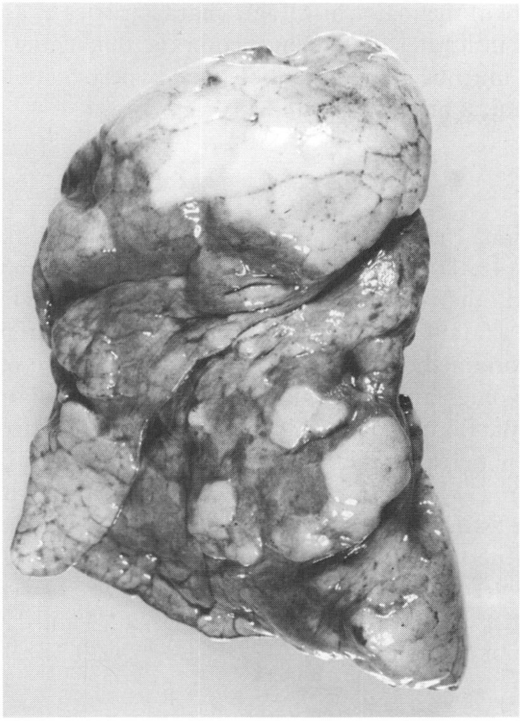

FIGURE 12.2
Gross appearance of lungs from an 18-year-old man who died suddenly of exercise- and cold-induced asthma. The lungs, which failed to collapse at autopsy, showed marked hyperinflation as well as areas of atelectasis.

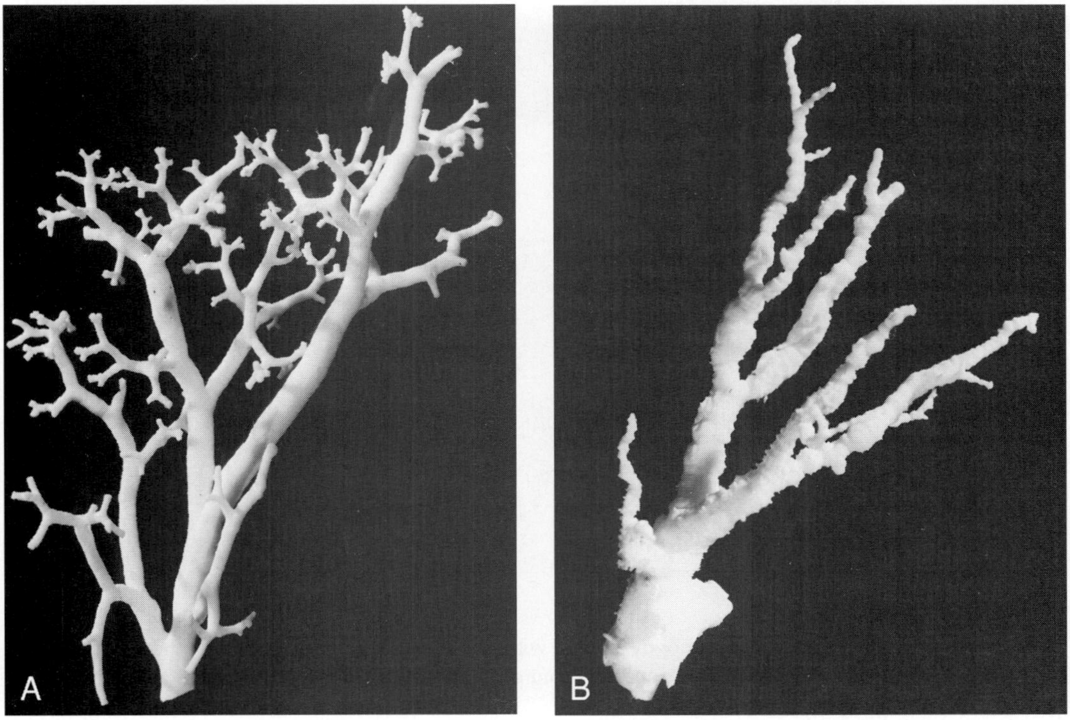

three or more of the major histologic characteristics of asthma: eosinophilic and lymphocytic infiltrates, basement membrane thickening, smooth muscle hypertrophy, and mucous gland and goblet cell hypertrophy in a person with an appropriate clinical history (68, 69).

Epithelium

In acute asthma the epithelium is shed as a result of inflammatory processes in the mucosa (43, 70). Major basic protein released from the cores of eosinophil granules and other eosinophil toxic proteins are thought to mediate this effect (71–73). In a fatal case it may be difficult to differentiate active epithelial loss from postmortem shedding due to autolysis. Layering of epithelial cells within the mucous plugs and interepithelial and subepithelial edema favor an antemortem event. Repeated episodes of exfoliation lead to hyperplasia of the epithelium with increased mitotic activity (74) and the appearance of cell proliferation markers (75). Electron microscopic studies of the bronchial mucosa taken during acute asthma reveal loss of epithelial cells, intercellular edema, exposure of epithelial nerves, and degranulating eosinophils in the subepithelial tissues (76, 77). Goblet cell hyperplasia is also a feature of the asthmatic epithelium (78, 79). It is seen at all levels of the airway (Figs. 12.4 and 12.5) and in nonsmokers as well as smokers.

Mucous Glands

Morphometric studies show that the mucous glands are larger in asthmatics than in normal individuals and that they can enlarge to the same degree as in chronic

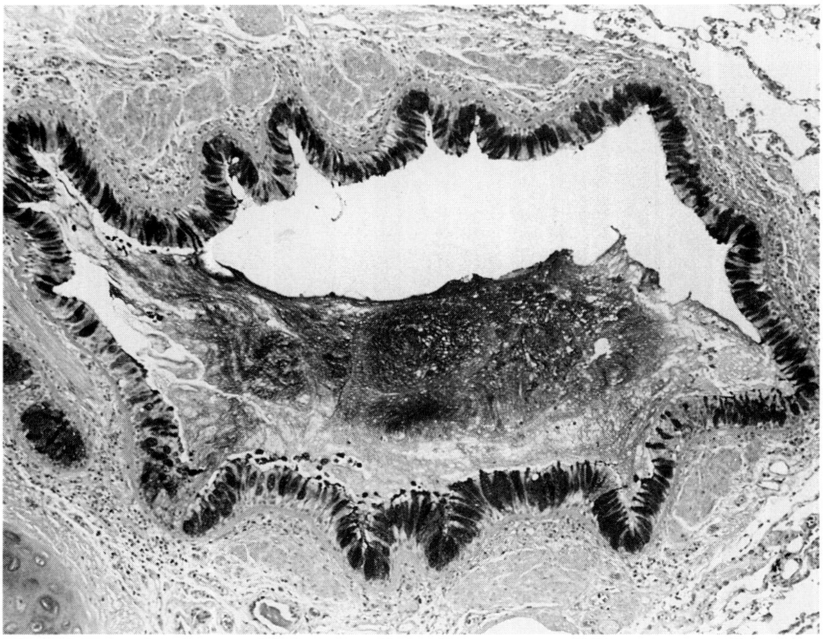

FIGURE 12.4
Section of cartilaginous airway stained with Alcian blue and PAS for mucin, showing marked goblet cell metaplasia and a mucous plug partially occluding the lumen of the airway in a person dying of asthma.

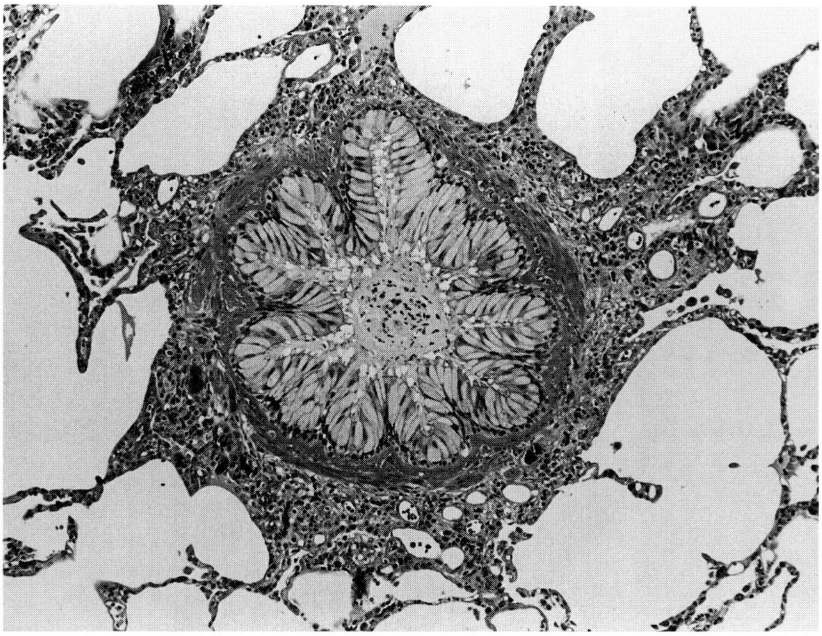

FIGURE 12.5
Transverse section of membranous bronchiole showing marked goblet cell metaplasia of the lining mucosa in a person dying of asthma. The airway also shows folding of the mucosa because of bronchoconstriction, mucous plugging, smooth-muscle hypertrophy, and a chronic inflammatory cell infiltrate in the airway adventitia.

cigarette smokers (78, 80, 81) (Fig. 12.6). They also extend farther down the bronchial tree. As in chronic bronchitis, the ratio of mucous to serous cells in the acini of the glands is increased (82).

The mucous gland ducts in asthma are markedly ectatic and form large pits where they enter the lumen (Fig. 12.7). Similar changes are seen in chronic bronchitis. The ectatic ducts may rupture during status asthmaticus or forced ventilation, producing interstitial emphysema and/or pneumothorax (69).

Mucous Plugs

A characteristic feature of fatal asthma is mucous plugs partially or completely occluding the airway lumen. They are most prominent in segmental and subsegmental airways but may be seen at any level from major bronchus to respiratory bronchiole. The mucous plugs contain periodic acid-Schiff (PAS) positive material mixed with inflammatory cells, remnants of lipid-based eosinophil mediators (Charcot-Leyden crystals), desquamated epithelial cells (Creola bodies), spiral mucous casts (Kurschmans spirals), and serum proteins (83). Mucous plugs in asthma may show spiral laminations (Fig. 12.8), indicating that their formation occurs in stages and is influenced by respiratory effort.

The viscoelastic properties of the mucus are altered in asthma. Viscosity is increased and clearability reduced (84–86). The changes in physical properties are due to alterations in the biochemical composition of the mucus and the presence of proteins and exfoliated epithelial cells (87).

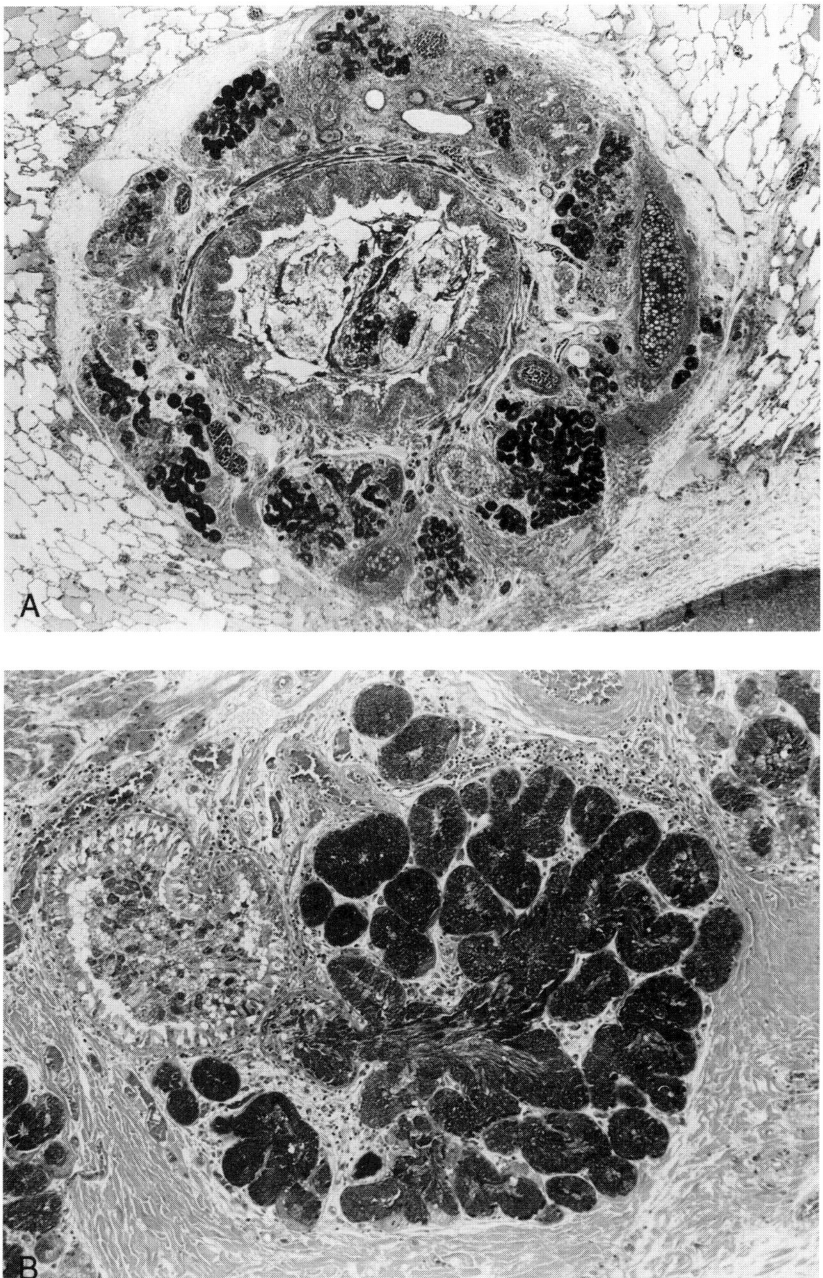

FIGURE 12.6

A. Section of cartilaginous airway stained with Alcian blue and PAS for mucin showing enlarged mucous glands encircling the airway with a mucous plug in the lumen. The mucous glands extend beyond the cartilaginous plates almost into the lung parenchyma. **B.** Higher-power view of mucous gland seen at bottom right. There is an increase in the size of the acini; mucous cells are more numerous than serous cells, and the acini can be seen connecting to a cystic gland duct at left.

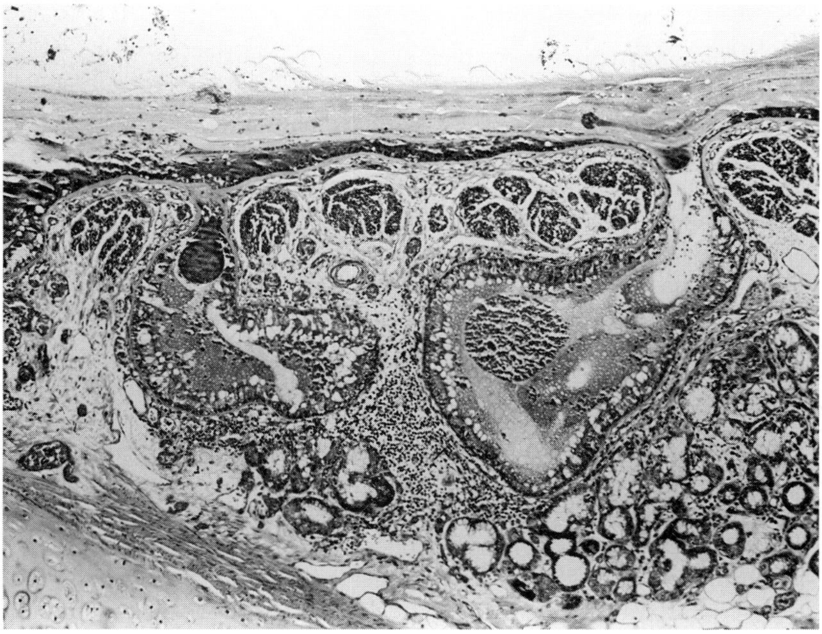

FIGURE 12.7
Fatal asthma. Longitudinal section of cartilaginous airway showing mucous glands together with two ectatic mucous gland ducts containing inspissated mucus. A mucous blanket is seen in the airway lumen.

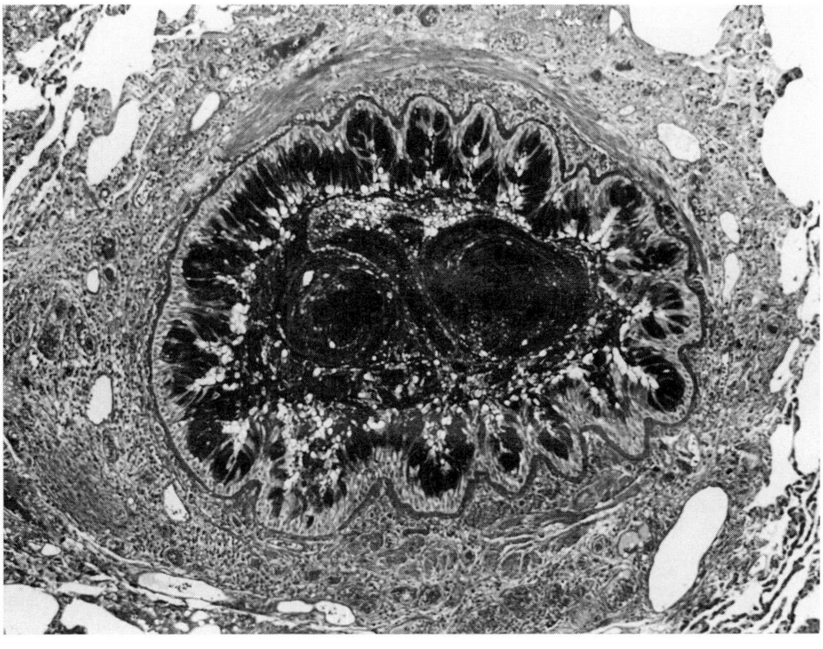

FIGURE 12.8
Section of large membranous bronchiole from patient with fatal asthma, stained with PAS and Alcian blue to demonstrate mucus. There is marked goblet cell metaplasia of the lining epithelium and a dense mucous plug containing two spiral bodies occluding the lumen.

Basement Membrane

Thickening of the basement membrane is one of the distinctive features of the asthmatic airway (88–90). By light microscopy the basement membrane region of the airway epithelium has a homogeneous pink glassy appearance and is thickest in the large cartilaginous airways and segmental bronchi (91) (Figs. 12.9 and 12.10). The basement membrane thickening extends into the mucous gland ducts. Immunohistochemical studies show that this layer is composed of collagen types I, III, and V together with fibronectin (90, 92). By contrast, the true basal lamina is composed predominantly of collagen types IV and VII, laminin, and heparin sulfate proteoglycans (93–95). The latter are unaltered in asthma (90). Electron microscopy has revealed that the lamina lucida and densa of the true basement membrane in asthma are normal and that the subepithelial collagenous layer (lamina reticularis) is thickened and composed of edematous collagen fibers with a plexiform arrangement of the fibrils (96). The subepithelial collagen is derived from myofibroblasts (90, 92, 96). Basement membrane thickening is seen in persons with other conditions characterized by chronic inflammation, such as nonasthmatic smokers (91) and those with chronic bronchitis and bronchiectasis. However, the basement membrane thickening in these states is never a prominent feature. The thickness of the basement membrane does not appear to be related to the severity of asthma or affected by treatment with corticosteroids (77, 97). Cessation of exposure is followed by return of normal basement membrane thickness in TDI-induced asthma (98).

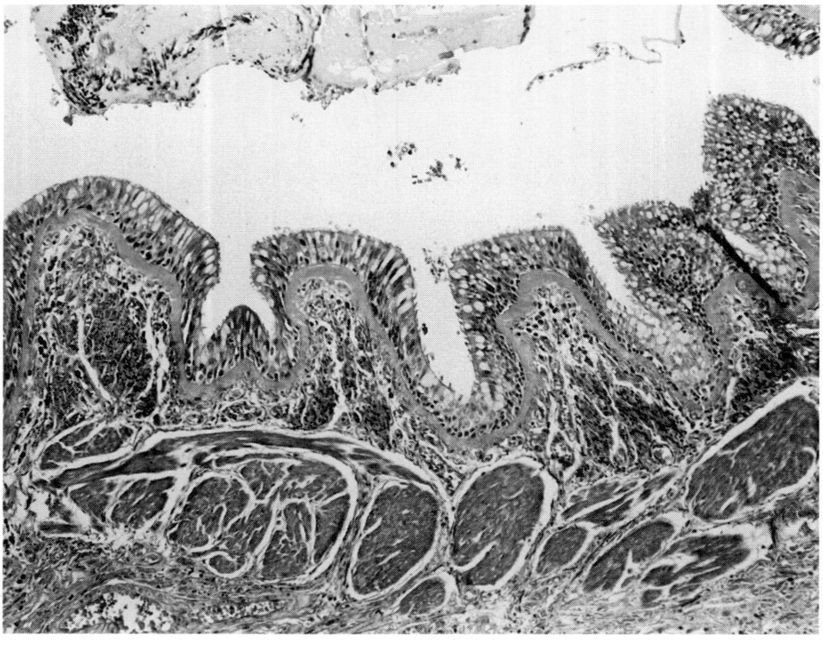

FIGURE 12.9
Section from airway showing epithelial hyperplasia and goblet cell metaplasia of the lining epithelium, basement membrane thickening, mucosal inflammatory cells, and large hypertrophic smooth muscle bundles in a patient with fatal asthma. Longitudinal elastic fibers are seen within the mucosal folds.

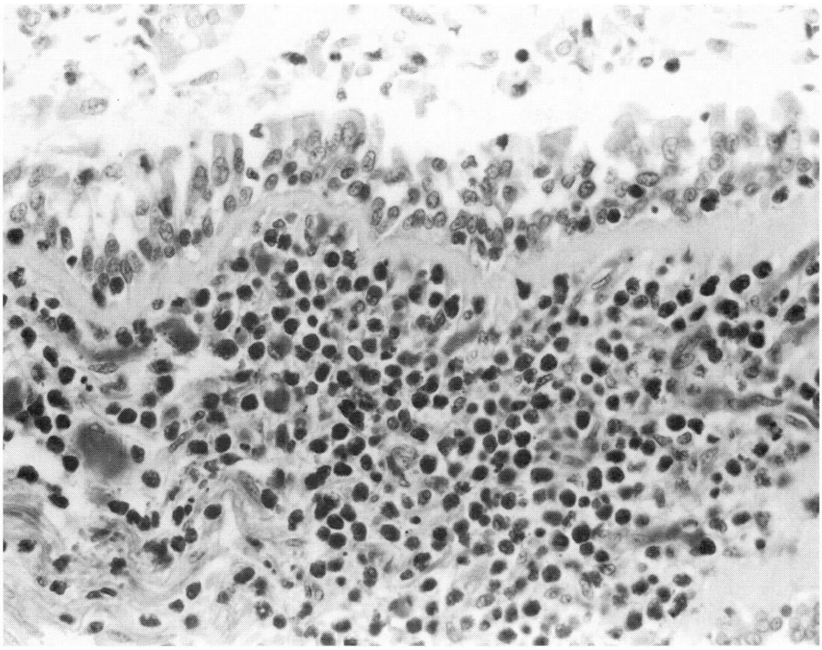

FIGURE 12.10
High magnification of bronchial mucosa showing epithelial disruption and exfoliation, basement membrane thickening, and a mixed inflammatory cell infiltrate in the mucosa, including eosinophils, lymphocytes, and mast cells in a patient with fatal asthma.

Elastic Fibers

In addition to basement membrane changes, the airways in asthma show a marked increase in the longitudinal mucosal elastic bundles (99). These structures originate in the posterior aspect of the trachea, radiate into 15 to 20 distinct subepithelial longitudinal bundles, and pass into the segmental bronchi (100). They terminate in the elastic fibers that support the mouths of the alveolar ducts. Their normal function is not known, but they may be involved in longitudinal stretching and recoil of the airways during respiration and in preventing airway collapse. They are rich in myofibroblasts and give rise to the prominent longitudinal mucosal folds seen in the asthmatic airway (Figures 12.3*B* and 12.9).

Smooth Muscle

An increase in the smooth muscle mass in asthma is another distinctive feature of the disease. Although to some extent the appearance is artifactual because of the marked bronchoconstriction in cases of fatal asthma (101), morphometric methods show that the increase is rea1 (78, 91, 102–104). There is an approximate twofold to fourfold increase in smooth muscle in the airways in fatal asthma (Fig. 12.11), and this increase is due to a combination of hypertrophy and hyperplasia (105, 106). The smooth muscle hypertrophy affects all levels of the airways but is most marked in the segmental cartilaginous airways and terminal bronchioles (Figures 12.9, 12.11–12.15). Because the normal smooth muscle in the airways is arranged in spiral overlapping bundles, hypertrophy of

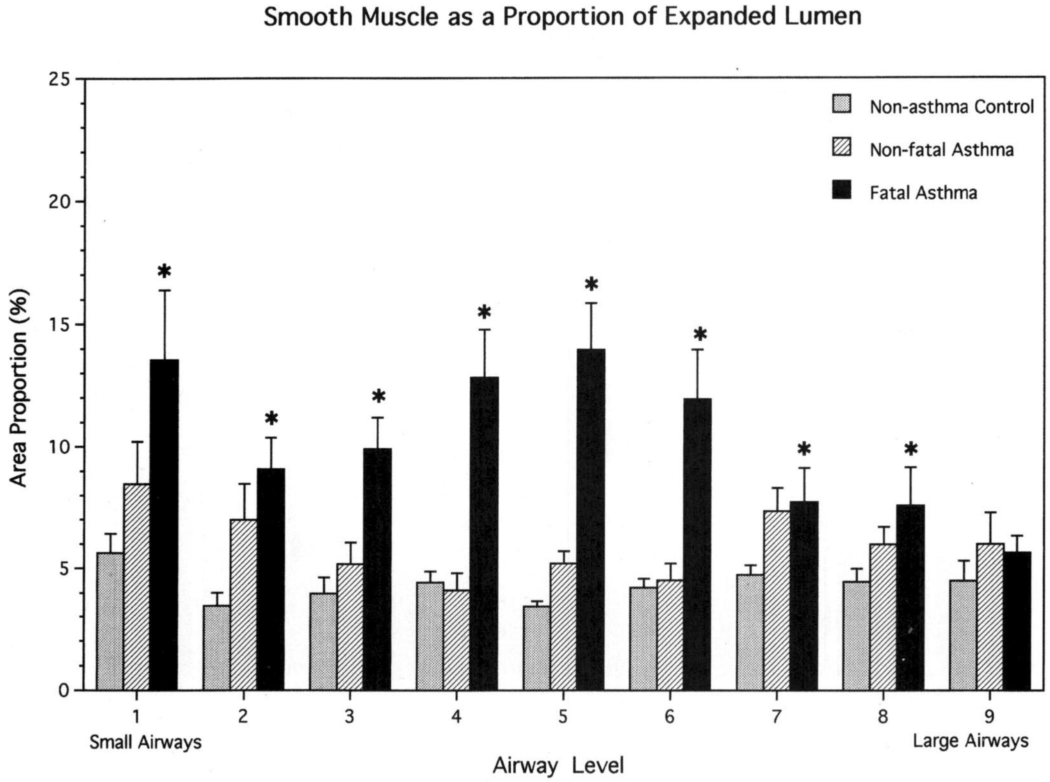

FIGURE 12.11
Histogram showing the proportion of smooth muscle in airways from 12 patients with fatal asthma compared with two control groups, a population of persons with asthma who died of other causes (nonfatal asthma) and a group consisting of persons who never had asthma and who died of nonrespiratory causes (nonasthma control). In the nonasthma control the proportion of smooth muscle in the airways from large to small is approximately constant. Fatal asthma produces a marked increase in smooth muscle with a bimodal distribution. Maximal increases in smooth muscle are seen in the segmental and subsegmental airways and in the small terminal bronchioles. Nonfatal asthma shows a less marked increase in smooth muscle than in the fatal asthma group, with no bimodal distribution, suggesting that persons with nonfatal asthma have a phenotype different from that of those who die of asthma.

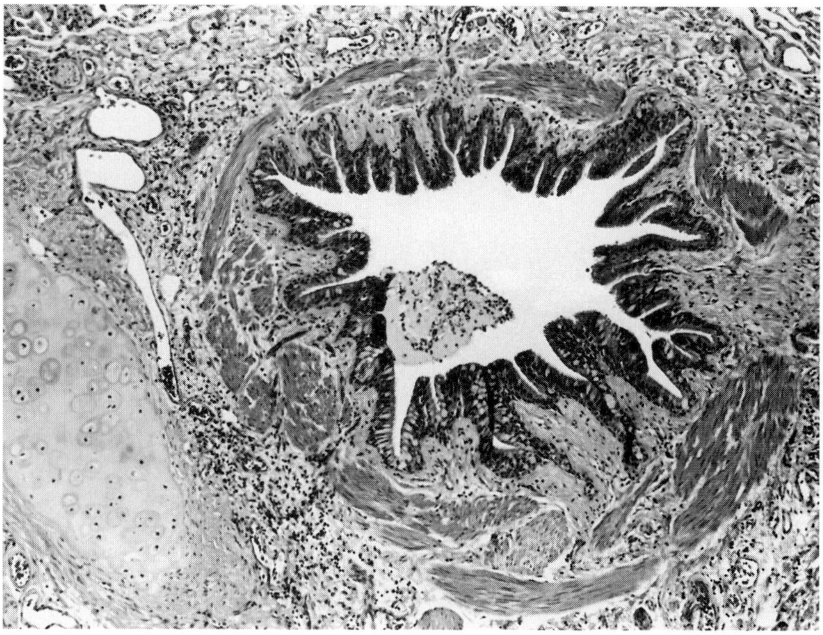

FIGURE 12.12
Cross-section of cartilaginous airway showing marked folding of the mucosa due to smooth muscle contraction in a person dying of asthma. The smooth muscle bundles are thickened and prominent.

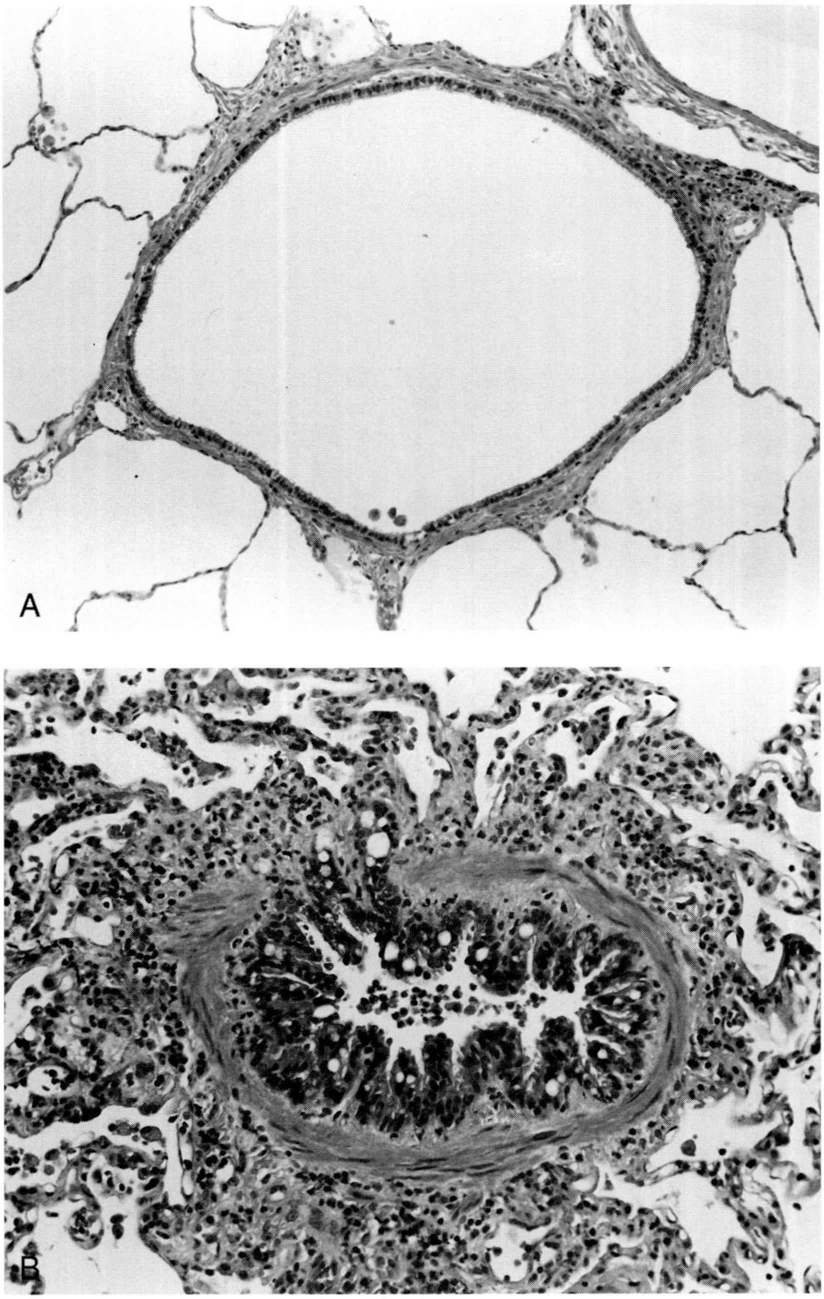

FIGURE 12.13
Membranous bronchioles from (A) normal nonasthmatic individual and (B) person dying of asthma. The normal bronchiole is fully distended, the epithelium is thin, and the smooth muscle is not prominent. The airway from the person who died of asthma shows marked bronchoconstriction with folded mucosa and thickened smooth muscle layer. There is also a marked chronic inflammatory cell infiltrate in the interstitium peripheral to the smooth muscle.

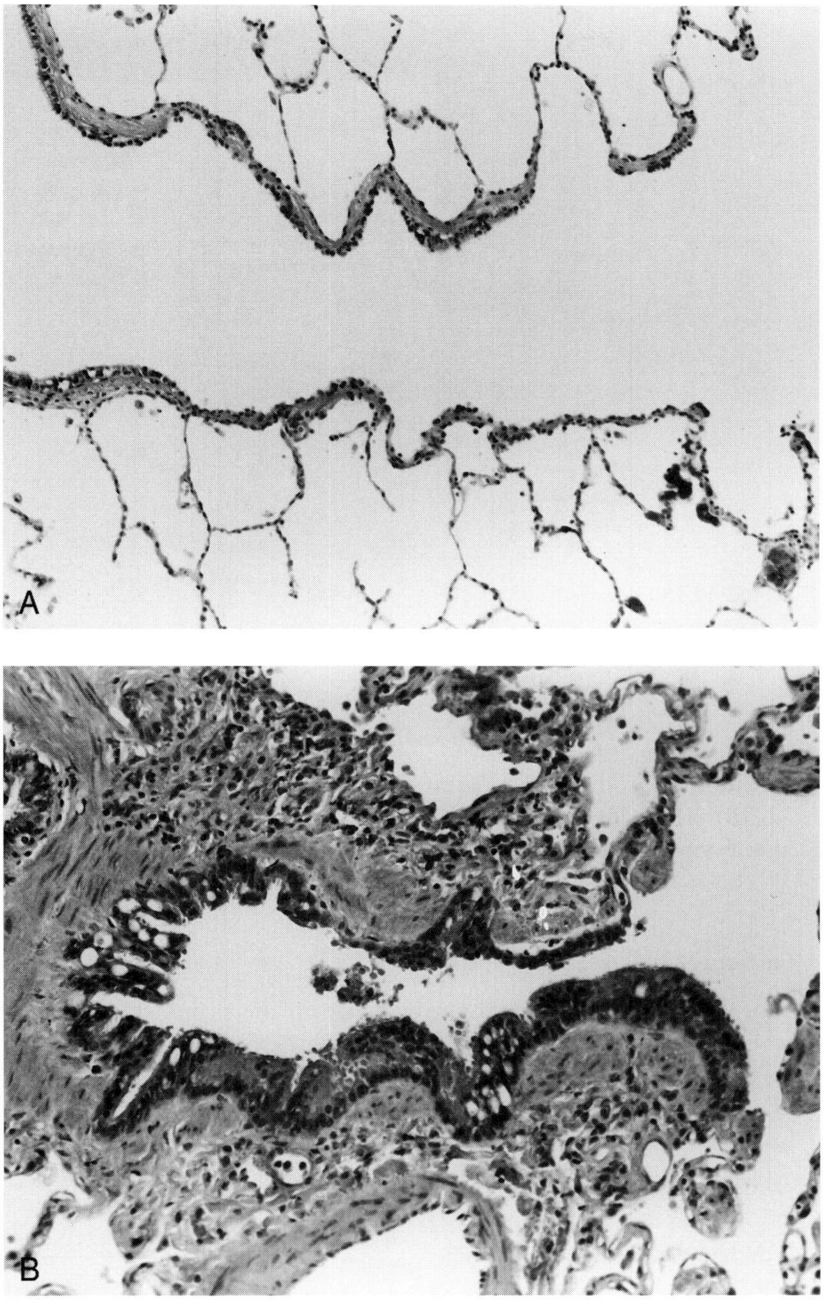

FIGURE 12.14
Longitudinal section of terminal bronchiole at junction with a respiratory bronchiole from (A) normal nonasthmatic individual and (B) person dying of asthma. The asthmatic airway shows marked thickening of the wall, primarily because of smooth-muscle hyperplasia, chronic inflammatory cells in the periphery, and marked epithelial and goblet cell hyperplasia.

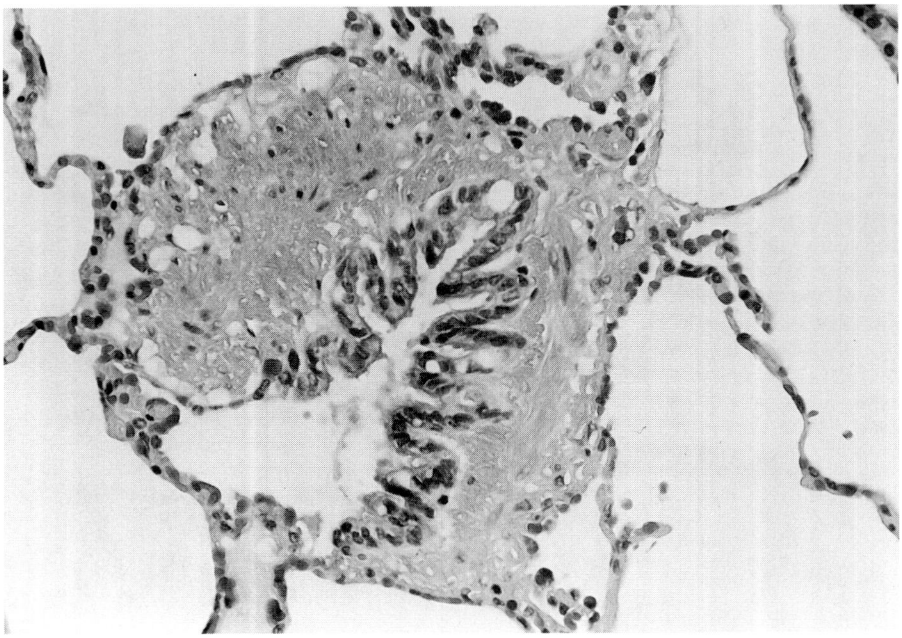

FIGURE 12.15
Transverse section of terminal bronchiole showing extreme smooth muscle hyperplasia in a patient with fatal asthma.

the bundles produces distinct areas of constriction in longitudinal section (Fig. 12.3*B*) (107). Smooth muscle hypertrophy is a major cause of the nonspecific airway hyperreactivity that characterizes asthma (107, 108).

Cartilage

Morphometric studies show an increase in the proportion of cartilage in the walls of asthmatic airways (102). Histologic examination of the cartilage plates shows increase in the perichondrium, distortion of the cartilage plates, and evidence of remodeling. These changes probably result from the increased mechanical forces on the airways during asthmatic episodes.

Bronchial and Pulmonary Arteries

Bronchial artery pathology is a feature of the asthmatic airway and is most severe in asthmatics who smoke (109). The lesions consist of hypertrophy and hyperplasia of the intimal longitudinal smooth muscle fibers, reduplication of the internal elastic lamina, and an increase in collagen and elastic fibers in the intima. The muscular media is not affected. The lesion may significantly reduce the vascular lumen. The changes are not specific for asthma and may be observed in cigarette smokers with chronic obstructive pulmonary disease. Their physiologic significance is not known. The pulmonary arterial circulation appears relatively unaffected in asthma.

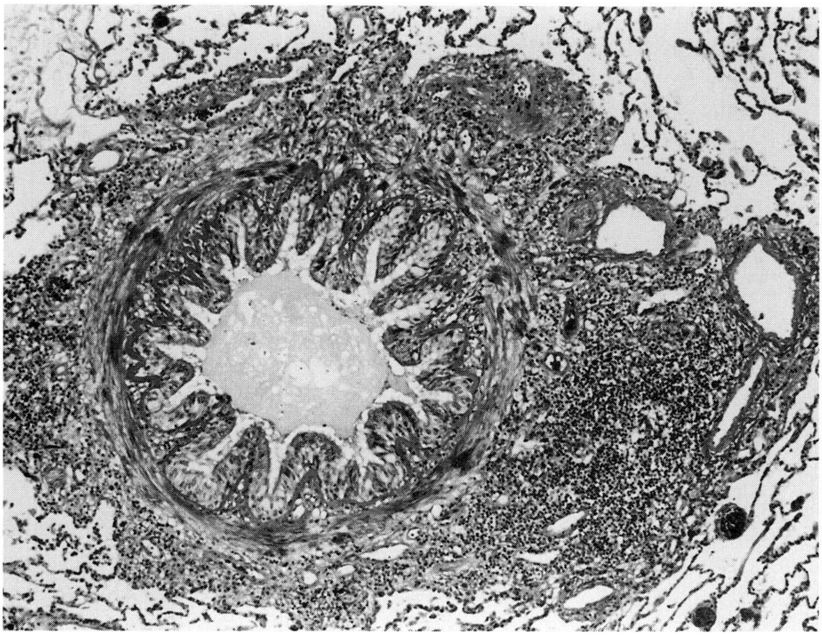

FIGURE 12.16
Cross-section of membranous bronchiole showing bronchoconstriction, mucous plugging, smooth-muscle hypertrophy, and a marked chronic inflammatory cell infiltrate peripheral to the smooth muscle in a patient with fatal asthma. The last feature is characteristic of the small airway inflammation in asthma.

Inflammatory Cells

Chronic lymphocytic inflammation is an invariable finding in the asthmatic airway. Depending on the stage and severity of the disease, a considerable number of cell types are recruited to the airways in asthma. These include lymphocytes (predominantly T cells) (59, 110, 111), macrophages (49, 77), mast cells, activated eosinophils, and neutrophils (59, 110–115) (Fig. 12.14). Lymphocytes and eosinophils are seen within the epithelium, in the submucosa (Fig. 12.10), and infiltrating the bronchial mucous glands of the larger conducting airways. They are not prominent within the smooth muscle layer. In the smaller airways these cells tend to lie peripheral to the smooth muscle, within the adventitia (Fig. 12.16). Mast cells are also observed within the epithelium, in the submucosa, and within the mucous glands. In addition, mast cells are prominent within the smooth muscle bundles. The inflammatory infiltrate tends to be patchy, so it is important to sample liberally and include both large and small airways. An increased inflammatory cell infiltrate has been observed in the minor salivary glands in patients with asthma (116). Cases of fatal asthma with few or no eosinophils in the airways have also been described (71). The cell count and its composition may be affected by corticosteroid use (51, 64, 77, 97, 117).

EVIDENCE FOR DEATH FROM ASPHYXIATION

To ascribe death to asthma, it is important to document features that indicate fatal asphyxiation due to acute airway obstruction. These features include hyperinflation and/or collapse on gross examination, pleural petechial hemorrhages, and difficulty in inflating the lungs because of mucous plugs and/or bronchoconstriction. Microscopically it is important to document luminal narrowing due to bronchoconstriction and mucous plugs. There is no evidence that bronchoconstriction and/or bronchorelaxation occurs postmortem or follows the introduction of fixatives (118). Therefore, the state of contraction of the airways on histologic sectioning is a good indication of the state of the airways immediately prior to death.

PATHOLOGIC FEATURES OF NONFATAL ASTHMA

The classic pathologic descriptions of asthma are derived from fatal cases. As fatal asthma comprises a very small proportion of all cases, their representation of asthma in general is questionable. Recent studies of lungs from asthmatics dying of other causes (nonfatal asthma) and bronchial biopsies from living asthmatics indicate that there may be more than one morphologic type of asthma (89, 91, 102).

Morphometric studies of the airways from persons with asthma but dying of other causes show quantitative and qualitative differences in airway wall remodeling (89, 91, 102, 107) (Fig. 12.11). Smooth muscle hypertrophy when present in nonfatal asthma shows a different distribution from that seen in fatal asthma. Whereas fatal asthma affects both the segmental airways and nonterminal bronchioles, nonfatal asthma appears to affect mainly the smaller airways (91, 102, 107) (Fig. 12.11). These observations led Ebina et al. (105, 107). to suggest that there may be distinct asthma phenotypes based on the distribution of smooth muscle along the airways.

The inflammatory cell profiles in the airway also appear to vary between nonfatal and fatal cases (51). Fatal asthma is characterized by fewer CD-3 T cells and greater numbers of eosinophils in the larger airways than in nonfatal asthma. Thickening of the basement membrane and eosinophilic infiltrates, however, appear to be similar for fatal and nonfatal asthma (43, 77).

PATHOLOGIC FEATURES OF OCCUPATIONAL ASTHMA

A single fatal case of occupational asthma has been reported by Fabbri et al. (119). The subject was a 43-year-old car painter with a history of isocyanate-induced asthma who died within an hour of exposure to a polyurethane paint containing TDI. Autopsy examination showed hyperinflated lungs and mucous plugs in the airways. Histologic examination revealed thickening of the basement membrane, extensive infiltration by eosinophils of the mucosa, diffuse mucous plugging of bronchioles, and smooth muscle hyperplasia, changes identical to those described for nonoccupational fatal asthma. A case of sudden death following exposure of an asthmatic to sulphur fumes has been described (120). The patient, a 76-year-old homemaker, was exposed to sulphur dioxide fumes released from a sulfide-containing derusting agent being used to open a clogged drain. She died within a few minutes of exposure. An autopsy showed bronchoconstriction, but mucous plugging was not a prominent feature. Sudden death from asthma without extensive mucous plugging has been described (121). It probably results from exposure to an intense bronchoconstrictive agent and/or systemic anaphylaxis.

Information on the histopathologic features of occupational asthma are largely derived from bronchial biopsy and bronchoalveolar lavage (BAL) studies of patients with exposure to TDI (48, 49, 98, 122) or western red cedar (123). BAL studies of isocyanate-induced asthma have shown a marked early and sustained increase in neutrophils followed by an increase in eosinophils (124). The chemotactic agents responsible for the leukocyte infiltration of the airways in occupational asthma are not known, but LTB4, a metabolite of the lipo-oxygenase pathway of arachidonic acid, has been identified in BAL lavage supernatant after TDI exposure (125). Histamine and leukotriene E4 are increased during the early asthmatic response to plicatic acid, a low-molecular-weight compound responsible for western red–cedar induced asthma (5).

The pathology of isocyanate-induced asthma appears to be similar to that of atopic asthma (98). Bronchial biopsies from subjects with TDI-induced asthma show increased numbers of eosinophils, mast cells, T lymphocytes, interepithelial edema, and thickening of the reticular layer of the basement membrane (49, 98, 122). In the study by Di Stefano et al. (122) there was a significant increase in mucosal mast cells in subjects who developed asthma after short-term exposure (2.4 ± 0.5 years) compared with subjects who developed asthma after long-term exposure (21.6 ± 3.1 years). Bronchial biopsies from persons with occupational asthma due to western red cedar have been compared with those of nonatopic and nonasthmatic control subjects. Both western red cedar asthma and atopic asthma were associated with increased numbers of T cells and activated eosinophils in the bronchial mucosa. There were no major histologic differences between atopic asthma and western red cedar asthma (123).

Total removal from exposure usually improves symptoms; however, those in whom the asthma persists show evidence of continued eosinophilic inflammation in the airways (126). Saetta et al. (98) showed a decrease in thickness of the basement membrane in seven patients with occupational asthma due to TDI following removal from exposure. These findings indicate that removal from exposure to a specific agent may result in regression of mesenchymal changes.

REACTIVE AIRWAYS DYSFUNCTION SYNDROME, OR IRRITANT-INDUCED ASTHMA

Clinical Features

RADS is characterized by persistent asthma after a single exposure to a high concentration of an irritant substance. The term was coined by Brooks et al. (127) in a paper describing 10 individuals who developed persistent asthmalike symptoms following accidental exposure to high concentrations of irritant vapors, fumes, gases, or smoke in places with poor ventilation. Although the disease has received general acceptance as a distinct form of asthma, recently this has been challenged (128). The spectrum of agents responsible for the syndrome is extensive (Table 12.4).

To be diagnosed with RADS the patient must have the following features:

1. There must be a well-documented exposure to a high concentration of an irritant substance, with symptoms developing within a short time (several minutes to several hours). Most patients require medical attention during or shortly after the acute injury.
2. The disease must originate from the time of exposure and persist for at least 3 months. Most documented cases persist for several years, with the longest recorded case being 12 years (127). An acute exacerbation of preexisting asthma does not qualify as RADS.

TABLE 12.4
Agents Reported to Cause Reactive Airway Dysfunction Syndrome

AGENT	REFERENCE
Hydrogen sulfide	Gandevia (129)
	Chan-Yeung et al.* (130)
Nitrogen dioxide	Gautrin et al. (131)
Sulphur dioxide	Alford et al. (132)
Ammonia	Bernstein and Bernstein* (133)
Chlorine	Donnelly and Fitzgerald (134)
	Gautrin et al.* (131)
Ethylene oxide	Deschamps et al.* (135)
Phosgene	Tarlo and Broker (136)
Ether	Taylor and Bernard (137)
Butadiene	Demeter and Dordascu (138)
TDI	Palcznski et al. (139)
Metam sodium (pesticide)	Cone et al. (140)
Sulfuric acid	Boulet (141)
Hydrochloric acid	Deschamps et al. (142)
Sodium hypochlorite (bleach)	Deschamps et al. (142)
Acetic acid	Kern (143)
Formaldehyde	Demeter and Cordasco (138)
Phosphoric acid	Angelillo (144)
Tear gas	Hu and Christiani (145)
Spray paint	Brooks et al.* (127)
Welding fumes	Brooks et al.* (127)
Smoke inhalation	Stenton et al. (146)

* Bronchial biopsies.
Adapted from Alberts AM, do Pico GA. Reactive airways dysfunction syndrome. Chest 1996;109:1618–1626.

3. There must be persistent asthmalike symptoms with objective documented evidence of nonspecific bronchial hyperreactivity to histamine or methylcholine.
4. Repeated exposures to lower levels of the substance that initiated the problem must not cause symptoms. The demonstration of specific IgE or IgG antibodies also negates this diagnosis.

Several investigators have drawn attention to cases with some but not all of the criteria for a diagnosis of RADS. These include those with pre-existing respiratory diseases or atopy, cases resulting from multiple exposures to lower levels of irritant chemicals, and cases that appear to have developed in combination with a nonspecific sensitizing agent, such as ozone (3). This suggests a continuous spectrum of disease under the umbrella of occupational asthma.

Population at Risk and Causative Agents

The population at risk includes all workers exposed to irritant chemicals, particularly those likely to be exposed to them at high concentrations in confined places (147). Approximately 10% of workers diagnosed with occupational asthma fulfill the criteria for RADS (3). Under appropriate circumstances a high proportion of affected workers may develop RADS. Harkonen et al. (148) describe a RADS-like syndrome developing in three of seven miners exposed to sulfur dioxide in a pyrite explosion.

A diverse group of agents have been reported to cause RADS (Table 12.4). The only feature they have in common is that they are irritant to the upper respiratory tract. They include acids, alkalis, oxidizing agents, organic solvents, smoke, fumes, and complex mixtures. The disease may follow exposure to a single agent or to combinations of irritant chemicals. For example, RADS was reported in three police officers exposed to fumes containing sodium hydroxide, silicone tetrachloride, and trichlorosilane from a roadside truck accident (149). Cone et al. (140) report 20 cases of RADS developing as a result of exposure to metam sodium, a pesticide, after a train derailment.

Pathogenesis

The pathogenesis of RADS is unknown; however, the sudden onset following exposure to an airway injury indicates that the process begins with acute epithelial injury. Three major theories have been advanced to explain the persistence of symptoms and the development of hyperreactive airway disease that persists for many years after the initial injury (150):

1. Recovery from epithelial injury leads to abnormal neural reinnervation and altered receptor threshold in the airways. According to this hypothesis, alterations in the nonadrenergic, noncholinergic nerves and their receptors would most likely be involved.
2. Injury to the epithelium and re-epithelialization lead to increased epithelial permeability and greater sensitivity to bronchoconstricting agents. This theory is supported by bronchial biopsy findings reported by Gautrin et al. (131) that show abnormalities of the epithelium several years after the initial acute exposure.
3. As a result of the acute airway injury, persistent chronic inflammation develops, altering airway reactivity. Evidence for this theory is provided by biopsy studies (Table 12.4).

PATHOLOGIC FEATURES

There have been no autopsy studies of RADS, and only a few patients have had biopsies (Table 12.4). Pathologic studies of the airways in persons dying of exposure to acute irritants, for example sulfur dioxide (151) and hydrogen sulfide (152), reveal massive epithelial ulceration, increased microvascular permeability, acute inflammation, and hemorrhagic pulmonary edema. It is likely that similar features are seen in patients who develop RADS; however, biopsies in the acute stage have not been undertaken.

Bronchial biopsies taken a year or more after the initial injury from patients exposed to diverse agents, including sodium hypochlorite, chlorine, hydrogen sulfide, spray paint, welding fumes, anhydrous ammonia, and ethylene oxide, are moderately consistent in their findings. In general they show epithelial changes, mild lymphocytic infiltrates in the mucosa, goblet cell hyperplasia, and epithelial dysplasia. Variable features are eosinophils, thickening of the basement membrane, and smooth muscle hyperplasia. How these tissue responses compare with classic asthma and other asthmalike syndromes is shown in Table

TABLE 12.5
Contrasts in Tissue Response in Asthma and Asthma-like Syndromes

FEATURE	FATAL ASTHMA	NONFATAL ASTHMA	OCCUPATIONAL ASTHMA	RADS	BYSINOSSIS
Epithelial					
Desquamation	+ + +	+	+	+	NK
Dysplasia	−	−	−	+	NK
Lymphocytes	+ +	+	+	+	NK
Eosinophils	+ + +	+ +	+ +	+ or −	−
Basement membrane thickening	+ + +	+ +	+ +	+ or −	NK
Goblet cell hyperplasia	+ + +	+ +	+ +	+	+ +
Mucous gland hyperplasia	+ + +	+	NK	NK	+ +
Smooth muscle hyperplasia	+ + +	±	±	+ or −	+
Blood eosinophilia	+ +	+ +	+ +	+ or −	−

NK, not known.

12.5. In summary, the pathology appears to differ from that of classic asthma, but more studies, particularly from persons dying with the disease, are required.

BYSSINOSIS

Clinical Features

Exposure to cotton dust, flax, and soft hemp can lead to several distinct but related clinical effects. These include mill fever, a form of organic dust toxic syndrome); chest tightness, cough, wheeze, and shortness of breath, to which the term byssinosis is usually applied; chronic bronchitis (chronic cough and phlegm after many years of exposure); and airway hyperresponsiveness (153). In classic cases of byssinosis the symptoms develop approximately 4 hours after exposure to cotton dust and are worst on Monday mornings. Pulmonary function monitoring shows a gradual across-shift decline in forced expiratory volume in 1 second (FEV_1), with a return to baseline values by the next day (154, 155). Duration and concentration of exposure are important determinants of byssinosis prevalence (156–158). The most substantial health problem associated with it is the potential for accelerated declines in lung function and irreversible chronic impairment (155). The effect of smoking appears to be additive with that of cotton dust exposure (159).

The number of persons at risk for these disorders is not known. Data from the 1970s suggest that approximately 500,000 workers may have been exposed to cotton and related dusts, 80% in textile industries (yarn and fabric manufacturers) and 20% in nontextile industries (ginning, warehousing, cottonseed processing, and manufacture of mattress padding) (160).

Intensive investigations to identify the causative agents in cotton dust have been only partially successful. The potency of various vegetable fibers to cause byssinosis, from worst to best, are cotton, flax, soft hemp, and sisal. Cotton plants consist of bract, leaf, vein, petiole, capsule, cotyledon, and pericarp. Moreover, the dust contains fungi, bacteria, other plants, and soil. The finding that washed cotton is less likely to cause byssinosis indicates that the agent is a surface contaminant and/or is water soluble (161). Biologically active agents identified in cotton dust include gram-negative bacterial endotoxin (162–165), proteases (166), cellulose (163), and other organic compounds (167). Postulated mechanisms whereby these agents may induce byssinosis include local histamine release, formation of antigen antibody reactions, direct and indirect effects of endotoxins and proteolytic enzymes, and nonspecific pharmacologic mediator release (168–170).

Pathologic Features

Postmortem studies have failed to reveal any distinctive pathologic features in persons employed in cotton mills or receiving compensation during life for byssinosis. Such findings as have been reported are relatively nonspecific. The possible exception to this is the observation of birefringent cotton fibers in a small proportion of cases and the presence of byssinosis bodies, which are thought to be iron-encrusted cotton fibers (171). The bodies are spherical and range up to 10 μm in diameter. They have a central black nidus surrounded by a clear halo up to 2 μm thick. They appear to be a marker of exposure.

Pratt et al. (172) and Edwards et al. (173) performed morphometric studies on lungs from workers with byssinosis and nonexposed controls and concluded that those with byssinosis had larger bronchial mucous glands and showed goblet cell metaplasia of the airways. Edwards et al. (173) found an increase in smooth muscle in the main bronchi but not in the segmental airways in persons with byssinosis but not in controls. When smoking history was taken into account, none of the studies showed any evidence that byssinosis was associated with emphysema (172–174). There is no evidence that cotton dust causes interstitial fibrosis, bronchiolitis, granulomas, asthma, or cor pulmonale (171–174). Contrast in tissue response between asthma, asthmalike syndromes, and byssinosis is shown in Table 12.5.

ORGANIC DUST TOXIC SYNDROME

Clinical Features

Exposure to organic dusts containing large quantities of micro-organisms can result in an acute systemic illness characterized by fever; malaise; aches and pains in the arms, legs, and lumbar region; and occasionally vomiting. Respiratory symptoms are not prominent, but some patients develop a dry cough and demonstrate fine basilar rales on auscultation. The symptoms develop within 4 to 8 hours of exposure. Organic dust toxic syndrome has a benign course with full recovery within 72 hours. Clinically it resembles the systemic syndromes associated with exposure to metal fumes (see Chapter 3). It is most commonly associated with exposures in the farming industry, particularly to moldy farm products containing spores from fungi and actinomyces (175, 176) but is also common in hog farmers (177), among whom exposure is primarily to bacteria rich in endotoxin (178). It differs from hypersensitivity pneumonitis in several important respects:

1. Organic dust toxic syndrome is associated with exposure to extremely high levels of micro-organisms, approximately 10 times those associated with hypersensitivity pneumonitis (176, 179).
2. A single exposure causes organic dust toxic syndrome, whereas repeated exposures over several weeks are required to develop hypersensitivity pneumonitis.

3. Organic dust toxic syndrome may occur in any individual without prior sensitization. Hypersensitivity pneumonitis, by contrast, affects a relatively small proportion of individuals exposed to organic dusts, and its clinical expression includes sensitization and immune responses.

The pathogenesis of organic dust toxic syndrome appears to entail a direct toxic effect of a component or components of the dust. A large number of bacterial and fungal constituents interact with specific receptors on inflammatory cells and/or directly activate complement (180, 181). These interactions are mostly nonimmune primary defense mechanisms to inhaled micro-organisms. Agents capable of initiating these direct responses include endotoxin, fungal β-1,3 glucan, bacterial *fmlp* peptides, teichoic acids, protodyne, bacterial heat shock proteins, gram-negative lipopolysaccharides (LPS) and bacterial derived interleukin I (182–186).

A study of BAL fluid in grain handlers exposed to an extract of grain dust supports the concept that one or more of these substances initiate the acute inflammatory response (187). The BAL fluid contained large numbers of neutrophils and increased levels of cytokines TNF-2, IL-1β, IL-6, and IL-8. An increase in serum IL-6 has been observed in workers exposed to hog house dust containing gram-negative LPS (186).

Pathologic Features

Because the disease is benign and usually self-limiting, information on the tissue response is very limited. The few reported cases with a lung biopsy may not represent the syndrome as a whole. In one report the patient, a farmer, was exposed to moldy dusts for approximately an hour while cleaning a silo (188). He developed chills, fever, and dry irritating cough in the evening. The next day he was decidedly worse, with extreme malaise, weakness, and distressing cough. Chest examination revealed crepitant rales but no evidence of bronchospasm. Chest radiograph showed reticular and fine nodular densities in the lower two-thirds of both lung fields. Bronchoscopy revealed hyperemic airway mucosa, and transbronchial biopsy showed massive exudate of neutrophils and macrophages in the alveolar spaces and bronchioles. Special stains showed large numbers of organisms, and culture grew at least five fungi, including *Fusarium* and *Penicillium* (188). The pathology in the severe cases thus appears to involve acute inflammation, hyaline membrane formation, and the demonstration of large numbers of heterogeneous (nonproliferating) organisms. Whether these features are characteristic of the usual case with a more benign outcome is not clear.

EXTRINSIC ALLERGIC ALVEOLITIS

Clinical Features and Pathogenesis

EAA, also called hypersensitivity pneumonitis, is a hypersensitivity reaction to a variety of organic antigens and a few simple inorganic chemical compounds (Table 12.6). EAA may be given a specific disease name when a particular antigen or occupation is the cause of the condition, for example, farmers' lung or pigeon breeders' lung, but the clinical and pathologic appearances tend to be fairly similar no matter what the cause. Some cases of EAA occur in persons who do not have a specific implicated occupation but who work in a building with a closed ventilating system that has become contaminated by micro-organisms

TABLE 12.6
Causes of Extrinsic Allergic Alveolitis (Hypersensitivity Pneumonitis)

DISEASE	SOURCE OF ANTIGEN	PROBABLE ANTIGEN
Vegetable Products		
Farmers' lung disease	Moldy hay	Thermophilic actinomycetes, *Aspergillus* spp., Thermoactinomyces *vulgaris, Micropolyspora faeni*
Bagassosis	Moldy pressed sugar cane (bagasse)	Thermophilic actinomycetes, Thermoactinomyces *sacchari, T. vulgaris*
Mushroom workers' disease	Moldy compost	Thermophilic actinomycetes? *M. faeni, T. vulgaris*
Suberosis	Moldy cork	*Pencillium* spp.
Malt workers' lung	Contaminated barley	*Aspergillus clavatus*
Maple bark disease	Contaminated maple logs	*Cryptostroma corticale*
Sequoiosis	Contaminated wood dust	*Graphium* spp., *Pullularia* spp.
Wood pulp workers' disease	Contaminated wood pulp	*Alternaria* spp.
Humidifier lung	Contaminated humidifiers, air conditioners, dehumidifiers	Thermophilic actinomycetes, thermoactinomyces *candidus, T. vulgaris, Penicillium* spp., *Cephalosporium* spp., amoebas
Familial hypersensitivity pneumonitis	Contaminated wood dust in walls	*Bacillus subtilis*
Cheese washers' disease	Cheese casings	*Penicillium* spp.
Wood trimmers' disease	Contaminated wood trimmings	*Rhizopus* spp., *Mucor* spp.
Thatched roof disease	Dried grasses and leaves	*Sacchoramonospora viridis*
Tea growers' disease	Tea plants	Unknown
Coffee workers' lung	Green coffee	Unknown
Streptomyces hypersensitivity pneumonitis	Contaminated fertilizer	*Streptomyces albus*
Caphalosporium hypersensitivity pneumonitis	Contaminated basement (sewage)	*Cephalosporium*
Sauna takers' disease	Sauna water	*Pullularia* spp.
Detergent workers' disease	Detergent	*B. subtilis*, enzymes
Paprika splitters' lung	Paprika dust	*Mucor stolonifer*
Summer hypersensitivity pneumonitis (Japan)	Contaminated houses, walls	*Trichosporon cutaneum*
Animal Products		
Pigeon breeders' disease	Pigeon droppings	Altered pigeon serum (probably IgA)
Duck fever	Duck feathers	Duck proteins
Turkey handlers' disease	Turkey products	Turkey proteins
Laboratory workers' hypersensitivity pneumonitis	Rat fur	Male rat urine
Pituitary snuff takers' disease	Pituitary powder	Bovine and porcine proteins
Insect Products		
Millers' lung	Wheat weevils	*Sitophilus granarius*
Reactive Simple Chemicals		
TDI hypersensitivity pneumonitis	TDI	Altered proteins (albumin + others)
TMA hypersensitivity pneumonitis	TMA	Altered proteins
MDI hypersensitivity pneumonitis	MDI	Altered proteins
Epoxy resin lung	Heated epoxy resin	Phthalic anhydride

MDI, diphenylmethane diisocyanate; TDI, toluene diisocyanate; TMA, trimetallic anhydride.

Reprinted with permission from Colby TV, Carrington CB. Interstitial lung disease. In: Thurlbeck WM, Churg AM, eds. Pathology of the lung. New York: Thieme Medical, 1995:651.

(humidifier lung) (189). Some patients show a pattern of EAA on biopsy, but no occupational or domestic cause of the disease can be discovered (190).

The prevalence in exposed workers has been difficult to estimate because of methodologic problems with disease recognition. The susceptible population may be large. Studies of acute outbreaks of EAA in office workers exposed to bacterial antigens show that up to 70% of exposed populations may develop the disease. In other circumstances the prevalence is much lower. A prevalence of 42 per 100,000 has been reported, using strict criteria for the diagnosis, in a population of Wisconsin dairy farmers (191).

Immunologically EAA appears to be a type III or type IV response to an inhaled antigen, and circulating serum precipitins to the antigen can be found in sensitized individuals. A role for precipitating antibodies with the formation of antigen–antibody complexes and the activation of complement is indicated in the acute phase reaction (192). The lymphocytosis (193) and granuloma formation in the later stages suggest a T cell–mediated hypersensitivity response (194). However, sensitization is common in farmers without disease; hence the presence of precipitating antibodies has low predictive value in recognition and little prognostic value for disease progression (195). Thus in a clinically typical case the finding of serum precipitins may be diagnostically useful, but inhalation challenge tests with the suspect antigen may be necessary to confirm the diagnosis.

EAA is usually separated into acute, subacute, and chronic forms. Acute EAA occurs within a few hours of exposure to the antigen, and symptoms last 18 to 24 hours and then disappear. The patient develops fever, chills, dyspnea, and malaise and may show a radiographic picture of diffuse airspace infiltrates. This radiographic and clinical picture must be separated from organic toxic dust syndrome and pulmonary mycotoxicosis (see previous section), which is caused by massive exposures to microbial agents such as fungal spores in hay. Organic toxic dust syndrome is not immunologically mediated and occurs in all exposed individuals, whereas acute EAA occurs only in sensitized individuals. The systemic symptoms of the two diseases may be identical.

Subacute EAA develops slowly over weeks to months, usually in the setting of multiple exposures to the offending antigen but without obvious acute episodes. The patient typically has shortness of breath and sometimes cough, sputum production, and malaise (196). Radiographic examination reveals interstitial infiltrates on plain film (Figs. 12.17 and 12.18) and either a ground-glass pattern or fine nodules in the centers of the lobules on high-resolution CT scan, the latter finding reflecting the centrilobular (bronchiolar) inflammatory process seen in EAA (197, 198).

EAA is defined as chronic when there is either radiographic or pathologic evidence of fibrosis. Both subacute and chronic forms typically show a restrictive pattern of pulmonary function, sometimes accompanied by evidence of airflow obstruction. The latter effect is presumably caused by the bronchiolitis seen in EAA, and the restrictive pattern reflects the interstitial infiltrate and fibrosis associated with the granulomas.

The treatment and prognosis of EAA are controversial, and disease caused by different antigens may have different outcomes. In theory the treatment of choice is removal from contact with the antigen and administration of steroids. Many cases show an excellent response to steroids, and we have seen dramatic improvements in pulmonary function after steroid treatment even when there is definite fibrosis in the biopsy. In general, though, fibrosis implies a worse prognosis (199). Whether workers who have no other possible occupation (typically farm workers) can be treated with steroids (or even not be treated at all) and maintain their occupation without further functional loss is disputed (191, 200–202).

Pathologic Features

Biopsy is rarely performed in cases of acute EAA, and the pathologic features are poorly defined in the literature (203, 204). Both hyaline membrane and an acute inflammatory infiltrate have been reported (203, 204); however, similar features are seen in organic toxic dust syndrome, a condition caused by massive acute exposures to a dust such as silo contents (203), and the distinction between the two may be difficult. It is our view that acute EAA should be diagnosed only if granulomas or granulomatous inflammation is seen in addition to the acute inflammatory changes.

The pathologist is far more likely to encounter biopsies from the subacute or chronic forms of EAA. Subacute and chronic EAA are forms of chronic interstitial pneumonia. Classic cases of subacute EAA show a triad of a diffuse chronic (lymphocyte and plasma cell) inflammatory infiltrates, bronchiolitis, and small nonnecrotizing granulomas or individual giant cells (190, 203, 205–209) (Figs. 12.19 and 12.20). The relative prominence of each of these features varies from case to case, and sometimes not all of the features are present. In our experience

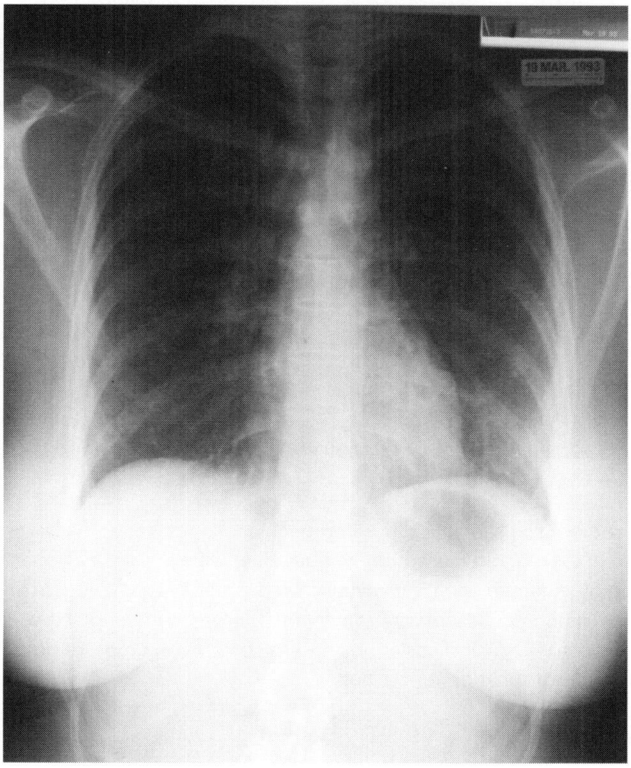

FIGURE 12.17
Chest radiograph showing lower-zone ground-glass to fine interstitial infiltrates in a patient with extrinsic allergic alveolitis.

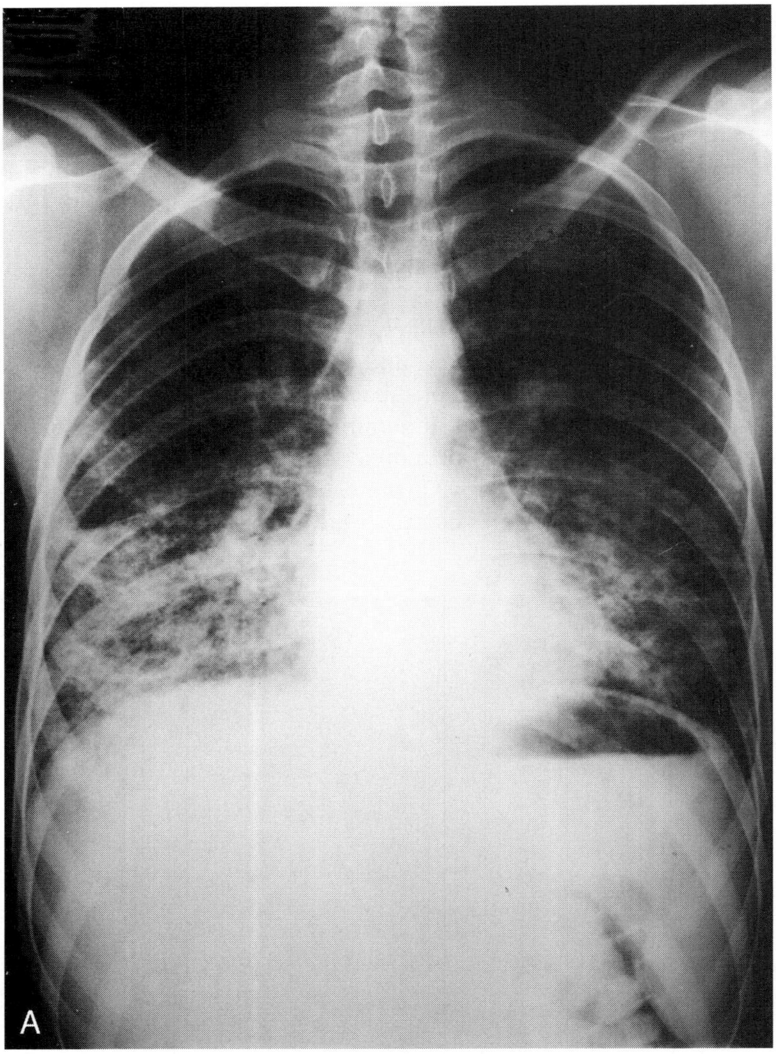

FIGURE 12.18

A. Chest radiograph showing diffuse parenchymal opacities in the lower and middle zones of the lung in a 19-year-old mushroom worker. **B.** Low-power view of open lung biopsy showing granulomatous inflammation surrounding and partially occluding a small airway. **C.** High-power view of the noncaseating granuloma. The adjacent lung showed a mild chronic interstitial pneumonia. Oral corticosteroids and removal from exposure produced complete resolution of the radiographic abnormalities.

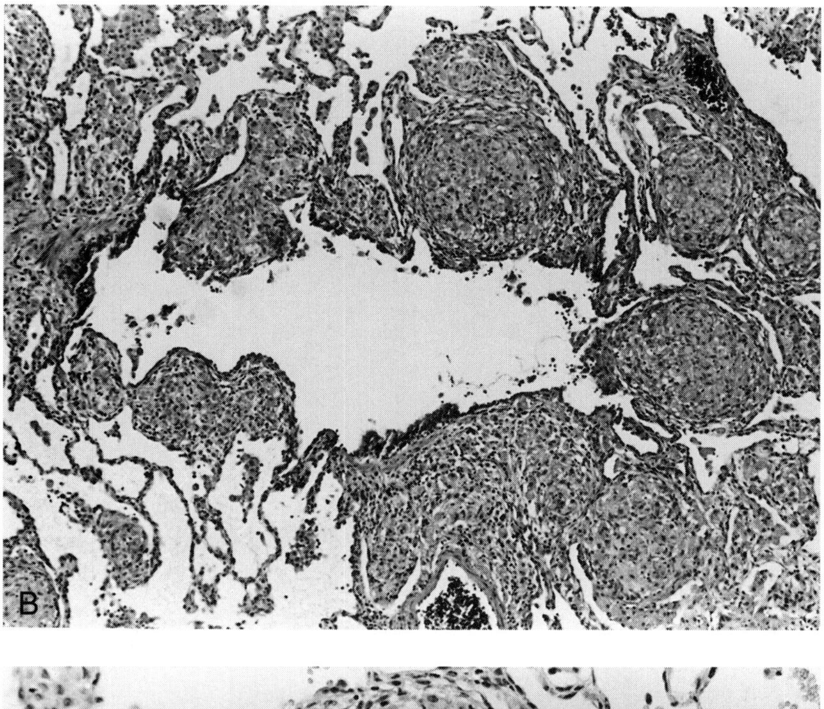

FIGURE 12.18 *(continued)*

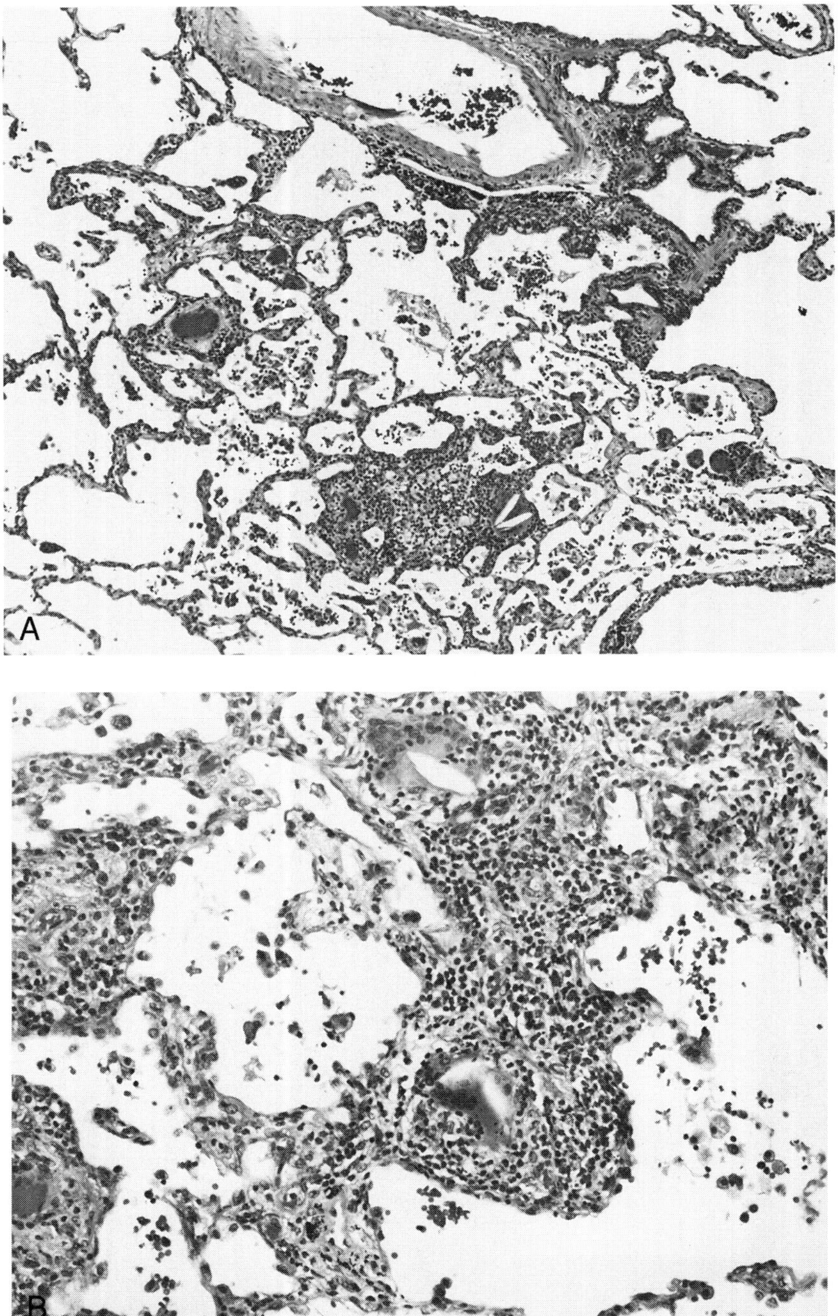

FIGURE 12.19

A. Low-power view of extrinsic allergic alveolitis (farmer's lung) showing mild interstitial chronic inflammatory infiltrate that appears most marked in and around the small airways. (×64.) **B.** Higher-power view demonstrating interstitial infiltrate and two individual giant cells with inclusions, a typical histologic appearance in extrinsic allergic alveolitis. (×400.)

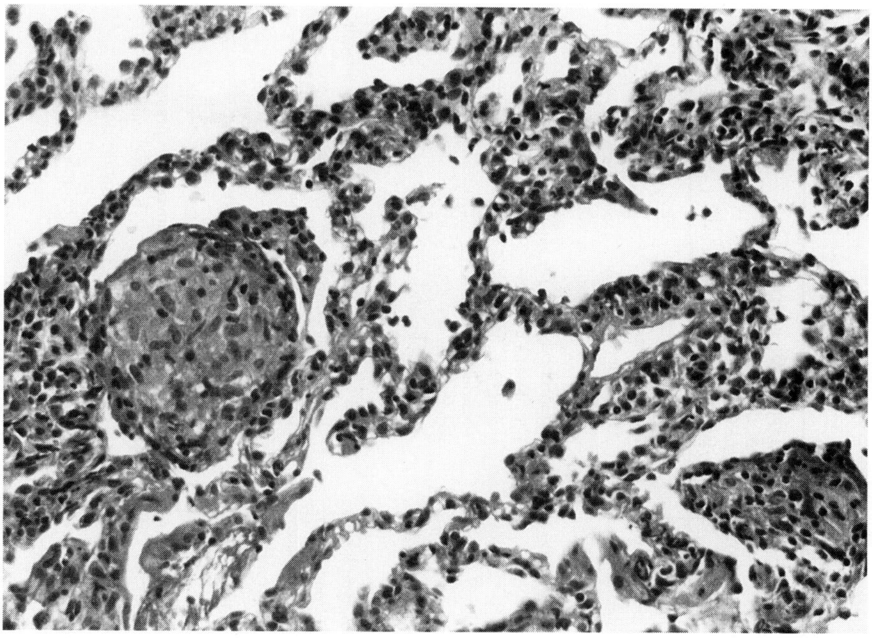

FIGURE 12.20
Transbronchial biopsy from a 26-year-old female employee of a mushroom farm. Symptoms included headache, malaise, dry cough, shortness of breath, fever, chills, sweats, and myalgia, which was worse on the afternoon of weekdays but not at weekends. Chest radiograph revealed diffuse reticulonodular markings, and pulmonary function testing demonstrated a severe restrictive ventilatory impairment (FVC 39% of predicted) and diminished diffusing capacity (54% of predicted). The biopsy shows a diffuse interstitial infiltrate of lymphocytes and plasma cells. A small noncaseating granuloma is also present. (Hematoxylin and eosin, ×150.)

the interstitial infiltrate in the milder cases tends to be more prominent around the small bronchioles, and the more distal portions of the lobule may be totally spared. However, quite marked and widespread interstitial infiltrates, which raise the possibility of lymphocytic interstitial pneumonia or even lymphoma, are sometimes seen in EAA.

The bronchiolitis of EAA is similarly variable in intensity and appearance. In some cases it manifests as a mild chronic inflammatory infiltrate in the bronchiolar wall (Figures 12.18 and 12.19) and in others appears as tufts of granulation tissue in the lumens of membranous and particularly respiratory bronchioles. The distinction from bronchiolitis obliterans with organizing pneumonia (BOOP), better called cytogenic organizing pneumonia, is occasionally difficult, although granulation tissue plugs are usually a minor component of EAA but a major component of BOOP (203).

The presence of nonnecrotizing interstitial granulomas or individual giant cells (Fig. 12.2) is extremely helpful in suggesting the correct diagnosis. The granulomas of EAA are often poorly defined, as opposed to the distinct nodular granulomas of sarcoidosis, and sometimes one sees only scattered individual giant cells (190, 203, 206). Giant cells may also be seen in the alveolar spaces. The giant cells or granulomas frequently contain crystalline material (calcium oxalate), cleftlike spaces (cholesterol), asteroid bodies, or bluish calcified Schau-

TABLE 12.7
Extrinsic Allergic Alveolitis: Differential Diagnosis

FEATURE	EAA	SARCOIDOSIS	BERYLLIOSIS	GRANULOMATOUS INFECTION	ASPIRATION, FOREIGN BODY, AND CHOLESTEROL GRANULOMAS	UIP
Granulomas	Variable in size and location; often ill-defined, noncohesive, noncaseating	Discrete epitheliod granulomas in peribronchial location; may be confluent; focal necrosis may be seen	Similar to sarcoid granulomas	Usually necrotizing; agent may be demonstrable in granuloma	Variable in size and location; necrosis uncommon	No
Giant cells, inclusions	Giant cells with birefringent and nonbirefringent inclusions; calcified Schauman bodies, Ca oxalate crystals, cholesterol clefts; may be independent of granulomas	Langhan's type, only seen in granulomas; birefringent calcium oxalate crystals common	Similar to sarcoid	Langhan's type	Foreign body type of inclusions clue to diagnosis (plant residue, mineral dust [talc], cholesterol clefts)	No
Inflammatory cells	Diffuse; lymphocytes and plasma cells predominate; occasional eosinophils; polymorphs in acute phase	Focal; lymphocytes predominate around granulomas	Similar to sarcoid	Focal; lymphocytes predominate around granulomas	Focal; predominantly lymphocytes and plasma cells	Patchy; variable intensity; lymphocytes and plasma cells
Bronchiolitis	Common (50%)	Rare to absent	Rare to absent	Variable	With aspiration, yes; other types, no	Rare
Fibrosis	Late stages only	Nodular	Nodular	Nodular	Nodular	Invariably present; may be predominant feature; patchy
Alveolitis, organizing pneumonia	Yes (65%), acute phase	No	No	Occasional	Occasional	Variable
Special studies	History of exposure; precipitating antibodies to suspected agent	Positive Kveim-Sutzback skin test; hypercalciuria, hypergamma-globulinaemia, increased ACE	History of exposure; positive skin test; microanalysis of lung tissue	Culture, special stains, PCR, etc.	Polarizing microscopy; in situ microanalysis.	May be associated with connective tissue disorder

mann bodies (Fig. 12.19). These nonspecific findings have no diagnostic or causative significance. Occasionally, as in maple bark disease, the causative agent can be identified in the granulomas (210). Demonstration of the antigen in the tissues by immunocytochemistry may also be usefu1 (189).

The frequency with which granulomas or individual giant cells are seen in EAA is uncertain: in the largest reported series (206) they were present in 75% of cases. Thus there clearly are cases that appear to be EAA on clinical grounds and in which a mild bronchiolocentric interstitial infiltrate is seen, but in which granulomas or giant cells cannot be found. In these circumstances care should be taken in rendering a diagnosis. The opposite setting, in which numerous well-defined granulomas predominate but little or no interstitial infiltrate is present, should raise the question of sarcoidosis (203) (Table 12.7).

In most biopsies, true interstitial fibrosis is not a feature of EAA; if fibrosis is present, at least in theory the disease falls into the chronic form (203). In practice some cases of chronic EAA show all the typical features of the subacute forms just described with the addition of minor degrees of fibrosis. In other cases the fibrosing process is quite dramatic, with marked diffuse interstitial scarring and none of the features of subacute EAA (203, 211) (Fig. 12.21). Such cases are easily confused with usual interstitial pneumonia (UIP), particularly if they show only nonspecific honeycombing (211); however, the fibrosis of severe chronic EAA is usually much more homogeneous than that of UIP, and Schaumann bodies, the calcified residua of granulomas, and giant cells or granulomas may be present (Fig. 12.21). Schaumann bodies and granulomas are extremely helpful, since they are not part of UIP and so limit the differential diagnosis to sarcoidosis, berylliosis, and EAA. The zonal distribution of fibrosis may also be useful:

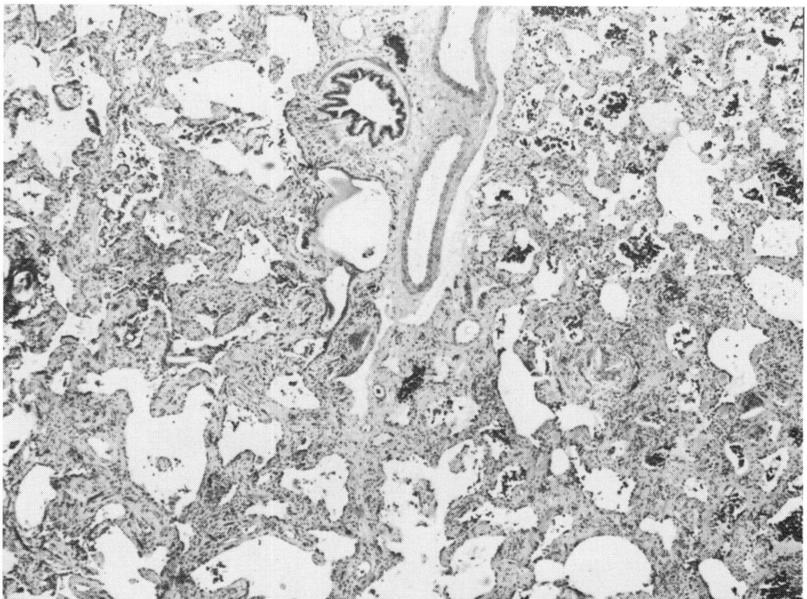

FIGURE 12.21
Chronic form of extrinsic allergic alveolitis in a pigeon fancier. Low-power view (A) showing homogeneous pattern of interstitial fibrosis and higher-power views showing (B) giant cells and poorly formed granulomas and (C) a Schaumann body. (A, ×40; B and C, ×400.)

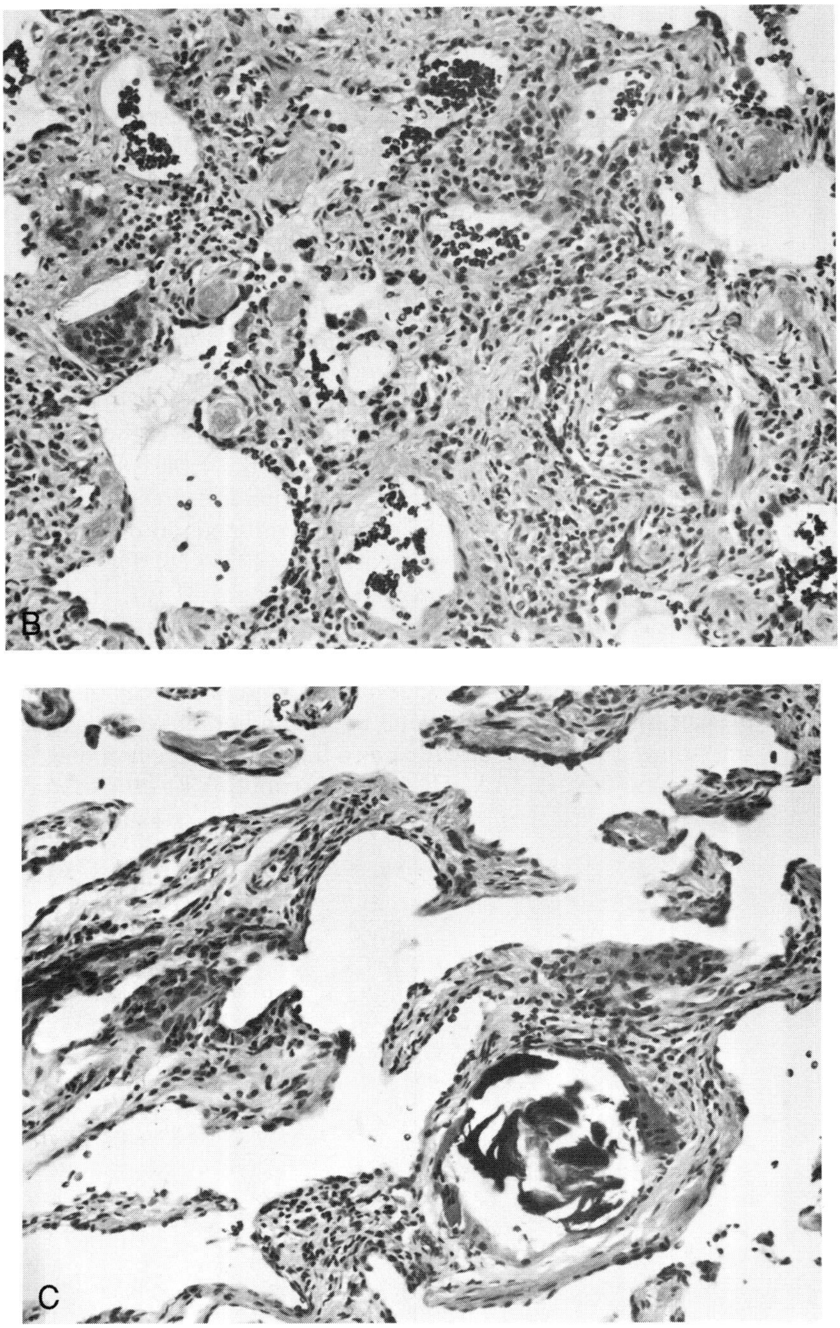

FIGURE 12.21 *(continued)*

while many cases of EAA show a lower zonal predominance, some are upper zonal (208), a finding that is strongly against a diagnosis of UIP. This distinction is important because in our experience and that of others (203), EAA patients whose biopsies appear quite fibrotic may show remarkable degrees of functional improvement with steroids, whereas steroids generally are ineffective in UIP.

The range of causative agents of EAA is extremely broad (Table 12.6), but the pathologic features appear to be the same whatever the offending antigen. Thus reference to the clinical history is important in rendering a specific causative diagnosis such as farmers' lung or pigeon breeders' lung, particularly when specific diagnostic features such as granulomas are lacking. In some cases the classic features of EAA are discovered on biopsy but no causative agent can be found by history; in this circumstance a diagnosis of EAA is still appropriate, and such patients appear to respond well to steroids (190).

BAL can also be helpful in suggesting EAA. The typical findings are a severalfold increase in total cells, with a relative increase in lymphocytes to 50 or 60% of total cells and with a decreased T4–T8 ratio (203). Neutrophils are increased in the acute stage of the disease (194), and mast cells, plasma cells, and eosinophils are increased in the subacute forms (212, 213).

REFERENCES

1. Fishwick D, Pickering CA. Byssinosis: a form of occupational asthma? Thorax 1992;47:401–403.
2. Bernstein DI. Clinical assessment and management of occupational asthma. In: Bernstein IL, Chan-Yeung M, Malo JL, Bernstein DI, eds. Asthma in the workplace. New York: Marcel Dekker, 1993:103–124.
3. Brooks SM, Bernstein IL. Reactive airways dysfunction syndrome or irritant-induced asthma. In: Bernstein IL, Chan-Yeung M, Malo JL et al., eds. Asthma in the workplace. New York: Marcel Dekker, 1993:533–549.
4. Karol MH, Tollerud DJ, Campbell TP, et al. Predictive value of airways hyperresponsiveness and circulating IgE for identifying types of responses to toluene diisocyanate inhalation challenge. Am J Respir Crit Care Med 1994;149:611–615.
5. Chan-Yeung M, Malo JL. Natural history of occupational asthma. In: Bernstein IL, Chan-Yeung M, Malo JL, Bernstein DI, eds. Asthma in the workplace. New York: Marcel Dekker, 1993:299–322.
6. Butcher BT, Karr RM, O'Neill CE, et al. Inhalation challenge and pharmacologic studies of TDI sensitive workers. J Allergy Clin Immunol 1979;64:146–152.
7. Mapp CE, Corono PC, De Marzo N, Fabbri L. Persistent asthma due to isocyanates: a follow-up study of subjects with occupational asthma due to toluene diisocyanate (TDI). Am Rev Respir Dis 1988;137:1326–1329.
8. Malo JL, Cartier A, Côté J, et al. Influence of inhaled steroids on recovery from occupational asthma after cessation of exposure: an 18-month double-blind crossover study. Am J Respir Crit Care Med 1996;153:953–960.
9. Axon EJ, Beach JR, Burge PS. A comparison of some of the characteristics of patients with occupational and nonoccupational asthma. J Occup Med 1995;45: 109–111.
10. Seta JA, Young RO, Bernstein IL, Bernstein DI. Compendium 3: The United States National Exposure Survey data base. In: Bernstein IL, Chan-Yeung M, Malo JL, Bernstein DI, eds. Asthma in the workplace. New York: Marcel Dekker, 1993: 627–624.
11. U.S. Department of Health and Human Services. Work-related lung disease surveillance report 1994. National Institute for Occupational Safety and Health publication 94–120, 1994:135.
12. Gannon PFG, Burge PS. The SHIELD scheme in the West Midlands Region, United Kingdom. Br J Ind Med 1993;50:791–796.
13. Meredith SK, Taylor VM, McDonald JC. Occupational respiratory disease in the United Kingdom: a report to the British Thoracic Society and Society of Occupational Medicine by the SWORD project group. Br J Ind Med 1991;48:292–298.

14. Malo JL. Compensation for occupational asthma in Québec. Chest 1990;98(Suppl 5):236S– 239S.
15. Blanc P. Occupational asthma in a national disability survey. Chest 1987;92: 613–617.
16. Becklake MR. Epidemiology: prevalence and determinants. In: Bernstein IL, Chan-Yeung M, Malo JL, Bernstein DI, eds. Asthma in the workplace. New York: Marcel Dekker, 1993:29–60.
17. Hoffman RE, Wood RC, Kreiss K. Building-related asthma in Denver office workers. Am J Public Health 1993;81:89–93.
18. Chan-Yeung M, Malo JL. Compendium 1: Table of the major inducers of occupational asthma. In: Berstein IL, Chan-Yeung M, Malo JL, Bernstein DI, eds. Asthma in the workplace. New York: Marcel Dekker., 1993:595–623.
19. Burge PS. New developments in occupational asthma. Br Med Bull 1992;48: 221–230.
20. Gerrard JW, Heiner DC, Ko CG, et al. Immunoglobulin levels in smokers and non-smokers. Ann Allergy 1980;44:261–262.
21. Burrows B, Halonen M, Barbee RA, Lebowitz MD. The relationship of serum immunoglobulin E to cigarette smoking. Am Rev Respir Dis 1981;124:523–529.
22. Wittig HJ, McLaughlin ET, Leifer KL, Belloit JD. Risk factors in the development of allergic disease: analysis of 2,190 patient records. Ann Allergy 1979;41:84–88.
23. Chan-Yeung M, Lam S. Occupational asthma. Am Rev Respir Dis 1986;133:686.
24. Pirson F, Charpin D, Sansonetti M, et al. Is intrinsic asthma a hereditary disease? Allergy 1991;46:367–371.
25. Sandford A, Weir T, Paré P. The genetics of asthma. Am J Respir Crit Care Med 1996;153:1749–1765.
26. Konig P, Godfrey S. Exercise-induced bronchial lability in monozygotic and dizygotic twins. J Allergy Clin Immunol 1974;54:280.
27. Townley RG, Guirgis H, Bewtra A, et al. IgE levels and methacholine inhalation responses in monozygous and dizygous twins. J Allergy Clin Immunol 1976;57:227.
28. Bignon JS, Aron Y, Ju LY, et al. HLA class II alleles in isocyanate-induced asthma. Am J Respir Crit Care Med 1994;149:71–75.
29. Mapp CE. Occupational asthma: interactions between genetic factors and adverse environment? Med Lav 1994;85:187–192.
30. Bai TR. Abnormalities in airway smooth muscle in fatal asthma. Am Rev Respir Dis 1990;141:552–557.
31. Whicker SD, Armour CL, Black JL. Responsiveness of bronchial smooth muscle from asthmatic patients to relaxant and contractile agonists. Pulm Pharmacol 1988; 1:25–31.
32. Reihsaus E, Innis M, MacIntyre N, Liggett SB. Mutations in the gene encoding for the b_2- adrenergic receptor in normal and asthmatic subjects. Am J Respir Cell Mol Biol 1993;8:334–339.
33. Turki J, Pak J, Green SA, et al. Genetic polymorphisms of the β_2-adrenergic receptor in nocturnal and nonnocturnal asthma. J Clin Invest 1995;95:1635–1641.
34. Halayko AJ, Stephens NL. Potential role for phenotypic modulation of bronchial smooth muscle cells in chronic asthma. Can J Physiol Pharmacol 1994;72:1448-1457.
35. Nicholson KG, Kent J, Ireland DC. Respiratory viruses and exacerbations of asthma in adults. BMJ 1993;307:982–986.
36. Johnston SL, Pattemore PK, Sanderson G, et al. Community study of role of viral infections in exacerbations of asthma in 9–11 year-old children. BMJ 1993;310: 1225–1228.
37. Busse W, Castleman W. Infections. Respir Crit Care Med 1995;151:S20–S21.
38. Hegele FG, Hayashi S, Bramley AM, Hogg JC. Persistence of respiratory syncytial virus genome and protein after acute bronchiolitis in guinea pigs. Chest 1994;105: 1848–1854.
39. Li JTC, O'Connell EJ. Viral infections and asthma. Ann Allergy 1987;59:321–331.

40. Gosset P, Tillie-Leblond I, Janin A, et al. Expression of E-selectin, ICAM-1 and VCAM-1 on bronchial biopsies from allergic and nonallergic asthmatic patients. Int Arch Allergy Immunol 1995;106:69–77.
41. Schleimer RP, Benenati SV, Friedman B, Bochner BS. Do cytokines play a role in leukocyte recruitment and activation in the lungs? Am Rev Respir Dis 1991;143: 1169–1176.
42. Goldstein RA, Paul WE, Metcalfe DD, et al. Asthma: NIH Conference. Ann Intern Med 1994;121:698–708.
43. Beasley R, Roche WR, Roberts JA, et al. Cellular events in the bronchi in mild asthma and after bronchial provocation. Am Rev Respir Dis 1990;139:806–817.
44. Laitinen A, Laitinen LA. Airway morphology: epithelium/basement membrane. Am J Respir Crit Care Med 1994;150:S14-S17.
45. Ferguson AC, Whitelaw M, Brown H, et al. Correlation of bronchial eosinophil and mast cell activation with bronchial hyperresponsiveness in children with asthma. J Allergy Clin Immunol 1992;90:609–613.
46. Kroegel C, Virchow JC Jr, Luttmann W, et al. Pulmonary immune cells in health and disease: the eosinophil leucocyte (part 1). Eur Respir J 1994;7:519–543.
47. Kay AB, Corrigan CJ. Eosinophils and neutrophils. Br Med Bull 1991;48:51–64.
48. Bentley AM, Maestrelli P, Saetta M, et al. Activated T-lymphocytes and eosinophils in the bronchial mucosa in isocyanate-induced asthma. J Allergy Clin Immunol 1992;89:821–828.
49. Bentley AM, Menz G, Storz CHR, et al. Identification of T lymphocytes, macrophages and activated eosinophils in the bronchial mucosa in intrinsic asthma. Am Rev Respir Dis 1992;146:500–506.
50. Azzawi M, Johnston PW, Majamdar S, et al. T lymphocytes and activated eosinophils in airway mucosa in fatal asthma and cystic fibrosis. Am Rev Respir Dis 1992;145:1477–1482.
51. Synek M, Beasley R, Frew AJ, et al. Cellular infiltration of the airways in asthma of varying severity. Am J Respir Crit Care Med 1996;154:224–230.
52. Zhang S, Mohammed Q, Burbidge A, et al. Cell cultures from bronchial subepithelial myofibroblasts enhance eosinophil survival in vitro. Eur Respir J 1996;9: 1839–1846.
53. Lai CKW, Holgate ST. The mast cell in asthma. In: Kay AB, ed. Clinical immunology and allergy: the allergic basis of asthma. London: Balliere Tindall, 1988:37–65.
54. Panettieri RA, Yadvish PA, Kelly AM, et al. Histamine stimulates proliferation of airway smooth muscle and induces c-fos expression. Am J Physiol 1990;259: 365–371.
55. Poulter LW, Janossy G, Power C, et al. Immunological/physiological relationships in asthma: potential regulation by lung macrophages. Immunol Today 1994;15: 258–261.
56. Szczeklik A, Nizankowska E, Serafin A, et al. Autoimmune phenomena in bronchial asthma with special reference to aspirin intolerance. Am J Respir Crit Care Med 1995;152:1753–1756.
57. Corrigan CJ, Kay AB. Role of T-lymphocytes and lymphokines. Br Med Bull 1992; 48:72–84.
58. Bradley LM, Yoshimoto K, Swain SL. IFN-g and IL-12 regulate the subsets of memory effector/helper T cells in vitro. J Immunol 1995;155:1713–1724.
59. Robinson DS, Hamid Q, Bentley A, et al. Activation of CD4+ T cells increased Th2-type cytokine mRNA expression and eosinophil recruitment in bronchoalveolar lavage after allergen inhalation challenge in patients with atopic asthma. J Allergy Clin Immunol 1993;92:313–324.
60. Walker C, Bode E, Boer LL, et al. Allergic and nonallergic asthmatics have distinct patterns of T-cell activation and cytokine production in peripheral blood and bronchoalveolar lavage. Am Rev Respir Dis 1992;146:109–115.
61. Del Prete G, De Carli M, Almerigogna F, et al. Human IL-10 is produced by both

type 1 helper (TH1) and type 2 helper (Th2) T cell clones and inhibits their antigen-specific proliferation and cytokine production. J Immunol 1993;150:353–360.

62. Fabbri LM, Boschetto P, Zocca E, et al. Bronchoalveolar neutrophilia during late asthmatic reactions induced by toluene diisocyanate. Am Rev Respir Dis 1987;136: 36–42.
63. Mapp CE, Saetta M, Maestrelli P, et al. Mechanisms and pathology of occupational asthma. Eur Respir J 1994;7:544–554.
64. Redington A, Howarth PH. Airway wall remodeling in asthma. Thorax 1997;52: 310–312.
65. Yanai M, Sekizawa K, Ohrui T, et al. Site of airway obstruction in pulmonary disease: direct measurements of intrabronchial pressure. J Appl Physiol 1992;72: 1016–1023.
66. Wiggs BR, Bosken C, Paré PD, Hogg JC. A model of airway narrowing in asthma and in chronic obstructive pulmonary disease. Am Rev Respir Dis 1992;145: 1251–1258.
67. Kuwano K, Bosken CH, Paré PD, et al. Small airways dimensions in asthma and in chronic obstructive pulmonary disease. Am Rev Respir Dis 1993;148:1220–1225.
68. Tough S, Green FH, James E, et al. Sudden death from asthma in 108 children and young adults. J Asthma 1996;33:179–188.
69. Cluroe A, Holloway L, Thomson K, et al. Bronchial gland duct ectasia in fatal bronchial asthma: association with interstitial emphysema. J Clin Pathol 1989;42: 1026–1031.
70. Laitinen LA, Heino M, Laitinen AR, et al. Damage of the airway epithelium and bronchial reactivity in patients with asthma. Am Rev Respir Dis 1985;131: 599–606.
71. Gleich GJ, Motojima S, Frigas E, et al. The eosinophilic leukocyte and the pathology of fatal bronchial asthma: evidence for pathologic heterogeneity. J Allergy Clin Immunol 1987;80:412–415.
72. Filley WV, Holley KE, Kephart GM, et al. Identification by immunofluorescence of eosinophil granule major basic protein in lung tissues of patients with bronchial asthma. Lancet 1982;2:11–16.
73. Frigas SE, Leogering DA, Gleich GJ, et al. Cytotoxic effects of the guinea pig major basic protein on tracheal epithelium. J Lab Invest 1980;42:35–43.
74. Dunnill MS. The pathology of asthma, with special reference to changes in the bronchial mucosa. J Clin Pathol 1960;13:27–33.
75. Demoly P, Basset-Seguin N, Chanez P, et al. Rapid communication: c-fos proto-oncogene expression in bronchial biopsies of asthmatics. Am J Respir Cell Mol Biol 1992;7:128–133.
76. Laitinen LA, Laitinen A, Haahtela T. Airway mucosal inflammation even in patients with newly diagnosed asthma. Am Rev Respir Dis 1993;147:697–704.
77. Jeffery PK, Godfrey RW, Adelroth E, et al. Effects of treatment on airway inflammation and thickening of basement membrane reticular collagen in asthma: a quantitative light and electron microscopic study. Am Rev Respir Dis 1992;145: 890–899.
78. Dunnill MS, Massarella GR, Anderson JA, et al. A comparison of the quantitative anatomy of the bronchi in normal subjects, in status asthmaticus, in chronic bronchitis and in emphysema. Thorax 1969;24:176.
79. Aikawa T, Shimura S, Sasaki H, et al. Marked goblet cell hyperplasia with mucus accumulation in the airways of patients who died of severe acute asthma attack. Chest 1992;101:916–921.
80. Takizawa T, Thurlbeck WM. Muscle and mucous gland size in the major bronchi of patients with chronic bronchitis, asthma and asthmatic bronchitis. Am Rev Respir Dis 1971;104:331–336.
81. Glynn AA, Michaels L. Bronchial biopsy in chronic bronchitis and asthma. Thorax 1960;15:142–153.
82. Jeffery PK. Comparative morphology of the airways in asthma and chronic obstructive pulmonary disease. Am J Respir Crit Care Med 1994;150:S6–S13.

83. Sanerkin NG, Evans DMD. The sputum in bronchial asthma: pathopneumonic patterns. J Pathol 1965;89:535–541.
84. Rubin BK. Therapeutic aerosols and airway secretions. J Aerosol Med 1996;9: 123–130.
85. Allegra L, Abraham WM, Chapman GA, Wanner A. Duration of mucociliary dysfunction following antigen challenge. J Appl Physiol 1983;55:726–730.
86. Pavia D, Bateman JRM, Sheahan NF, et al. Tracheobronchial mucociliary clearance in asthma: impairment during remission. Thorax 1985;40:171–175.
87. List SJ, Findlay BP, Forstner GG, Forstner JF. Enhancement of the viscosity of mucin by serum albumin. Biochem J 1978;175:565–571.
88. Jeffery PK. Histological features of the airways in asthma and COPD. Respiration 1992;59(Suppl 1):13–16.
89. Sobonya RE. Quantitative structural alterations in long-standing allergic asthma. Am Rev Respir Dis 1984;130:289–292.
90. Roche WR, Beasley R, Williams JH, et al. Subepithelial fibrosis in the bronchi of asthmatics. Lancet 1989;1:520–524.
91. Green FHY, Perry S, Karkhanis A, et al. The role of smoking and asthma in airway wall remodeling. Am J Respir Crit Care Med 1997;155:A896.
92. Brewster CE, Howarth PH, Djukanovic R, et al. Myofibroblasts and subepithelial fibrosis in bronchial asthma. Am J Respir Cell Mol Biol 1990;3:507–511.
93. Wetzels RHY, Robben HCM, Leigh AM, et al. Distribution patterns of type VII collagen in normal and malignant tissues. Am J Pathol 1991;139:451–459.
94. Timple R. Structure and biological activity of basement membrane proteins. Eur J Biochem 1989;180:487–502.
95. Paulsson M. Basement membrane proteins: structure, assembly and cellular interactions. Crit Rev Biochem Mol Biol 1992;27:93–127.
96. Evans MJ, Guha SC, Cox RA, et al. Attenuated fibroblast sheath around the basement membrane zone in asthma. Am J Respir Cell Mol Biol 1993;8:188–192.
97. Djukanovíc R, Wilson JW, Britten KM, et al. Effect of an inhaled corticosteroid on airway inflammation and symptoms in asthma. Am Rev Respir Dis 1992;145: 669–674.
98. Saetta M, Di Stefano A, Maestrelli P, et al. Airway mucosal inflammation in occupational asthma induced by toluene diisocyanate. Am Rev Respir Dis 1992;145: 160–168.
99. Carrol N, Green F, James A. Longitudinal elastic bundles in fatal and nonfatal asthma. Am J Resp Crit Care Med 1996;153:A867.
100. Monkhouse WS, Whimster WF. An account of the longitudinal mucosal corrugations of the human tracheo-bronchial tress, with observations on those of some animals. J Anat 1976;122:681–695.
101. Perry SF, Harji S, Karkhanis A, Green FHY. Do asthmatic lungs have more smooth muscle than normal lungs? Respir Crit Care Med 1994;149:A583.
102. Carroll N, Elliott A, Morton A, et al. The structure of large and small airways in nonfatal and fatal asthma. J Am Rev Respir Dis 1993;147:405–410.
103. Saetta M, Di Stefano A, Rosina C, et al. Quantitative structural analysis of peripheral airways and arteries in sudden fatal asthma. Am Rev Respir Dis 1991;143: 138–143.
104. Hossain S. Quantitative measurement of bronchial muscle in men with asthma. Am Rev Respir Dis 1973;107:99–109.
105. Ebina M, Takakashi T, Chiba T, et al. Cellular hypertrophy and hyperplasia of airway smooth muscles underlying bronchial asthma. Am Rev Respir Dis 1993;148: 720–726.
106. Heard BE, Hossain S. Hyperplasia of bronchial muscle in asthma. J Pathol 1973; 110:319–331.
107. Ebina M, Yaegashi H, Chiba R, et al. Hyperreactive site in the airway tree of asthmatic patients revealed by thickening of bronchial muscles. Am Rev Respir Dis 1990;141: 1327–1332.

108. James AL, Paré PD, Hoss JC. The mechanics of airway narrowing in asthma. Am Rev Respir Dis 1989;139:242–246.
109. Green FHY, Carroll N, James A, et al. The bronchial arteries in asthma. Am J Resp Crit Care Med 1996;153:A818.
110. Azzawi M, Bradley B, Jeffery PK, et al. Identification of activated T lymphocytes and eosinophils in bronchial biopsies in stable atopic asthma. Am Rev Respir Dis 1990;142:1407–1413.
111. Hamid Q, Song Y, Kotsimbos TC, et al. Small airways inflammation in asthma. J Allergy Clin Immunol (in press).
112. Bousquet J, Chanez P, Lacoste JY, et al. Eosinophilic inflammation in asthma. N Engl J Med 1990;323:1033–1039.
113. Djukanovíc R, Roche WR, Wilson JW, . Mucosal inflammation in asthma. Am Rev Respir Dis 1990;142:434–457.
114. Djukanovíc R, Wilson JW, Britten KM, et al. Quantitation of mast cells and eosinophils in the bronchial mucosa of symptomatic atopic asthmatics and healthy control subjects using immunohistochemistry. Am Rev Respir Dis 1990a;142: 863–871.
115. Sur S, Crotty TB, Kephart GM, et al. Sudden-onset fatal asthma: a distinct entity with few eosinophils and relatively more neutrophils in the airway submucosa? Am Rev Respir Dis 1993;148:713–719.
116. Wallaert B, Janin A, Lassalle P, et al. Airway-like inflammation of minor salivary gland in bronchial asthma. Am J Respir Crit Care Med 1994;150:802–809.
117. Lundgren R, Söderberg M, Hörstedt P, Stenling R. Morphological studies of bronchial mucosal biopsies from asthmatics before and after ten years of treatment with inhaled steroids. Eur Respir J 1977;1:883–889.
118. James AL, Hogg JC, Dunn LA, et al. The use of the internal perimeter to compare airway size and to calculate smooth muscle shortening. Am Rev Respir Dis 1988; 138:136–139.
119. Fabbri LM, Danieli D, Crescioli S, et al. Fatal asthma in a subject sensitized to toluene diisocyanate. Am Rev Respir Dis 1988;137:1494–1498.
120. Huber AL, Loving TJ. Fatal asthma attack after inhaling sulfur fumes. JAMA 1991; 266:2225.
121. Reid LM. The presence or absence of bronchial mucus in fatal asthma. J Allergy Clin Immunol 1987;1980(Suppl):415–416.
122. Di Stefano A, Saetta M, Maestrelli P, et al. Mast cells in the airway mucosa and rapid development of occupational asthma induced by toluene diisocyanate. Am Rev Respir Dis 1993;147:1005–1009.
123. Frew AJ, Chan H, Lam S, Chan-Yeung M. Bronchial inflammation in occupational asthma due to Western red cedar. Am J Respir Crit Care Med 1995;151:340–344.
124. Fabbri LM, Seatta M, Maestrelli P, Mapp C. Airway inflammation in isocyanate-induced asthma. In: Chretien J, Dusser D, eds. Lung biology in health and disease: environmental impact on the airways: from injury to repair, vol 93. New York: Marcel Dekker, 1987:287–297.
125. Zocca E, Fabbri LM, Boschetto P, et al. Leukotriene B4 and late asthmatic reactions induced by toluene diisocyanate. J Appl Physiol 1990;68:1576–1580.
126. Paggiaro P, Bacci E, Paoletti P, et al. BAL and morphology of the airways after cessation of experiments in asthma subjects sensitized to toluene diisocyanate. Chest 1990;98:536–542.
127. Brooks SM, Weiss MA, Bernstein IL. Reactive airways dysfunction syndrome (RADS): persistent asthma syndrome after high level irritant exposures. Chest 1985;88:376–384.
128. Glindmeyer H, Lefante J, Freyder L, et al. Relative rate of new onset asthma among workers exposed to irritant chemicals. Am J Respir Crit Care Med 1997;155:A258.
129. Gandevia B. Occupational asthma. Med J Aust 1970;2:332–335.
130. Chan-Yeung M, Lam S, Kennedy SM, Frew AJ. Persistent asthma after repeated ex-

posure to high concentrations of gases in pulp mills. Am J Respir Crit Care Med 1994;149:1676–1680.
131. Gautrin D, Boulet LP, Boutet M, et al. Is reactive airways dysfunction syndrome a variant of occupational asthma? J Allergy Clin Immunol 1994;93:12–22.
132. Alford PT, McLees BD, Case LD, et al. Reactive airways dysfunction syndrome (RADS) in workers post exposure to sulfur dioxide (SO_2). Chest 1988;94:87S.
133. Bernstein IL, Bernstein DI. Reactive airways disease syndrome (RADS) after exposure to toxic ammonia fumes. J Allergy Clin Immunol 1989;83:173.
134. Donnelly SC, Fitzgerald MX. Reactive airways dysfunction syndrome (RADS) due to chlorine gas exposure. Ir J Med Sci 1990;159:275–277.
135. Deschamps D, Rosenberg N, Soler P, et al. Persistent asthma after accidental exposure to ethylene oxide. Br J Ind Med 1992;49:523–525.
136. Tarlo SM, Broker I. Irritant-induced occupational asthma. Chest 1989;96: 297–300.
137. Taylor RF, Bernard GR. Airway complications from free-basing cocaine. Chest 1989;95:476– 477.
138. Demeter SL, Cordasco EM. Reactive airways dysfunction syndrome: a subset of occupational asthma. J Disability 1990;1:23–39.
139. Palczynski C, Gorski P, Jakubowski J. The case of TDI-induced reactive airway dysfunction syndrome with the presence of specific IgE antibodies. Allergol Immunopathol 1994;22: 80–82.
140. Cone JE, Wugofski L, Balmes JR, et al. Persistent respiratory health effects after a metam sodium pesticide spill. Chest 1994;106:500–508.
141. Boulet LP. Increases in airway responsiveness following acute exposure to respiratory irritants. Chest 1988;94:476–481.
142. Deschamps D, Soler P, Rosenberg N, et al. Persistent asthma after inhalation of a mixture of sodium hypochlorite and hydrochloric acid. Chest 1994;105: 1895–1896.
143. Kern DG. Outbreak of the reactive airways dysfunction syndrome after a spill of glacial acetic acid. Am Rev Respir Dis 1991;144:1058–1064.
144. Angelillo VA. Reactive airways dysfunction syndrome (RADS): a report of three cases. Respir Care 1992;37:254–257.
145. Hu H, Christiani D. Reactive airways dysfunction after exposure to teargas. Lancet 1992;339:1535 (letter).
146. Stenton SC, Kelly CA, Walters EH, et al. Induction of bronchial hyperresponsiveness following smoke inhalation injury. Br J Dis Chest 1988;82:436–438.
147. Alberts AM, do Pico GA. Reactive airways dysfunction syndrome. Chest 1996;109: 1618–1626.
148. Harkonen H, Nordman H, Korhonen O, et al. Long-term effects of exposure to sulfur dioxide. Am Rev Respir Dis 1983;128:890–893.
149. Promisloff RA, Phan A, Lenchner GS, et al. Reactive airway dysfunction syndrome in three police officers following a roadside chemical spill. Chest 1990;98:928–929.
150. Alberts WM, Brooks SM. Occupational asthma: serious consequences for workers and employers. Postgrad Med 1995;97:93–98.
151. Charan NB, Myers CG, Lakshminarayan S, Spencer TM. Pulmonary injuries associated with acute sulfur dioxide inhalation. Am Rev Respir Dis 1979;119:555–560.
152. Green FHY. Health problems associated with inhalation of toxic gases. In: Prior MG, Roth SH, Green FHY, et al., eds. Proceedings International Conference on Hydrogen Sulfide Toxicity, Alberta: University of Alberta Press, 1990:157–170.
153. Merchant JA, Bernstein IL. Cotton and other textile dusts. In: Bernstein IL, Chan-Yeung M, Jalo JL, Bernstein DI, eds. Asthma in the workplace. New York: Marcel Dekker, 1993:551–576.
154. Merchant JA, Lumsden JC, Kilburn KH, et al. Dose response studies in cotton textile workers. J Occup Med 1973;15:222–230.
155. Castellan RM. Cotton dust. In: Schenker M, Balmes J, eds. Occupational and environmental respiratory disease. St. Louis: Mosby, 1996:401–419.

156. Molyneux MKB, Tombleson JBL. An epidemiological study of respiratory symptoms in Lancashire mills, 1963–1966. Br J Ind Med 1970;27:225–234.
157. Fox AJ, Tombleson BJL, Watt A, et al. A survey of respiratory disease in cotton operatives: 2. Symptoms, dust estimations and the effect of smoking habit. Br J Ind Med 1973;30:48–53.
158. Merchant JA, Lumsden JC, Kilburn KH, et al. An industrial study of the biological effects of cotton dust and cigarette smoke exposure. J Occup Med 1973;15: 212–221.
159. Beck GJ, Schachter EN. The evidence for chronic lung disease in cotton textile workers. Am Statistician 1983;37:404–412.
160. Merchant JA. Byssinosis. In: Merchant JA, Boehlecke BA, Pickett-Harner M, eds. Occupational respiratory diseases. National Institute for Occupational Safety and Health Pub 86–102. Washington: U.S. Government Printing Office, 1986:533–568.
161. Merchant JA, Lumsden JC, Kilburn KH, et al. Pre-processing cotton to prevent byssinosis. Br J Ind Med 1973b;30:237–247.
162. Kennedy SM, Christiani DC, Eisen EA, et al. Cotton dust and endotoxin exposure-response relationships in cotton textile workers. Am Rev Respir Dis 1987;135: 194–200.
163. Milton DK, Godleski JJ, Feldman HA, Greaves IA. Toxicity of intratracheally instilled cotton dust, cellulose and endotoxin. Am Rev Respir Dis 1990;142:184–192.
164. Castellan RM, Olenchock SA, Kinsley KB, Hankinson JL. Inhaled endotoxin and decreased spirometric values: an exposure-response relation for cotton dust. N Engl J Med 1987;317:605–610.
165. Holt PG. Current trends in research on the etiology and pathogenesis of byssinosis. Am J Ind Med 1987;12:711–716.
166. Milton DK, Chawla RK. Cotton dust contains proteases and elastases not inhibited by alpha-1-protease inhibitor. Am J Ind Med 1986;9:247–260.
167. Edwards J. International conference on byssinosis: mechanisms of disease induction. Chest 1981;79(4 Suppl):38S–43S.
168. Chinn DJ, Cinkotai FF, Lockwood MG. Airborne dust: its protease content and byssinosis in willowing mills. Ann Occup Hyg 1976;19:101–108.
169. Rylander R. The role of endotoxin for reactions after exposure to cotton dust. Am J Ind Med 1987;12:687–697.
170. Rylander R. Role of endotoxins in the pathogenesis of respiratory disorders. Eur J Respir Dis Suppl 1987;154:136–144.
171. Rooke GB. The pathology of byssinosis. Chest 1981;79:675–715.
172. Pratt PC, Vollmer RT, Miller JA. Epidemiology of pulmonary lesions in nontextile and cotton textile workers: a retrospective autopsy analysis. Arch Environ Health 1980;35:133–138.
173. Edwards C, Macartney J, Rooke G, Ward F. The pathology of the lung in byssinotics. Thorax 1975;30:612–623.
174. Moran TJ. Emphysema and other chronic lung disease in textile workers: an 18-year autopsy study. Arch Environ Health 1983;38:267–277.
175. Rask-Andersen A. Allergic alveolitis in Swedish farmers. Ups J Med Sci 1989;94: 271–285.
176. Malmberg P, Rask-Andersen A, Rosenhall L. Exposure to microorganisms associated with allergic alveolitis and febrile reactions to mold dust in farmers. Chest 1993;103:1202–1209.
177. Donham KJ. Health effects from work in swine confinement buildings. Am J Ind Med 1990;17:17–25.
178. Crook B, Robertson JF, Glass SA, et al. Airborne dust, ammonia, microorganisms and antigens in pig confinement houses and the respiratory health of exposed farm workers. Am Ind Hyg Assoc J 1991;52:271–279.
179. Lacey J, Lacey ME. Spore concentrations in the air of farm buildings. Trans Br Mycol Soc 1964;47:547–552.

180. Norn S. Microorganism-induced or enhanced mediator release: a possible mechanism in organic dust-related diseases. Am J Ind Med 1994;25:91–95.
181. Richerson HB. Unifying concepts underlying the effects of organic dust exposures. Am J Ind Med 1990;17:139–142.
182. Abel G, Czop JK. Stimulation of human monocyte beta-glucan receptors by glucan particles induces production of TNF-alpha and IL-1 beta. Int J Immunopharmacol 1992;14:1363–1373.
183. Peetermans WE, Raats CJ, Langermans JA, Van Furth R. Mycobacterial heat-shock protein 65 induces proinflammatory cytokines but does not activate human mononuclear phagocytes. Scand J Immunol 1994;39:613–617.
184. Dinarello CA. The biological properties of interleukin-1. Eur Cytokine Netw 1994; 5:517–531.
185. Malmberg P. Health effects of organic dust exposure in dairy farmers. Am J Ind Med 1990;17:7–15.
186. Zhiping W, Malmberg P, Larsson BM, et al. Exposure to bacteria in swine-house dust and acute inflammatory reactions in humans. Am J Respir Crit Care Med 1996;154:1261–1266.
187. Clapp WD, Becker S, Quay J, et al. Grain dust-induced airflow obstruction and inflammation of the lower respiratory tract. Am J Respir Crit Care Med 1994;150: 611–617.
188. Emanuel DA, Wenzel FJ, Lawton BR. Pulmonary mycotoxicosis. Chest 1975;67: 293–297.
189. Fink JN, Banaszak EF, Baroriak JJ, et al. Interstitial lung disease due to contamination of forced air systems. Ann Intern Med 1976;84:406–413.
190. Coleman A, Colby TV. Histologic diagnosis of extrinsic allergic alveolitis. Am J Surg Pathol 1988;2:514–518.
191. Rose C, King TE. Controversies in hypersensitivity pneumonitis. Am Rev Respir Dis 1992;145:1–2.
192. Fournier E, Tonnel AB, Gosset PH, et al. Early neutrophil alveolitis after antigen inhalation in hypersensitivity pneumonitis. Chest 1985;88:563–566.
193. Godard P, Clot J, Jonquet O, et al. Lymphocyte subpopulations in bronchoalveolar lavages of patients with sarcoidosis and hypersensitivity pneumonitis. Chest 1981; 80:447–452.
194. Cormier Y, Belanger J, Leblanc P, et al. Lymphocyte subpopulations in extrinsic allergic alveolitis. Ann N Y Acad Sci 1986;465:370–377.
195. Cormier Y, Belanger J. The fluctuant nature of precipitating antibodies in dairy farmers. Thorax 1989;44:469–473.
196. Sanderson W, Kullman G, Sastre J, et al. Outbreak of hypersensitivity pneumonitis among mushroom farm workers. Am J Ind Med 1992;22:859–872.
197. Cormier Y, Belanger J, Tardif A, et al. Relationships between radiographic change, pulmonary function and bronchoalveolar lavage fluid lymphocytes in farmer's lung disease. Thorax 1986;41:28–33.
198. Silver SF, Muller ML, Miller RR, Lefcoe MS. Hypersensitivity pneumonitis: evaluation with CT. Radiology 1989;173:441–445.
199. Perez-Padilla R, Salas J, Chapela R, et al. Mortality in Mexican patients with chronic pigeon breeder's lung compared with those with usual interstitial pneumonia. Am Rev Respir Dis 1993;148:49–53.
200. Cormier Y, Desmeules M. Treatment of hypersensitivity pneumonitis: contact avoidance vs. corticosteroid treatment. Can Respir J 1994;1:223–228.
201. Lalancette M, Carrier G, Laviolette M, et al. Farmer's lung: long-term outcome and lack of predictive value of bronchoalveolar lavage fibrosing factors. Am Rev Respir Dis 1993;148:216–221.
202. Kokkarinen JI, Tukiainen HO, Terho EO. Recovery of pulmonary function in farmer's lung. Am Rev Respir Dis 1993;147:793–796.
203. Colby TV, Carrington CB. Interstitial lung disease. In: Thurlbeck WM, Churg A, eds. Pathology of the lung. 2nd ed. New York: Thieme, 1995:650–657.

204. Barrowcliff DF, Arblaster PG. Farmer's lung: a study of an acute fatal case. Thorax 1968;23–490–500.
205. Liippo KK, Anttila SL, Tainkina-aho O, et al. Hypersensitivity pneumonitis and exposure to zirconium silicate in a young ceramic tile worker. Am Rev Respir Dis 1993;148:1089–1092.
206. Reyes CN, Wenzel FJ, Lawton BR, Emanuel DA. The pulmonary pathology of farmer's lung disease. Chest 1982;81:142–146.
207. Salvaggio JE, Karr RM. Hypersensitivity pneumonitis: state of the art. Chest 1979; 75:270–275.
208. Seal RME. Pathology of extrinsic allergic bronchiolo-alveolitis: alveolar interstitium of the Lung. Prog Resp Res 1974;8:66–73.
209. Sutinen S, Reijula K, Huhti E, Karkola P. Extrinsic allergic bronchiolo-alveolitis: serology and biopsy findings. Eur J Respir Dis 1983;64:271–282.
210. Emanuel DA, Wenzel FJ, Lawton BR. Pneumonitis due to Cryptostroma corticholi (maple bark disease). N Engl J Med 1966;274:1413.
211. Greenberg PA, Pien LC, Patterson R, et al. End-stage and ultimately fatal disease in a bird fancier. Am J Med 1989;86:119–122.
212. Drent M, Wagenaar S, van Velzen-Blad H, et al. Relationship between plasma cell levels and profile of bronchoalveolar lavage fluid in patients with subacute extrinsic allergic alveolitis. Thorax 1993;48:835–839.
213. Haslam PL, Dewar A, Butchers P, et al. Mast cells, atypical lymphocytes and neutrophils in bronchoalveolar lavage in extrinsic allergic alveolitis: comparison with other interstitial lung diseases. Am Rev Respir Dis 1987;135:35–47.

CHAPTER 13

Miscellaneous Conditions

❖ Andrew Churg
❖ Francis H. Y. Green

PULMONARY LESIONS ASSOCIATED WITH INTRAVENOUS DRUG ABUSE AND IATROGENIC CONDITIONS

Intravenous drug abusers develop a wide range of pulmonary lesions (1) (Table 13.1), the most common of which are infections, especially AIDS and abscesses. These reactions may be seen with intravenous abuse of any type of drug and are not considered further in this chapter. However, a number of the clinical and radiographic abnormalities listed in Table 13.1 and their corresponding pathologic changes listed in Table 13.2 appear to be caused by intravenous delivery of particulate matter to the lung, typically from abuse of drugs intended for oral use. Such lesions in one sense are a form of pneumoconiosis, often called intravenous talcosis or talc granulomatosis (2–5).

Many drugs intended for oral use contain fillers, which may be talc, microcrystalline cellulose, or cornstarch (Table 13.3). These insoluble particles evoke a variety of thrombotic and fibrotic lesions in the lung. The frequency of such reactions in drug abusers is uncertain; Paré et al. (2) and Tomashefski and Hirsch (6) point out that heroin is usually cut with a soluble filler such as lactose or maltose, which leaves no visible traces. Arnett et al. (7) claim that only about 1% of drug abusers inject drugs intended for oral consumption. Hopkins and Taylor (3) found granulomas in only 15 of 100 lungs from heroin addicts. Our own experience, however, is that refractile particles in and around small vessels are virtually universal findings in lungs from patients with histories of intravenous drug abuse. These particles may evoke no obvious reaction when present in small numbers, but they provide a valuable clue when a question of drug abuse arises.

Talc, microcrystalline cellulose, and cornstarch are all birefringent when viewed with polarized light, but starch can be identified by its round shape and Maltese cross pattern. Talc forms large irregular plates that are strongly birefringent (Figs.13.1–13.3) and are often a very pale yellow in hematoxylin and eosin–stained sections. If necessary the identity of the particles is easily confirmed by examination of digested tissue or properly prepared sections with energy-dispersive x-ray spectroscopy (8–10). Microcrystalline cellulose forms long

TABLE 13.1
Pulmonary Complications of Intravenous Drug Abuse

Infections (including AIDS)
Pneumonias
Abcesses
Mycotic aneurysms
Septic emboli
Adult respiratory distress syndrome
Pulmonary hypertension
Diffuse interstitial fibrosis
Complicated pneumoconiosis (progressive massive fibrosis) and similar lesions

TABLE 13.2
Pathologic Lesions Caused by Intravenous Injection of Drugs Intended for Oral Use

Vascular, perivascular, and interstitial foreign body granulomas
Angiothrombotic lesions
Diffuse interstitial fibrosis
Massive fibrosislike lesions (complicated pneumoconioses)
Emphysema

TABLE 13.3
Particulate Components of Various Drugs Intended for Oral Use and Commonly Injected Intravenously

PARTICLE	DRUGS
Talc	Methylphenidate HCl (Ritalin)
	Tripelennamine HCl (Pyribenzamine)
	Methadone
	Propoxyphene (Darvon)
	Meperidine (Demerol)
	Benzedrine
	Dilaudid
Microcrystalline cellulose	Pentazocine (Talwin)
	Methaqualone (Quaalude)
	Percodan
	Acetaminophen, aspirin with codeine
	Phenobarbital
Cornstarch	Barbiturates
	Paragoric
	Tripelennamine HCl (Pyribenzamine)
	Pentazocine (Talwin)

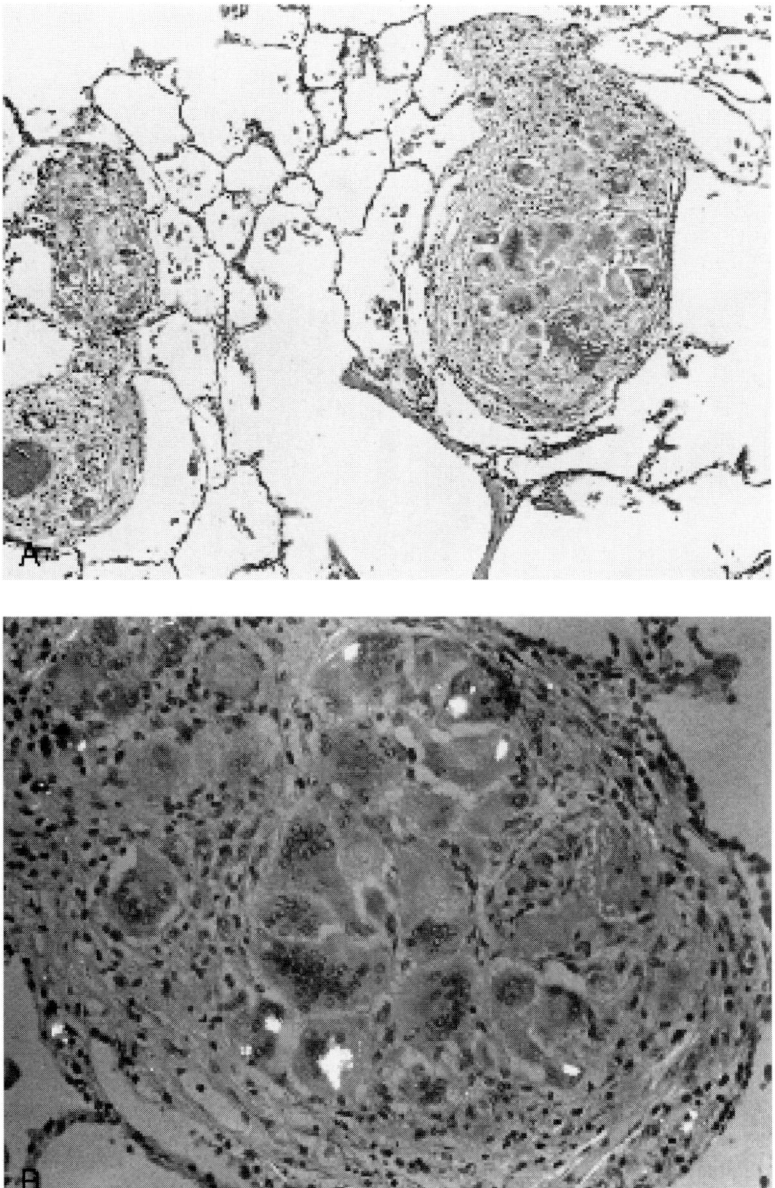

FIGURE 13.1

Foreign-body granulomas in intravenous drug abusers. Note the birefringent particles in **B**. (**A** ×645, **B** ×160; polarized light.)

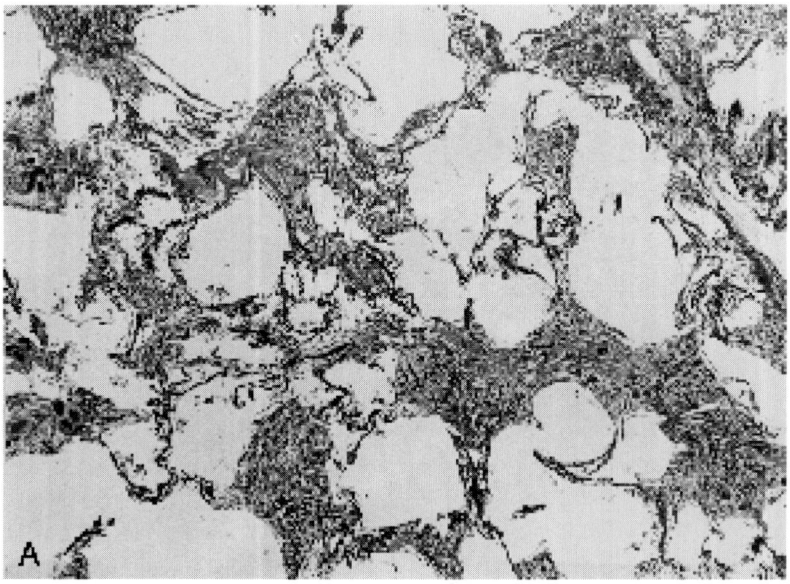

FIGURE 13.2
Interstitial fibrosis secondary to intravenous drug abuse. Note numerous giant cells (**B**) and birefringent foreign particles (**C**) in the fibrous tissue and the lack of particles and cells in the airspaces, which indicate intravenous particle delivery. (**A** ×25, **B** ×64, **C** ×160; polarized light.)

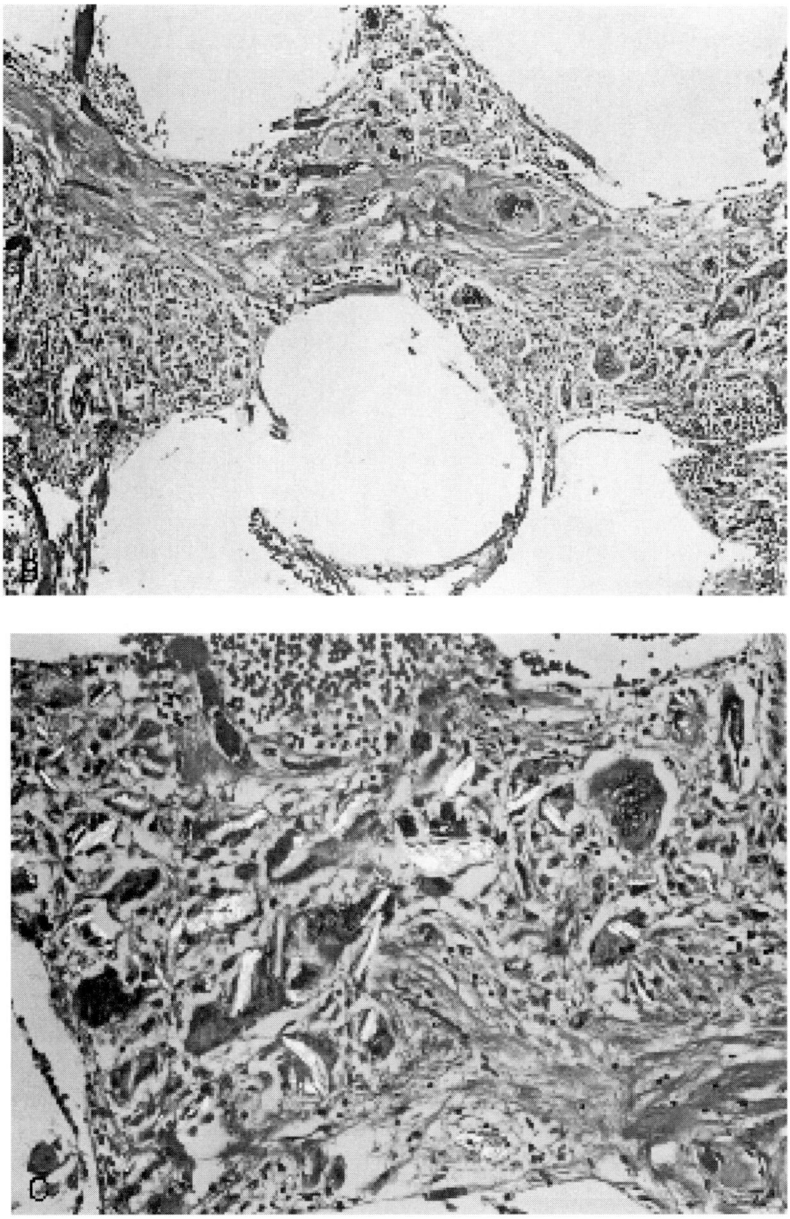

FIGURE 13.2 *(continued)*

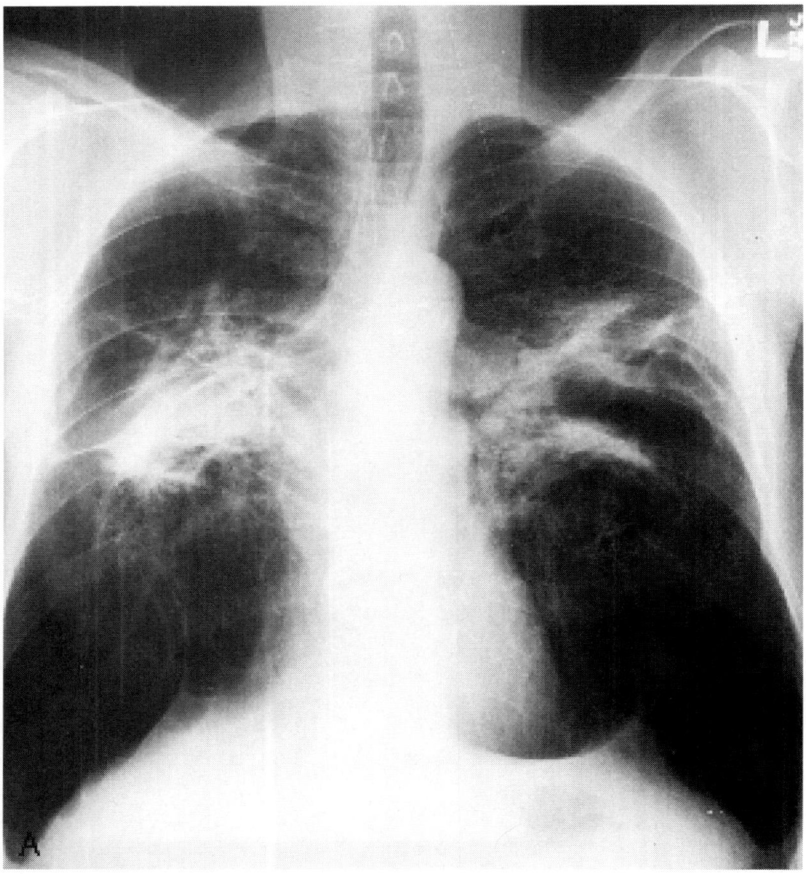

FIGURE 13.3
Massive fibrosis secondary to intravenous drug abuse. Patient had a long history of heroin abuse followed by intravenous methadone abuse. He developed bilateral mass lesions (**A**) and died of respiratory failure. Autopsy showed the mass lesions to consist of irregular rock-hard areas of contraction and fibrosis of the pulmonary parenchyma (**B**); microscopically the lesions consisted of masses of collagen intermixed with giant cells and birefringent particles (**C**). Analysis of the tissue showed that most of the particles were talc, probably derived from the methadone tablets (**C** ×64; polarized light).

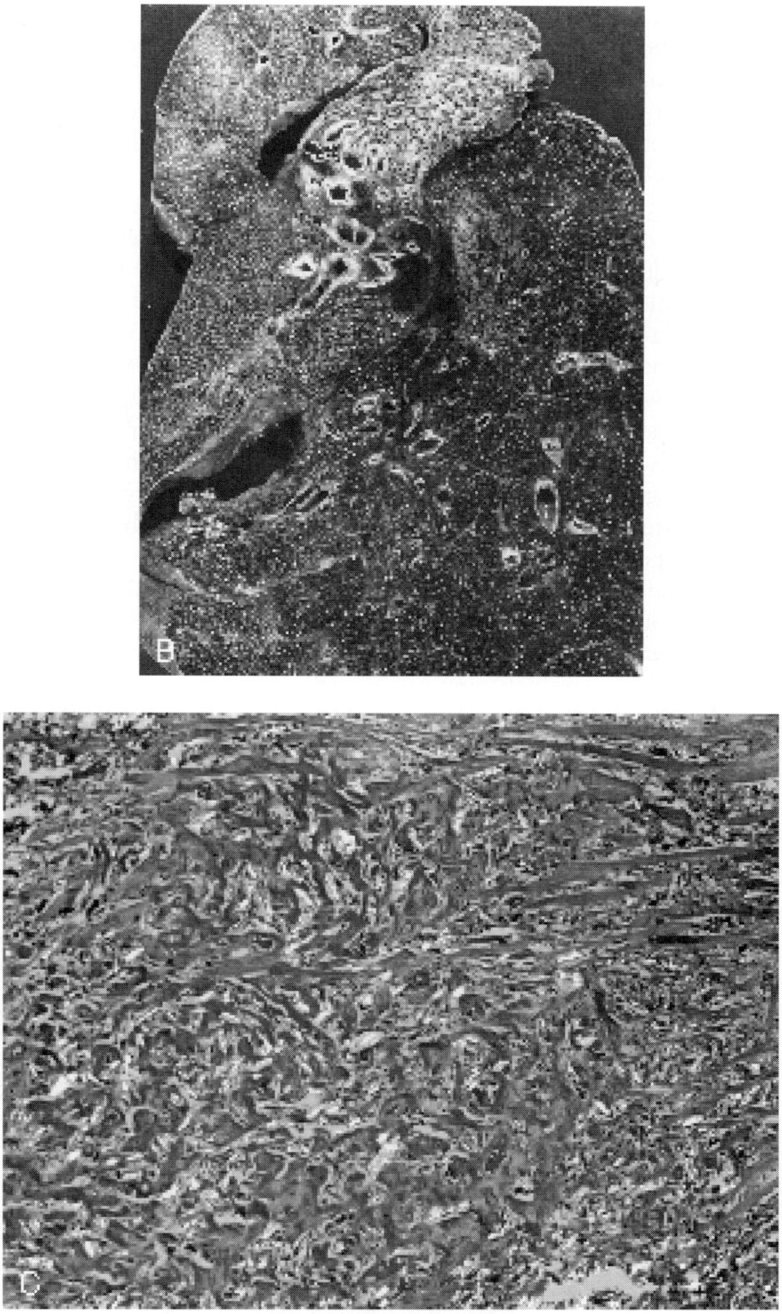

FIGURE 13.3 (*continued*)

crystals that stain with digested periodic acid-Schiff (PAS), methenamine silver, and Congo red (11, 12).

Particle sizes vary considerably from case to case, but individual particles as long as 23 μm have been reported (12). When the question of inhalation versus intravenous origin arises, the presence of large numbers of particles greater than 5 μm in diameter is strong evidence for an intravenous delivery route, since most inhaled particles larger than 5 μm are trapped in the upper respiratory tract (13).

These particles produce several types of reactions: vascular thromboses, foreign body granulomas, interstitial fibrosis, massive fibrosis, and emphysema. The foreign body granulomas can be associated with the vascular changes, the interstitial changes, or both, and the processes shade off one into the other. Animal experiments suggest that the granulomas and fibrosis are seen only with talc and cellulose (14).

The thrombotic process has been called angiothrombosis (6, 15). A variety of lesions can be found, including intravascular and perivascular granulomas containing foreign particles (Fig. 13.1), fibrotic intimal plaques, the weblike bands typical of many types of recanalized thrombi, and lesions composed of small capillary channels, which very much resemble the plexiform lesions of primary pulmonary hypertension (Fig. 13.4, *A* and *B*). Extensive destruction of the vessel elastic laminae is common (Fig. 13.4C). Dilated small vessels, similar to the so-called dilation or angiomatoid lesions of primary pulmonary hypertension, are also sometimes seen. Whether the plexiform and dilation lesions are morphologically identical to those of primary pulmonary hypertension is a matter of dispute (6, 11). However, even if granulomas are absent, refractile particles are found embedded in the drug-induced lesions, so the etiology is usually obvious.

The functional consequence of widespread pulmonary arterial thrombosis is pulmonary hypertension, which is frequently fatal (6, 7, 16, 17). Even in patients without evidence of pulmonary hypertension, isolated decreases in diffusing capacity are extremely common (2, 18); Overland et al. (18), for example, found a decreased diffusing capacity in 42% of a group of 512 addicts. This change is

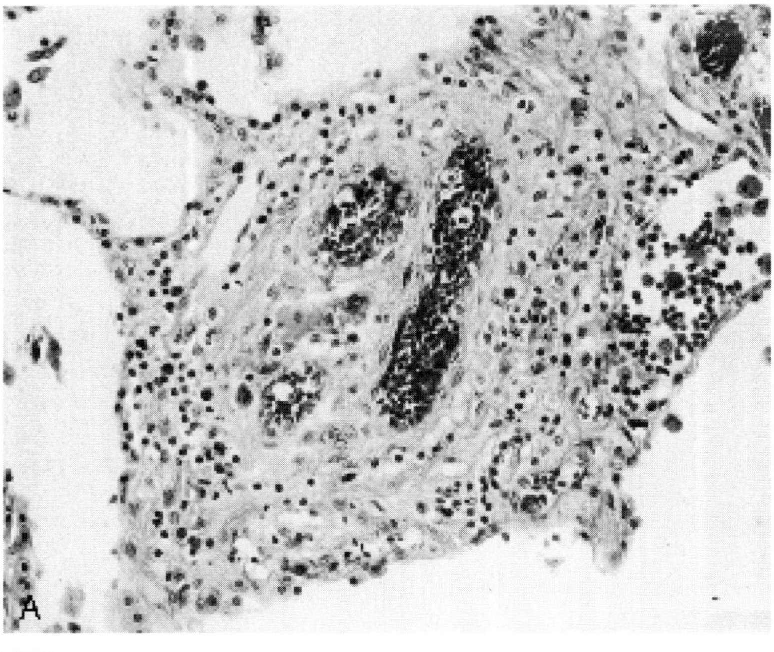

FIGURE 13.4

Vascular lesions in intravenous drug abusers. **A.** A multichannel lesion with features suggesting both a plexiform lesion and an organized thrombus. **B.** Elastic stained section demonstrating giant cells; foreign particles could also be seen by polarized light. Birefringent particles in and around the vessels should alert the pathologist to the possibility of intravenous drug abuse. **C.** Elastic stain showing granulomas that have partially destroyed the wall of a small pulmonary artery. (**A, B, C** ×160.)

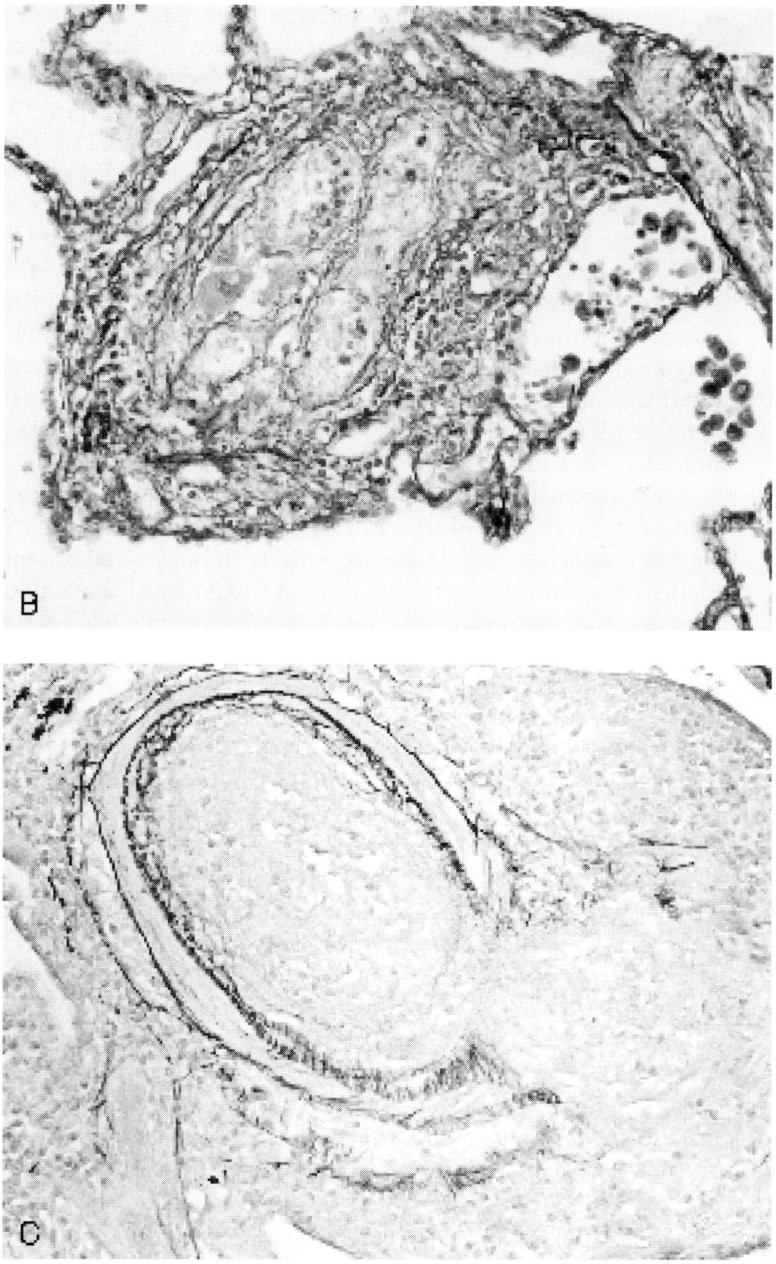

FIGURE 13.4 (*continued*)

believed to be caused by loss of vascular volume secondary to numerous microscopic thrombi.

When a granulomatous and fibrotic reaction to these particles is found in the interstitium, the process is often called talc granulomatosis (2–5). Experimental animal studies indicate that these lesions are evoked by migration of particles through vessel walls (14). Arnett et al. (7) suggest that the final location of the particles is important in determining the type of reaction: when the particles end up in the interstitium, arterial thrombi do not develop.

The interstitial granulomas consist of giant cells and quite variable numbers of mineral particles (Fig. 13.1); larger and more fibrotic lesions appear to be associated with greater local particle loads. With time the process may come to resemble the interstitial fibrosis of inhalational talcosis (Fig. 13.2), but the large particle size, the absence of ferruginous bodies formed on talc (see Chapters 8 and 9), and the absence of particles in alveolar spaces are clues that this is not an inhalational disease.

Another phenomenon similar to inhalational pneumoconiosis is large mass lesions composed of huge numbers of particles with giant cells and extensive fibrotic response (8) (Fig. 13.3). These lesions, which are in effect complicated pneumoconioses (progressive massive fibrosis), are typically upper zonal and may be bilateral (2, 4, 5, 8) (Fig. 13.3*A*). When patients are graded by number of tablets injected, the mass lesions are found in those at the very high end of the scale (2). Patients with diffuse fibrosis and mass lesions usually have marked functional impairment.

More recently it has been observed that some intravenous drug abusers develop severe airflow obstruction that cannot be accounted for by asthma or cigarette smoking; this syndrome appears to be most commonly associated with methylphenidate (Ritalin) abuse (19–21). Clinically and radiographically these patients have features of emphysema, and a pathologic picture very similar to that of panlobular emphysema has been seen at autopsy (8, 21). Emphysema is fairly common in lungs that also contain massive fibrotic lesions, suggesting that huge particle loads are important in its pathogenesis, perhaps because of the intense inflammatory response and consequent proteolytic enzyme release associated with the large numbers of embolized particles. Refractile particles and small granulomas may be found in many other organs at autopsy (22) and can also be seen in the optic fundus during life (2).

Not all foreign particles that arrive in the lung via the intravenous route are derived from drug abuse. Occasionally material from medical procedures is embolized. Cotton fibers released during cardiac catheterization (23) and fragments of Polytef, a particulate form of pyrolyzed Teflon that is injected periurethrally to control urinary incontinence (24) have been reported in the lung. Both cotton and Polytef are highly birefringent, have a characteristic appearance (23, 24), and can be recognized in tissue sections. These particles can induce intravascular and perivascular granulomatous reactions similar to those just described for drug fillers. The microscopic appearances of particles introduced into the circulation by surgical and catheterization procedures have recently been reviewed by Walley et al. (25).

PARAQUAT POISONING

Paraquat (1,1′-demethyl-4,4′ dipyridylium dichloride) is a weed killer widely used throughout the world. Paraquat poisoning is seen after accidental ingestion and occasionally after extensive skin contact (26); in some countries paraquat is also a fairly common suicide agent (27). Paraquat affects a variety of organs but is preferentially concentrated in the lung. The exact pattern of pulmonary response and the cause of death in fatal cases appears to depend on dose. When high doses of highly concentrated (20%) paraquat are ingested, acute myocarditis, renal tubular necrosis, and centrolobular hepatic necrosis are seen; they are the major causes of deaths within 5 days (28). Inflammation and ulceration of the oral cavity, pharynx, and esophagus may also be found acutely (28,

29). Most individuals surviving longer than 5 days have ingested smaller amounts of the chemical (28); those deaths are from respiratory failure (29–32).

The pathologic features of paraquat poisoning have been the subject of some dispute, although the problem is mostly one of interpretation, since the morphologic changes are generally agreed on. It appears from both human cases and animal experiments that the earliest microscopic lesions are those of acute diffuse alveolar damage (adult respiratory distress syndrome). They include massive pulmonary edema rich in fibrin, hemorrhage, necrosis of type I alveolar lining cells, and the formation of hyaline membranes (29–34). An interstitial inflammatory infiltrate is sometimes present. Grossly such lungs have a red color and firm consistency with obliteration of the normal pulmonary markings (Fig. 13.5, *A* and *B*). Neither the gross nor the microscopic appearances are specific at this point.

In humans and animals surviving the acute phase, paraquat poisoning has a variety of appearances. One is diffuse fibrosis with obliteration of airspaces (Fig. 13.5, *C* and *D*). Microscopically this process starts as a rather myxoid in situ organization of the fibrinous material in the alveolar spaces; with time the intra-

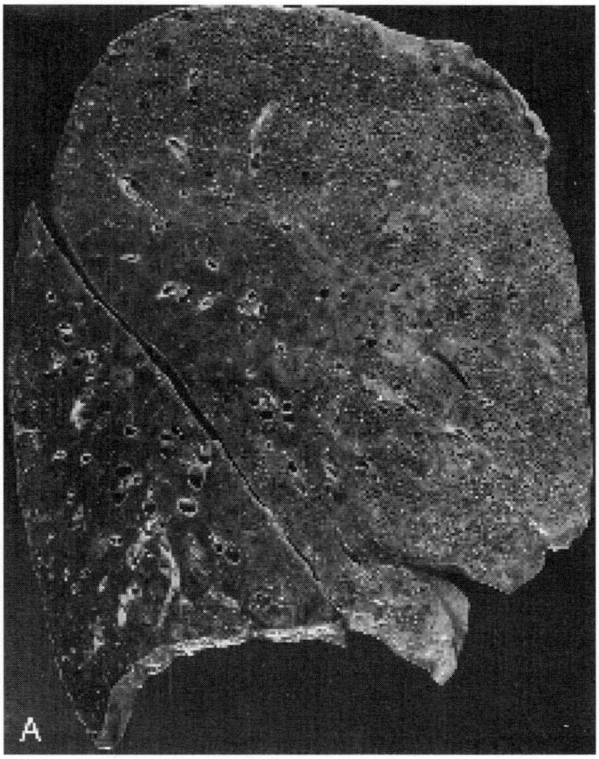

FIGURE 13.5

Lung tissue from a gardener who accidentally ingested paraquat and died approximately 4 weeks later. **A.** The gross specimen shows the loss of parenchymal markings typical of any form of diffuse alveolar damage. **B.** The higher power also illustrates the honeycomb change often seen in diffuse alveolar damage of relatively long standing. The latter should not be confused with diffuse interstitial fibrosis (usual interstitial pneumonia). **C** and **D.** The characteristic lesion of paraquat poisoning: obliteration of the airspaces by relatively acellular myxoid or fibrous tissue. **E** and **F.** Microscopic appearance of the honeycombed areas. (**C** ×40, **D** ×160, **E** ×40, **F** ×80.)

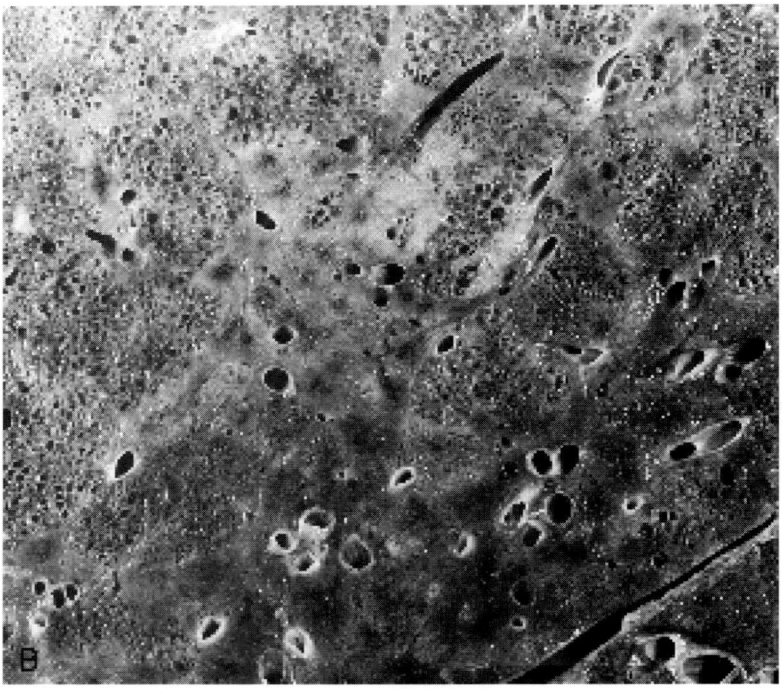

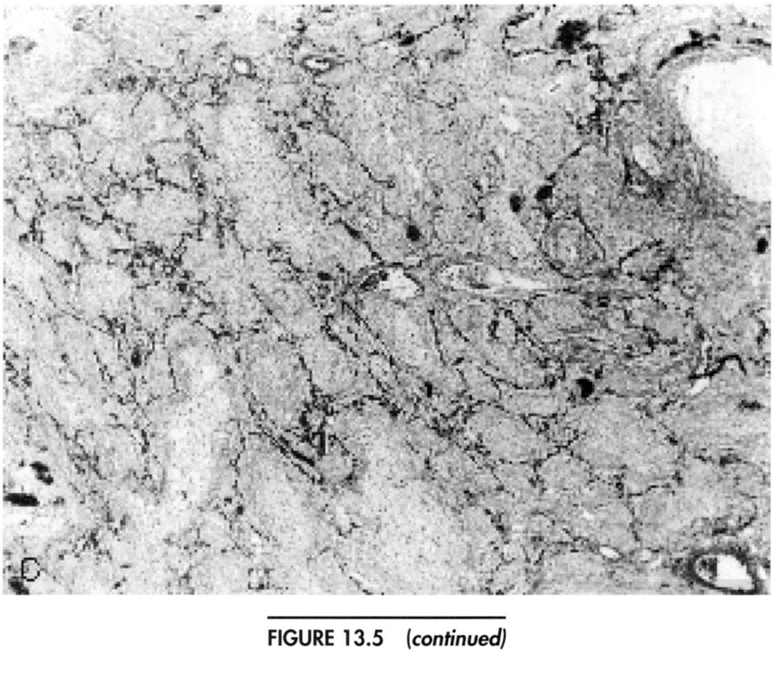

FIGURE 13.5 *(continued)*

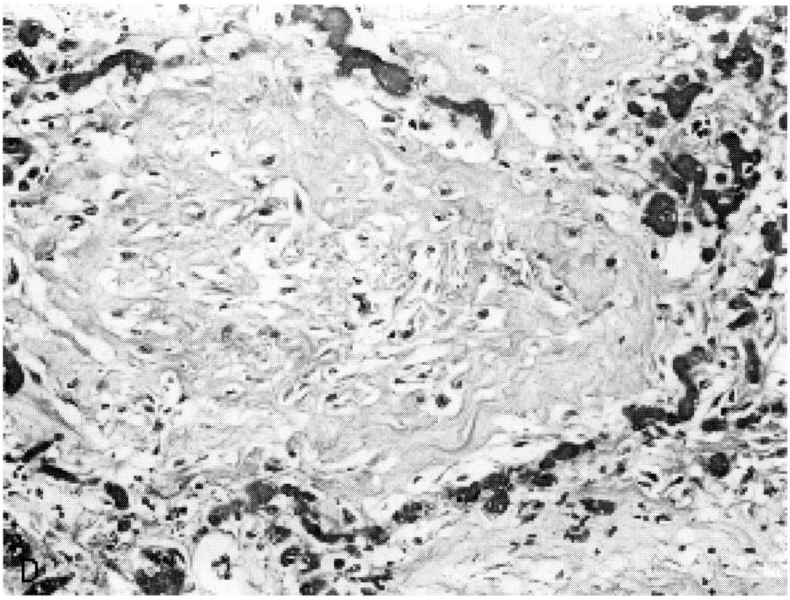

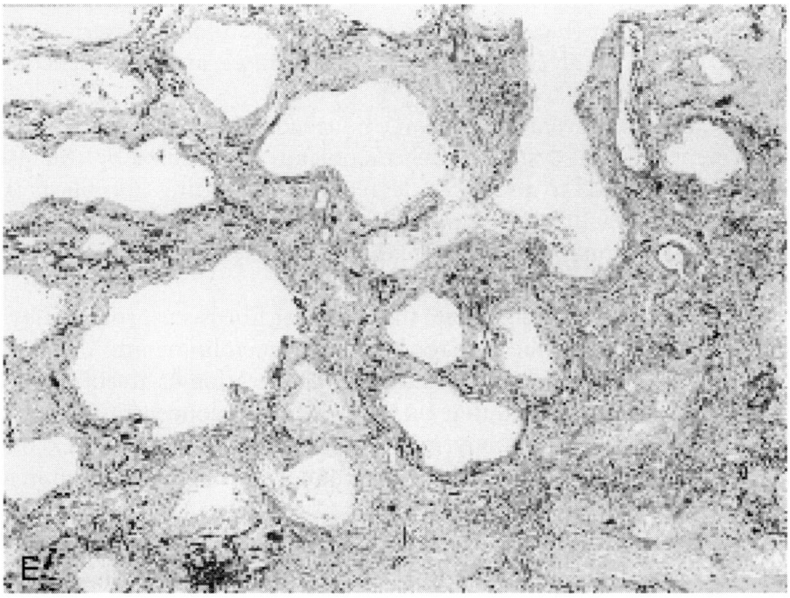

FIGURE 13.5 (*continued*)

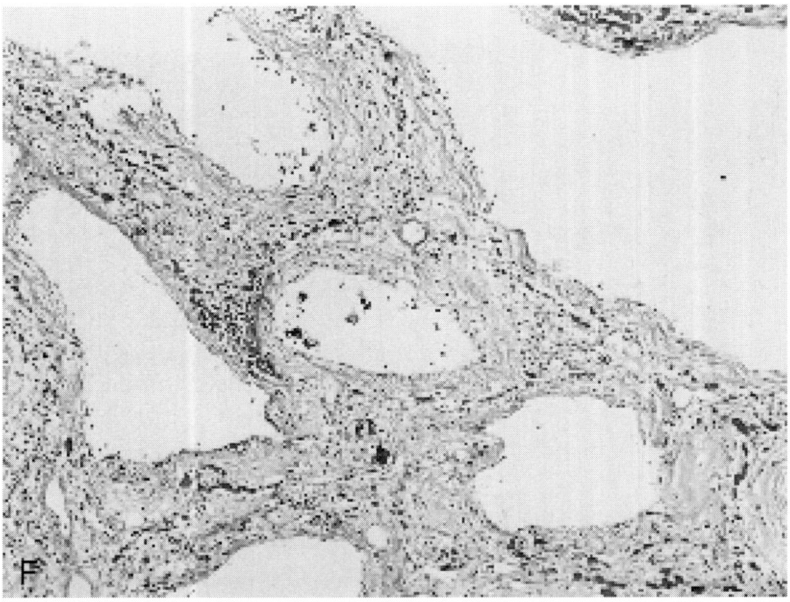

FIGURE 13.5 *(continued)*

alveolar material becomes more eosinophilic and appears as fibrous tissue, often containing very few cells (Fig. 13.5*D*). The underlying alveolar wall architecture may be remarkably well preserved (29, 35), even when extensive intra-alveolar fibrosis is present (Fig. 13.5, C and *D*). This histologic pattern is rarely seen in organizing diffuse alveolar damage of other causes, and its presence should bring paraquat poisoning to mind.

The lungs may eventually become honeycombed (Fig. 13.5, *E* and *F*), with development of small cysts that microscopically are formed by collapsed alveolar walls accompanied to a variable degree by proliferating fibroblasts (Fig. 13.5, *E* and *F*). Metaplastic epithelial changes, particularly in small airways, are also common. The honeycomb pattern and the diffuse consolidative pattern often exist within the same lung (Fig. 13.5*B*).

Experimental studies indicate that alveolar fibrosis is produced by fibroblasts that migrate through the damaged basement membrane into the alveolar spaces and may be compounded by a failure of regeneration of alveolar lining cells (33, 34). It has been suggested that therapy with high concentrations of oxygen and a mechanical respirator may make lesions worse (27, 30, 31), but the basic changes are undoubtedly caused by paraquat, since they are seen in animals under normobaric conditions (34).

There has been considerable discussion about whether paraquat lung is interstitial fibrosis (fibrosing alveolitis) or some other process entirely (30, 31, 34). The formation of dense intra-alveolar fibrosis appears to be unique to paraquat toxicity. However, the edema, hyaline membranes, and cellular granulation tissue that fill alveolar spaces are found in diffuse alveolar damage of any cause (36). The picture of honeycomb cysts is the one that has most frequently been confused with diffuse interstitial fibrosis of the type seen in usual interstitial pneumonia (UIP, or fibrosing alveolitis), not only in the case of paraquat but in many instances of adult respiratory distress syndrome caused by fumes (see Chapter 3). It is clear that this process is merely another type of organization of diffuse alveolar damage (37) and not a form of chronic interstitial fibrosis at all. In light of current knowledge it thus appears that paraquat lung is a peculiar variant of diffuse alveolar damage (adult respiratory distress syndrome).

VINYL CHLORIDE AND POLYVINYL CHLORIDE

At room temperature vinyl chloride monomer (VCM) is a flammable gas with a pleasant odor. Polymerization of VCM produces polyvinyl chloride (PVC). In this form PVC is a white powder consisting of particles with an average diameter less than 5 μm. PVC is an important base material for the plastics industry. VCM is also used to produce other resins, as a chemical intermediate, and as a solvent. Exposure to VCM occurs in industries associated with the manufacture of PVC resins, organic chemicals, and rubber (38). Exposure to both VCM and PVC is common in PVC polymerization facilities. A further hazard is posed by pyrolysis products from heated PVC wrapping film. The latter contains up to 30% additives and plasticizers that when heated, release hydrogen chloride and di-2-ethylhexyl adipate (39).

VCM is a human and animal carcinogen. Neoplastic effects have been demonstrated in animals at concentrations less than 10 ppm (40). In rats VCM exposure results in the formation of highly persistent etheno-DNA adducts, with much greater adduct levels in liver than in other organs (41). In humans angiosarcoma of the liver is definitely associated with exposure to VCM (41–49), and some but not all studies report increases in tumors of the brain, lung, and lymphohematopoietic system (41–49). Workers exposed to VCM and PVC are also at increased risk for several nonneoplastic and preneoplastic conditions, including hepatitis, dermatitis, a digital arthritis resembling Reynauds phenomenon, thrombocytopenia, acro-osteolysis, and probably systemic sclerosis (41, 46, 50). Abnormal sputum cytology has been reported in workers in the Italian VCM and PVC industries (51).

PVC dust may also be carcinogenic to humans, although the frequent presence of small amounts of VCM contaminant makes this a somewhat difficult proposition to evaluate. An increase in angiosarcoma of the liver has been reported in workers using PVC products (41, 48, 52). Recent studies failed to find increases in the incidence of lung cancer (47, 48).

Pulmonary function studies of workers exposed to both VCM and PVC dust have demonstrated obstructive patterns in approximately 50% of workers (40). However, pulmonary function was reported as normal in 104 male workers exposed to PVC dust alone (53). By contrast, radiographic abnormalities appear to be more common in workers exposed to PVC dust. Lilis et al. (40) studied three groups of vinyl chloride polymerization workers exposed to both VCM and PVC and recorded radiographic abnormalities in 22.7, 20.4 and 4.3% of the workers. The abnormalities were predominantly reticular opacities in the lower and mid zones. Nodular opacities were seen less frequently. There was a statistically significant increase in radiographic abnormalities with increasing duration of exposure. Other studies note a lower prevalence of disease. A U.K. study of 818 current and past workers in a PVC manufacturing plant showed radiographic abnormalities in 2.9% (54), and a radiologic survey of 733 individuals exposed to PVC dust in an Italian factory showed a 3.6% prevalence of pneumoconiosis (55). The latter study provided evidence that the radiographic abnormalities were produced by the PVC dust rather than the VCM gas, as no cases of pneumoconiosis were observed in 485 individuals who worked in areas free of PVC dust. These conclusions are supported by a more recent report of Ng et al. (56), who examined a group of workers using PVC that had only negligible VCM contamination; they found that the prevalence of fine radiographic opacities, decrements in pulmonary function, and the degree of reversible airflow obstruction all paralleled the level of PVC exposure.

Only a few reports describe the pathologic findings associated with VCM or PVC exposure. In the case reported by Arnaud et al. (57), the chest radiograph showed a diffuse micronodular infiltrate. Drill biopsies of the lung revealed diffuse infiltration of the interstitium, with histiocytes and multinucleated giant cells with finely vacuolated cytoplasm. There was mild associated fibrosis and smooth muscle hyperplasia. The histiocytic vacuoles were PAS and Alcian blue negative and did not polarize. Electron microscopy revealed numerous granules 0.3 to 0.4 μm in size within phagolysosomes. These granules were identical in appearance to a sample of PVC powder viewed by electron microscopy. The histologic appearances in the case reported by Szende et al. (58) were identical. Antti-Poika et al. (59) also identified particulate-laden macrophages in a biopsy from a patient with PVC exposure; the particulates stained red with Sudan IV after treatment of the sections with alcohol and acetone, a procedure claimed to produce specific staining of PVC (59). Similar lesions have also been produced in animals exposed to PVC dust (60, 61).

A series of three cases reported by Cordasco et al. (49) showed diffuse interstitial pulmonary fibrosis with a DIP-like reaction on lung biopsy. Exposures were to different VCM and PVC products in each case, and it is not at all clear whether these cases represent specific disease entities or examples of idiopathic pulmonary fibrosis occurring in exposed workers (39). Studnicka et al. (50) reported foreign body granulomas containing particles consistent with PVC in a patient with radiographic interstitial infiltrates. Interstitial fibrosis (62) and changes in small airways and alveolar lining cells (63, 64) have been reported in animals exposed to high concentrations of VCM.

Exposure to PVC fumes, such as occurs during the wrapping of meats with PVC film, can result in a form of occupational asthma (65, 66) (see Chapter 12) and chronic bronchitis. It is likely that these conditions are related more to pyrolysis products of the plasticizers than to degradation products of the PVC itself (39, 67).

HAIR SPRAY PREPARATIONS

Despite widespread use of hair sprays and presumed moderate to heavy exposures in certain occupational groups such as hairdressers and beauticians, very few well-documented cases of lung disease associated with exposure to hair spray aerosols have been reported. The most convincing cases include a history of heavy use of hair sprays, evidence of clinical and radiologic improvement following exposure cessation, and histologic confirmation of lung disease (68–72). These cases suggest that hair spray aerosols produce disease in humans, although attempts to reproduce the disease in animals thus far have failed (67) and the issue is far from resolved. Experimental studies using human volunteers indicate that hair sprays induce short-term effects on mucociliary transport (73) and bronchoconstriction in hyperreactive subjects but not in normal controls (74).

Reported clinical features are variable; although symptoms are usually absent, some patients have chest tightness and nonproductive cough or dyspnea. In nonsmokers a primarily restrictive lung disease is usually seen (72), whereas in smokers obstructive ventilatory impairment may predominate (71). Prolonged exposure to hair spray is associated with a micronodular pattern of homogeneous rounded densities 1 mm or less in diameter without a reticular component or calcification (72). This radiographic pattern is relatively distinctive, shared only with alveolar microlithiasis, intravenous talcosis, and oil embolism after lymphangiography (72). Other case reports describe less distinctive reticulonodular infiltrates and hilar lymphadenopathy on chest radiograph (69, 70, 72). Abstinence from further exposure and administration of corticosteroids may produce reversal of radiographic and functional abnormalities (72).

The predominant histopathologic features are giant-cell or sarcoidlike granulomas in the lungs and draining lymph nodes with vacuoles surrounded by foamy macrophages (71, 72). Diffuse interstitial pulmonary fibrosis and emphysema have also been reported (70, 71). The granulomas may predominate around small airways (72). One case report described the histopathologic findings as consistent with a hypersensitivity pneumonitis (68), but no evidence was presented to support hypersensitivity. All of the histopathology reported to date is more consistent with foreign body (macrophagic) reaction to the oils and other high-molecular-weight components of hair spray. This statement is supported by electron microscopic studies that showed accumulations of vacuolated macrophages with lamellar material attached to cell membranes and within secondary lysosomes (69, 71).

The agent or agents responsible for these lesions are not known. Hair sprays contain a large number of macromolecular chemicals in a propellant capable of generating a highly respirable aerosol (75). The active agents include polyvinylpyrrolidone (PVP), polyvinyl acetate (PVA), dimethyl hydantoin formaldehyde resin, alcohols, perfumes, aromatic oils, lanolin, shellac, and ethyl and carboxymethyl cellulose (67, 69). The aromatic oils in hair spray are the most likely cause of the granulomatous reaction. Formerly some preparations contained vinyl chloride, although this was discontinued in view of its carcinogenic properties. Some of these substances stain positively with PAS; hence use of this stain, although nonspecific, may be helpful in arriving at a diagnosis.

EXPOSURE TO OIL MISTS

Exposure to mineral oil mists is relatively common in the mechanical engineering, mining, printing, and construction industries (76). Exposures may also occur in the synthetic textiles industry, in which mineral oils are used as fiber lubricants (77). Less common occupational exposures include aspiration of diesel oil–contaminated seawater (67) and inhalation of liquid paraffin by a trainee circus fire eater (78).

Mineral oils may be natural or synthetic. They contain a number of additives, including emulsifiers, corrosion inhibitors, extreme pressure additives, germicides, antifoamers, and colorants (76). Emulsified oils are usually contaminated with bacteria and occasionally with fungi. Rare cases of occupational asthma and chronic bronchitis have been described in workers exposed to cutting oil mists (76, 79), and a recent report (80) describes several cases of extrinsic allergic alveolitis associated with bacterial contamination of metalworking fluids. However, the major hazard associated with oil mists is exogenous lipid pneumonia (81–87). This has been described after exposure to a variety of oil vapors, including cutting oils used for metal lathing, oils used as insect sprays, oils being removed from metal parts, and even oil mists produced in fires.

Clinical and radiographic changes are uncommon in most workers with oil exposure. In those with clinical symptoms the presenting features are variable, and no pattern is characteristic. The most common symptom is cough, which may be accompanied by sore throat, fever, chills, dyspnea, chest pain, hemoptysis, fatigue, and weight loss. The radiographic pattern is variable. Airspace consolidation, interstitial infiltrates, or ill-defined nodular opacities may be seen. Computed tomography and magnetic resonance imaging may show signal intensities characteristic of fat (88, 89).

Experimental studies indicate that relatively long exposures to high concentrations (100 mg/m↑3↓) of oil mists are necessary to produce lipid granulomas (77). Most human cases resulted from extremely high acute exposures. Heavy exposure to relatively light oil such as liquid paraffin or diesel fuel is reported to produce clinical features of an acute chemical pneumonitis (78). The pathogenesis of the acute reaction is not understood but may involve extraction of lipid from plasma membranes by the aspirated oil.

The acute lesions evolve into a chronic granulomatous reaction that may be diffuse or appear as a localized fibrotic mass on gross examination. Histopathologically the chronic lesions are characterized by large clear vacuoles with surrounding giant cells, macrophages with large lipid vacuoles, organizing pneumonia, or fibrosis (81–83). These features are identical to the pathologic changes found in individuals who chronically aspirate mineral oil (84, 86, 87). Exogenous lipid pneumonia can be differentiated from the endogenous form by histopathologic features and fat stains. In endogenous lipid pneumonia the macrophages have a finely vacuolated, foamy appearance with small (less than 0.5 μm) vacuoles of uniform size (82, 84). In the exogenous form the vacuoles are of variable size and include larger (more than 5 μm) vacuoles that compress the nucleus at the cell boundary (90). Mineral oil droplets can be demonstrated in cytologic specimens (85). Bronchoalveolar (BAL) fluid recovered from patients with lipoid pneumonia may be whitish and turbid because of its content of lipid. Mineral oils can be identified in frozen sections or BAL fluid with oil red O, Sudan IV, Sudan III, and Sudan black B stains and with fluorescent stains; however, they do not stain with May-Grunwald-Giemsa, Papanicolaou, or PAS (90). Thin-layer chromatography combined with infrared spectrophotometry has been used to characterize paraffin oil and oil sprays (91–93).

PULMONARY HEMORRHAGE

Some degree of hemorrhage may be seen in the lungs in cases of acute respiratory distress syndrome of inhalational origin, but the hemorrhage is usually a minor component, as is true of acute respiratory distress syndrome of other causes. However, rare cases of massive pulmonary hemorrhage have been reported after exposure to trimellitic anhydride (TMA) sprayed on hot metal in confined areas (94, 95), and a case of hemorrhage associated with spraying a hexamethylene di-isocyanate-containing paint on hot metal has also been reported (96). With both types of exposure hemorrhage is believed to be related to circulating antibodies directed against TMA or isocyanate complexed to albumin (94, 96).

FERRUGINATION OF ELASTIC FIBERS SECONDARY TO HEMORRHAGE

Long-standing repeated intrapulmonary hemorrhage may lead to interstitial fibrosis with accompanying encrustation of elastic fibers by hemosiderin and oc-

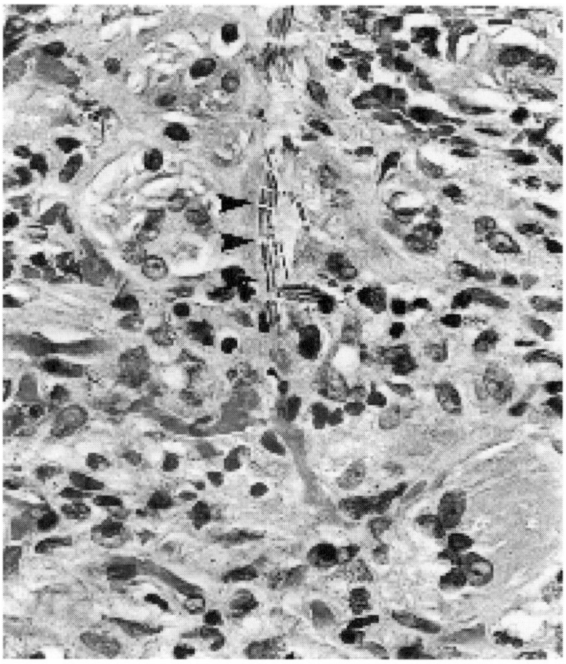

FIGURE 13.6
Ferruginated elastic fiber (*arrowheads*) mimicking an asbestos body in a case of chronic pulmonary hemorrhage, so-called endogenous pneumoconiosis. (×400.)

casionally a giant cell reaction to the encrusted fibers. This process can produce structures that very much resemble ferruginous bodies (Fig.13.6), and the combination of these fake ferruginous bodies and interstitial fibrosis is sometimes mistaken for a pneumoconiosis caused by inhaled particles; the lesion has been called endogenous pneumoconiosis (87). Clues to the diagnosis are ferrugination of the circular elastic fibers of vessel walls as well as linear elastic fibers of the interstitium and both recent and old hemorrhage, the latter evidenced by hemosiderin-laden macrophages. Arterial and/or venous changes of pulmonary hypertension are commonly present as well. This type of reaction has been reported in idiopathic pulmonary hemosiderosis and in pulmonary hypertension of various origins, including mitral stenosis and pulmonary veno-occlusive disease (97).

REFERENCES

Intravenous Drug Abuse

1. Stern WZ, Subbarao K. Pulmonary complications of drug addiction. Semin Roentgenol 1983;28:183–197.
2. Paré JAP, Fraser RG, Hogg JC, et al. Pulmonary 'mainline' granulomatosis: talcosis of intravenous methadone abuse. Medicine 1979;58:229–239.
3. Hopkins GB, Taylor DG. Pulmonary talc granulomatosis. Am Rev Respir Dis 1970; 101:101–104.
4. Sieniewicz DJ, Nidecker AC. Conglomerate pulmonary disease: a form of talcosis in intravenous methadone abusers. Am J Roentgenol 1980;135:697–702.
5. Genereux GP, Emson HE. Talc granulomatosis and angiothrombotic pulmonary hypertension in drug addicts. J Can Assoc Radiol 19744 25:87–93.

6. Tomashefski JF, Hirsch CS. The pulmonary vascular lesions of intravenous drug abuse. Hum Pathol 1980;11:133–145.
7. Arnett EN, Battle WE, Russo JV, Roberts WC. Intravenous injection of talc-containing drugs intended for oral use; a cause of pulmonary granulomatosis and pulmonary hypertension. Am J Med 1976;60:711–718.
8. Crouch E, Churg A. Progressive massive fibrosis of the lung secondary to intravenous injection of talc: a pathologic and mineralogic analysis. Am J Clin Pathol 1983;80: 520–526.
9. Crouch E, Churg A. Ferruginous bodies and the histologic identification of mineral dust exposure. Am J Surg Pathol 1984;8:109–116.
10. Ghadially FN, Murphy F, LaLonde JMA. Diagnosis of pulmonary talcosis by electron-probe x-ray analysis. J Submicrosc Cytol 1984;16:773–777.
11. Zeltner TB, Nussbaumer U, Rudin O, Zimmermann A. Unusual pulmonary vascular lesions after intravenous injections of microcrystalline cellulose: a complication of Pentozacine tablet abuse. Virchows Arch A Pathol Anat Histopathol 1982;395: 207–216.
12. Tomashefski JF, Hirsch CS, Jolly PN. Microcrystalline cellulose pulmonary embolism and granulomatosis: a complication of illicit intravenous injections of Pentazocine tablets. Arch Pathol Lab Med 1981;105:89–93.
13. Abraham JL, Brambilla C. Particle size for differentiation between inhalation and injection pulmonary talcosis. Environ Res 1980;21:94–96.
14. Puro HE, Wolf PJ, Skirgaudas J, Vazquez J. Experimental production of human "blue velvet" and "red devil" lesions. JAMA 1966;197:152–154.
15. Hopkins GB. Pulmonary angiothrombotic granulomatosis in drug offenders. JAMA 1972;221:909–912.
16. Lewman LV. Fatal pulmonary hypertension from intravenous injection of methylphenidate (Ritalin) tablets. Hum Pathol 1972;3:67–70.
17. Robertson CH, Reynolds RC, Wilson JE. Pulmonary hypertension and foreign body granulomas in intravenous drug abusers. Am J Med 1976;61:657–684.
18. Overland ES, Nolan AJ, Hopewell PC. Alteration of pulmonary function in intravenous drug abusers. Am J Med 1980;68:231–237.
19. Schmidt RA, Glenny RW, Godwin JD, et al. Panlobular emphysema in young intravenous Ritalin abusers. Am Rev Respir Dis 1991;143:649–656.
20. Pare JP, Cote G, Fraser RS. Long term follow-up of drug abusers with intravenous talcosis. Am Rev Respir Dis 1989;139:233–241.
21. Sherman CB, Hudson LD, Pierson DJ. Severe precocious emphysema in intravenous methylphenidate (Ritalin) abusers. Chest 1987;92:1085–1087.
22. Mariani-Costantini R, Jannotta FS, Johnson FB. Systemic visceral granulomatosis associated with miliary tuberculosis in a drug addict. Am J Clin Pathol 1982;78: 785–789.
23. Dimmick JE, Bove KE, McAdams AJ, et al. Fiber embolization: a hazard of cardiac surgery and catheterization. N Engl J Med 1975;292:685.
24. Mitterman RE, Marraccini JV. Pulmonary Teflon granulomas following periurethral Teflon injection for urinary incontinence. Arch Pathol Lab Med 1983;107:611–612.
25. Walley VM, Stinson WA, Upton RT, et al. Foreign materials found in the cardiovascular system after instrumentation or surgery (including a guide to their light microscopic identification). Cardiovasc Pathol 1993;2:157–185.

Paraquat

26. Levin PJ, Klaff LJ, Rose AG, Ferguson AD. Pulmonary effects of contact exposure to paraquat: a clinical and experimental study. Thorax 1979;34:150–160.
27. Smith P, Heath D. Paraquat. CRC Crit Rev Toxicol 1976;4:411–445.
28. Parkinson C. The changing pattern of paraquat poisoning in man. Histopathol 1980; 4:171–183.
29. Copland GM, Kolin A, Shylman HS. Fatal pulmonary intra-alveolar fibrosis after paraquat ingestion. N Engl J Med 1974;291:290–292.

30. Smith P, Heath D. Paraquat lung: a reappraisal. Thorax 1974;29:643–653.
31. Thurlbeck WM, Thurlbeck SM. Pulmonary effects of paraquat poisoning. Chest 1976;69(Suppl): 276–280.
32. Rebello G, Mason JK. Pulmonary histological appearances in fatal paraquat poisoning. Histopathol 1978;2:53–66.
33. Fukuda Y, Ferrans VJ, Schoenberger CI, et al. Patterns of pulmonary structural remodeling after experimental paraquat toxicity. Am J Pathol 1985;118:452–475.
34. Smith P, Heath D, Kay JM. The pathogenesis and structure of paraquat-induced pulmonary fibrosis in rats. J Pathol 1974;114:57–67.
35. Toner PG, Vetters JM, Spilg WGS, Harland WA. Fine structure of the lung lesion in a case of paraquat poisoning. J Pathol Bacteriol 1970;102:182–185.
36. Pratt PC, Vollmer RT, Shelburne JD, Crapo JD. Pulmonary morphology in a multihospital collaborative extracorporeal membrane oxygenation project: 1. Light microscopy. Am J Pathol 1979;95:191–214.
37. Churg A, Golden J, Fligiel S, Hogg JC. Bronchopulmonary dysplasia in the adult. Am Rev Respir Dis 1983;127:117–120.

Vinyl Chloride

38. National Institute for Occupational Safety and Health. Occupational diseases: a guide to their recognition. NIOSH pub 77–181, 1977:219.
39. Brooks SM. Pulmonary manifestations of vinyl and polyvinyl chloride. Chest 1988; 88:262–263.
40. Lilis R, Anderson H, Miller A, Selikoff IJ. Pulmonary changes among vinyl chloride polymerization workers. Chest, 1976;69:299–303.
41. Wagoner JK. Toxicity of vinyl chloride and poly (vinylchloride): a critical review. Environ Health Perspect, 1983;52:55–66.
42. Swenberg JA, Fedtke N, Ciroussel F, et al. Etheno adducts formed in DNA of vinyl chloride-exposed rats are highly persistent in liver. Carcinogenesis 1992;13: 727–729.
43. Waxweiller RJ, Stringer W, Wagoner JK, et al. Neoplastic risk among workers exposed to vinyl chloride. Ann N Y Acad Sci 1976;77:40–48.
44. Viola PL, Biogotti A, Caputo A. Oncogenic response of rat skin, lungs and bones to vinyl chloride. Cancer Res 1977;33:516–5197.
45. Buffler PA, Wood S, Eifler MA, et al. Mortality experience of workers in a vinyl chloride monomer production plant. J Occup Med 1979;22:195–203.
46. Laplance A, Clavel-Chapelon F, Contassot JC, Lanouziere C. Exposure to vinyl chloride monomer: results of a cohort study after a seven year follow up. Br J Ind Med 1992;49:134–137.
47. Piratsu R, Belli S, Brucno C, et al. La mortalita dei produttori de chloruro di vinile in Italia. Med Lav 1991;82:388–423.
48. Simonato L, L'Abbe KA, Andersen A, et al. A collaborative study of cancer incidence and mortality among vinyl chloride workers. Scand J Work Environ Health 1991;17: 159–169.
49. Cordasco EM, Demeter SL, Kerkay J, et al. Pulmonary manifestations of vinyl and polyvinyl chloride (interstitial lung disease). Chest 1980;78:828–834.
50. Studnicka MJ, Enzinger G, Drlicek M, et al. Pneumoconiosis and systemic sclerosis following 10 years of exposure to polyvinyl chloride dust. Thorax 1995;50:5: 583–585.
51. Maltoni C. Precursor lesions in exposed populations as indicators of occupational cancer risk. Ann N Y Acad Sci 1976;277:444–447.
52. Barnes AW. Vinyl chloride and the production of PVC. Proc R Soc Med 1976;69: 277–288.
53. Chivers CP, Lawrence-Jones C, Paddle GM. Lung function in workers exposed to polyvinyl chloride dust. Brit J Ind Med 1980;37:147–155.
54. Soutar C, Copland L, Thornley P, et al. An epidemiologic study of respiratory disease in workers exposed to polyvinylchloride dust. Chest 1988;80(Suppl):60S.

55. Mastrangelo G, Manno M, Marcer G, et al. Polyvinyl chloride pneumoconiosis: epidemiological study of exposed workers. J Occup Med 1979;22:540–542.
56. Ng TP, Lee HS, Low YM, et al. Pulmonary effects of polyvinyl chloride dust exposure on compounding workers. Scan J Work Environ Health 1991;17:53–59.
57. Arnaud A, Pommier de Santi P, Garbe L, et al. Polyvinyl chloride pneumoconiosis. Thorax 1978;83:19–25.
58. Szende B, Lapis K, Nemes A, Pinter A. Pneumoconiosis caused by the inhalation of polyvinyl chloride dust. Med Lav 1970;66:433–436.
59. Antti-Poika M, Nordman H, Nickets J, et al. Lung disease after exposure to polyvinyl chloride dust. Thorax 1986;41:566–567.
60. Argarwal DK, Kaw JL, Srivastava SO, Seth PK. Some biochemical and histopathological changes induced by polyvinyl chloride dust in rat lung. Environ Res 1978;16: 333–344.
61. Frongia N, Spinazzola A, Bucarelli A. Experimental lung damage from prolonged inhalation of airborne PVC dust. Med Lav 65:322–342, 1974.
62. Prodan L, Suciu I, Pislaru V, et al. Experimental chronic poisoning with vinyl chloride (monochloroethene). Ann N Y Acad Sci 1975;246:159–163.
63. Suzuki Y. Nonneoplastic effects of vinyl chloride in mouse lung. Environ Res 1980; 22:235–253.
64. Suzuki Y. Pulmonary tumors induced in mice by vinyl chloride monomer. Environ Res 1978;16:285–300.
65. Faulk H, Portnoy S. Respiratory tract illness in meat wrappers. JAMA 1976;235: 915–917.
66. Andrasch RH, Bardana EJ, Koster F, Pirofsky B. Clinical and bronchial provocation studies in patients with meat wrappers asthma. J Allergy Clin Immunol 1976;158: 299–298.
67. Woodhead M, Parkes WR. Disorders caused by other organic agents. In: Occupational lung disorders. 3rd ed. London: Butterworths, 1994:778–793.

Hair Spray

68. Stringer GC, Hunter SW, Bonnabeau RC. Hypersensitivity pneumonitis following prolonged inhalation of hair spray. JAMA 1977;238:887–889.
69. Gebbers JO, Tetzner C, Burkhardt A. Alveolitis due to hair spray. Virchow Arch 1979;382:323–338.
70. Bergmann M, Flance IJ, Cruz PT, et al. Thesaurosis due to inhalation of hair spray. N Engl J Med 1962;266:750–755.
71. Wright JL, Cockcroft DW. Lung disease due to abuse of hairspray. Arch Pathol Lab Med 1981;105:363–366.
72. Schraufnagal DE, Paré JAP, Wang NS. Micronodular pulmonary pattern: association with inhaled aerosol. Am J Roentgenol 1981;137:57–63.
73. Friedman M, Dougherty R, Nelson SR, et al. Acute effects of an aerosol hair spray on tracheal mucociliary transport. Am Rev Respir Dis 1977;116:281–286.
74. Schleuter DP, Soto RJ, Baretta ED, et al. Airway response to hair spray in normal subjects and subjects with hyperactive airways. Chest 1979;75:544–548.
75. Gross J, Gulden W. Holographische teilchen grossenan Analyse von Sprays verschiedener Zusammensetzung und Bestimmung der Teilchendichte in einem Modell des menschlichen Atemtraktes. Aerosol Rep 13:137–148, 1974.

Oils

76. Jarvholm B. Cutting oil mist and bronchitis. Eur J Respir Dis 118:79–83, 1982.
77. Stula EF, Kwon BK. Pulmonary pathology from inhalation of a complex mineral oil mist in dogs, rats, mice and gerbils. Am Ind Hyg Assoc J 1978;39:393–399.
78. Beerman B, Christensson T, Moller P, Stillstrom A. Lipoid pneumonia: an occupational hazard of fire eaters. Br Med J 1984;298:1728–1729.
79. Hendy MS, Beattie BE, Burge PS. Occupational asthma due to an emulsified oil mist. Br J Ind Med 1985;42:51–54.

80. Berstein DI, Lummus ZL, Santilli G, et al. Machine operator's lung: a hypersensitivity pneumonitis disorder associated with exposure to metalworking fluid aerosols. Chest 1985;108:636–641.
81. Foe RB, Bigham RS. Lipid pneumonia following occupational exposure to oil spray. JAMA 1954;155:33–34.
82. Weissman H. Lipoid pneumonia. Am Rev Tuberc 1951;64:572–576.
83. Seidel J. Mucolytic therapy for lipid pneumonia. JAMA 1959;171:1810–1813.
84. Katzenstein AL, Askin FB. Surgical pathology of non-neoplastic lung disease. Philadelphia: WB Saunders, 1982.
85. Weill H, Ferrans VJ, Gay RM, Siskind MM. Early lipoid pneumonia. Am J Med 1964;36:370–376.
86. Perrot LJ, Palmer H. Fatal hydrocarbon lipoid pneumonia and pneumonitis secondary to automatic transmission fluid ingestion. J Forensic Sci 37:1422–1427, 1992.
87. Hugosson CO, Riff EJ, Moore CCM, et al. Lipoid pneumonia in infants: a radiological–pathological study. Paediat Radiol 1991;21:193–197.
88. Carrillon Y, Tixier E, Revel D, Cordier JF. MR diagnosis of lipoid pneumonia. J Comp Assist Tomogr 1988;12:876–877.
89. de Oliveira GA, Del Caro SR, Bender Lamego CM, et al. Radiographic plain film and CT findings in lipoid pneumonia in infants following aspiration of mineral oil used in the treatment of partial small bowel obstruction by *Ascaris Lumbricoides*. Pediatr Radiol 1985;15:157–160.
90. Lauque D, Dongay G, Levade MD, et al. Bronchoalveolar lavage in liquid paraffin pneumonitis. Chest 1990;98:1149–1155.
91. Corrin B, Crocker PR, Hood BJ, et al. Paraffinoma confirmed by infrared spectrophotometry. Thorax 1987;42:389–390.
92. Levade T, Salvayre R. Chemical analysis of the bronchoalveolar washing fluid in the diagnosis of liquid paraffin pneumonia. J Clin Chem Clin Biochem 1987;25:45–48.
93. Penes MC, Vallon JJ. GC/MS detection of paraffins in a case of lipoid pneumonia following occupational exposure to oil spray. J Anal Toxicol 1990;14:372–374.

Pulmonary Hemorrhage

94. Patterson R, Addington W, Bannser AS, et al. Antihapten antibodies in workers exposed to trimellitic anhydride fumes: a potential immunopathogenetic mechanism for the trimellitic anhydride pulmonary disease-anemia syndrome. Am Rev Respir Dis 1979;120:1259–1267.
95. Admad D, Morgan WKC, Patterson R, et al. Pulmonary hemorrhage and hemolytic anemia due to trimellitic anhydride. Lancet 1979;2:326–328.
96. Patterson R, Nugent KM, Harris KE, Eberle ME. Immunologic hemorrhagic pneumonia caused by isocyanates. Am Rev Respir Dis 1990;141:226–230.

Ferrugination of Elastic Fibers

97. Spencer H. Pathology of the lung. 3rd ed. Oxford, UK: Pergamon Press, 1977.

CHAPTER 14

Legal Aspects for the Pathologist

❖ Stephen I. Richman
❖ Carl J. Smith, Jr.

INTRODUCTION

The first edition of this chapter observed that estimates of the incidence of occupational lung disease varied greatly. However, while the true picture was recognized to be unclear, it was stated that occupational lung disease was, and should be, a significant public health concern and that compensation for its victims and their survivors was, and must be, a major social and economic concern.

A recent report by the National Institute of Occupational Safety and Health (NIOSH) summarizes national and state pneumoconiosis mortality. In the 25 years from 1968 to 1992 pneumoconiosis caused the deaths of 100,890 workers in the United States. According to the report, coal workers' pneumoconiosis and silicosis accounted for the most substantial portion of those deaths, 60 and 15%, respectively. The incidence of asbestos-related deaths was reported at 10% (1).

While long-recognized diseases, such as coal workers' pneumoconiosis, silicosis, and asbestosis, account for the vast majority of pneumoconiosis deaths reported by NIOSH, the pathologist involved in the legal system to determine compensation is also intellectually challenged by the recognition of new relations among occupations, toxic exposures, and the development of disease. Would the relation to occupation and exposure be readily apparent to the pathologist who finds pneumoconiosis in a dental technician? The recognition that pneumoconiosis is a hazard for such workers as a result of their exposure to dust from processing cobalt, chromium, and molybdenum alloys is relatively recent (2).

Another area in which new relations among occupations, toxic exposures, and disease are constantly being recognized is occupationally related asthma. The term *occupationally related asthma* comprehends both asthma initiated ("caused") by workplace agents and pre-existing nonoccupational asthma that is aggravated by factors in the workplace. The 1995 consensus statement of the American College of Chest Physicians reports, "Occupational asthma has become the most common form of occupational lung disease in many industrialized countries." While occupationally related asthma is a challenge primarily for the clinician, the consensus statement points out that pathologic investigation should provide much needed information to fill the void in knowledge about the differences between various syndromes and the role of therapy (3). A discussion of the complex medicolegal issues inherent in cases of occupationally related asthma is provided by Richman (4).

Even in cases of easily recognized occupational lung diseases, such as silicosis and coal workers' pneumoconiosis, difficult questions of the possible relation to other diseases may confront the pathologist. While concluding that the existence of a causal relation between exposure to silica and the development of cancer has not been proven, Morgan and Seaton (5) state that an increased risk does seem likely to exist, probably through a synergistic effect with other carcinogens.

No less hotly debated is the possible causal relationship between coal dust exposure and the development of clinically significant emphysema. In 1979 Kleinerman et al. (6) stated that focal emphysema was a specific entity and an integral part of the simple lesion of coal workers' pneumoconiosis. At that time it was also stated that the major causative factor in the development of centriacinar emphysema was cigarette smoking (6). Because focal emphysema and centriacinar emphysema are difficult to distinguish in the presence of coal workers' pneumoconiosis, most autopsy studies do not try to assess the two entities separately (7). However, in their 1992 state of the art article, Wright et al. (8) write that coal dust can produce centriacinar emphysema independent of cigarette smoking but the extent of emphysema is correlated in a broad sense with both the dust load in the lungs and the presence of simple coal workers' pneumoconiosis. Whether any form of emphysema due to coal dust exposure in a nonsmoking miner can produce clinically significant respiratory symptoms or impairment is in controversy (9, 10) (see Chapters 4 and 6).

This chapter examines the role of the pathologist as an expert consultant and witness in the two legal systems, workers' compensation and product liability, that provide remedies to the victims of occupational lung disease and their survivors.

CLAIMS FOR BENEFITS UNDER WORKERS' COMPENSATION LAWS

Workers' compensation is the system of laws under which employees are compensated by their employers for occupational injury or disease. In the United States workers' compensation has traditionally been the function of the individual states. Now, in addition to state workers' compensation programs, there are federal programs for special classes of workers (e.g., longshore and harbor workers, federal employees). The federal black lung program for coal miners is the unique example of a workers' compensation program dealing exclusively with lung disease.

Before the 1930s occupational lung disease as a cause of disability or death was ignored by the United States workers' compensation system. In 1932 the building of a tunnel through a mountain of quartz at Gauley Bridge, West Virginia, brought death to hundreds of workers from massive exposure to silica dust (11, 12). Public shock over the Gauley Bridge disaster motivated state legislatures to extend workers' compensation coverage to include total disability and death due to silicosis and to other specific types of occupational lung disease, including "anthracosilicosis" and asbestosis (13). In 1968 another West Virginia disaster, the mining explosion at Farmington, precipitated the federal black lung program (14). While some state workers' compensation laws still contain limiting provisions, such as restrictive statutes of limitation, exposure requirements, and narrow definitions, all states have made substantial progress toward complete inclusion of occupational diseases in their workers' compensation programs (15). Coverage has so expanded that according to the Labor Department's so-called Selikoff report, upward of 90% of the workers' compensation claims filed in its survey were approved (16).

Underlying workers' compensation is the concept of a "no-fault" liability insurance system in which employees trade off their common law right to sue their employers for damages in exchange for income and medical benefits and (in some jurisdictions) rehabilitation services (17, 18). The defenses of contributory negligence, assumption of risk, and the fellow-servant rule (which often blocked an employee's claims when a worker's injury resulted from his or her own negligence, from his or her voluntarily taking a known risk, or from the actions of fellow workers) were abolished under the workers' compensation as part of the trade-off (19). Importantly for those who suffer from some types of occupational lung diseases, because of their long periods of incubation, time limitations on institution of suit (statutes of limitations) do not commence to run until the claimant knows or should know that disability or death in fact was due to a disease that was occupational (20, 21).

Under workers' compensation law the claimant is required to prove that the employee's disability or death arose out of his or her employment (22). Legal definitions of disability may vary significantly, but disability usually means loss of earning power due to occupation-related injury or disease (23).

In most of the United States workers' compensation benefits equal two-thirds of a worker's wages before injury (23, 24). By providing for less than complete compensation for wage loss, the system in theory creates incentives for healthy workers to avoid injury and for injured workers to return to work (25–27). However, it is doubtful that these socioeconomic objectives are attained in cases of occupational lung disease, because the population of such claimants is composed disproportionately of retired workers or their survivors and because avoidance of toxic exposures is difficult when the risk entails either unperceived exposure to chronic conditions or unanticipated episodes of acute exposure.

It was reported that in 1981 the average value of disability benefits for occupational lung disease under Pennsylvania's workers' compensation law was $200,000; under the federal black lung law it was approximately $125,000 to $150,000 (28). Our own experience and investigation indicate that these values have remained relatively constant.

In the United States disputed questions, including formidable ones of diagnosis, causation, and disability, are decided by litigation in an adversary proceeding. Evidence from lay and expert witnesses is presented, subject to cross-examination, to adjudicators employed by the compensation agency. Respiratory problems in particular are often unrelated causally to worksite exposures and frequently exhibit clinical symptoms indistinguishable from "ordinary diseases of life" (29). Consequently, 90% of respiratory disease claims are litigated (30). In more than 75% of the litigated cases, a controverted issue is causation; these issues involve "very complex scientific testimony and a costly battle of experts" (31).

In Pennsylvania workers' compensation cases, the law limits the attorney's fee, which a winning claimant may have to pay, to 20% of the total benefits (32). The successful claimant can therefore expect to receive approximately 80% of the value of this claim. In the defense of those claims, the employer or insurer will pay approximately $7000 by way of legal and medical fees and expenses. In federal black lung cases the employer or insurer also pays the fees of the successful claimant's attorney (33).

Compensation schemes vary from country to country. The following comments illustrate the variation in definitions of disability, requirements for compensation, and benefits received. These illustrations are based on the excellent text by Barth and Hunt (34).

In Belgium disability benefits are based on either wage loss or impairment according to a scale extending from total to 1% disability. The impaired worker who can perform his or her regular job is entitled to scaled-down benefits, which are determined by the extent of the disabling impairment.

In Denmark workers' compensation covers disabilities due to injuries and illnesses arising out of and in the course of employment that reduce or limit the capacity to work. A worker who suffers occupational injury or disease that reduces earnings by 5% or more is entitled to an industrial injuries benefit. A worker who has a 100% loss of earning capacity receives an "annual pension" of two-thirds of previous earnings. For partial disability, benefits are also determined as two-thirds of loss of earning capacity. No benefit is payable when the disability is determined to be 0 to 5%.

Most West German workers are covered by compulsory sickness insurance. A covered person who falls ill, whether the illness is work connected or not, is entitled to full earnings (100% wage replacement) for up to 6 weeks. If after the period of temporary total disability the worker is at least 20% disabled for 13 weeks or more, he or she is eligible for a permanent disability award. For covered persons disabled for causes not connected to work disability must be at least 50% for the person to receive an invalid's pension. Disability is based on the loss of earning capacity rather than on physical impairment only. In permanent disability cases compensation is awarded as two-thirds of the evaluated level of disability (subject to a maximum ceiling).

A Swiss worker who is occupationally injured or ill is eligible for benefits to replace 80% of lost wages. These benefits continue until he or she returns to work or the condition stabilizes. The individual who sustains a permanent disability that will affect earning capacity is entitled to a pension that is scaled to the extent of disability.

In the Canadian province of Ontario, for temporary total disability an injured or ill worker receives 75% of his or her weekly wage up to a maximum. In cases of permanent disability determinations of the extent of disability are made after maximum recovery has occurred. If the disability is rated as no more than 10%, a lump sum is paid. Benefits are based on a board-determined rating of disability, which takes into account the worker's socioeconomic condition and the physician's evaluation, rather than impairment alone.

SUITS FOR DAMAGES UNDER PRODUCT LIABILITY LAWS

In the United States the chief means by which victims are compensated by the supplier of a defective and unreasonably dangerous product is a civil suit for damages based on the law of product liability. If the harm befell the victim because of employment and if the supplier was *not* the victim's employer, the supplier is sometimes called a *third party*; and the suit against it is sometimes called a *third-party claim*.

The law of product liability is grounded on a codification of the common law of torts as reported in Section 402A of the Restatement (Second) of Torts. By it "strict liability" attaches to the person who markets a product that, though useful and desirable, is inherently unsafe if its user or consumer is not given proper warning of the product's dangers. The "strict" liability of the supplier to the victim is justified by the public policy belief that the burden of harm caused by the product should be placed on those who market it and should be treated as a cost of doing business against which liability insurance can be obtained (35).

Under the law of product liability a supplier of toxic materials is required to warn of dangers involved in handling the materials; the failure to give adequate warning renders the material *unreasonably dangerous* and its supplier liable in damages to the unwarned victim harmed by the material (36). Liability attaches to failure to provide adequate warning even if at the time of manufacture the manufacturer could not have known of the product's hazards. In asbestos-related lawsuits most plaintiffs allege that the supplier failed to perform this duty to warn of the hazards from inhalation of asbestos fiber originating from asbestos-containing products (37). In suits against Manville Corporation, a leading producer of asbestos, it has been conclusively determined in the courts that asbestos materials are *unreasonably dangerous* as a matter of law because asbestos fibers cause asbestosis and mesothelioma and because adequate warning about those health risks was not given by Manville Corporation (38, 39).

In cases of "creeping disease" (i.e., disease that may not become apparent for many years after the onset of exposure) contracted from exposure to hazardous substances, the statute of limitations begins to run only when the plaintiff knows or should have known both that he or she has been injured and that the injury was caused by another's conduct (40, 41).

The toxic product liability claim is usually adjudicated at a trial in which the issues are decided by a judge and jury. Once the product liability issue of adequate warning is reached and passed, the remaining disputed questions are the same as those tried and decided in the workers' compensation proceeding; namely, the formidable ones of diagnosis, causation, and disability. As previously stated, these issues involve very complex scientific testimony and a costly battle of experts.

The preponderance of product liability lawsuits are for workplace incidents, and their role in compensating for workplace disease is growing (39). Product liability lawsuits have been brought against suppliers of a large number of products believed to be toxic, including silica, formaldehyde, cobalt, and so on. Suppliers of asbestos materials have received the most notoriety.

In a dated but still pertinent report the Rand Corporation noted: "Approximately 24,000 people had filed product liability lawsuits claiming asbestos-related injury as of March, 1983. Many times that number have been exposed to asbestos, and the potential liability of the defendant firms may run into the billions of dollars." About $1 billion in compensation and litigation expenses was spent on asbestos product liability litigation through the end of 1982. The average total compensation per claim paid by all defendants and their insurers was approximately $60,000, of which the plaintiff received an average of $35,000 after deducting $25,000 for legal fees and expenses. The Rand Corporation went on to provide this interesting analysis of the data: "For every $2.71 of expenses by defendants and insurers, defense litigation expenses are an estimated $1, plaintiff's litigation expenses are an estimated $0.71, and the plaintiff receives $1. The plaintiff, then, receives an estimated 37% of the total expenses" (42).

THE PATHOLOGIST'S ROLE AS MEDICOLEGAL CONSULTANT

Preparation of Specimens and Reports

The pathologist's involvement with either a workers' compensation claim or a product liability lawsuit may originate because he or she examined surgical specimens or performed autopsies. The pathologist's involvement in a legal case may also originate from an attorney's request for consultation regarding pathologic studies done by another pathologist. Regardless of type of legal proceeding or origin of case involvement, the principal roles of the pathologist as a medicolegal consultant are (*a*) to describe and diagnose all significant pathology, (*b*) to prove or disprove a causal relationship between the significant pathology and impairment or death, (*c*) to identify and explain the causation of the significant pathology, and sometimes (*d*) to evaluate impairment and disability.

When a pathologist handles original specimens, the responsibility for preparing a descriptive report of gross specimens received and of necropsies performed (43) must be carried out in a detailed and explicit way, recognizing that the reported description will probably become the only available evidence of gross appearances. If surgical biopsy material is involved, the pathologist must ensure that each specimen is accompanied by pertinent clinical information (43, 44).

Microscopic slides and paraffin blocks must be adequately and permanently identified and properly indexed and stored to maintain their diagnostic value (43). When a pathologist identifies a structure with particular diagnostic importance (i.e., asbestos bodies in a case of asbestosis or a granuloma in a case of suspected berylliosis), it is advisable to delineate the lesion with an indelible marker so that the identity of the structure can be confirmed by other pathologists. The pathologist should realize the value of microanalytic studies and their interpretation and know when they should be performed in support of a diagnosis. Histologic sections should be of a size and number and from sites representative of the gross conditions. It is also important to take adequate samples from sites away from the lesion, particularly areas of apparently normal lung, as these may hold clues to occupational exposures and disease origin (see Chapter 2).

When functioning as a medicolegal consultant, the pathologist should be more than prosector and histologist. He *must* study and evaluate the available evidence of clinical history, occupational history, environmental history, and the history of smoking and other social habits that may be relevant (45, 46). It is the pathologist's duty to make the referring attorney aware of his or her information requirements. It is the duty of the referring attorney, who has access to legal processes for gathering facts, to furnish the pathologist consultant with all needed data. Stating opinions in regard to the causes of death or disability without acquiring knowledge of a victim's clinical, occupational, social, and environmental history is by our own observations a frequent and regrettable practice followed by some pathologists, who ignore vital data and base their opinions exclusively on the pathologic materials. Although this practice may be appropriate in some instances (e.g., where the issue is purely one of a histologic diagnosis, such as in a case of mesothelioma), very often it leads to serious errors.

In studying the clinical history the pathologist should include the reported interpretations of chest radiographs, electrocardiographic records, tests of pulmonary function, and other relevant laboratory data. The pathologist who considers his or her knowledge of these matters wanting should candidly acknowledge these limitations to the referring attorney and request additional consultations with appropriate medical specialists (e.g., in radiology, cardiology, or pulmonology). In certain survivor claims, in which entitlement may be based on either death or disability due to occupational disease, we often retain as medicolegal consultants both a pathologist and a pulmonologist, and we request them to consult each other. The pathologist who is asked to render an opinion as to disability may require additional consultation to feel qualified and comfortable with the principles of physiology required for competent expressions of opinion on impairment and disability. In performing the investigation the pathologist should acquire familiarity with the reported studies that correlate pathologic findings, radiologic appearances, and measured pulmonary function.

Where there is any uncertainty as to the causation of the pathologic findings, historical and clinical investigation is essential (Naeye RL, personal communication, July 6, 1985). The tendency of pathologists to sample the "worst" areas they see at autopsy may mislead the consulting pathologist to the conclusion that the pathology is more severe than is actually the case; but if there are also physiologic data available, this sampling error can often be identified (Naeye RL, personal communication, July 6, 1985).

The pathologist should also be aware that for detection of certain diseases the histopathologic evaluation may be either more or less sensitive than either pulmonary function or radiology. For example, silicosis and coal workers' pneumoconiosis may be apparent to the pathologist in the absence of radiographic evidence of disease (6, 47). Conversely, with diseases such as asthma or byssinosis, which result largely from airway reactivity, the pathologist may find no morphologic correlates (48). This underscores the need for review of the clinical information.

The consulting pathologist should also learn about the prevalences and causative associations of diseases established by epidemiology. In the study of the occupational and environmental history the pathologist should identify and comprehend the importance of relevant exposures to toxic pollution. Consultation with a chemist, toxicologist, or industrial hygienist may be required for such knowledge, and the pathologist should make the need known to the referring attorney.

Using *all* of the collected information, the consulting pathologist prepares his opinions as to diagnosis, causation, and disability. "Diagnoses... shall be expressed in acceptable terminology of a recognized disease nomenclature" (46). This requirement is especially important in litigation. Lawyers and adjudicators are very likely to be confused by the pathologic babel that occurs when standard diagnostic criteria and nomenclature (e.g., as in coal workers' pneumoconiosis [6] and in asbestos-related diseases [49]) are not used. As legal counsel we have frequently seen pathologists ignore or reject the published standards and instead employ peculiar nomenclatures and diagnostic criteria in a regrettable tactic calculated to confuse. According to Naeye, the consulting pathologist not only needs to know the published medical criteria and nomenclatures for making the diagnosis, he or she should follow them in expressing opinions or else should provide justification based on his or her own independent research (Naeye RL, personal communication, July 6, 1985).

After completion of all consultations and study of all records and materials, the consulting pathologist can compose the report. This report should identify in vivo and postmortem records and materials that were studied or considered. It should describe histologic findings with measured precision and in detail. Microphotographs of lesions, especially when a standard or control photograph is available for comparison, can be an effective way to present pathologic findings and conclusions. The report might cite appropriate references of authorities to support the conclusions reached. The ultimate conclusions as to diagnosis, causation, or disability should be declared by opinions expressed with "reasonable medical certainty", and reasonable medical certainty *must* include *logical* deduction from the data available and a comparison with the known literature on the subject (N. L. Lapp, personal communication, August 18, 1982: "You and I have both seen pathologists who described minimal, if any, changes typical of coal workers' pneumoconiosis and from that have made an extraordinary leap of logic to a totally disabling disease...").). Where there is disagreement between the reporting pathologist and another physician who expresses a contrary opinion, that disagreement should be forthrightly stated and the reason for it supported.

The report is often not confidential and is usually available to all parties of the proceeding. It may be admitted into evidence and unsupplemented by oral testimony, constitute the plenary statement of the physician. If the author of the report does give oral testimony at a deposition or hearing, any ambiguities or errors in the report will be used to discredit its author's opinions. Therefore, special attention must be assigned to preparation of the report. Requests from the referring attorney for amplification are common and should not be regarded as slighting or offensive. Completeness, accuracy, and unequivocality in a report intended for use in a legal proceeding are absolutely essential.

Problems of Legal versus Medical Criteria

In formulating opinions, the consulting pathologist must also take into account the *legal* criteria as provided by the referring attorney, because the legal and medical criteria may conflict. The conflict between the legal and the medical definitions of pneumoconiosis merits special attention.

According to most authorities, the only clinically significant chronic respiratory diseases established by science to be attributable to inhalation of coal dust are coal workers' pneumoconiosis and silicosis, which are types of pneumoconiosis (50). They assert that the causative connection between coal mining and clinically significant chronic obstructive lung disease (asthma, chronic bronchitis, and emphysema) has not been established (51). In the late 1960s, however, medical opinion was sharply divided over the effects of inhaled coal mine dust on the development of chronic bronchitis and emphysema. Some physicians thought that all chronic respiratory disease in coal miners should be regarded as included in a condition they called black lung; (51) *black lung* is not, however, a medical term (50).

The subsequent development of the federal black lung program provides a fascinating example of the problems encountered in reconciling legal and medical criteria (51). In March 1969 militant striking coal miners shut down the mines of West Virginia until that state's legislature passed a law that not only recognized black lung as an occupational disease but also expressly entitled any coal miner who had worked 10 years or more in the mines and who suffered from any respiratory impairment to be eligible for workers' compensation.

Using the political momentum gained in West Virginia, the miners carried to

Washington their demand to be compensated for the respiratory distress symptoms they called black lung. Congressman Kenneth Heckler of West Virginia and Carl D. Perkins of Kentucky moved to amend the pending Coal Mining Safety Bill to include a black lung benefit program like that just enacted in West Virginia. Senators Jennings Randolph and Robert Byrd of West Virginia also offered an amendment to provide compensation for disabled miners, although their bill compensated only for disability due to coal workers' pneumoconiosis and not for black lung. Most other senators and representatives gave little attention to the complex medical issue; they assumed that coal workers' pneumoconiosis and black lung were one and the same entity. In House debate Congressman John Dent put it this way: "Pneumoconiosis or black lung or whatever you want to call it" (52).

Byrd later offered this clarification: "Let us stop quibbling with dying men as to whether their lungs are riddled with black lung or whether they are affected with asthma, or silicosis or chronic bronchitis" (53).

The law that did pass in 1969 contained, in Title IV, Black Lung Benefits, the expressed intent of Congress to provide benefits to coal miners "who are totally disabled due to pneumoconiosis" (54). It also contained this compromised definition of *pneumoconiosis*: "a chronic dust disease of the lung arising out of employment in an underground coal mine" (55).

By 1972 most well-informed physicians were denying that coal mining caused clinically significant pulmonary disease, except for coal workers' pneumoconiosis, silicosis, and their complications. But physicians who attended miners in union clinics disagreed. They asserted that coal mining caused *black lung*, which they regarded as a separate disease composed of a complex of medical disorders that included not only pneumoconiosis (as medically defined) but also chronic bronchitis, emphysema, and asthma. In the 1972 Congressional debate, attention was focused on the definition of disability; the definition of pneumoconiosis was ignored. Therefore, *pneumoconiosis* continued to mean, ambiguously, *a chronic dust disease of the lungs arising out of employment in a coal mine*. The 1972 act added a requirement that compelled a diagnosis of pneumoconiosis notwithstanding a negative chest radiograph, "if other evidence demonstrates the existence of a totally disabling respiratory or pulmonary impairment" (56). Opposing the requirement, Congressman John Ashbrook of Ohio argued vigorously but unsuccessfully that it is virtually impossible to have disabling coal workers' pneumoconiosis in the face of a negative chest radiograph and that the cause of impairment in such a case could be "emphysema, asthma, chronic bronchitis, or a combination of any conditions other than pneumoconiosis" (57).

Congress rejected the argument. By doing so, it also rejected "prevailing opinion among pathologists, epidemiologists and internists" (51). Accordingly, regulations issued by the Secretary of Health, Education, and Welfare defined pneumoconiosis not only as a "chronic dust disease of the lung arising out of the Nation's coal mines", but also as *any* totally disabling chronic respiratory or pulmonary impairment unless it is established that the impairment "did *not* arise out of, or in connection with, employment in a coal mine" (58). The definition of pneumoconiosis based on respiratory or pulmonary impairment, which did not require lung tissue reaction to inhaled dust, was formally codified by the amendments contained in the 1977 act (59). It redefined pneumoconiosis to mean "a chronic dust disease of the lung and its sequelae, including respiratory and pulmonary impairments, arising out of a coal mine employment" (60). The report of the Senate Committee on Human Resources candidly explained: "The

Committee bill expands the definition of pneumoconiosis to include ... respiratory and pulmonary impairments arising out of coal mine employment" (61). This statutory definition of pneumoconiosis is still in effect.

The current regulatory definition of pneumoconiosis expands the disease even further to include, along with coal workers' pneumoconiosis and silicosis, anthracosilicosis, anthracosis, anthrasilicosis, massive pulmonary fibrosis, and silicotuberculosis arising out of coal mine employment. A disease "arising out of coal mine employment" includes any chronic pulmonary disease resulting in respiratory or pulmonary impairment that is significantly related to or substantially aggravated by dust exposure in coal mine employment (62).

Other examples of conflict between the legal and medical criteria in the definition of pneumoconiosis can be cited. Because anthracosis is pneumoconiosis according to the federal black lung regulation (62), if the pathologist intends only to describe a condition of carbonaceous pigmentation and not to diagnose a disease, he should avoid the term *anthracosis* and instead provide a verbal description of the condition.

The word *macule* is yet another example. To some it means merely an area "distinguished by color from its surroundings" (63); but to others means the pathognomonic lesion of early-stage coal workers' pneumoconiosis (6). If the latter is intended, declares Green, the pathologist should describe the lesion as a coal dust macule based on the typical light microscopic appearances of coal mine dust (see Chapter 6). The pathologist should also make a determination as to whether focal emphysema is present or absent. In this way the lesion can be distinguished from the aggregates of black pigment in the walls of the respiratory bronchioles common to urban dwellers and heavy smokers (F. Green, personal communication, May 1988).

Another area of discrepancy between medical and legal criteria can arise in the determination of causation. For example, assuming that "bronchogenic carcinoma" is the correct pathologic diagnosis in the case of a person who both was a heavy smoker and was exposed to asbestos products and other carcinogens, unresolved scientific questions may yet preclude an expression of opinion as to causation with reasonable medical certainty (64, 65). Some contend that in such cases any asbestos exposure, no matter how slight, should by law be presumed to be causative unless a contrary origin is proved with reasonable medical certainty. A legal presumption of this type was proposed in one of the asbestos statutes introduced in Congress (66). However, according to Weill, "[it] is not possible ... to conclude that any ... [asbestos] exposure, no matter how trivial, is causally associated with the development of [bronchogenic carcinoma]" (67). Because of scientific uncertainty regarding the causation of bronchogenic carcinoma, the proposed statute's enactment may result in unfairly blaming asbestos for bronchogenic carcinoma even when asbestos exposure was insignificant relative to exposure to other known carcinogens.

The consulting pathologist may be asked for an opinion regarding the cause of disability or death when more than one dread disease affects the same patient. Take, for example, the extremely dyspneic cigarette-smoking insulator whose diagnoses include bronchogenic carcinoma, centrilobular emphysema, asbestosis, and severe coronary artery disease with congestive heart failure. In formulating an opinion, should the consulting pathologist merely list all of the diagnoses as identified causes of disability or death and thereby ignore the relative contribution of each?

The consulting pathologist must be made aware of the applicable legal standard of causation, and the opinion must conform to it. When death or disability is due to multiple diseases, of which one creates liability, the question is perplexing. When is the contribution of the single *compensable* disease large enough to permit the finding that it caused the death or disability? In cases of workers' compensation, the issue is far from settled (68). Depending on the jurisdiction wherein the case arises, the law is interpreted variably. Under federal black lung law pneumoconiosis is a substantial contributing cause of death if it actually hastens the miner's death (69). For an occupational disease to be compensable under Pennsylvania's workers' compensation law, it must be *"a substantial" contributing cause* of death or disability (whatever that means) (70).

In a product liability lawsuit, however, the legal standard of causation is a settled matter. The standard is whether the identified pathology was "a *substantial* factor" in causing death or disability (36) or was a competent producing cause of disability or death (38).

THE PATHOLOGIST'S ROLE AS EXPERT WITNESS

In worker's compensation and in product liability cases, much of the scientific evidence is greatly beyond the ken of most adjudicators. Because of this, litigants employ expert witnesses who know the medicine and who can explain the case understandably. Under the *federal rules of evidence*, "If scientific, technical or other specialized knowledge will assist the trier of fact to understand the evidence or to determine a fact in issue, a witness qualified as an expert by knowledge, skill, experience, training or education may testify thereto in the form of an opinion or otherwise" (71). The "battle of experts" has in consequence become a standard part of occupational lung disease litigation. Only through expert testimony can a litigant successfully present his or her contention with respect to the issues of diagnosis, causation, or disability.

The findings and opinions of the pathologist as expert witness are presented by oral testimony given under oath. The opposing party has a full right to cross-examine the expert witness as to all matters covered in direct examination. The setting for testimony may be the hearing room or courtroom in the presence of the adjudicator or it may be the physician's office by way of stenographic or videotape deposition that is later read or shown to the adjudicator in the hearing room or courtroom.

Because a decision in a case is often reached by adopting a particular expert's opinion, it is important that the trier of fact be informed of the professional qualifications of the expert. According to Belli, a famous trial lawyer, one must impress the jury with and by the witness's credentials. "The more experience the expert has and the more widely recognized he or she is as an authority in the field, the more impressed the members of the jury will be; they will then accord such testimony more weight" (72). Therefore, the expert witness should be prepared to provide, without modesty or exaggeration, an accurate and complete description of his or her professional qualifications.

The opinion expressed by an expert witness may be based on any source, including such hearsay sources as hospital records, reports of other physicians, statements elicited from the disease's victim, and acknowledged scientific treatises; *provided* that the source is inherently reliable and of the kind customarily relied on by experts in forming their opinions (72, 73). However, an expert's opinion that is based on false facts is not competent (74).

Either in preparation for trial or during the presentation of testimony at trial, the expert witness may desire to review the information on which his or her opinions are based. The expert witness is permitted to refer to any matters, including radiographs, pathology materials, and even his or her own report, to refresh his or her memory. However, once referenced, the information is subject to the cross-examiner's full right to examine and use it. Occasionally embarrassment occurs when inspection at trial of the expert's file results in disclosure of forgotten contents that the witness would have preferred to keep private.

Learned treatises are often invoked to corroborate or to impeach the expert's attested opinions. The federal rules of evidence provide: "To the extent called to the attention of an expert witness upon cross-examination or relied upon by him in direct examination, statements contained in published treatises, periodicals, or pamphlets on a subject of history, medicine or other science or art, established as a reliable authority by the testimony or admission of the witness ... may be read into evidence..."(75). Skillful use of learned treatises on behalf of a litigant by its expert witness and attorney can be an effective way to demonstrate that the opinions expressed by the expert reflect positions and views that are well established and correct and that the contrary views of the opposing expert are not.

The expert should, if possible, declare that he or she holds the opinion with a *reasonable degree of* medical certainty. "I think," and "I believe" are acceptable as shorthand recitals of the standard of reasonable medical certainty. However, opinions given as "probably," as "might be," or as "could be" are not competent expressions because they are too equivocal and conjectural. An opinion based on mere possibility is clearly improper (76, 77).

The traditional legal formulations may not harmonize with the new formulations of epidemiology. This point is well illustrated where lung cancer is seen in a smoking asbestos worker exposed to other carcinogens. According to Enterline (64), an opinion about the tumor's origin cannot be stated *with certainty*, because to attribute with certainty lung cancer to asbestos would falsely imply that the asbestos exposure somehow blocked the possible effects of all other cancer-causing agents; but an opinion *can* be expressed *relatively* as a mathematical probability for each carcinogenic agent to which the worker had been exposed. At what point medicine's *probability* becomes equivalent to law's *reasonable medical certainty* is yet to be addressed by the courts. Until it is, the problem will certainly perplex the knowing and conscientious medical expert.

When his or her opinions are informed, honest, and forthright, the pathologist who is properly prepared should not be apprehensive about performing as expert witness and giving oral testimony. Nor should he or she be timid in criticism of other physicians when it is certain that their opinions are not informed, honest or forthright.

The late C. L. Anderson, a pulmonologist at Western Pennsylvania Hospital in Pittsburgh who had wide experience as an expert witness, offered some advice: On cross-examination, do not be misled by hypotheticals; stick to what is known medically, do not be persuaded by "what might be" or "what could be"; stay with "what is"; avoid the fate of the unwary physician led by the cunning cross-examiner down the path to an improbable disease state (CL Anderson, personal communication, July 21, 1982). Keeping in mind the specific medicolegal issues about which he or she has been consulted, the pathologist, in giving testimony, should avoid digression, remain relevant, and explicate points comprehensibly. And be convincing! "However learned and honest the person may be, it must always be remembered that it is not just what the expert knows, it is also what the [referee, judge, or] jury understands and believes the expert knows" (72).

The outcome of occupational lung disease litigation is frequently determined as much by medical points as by legal points. The attorney who is an experienced and successful litigator of these cases knows generally the medicine of lung disease and is particularly well read on the medical aspects of the case with which he or she is immediately involved. Because the role of the expert witness is so important to the result, the pathologist who would be a medical consultant should anticipate cross-examination by an informed attorney. For the pathologist who is informed about the subject of testimony, being an expert witness should not create concern, because the medical and scientific training of a pathologist yield an enormous advantage over an adversary trained in the law.

REFERENCES

1. National Institute of Occupational Safety and Health. Work related lung disease surveillance report. NIOSH pub 96–134, 1996.
2. Selden AI, Persson B, Bomberger-Dankvardt SI, Winström LE, et al. Exposure to cobalt chromium dust and lung disorders in dental technicians. Thorax 1995;50:769.
3. Chan-Yeung M, Brooks S, Alberts WM, et al. ACCP consensus statement. Chest 1995;108:1084–1117.
4. Richman SI. Legal treatment of the asthmatic worker: a major problem for the nineties. J Occup Med 1990;32:6027–6031.
5. Morgan WKC, Seaton A. Occupational lung diseases. 3rd ed. Philadelphia: WB Saunders, 1995.
6. Kleinerman J, Green F, Harley R, Taylor C, et al. Pathology standards for coal workers' pneumoconiosis. Arch Pathol Lab Med 1979;103:375–385.
7. Churg A, Green FHY. Pathology of occupational lung disease. New York: Igaku-Shoin, 1988:144.
8. Wright JL, Cagle P, Churg A. State of the art, diseases of the small airways. Am Rev Respir Dis 1992;146:247.
9. Seaton A. Coal mining, emphysema and compensation [Editorial]. Br J Ind Med 1990;47:433–435.
10. Lapp NL, Morgan WKG, Zaldivar G. Airways obstruction, coal mining and disability. Occup Env Med 1994;51:234–238.
11. Trasko VM. Socioeconomic Aspects of the Pneumoconioses. Arch Environ Health 1964;9:521–528.
12. Page J, O'Brien M. Bitter wages. New York: Grossman, 1973:59–63.
13. Pennsylvania Occupational Disease Act 284, June 21, 1939. Public Law 566.
14. Solomons ME. Workers compensation for occupational disease victims. Albany Law Rev 1977;41:195–249.
15. National Association of Insurance Commissioners. Occupational disease issues: report of the NAIC Occupational Disease Advisory Committee. NAIC, 1985:5.
16. Selikoff IJ. Disability compensation for asbestos-associated disease in the United States. Report to the U.S. Department of Labor, 1982.
17. U.S. Department of Labor. An interim report on occupational diseases. Washington: U.S. Government Printing Office, 1980:66.
18. Johnson WG. Compensation for occupational illness. Ann N Y Acad Sci 1981;363: 205–217.
19. Pennsylvania Workers' Compensation Act. No. 338, Public Law 736, §201, June 2, 1915.
20. National Association of Insurance Commissioners. Occupational disease issues: report of the NAIC Occupational Disease Advisory Committee. NAIC, 1985.
21. Stander I. Guide to Pennsylvania workers' compensation. 2nd series. Philadelphia: Pennsylvania Law Journal-Reporter, 1984:230–236.

22. Pennsylvania Workers' Compensation Act. No. 338, Public Law 736, §301.
23. Richman SI. Meanings of impairment and disability: the conflicting social objectives underlying the confusion. Chest 1980;78(Suppl):367–371.
24. Pennsylvania Workers' Compensation Act. No. 338, Public Law 736, §306.
25. Worrall JD. Compensation costs, injury rates, and the labor market. In: Worrall JD, ed. Safety and the work force. Ithaca, NY: ILR Press, 1983:11, 61—86, 154—160.
26. Butler RJ. Wage and injury rate response to shifting levels of workers compensation. In: Worrall JD, ed. Safety and the work force. Ithaca, NY: ILR Press, 1983:11, 61—86, 154—160.
27. Chelius JR. The incentive to prevent injuries. In: Worrall JD, ed. Safety and the work force. Ithaca, NY: ILR Press, 1983:11, 61—86, 154—160.
28. Newmeyer GE. Cost of the black lung program. Mining Congr J 1981;67:74–75.
29. U.S. Department of Labor. An interim report on occupational diseases. Washington: U.S. Government Printing Office, 1980:68.
30. U.S. Department of Labor. Proceedings of the Interdepartmental Workers' Compensation Task Force: is there a better way? Report to the president and the congress. Washington: U.S. Government Printing Office, 1977:19.
31. Victor RB. Workers' compensation and occupational diseases: incentive for prevention. In: Theberge LJ, Hollenshead NH, et al., eds. Proceedings of the Conference on Workers' Compensation and Workplace Liability. Washington: National Center for the Public Interest, 1981:367–71.
32. Pennsylvania Workers' Compensation Act. No. 338, Public Law 736, §442.
33. 43 Federal Register 36772. 20 Code of Federal Regulations §725.367. Aug 18, 1978.
34. Barth PS, Hunt WA. Workers' compensation and work-related illnesses and diseases. Cambridge, MA: MIT Press, 1980:207–245.
35. American Law Institute. Restatement (Second) of Torts. St. Paul: West, §402A, comment b. 1965.
36. Borel v Fibreboard Paper Products Corp, 493 F.2d 1076 (5th Cir, 1973).
37. Parker GE. Occupational disease: the asbestos experience. Mining Congr J 1982; 19–24.
38. Flatt v Johns-Manville Sales Corp, 488 F. Suppl 836 (ED Tex, 1980).
39. Bertrand v Johns-Manville Sales Corp, 529 F Suppl 539 (D Minn, 1982).
40. Pastierik v Duquesne Light Co, 491 A.2d 841 (Pa Super, 1985).
41. McGowen v University of Scranton, 759 F.2d 287 (3rd Cir, 1985).
42. Kakalik JS, Ebener PA, et al. Costs of asbestos litigation. The Institute for Civil Justice. Santa Monica: Rand, 1984.
43. AMH/85. Accreditation manual for hospitals. Chicago: Joint Commission Accreditation of Hospitals, 1984:107–111.
44. Pennsylvania Code, 28 §135.15. Harrisburg: Commonwealth of Pennsylvania, 1983.
45. U.S. Dept of the Army, Navy and Air Force. Autopsy manual. §1, 1960.
46. Katzenstein AA, Askin FB. surgical pathology of non-neoplastic lung disease. Philadelphia: WB Saunders, 1982:103.
47. Craighead JE, Vallyathan NV. Cryptic pulmonary lesions in workers occupationally exposed to dust containing silica. JAMA 1980;244:1939–1941.
48. Parkes WR. Occupational lung disorders. ed 2. London: Butterworths, 1982: 359–414.
49. Pneumoconiosis Committee of the College of American Pathologists. Asbestos-associated diseases: the pathology of asbestos-associated diseases of the lungs and pleural cavities: diagnostic criteria and proposed grading scheme. Arch Pathol Lab Med 1982;106:544–596.
50. Renzetti AD, Jr. Medical aspects of impairment and disability. In: Renzetti AD Jr, Richman SI, eds. Current medical methods in diagnosing coal workers' pneumoconiosis and a review of the medical and legal definitions of related impairment and disability: Final report to the U.S. Department of Labor. Philadelphia: Franklin Research Center, 1983.

51. Fox DM, Stone JF. Black lung: miners' militancy and medical uncertainty, 1968–1972. Bull Hist Med 1980;54:45–63.
52. Legislative history of the Federal Coal Mine Health and Safety Act of 1969 (Public Law 91–173, as amended through 1974, including black lung amendments of 1972.) Prepared for the Subcommittee on Labor of the Committee on Labor and Public Welfare, United States Senate, 94th Congress, 1st session. Washington: U.S. Government Printing Office, 1975. Statement of the managers on the part of the House, p. 1622
53. Senate Report No. 97–743. 92nd Congress, 2nd session. U.S. Cong & Admin News 1972:2305–2307.
54. Black Lung Benefits Act, Public Law 91-173, Title IV, §401, Dec 30, 1969, 83 Stat. 792.
55. Black Lung Benefits Act [Ref. 54] §402(b).
56. Black Lung Benefits Act of 1972, Public Law 92-303, §4(c), May 19, 1972, 86 Stat. 153, 154.
57. Legislative history of the Federal Coal Mine Health and Safety Act of 1969 (Public Law 91–173, as amended through 1974, including black lung amendments of 1972.) Prepared for the Subcommittee on Labor of the Committee on Labor and Public Welfare, United States Senate, 94th Congress, 1st session. Washington: U.S. Government Printing Office, 1975. Statement of the managers on the part of the House, p.1817.
58. 36 Federal Register 20641. 20 Code of Federal Regulations §410.401, 410.414. Sept 30, 1972.
59. Black Lung Benefits Reform Act of 1977, Public Law 95-239, §2, March 1, 1978, 92 Stat. 95.
60. Black Lung Benefits Reform Act of 1977. [Ref. 59] §2(b).
61. Committee on Education and Labor, House of Representatives, 96th Congress. Black Lung Benefits Reform Act and Black Lung Benefits Revenue Act of 1977 (Committee Print). Washington: U.S. Government Printing Office, 1977:623.
62. 45 Federal Register 13678. 20 Code of Federal Regulations §718.201. Feb 29, 1980.
63. Dorland's Illustrated Medical Dictionary. ed 26. Philadelphia: WB Saunders, 1981.
64. Enterline PE. Attributability in the fact of uncertainty. Chest 1980;78(Suppl): 377–379.
65. Health Consequences of Smoking—Cancer. A report of the surgeon general. Washington: U.S. Government Printing Office, 1982:17–18, 21–63.
66. H.R. 5735, §5(b)(3) (Miller Bill).
67. Weill H. Basis for clinical decision making. Chest 1980;78(Suppl):382–383.
68. National Association of Insurance Commissioners. Occupational disease issues: report of the NAIC Occupational Disease Advisory Committee. NAIC, 1985:29.
69. Lukosevicz v Director, Office of Workers' Compensation Programs, 888 F.2d 1001 (3rd Cir 1989).
70. Kusenko v Republic Steel Corporation, 484 A.2d 374 (Pa, 1984).
71. Federal Rule of Evidence 702. Jan 2, 1975.
72. Belli MM. The expert witness. Trial, July 1982;35–37.
73. Federal Rule of Evidence 703. Jan 2, 1975.
74. Lamoreaux v Workers' Compensation Appeal Board (Celotex Corporation), 497 A.2d 1388 (Pa, 1985).
75. Federal Rule of Evidence 803(18). Jan 2, 1975.
76. Philadelphia College of Osteopathic Medicine v Workers' Compensation Appeal Board (Lucas), 465 A.2d 132 (Pa, 1983).
77. Lewis v Workers' Compensation Appeal Board (Pittsburgh Board of Education), 508 Pa. 360, 498 A.2d 800, 1985.

Index

Italic page numbers indicate figures; page numbers followed by t indicate tables.

S

T

U

V

W

X

Z